THE SOCIAL MEDICINE READER

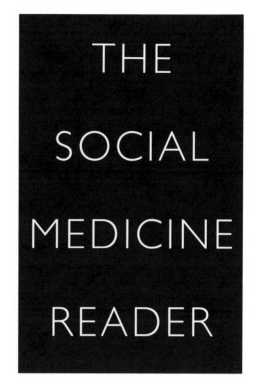

THE SOCIAL MEDICINE READER

Gail E. Henderson

Nancy M. P. King

Ronald P. Strauss

Sue E. Estroff

Larry R. Churchill

Editors

DUKE UNIVERSITY PRESS DURHAM & LONDON 1997

This work has been published with the aid
of a University Research Council grant
administered through the Offices of Research
Services of the University of North Carolina at
Chapel Hill, and support from the Department
of Social Medicine, School of Medicine, at the
University of North Carolina at Chapel Hill.
Printed in the United States of America on
acid-free paper ∞   Designed by Mary Mendell
Typeset in Melior by Keystone Typesetting, Inc.
Library of Congress Cataloging-in-Publication Data
appear on the last printed page of this book.
Second printing, 1998

Contents

∎

—

Preface

■

The five editors of this reader are faculty members of the Department of Social Medicine, at the University of North Carolina School of Medicine. Their varied backgrounds (sociology, law, dentistry, anthropology, psychiatry, philosophy, and ethics) reflect the interdisciplinary character of the department. Founded in 1977, the Department of Social Medicine is comprised of physicians and scholars in the social sciences, humanities, and public health. Its teaching mission is to inform the work and thought of physicians and other health workers on the social conditions and characteristics of patients, causes of illness, and barriers to effective care; and the responsibilities of the medical profession and other medical institutions.

The term "social medicine" has long been associated with public health and politics. In the nineteenth century, European physician-activists began to see scientific medicine as an antidote to the social ills brought about by the industrial revolution. To them, medicine's natural jurisdiction was the poor. Medicine, according to the best known activist and originator of modern pathology, Rudolph Virchow, was essentially a social science. During the twentieth century, medicine's attention to social problems in the United States has been articulated through various philanthropic efforts, public health movements, and community-oriented primary care.

In medical schools, teaching and research focusing on the topics covered in this reader have occurred in a variety of venues, through family or community medicine departments, departments of medical humanities or sociomedical sciences, and public health. Each of these perspectives provides one important way of addressing the issues. However, only the combination of these fields and disciplines can provide a rich and comprehensive understanding of the relationships among medicine, the health of a population, and the society that produces them.

This reader is based on the syllabus of our year-long course, "Medicine and Society," which has been taught at the University of North Carolina since 1978. Because of the pivotal role played by the generations of scholars who have taught in the course, we acknowledge them by name, and thank them for their contributions. Arthur Axelbank, M.D., Dan Beauchamp, Ph.D., James W. Begun, Ph.D., Deborah Bender, Dr.P.H., Allan Brandt, Ph.D., James A. Bryan II, M.D., Watson A. Bowes, M.D., James P. Browder, M.D., Ph.D., Timothy Carey, M.D., M.P.H., Betty Compton, F.N.P., Alan W. Cross, M.D., Gordon H. Defriese, Ph.D., Mia Doron, M.D., Judith Farquhar, Ph.D., John Frey, M.D., Janet Gunn, Ph.D., Seymour Halleck, M.D., Ph.D., Harvey J. Hamrick, M.D., Russell P. Harris, M.D., Axalla Hoole, M.D., T. Robert Konrad, Ph.D., Paul Kory, M.D., Ernest Kraybill, M.D., Frank Loda, M.D., Donald L. Madison, M.D., Campbell McMillan, M.D., Michael McVaugh, Ph.D., Harold Meyer, M.D., Melanie Mintzer, M.D., Joseph P. Morrissey, Ph.D., Virginia Nichols, M.D., Jeffrey Obler, Ph.D., Donald Patrick, Ph.D., C. Glenn Pickard, M.D., Faye Pickard, R.N., Maria Portilla, M.D., Laurie Price, Ph.D., Roberta Riportella, Ph.D., Robert Rhyne, M.D., Patricia Rieker, Ph.D., John Roberts, M.D., Desmond K. Runyan, M.D., Dr.P.H., Barry Saunders, M.D., Susan Schooley, M.D., Joel Schwartz, Ph.D., Susan Skochelak, M.D., Joyce Sparling, Ph.D., Margo Stein, Ph.D., Alan Stern, Ph.D., Maxine Stern, Ph.D., Scott Stroup, M.D., Mary Sugioka, M.D., Isaac M. Taylor, M.D., Keith Wailoo, Ph.D., and Glenn Wilson, M.A.

Thanks are also due to the first chair of the Department of Social Medicine, Glenn Wilson, who oversaw the beginning of the course and syllabus that became the foundation of this volume. Course directors Larry Churchill, Gail Henderson, Nancy King, and Keith Wailoo, have refined the direction and focus of the course over the years. Secretarial and administrative support during the intervening years were provided by Judy Benoit, Sally Council, Becky Eatmon, Martha Edwards, Kay Hill, Jackie Jones, Kathy Leutze, Carolyn McIntyre, and Sally Powell. Preparation of the manuscript was ably handled by Carolyn McIntyre. At Duke University Press, the following people provided guidance and support: Miriam Angress, Steve Cohn, Peter Guzzardi, and Rachel Toor. Maura High's thoughtful editing improved the manuscript considerably.

Introduction

∎

The Social Medicine Reader had its origins almost two decades ago in a required year-long course taught to first-year medical students by social scientists, humanities scholars, and physicians. The goal of the course was to show that medicine and medical practice have a profound influence on—and are influenced by—social, cultural, political, and economic forces. Scholars from many fields are interested in these interactions, but knowing about them is more than a matter of simple interest to physicians and other health care providers—it is essential. Teaching this perspective requires integrating medical and nonmedical materials and viewpoints. This reader, therefore, arises not from one or two academic disciplines, but from many fields within social sciences, humanities, and medicine.

Over the years, students in our course have influenced our approach as much as our scholarly orientations. Early on, we struggled to make these issues compelling to students when they were preoccupied by heavy course loads and exams in the basic medical sciences. Who has time to read a short story when muscles have to be memorized for anatomy? Through many trials and many errors, and with the sometimes blunt feedback of dozing and disengaged students, we learned how to make poetry compete with pathology, to make social issues as important as

anatomy for these future clinicians. First-year medical students still have to cope with sleep deprivation and anxiety, but their approach to social medicine is no longer, "Why do I have to think about this stuff?" but more "How can I best grapple with all of these complicated issues?"

Students, like the rest of us, tend to seek certainty and avoid ambiguity, but they also bring curiosity, intensity, and sophistication to the issues we and they raise in this class. As the medical student body has become more diverse—almost half are women and nearly one-third are from minority groups—and as health care and social issues have become more volatile and political, the course and its tone and content have also evolved. Students may still worry about their pathology exams, but their concerns about ethics, end-of-life decision making, health care for the uninsured, and how gender and race influence health, illness, and medical care are nearly as prominent.

The motivations and perspectives of medical students in our classes reflect their generations and experiences—more and more of them have been out in the world before beginning the rigors of medical training. More are parents. Their life experiences affect how they respond to issues such as maternal-fetal conflicts in medicine. In one of our classes, an obstetrician-gynecologist and two ethicists describe and discuss a crisis with a woman who repeatedly refuses a Cesarean delivery despite the increasing distress of the fetus. The ob-gyn gives the medical story, which is punctuated by commentary from the ethicists who advocate either court-ordered intervention or respecting the woman's bodily privacy. At the end of the session, the students express their views via secret ballot, and the ob-gyn relates the outcome of the case. The vote has been close for over a decade; but the character of discussion of the issues has changed considerably over time. Clearly, the politics of reproduction, public debate about the welfare of children, and new attitudes about rights and responsibilities influence the students' response, and in turn shape how we challenge them to wrestle with these controversies.

Health care financing and organization have also evolved over the years. A decade ago we staged a mock hospital board meeting on the subject of a new HMO that planned to come to town. At the meeting were the hospital administrator, a labor union representative, a corporate executive, a local physician, an insurance executive, and a public health advocate. There were dire predictions and uncertainties in the scripts that each student argued. Several years ago, we replaced this outdated scenario with a similar exercise that enacted a Senate hearing on health care reform legislation like that proposed by President Clinton in 1993. This too became outdated. For the past two years, we have held a mock roundtable discussion for the U.S. Government Accounting Office on what to do about the millions of persons who are without health insurance. The roles have changed. We have added a governor, a Medicare and Medicaid advocate, and a small business representative. The hospital administrator now works for a public hospital corporation. The issues remain hotly debated and revolve around responsibility, limit setting, fairness, and who should pay how much for whom. It is difficult to come to any sort of resolution or devise any policy that gains broad enough support, but the effort to reach consensus provides valuable lessons on the shape of medicine outside the clinic or hospital walls.

With health care and health so prominent in the political, personal, and financial discourse of the day, this book provides a starting point for informed, critical analysis among individuals whose chosen life work is the care of patients. *The Social Medicine Reader* represents the most engaging, provocative, and informative materials and issues we have traversed with our students. They appeal to head and heart, sensibility and sentiment, intellect and cherished beliefs about life and death, justice and injustice, and science and society.

It is important to pull together diverse views on these issues now, when we are being flooded with new studies on the complex links between medicine and society. Even the most technical sciences, like molecular biology and genetics, have been shown to be shaped by politics and culture. Many of these new studies come from fields outside of biomedicine, such as comparative literature, philosophy, social history, and women's and gender studies. The language they use is often unfamiliar to biomedical practitioners, who are confronted, ironically, in the postmodernist era with a vocabulary that can be as daunting and technical as their own.

At the same time that literary and critical studies enrich (and perhaps complicate) our views of medicine in society, there is a proliferation of research in areas known as health services research, clinical epidemiology, health outcomes and cost effectiveness research, and quality of life research. These studies take the opposite tack from cultural studies. They are empirical investigations, basing conclusions on statistical analyses of randomized controlled trials. Questions such as which treatments work, to what extent, and for which types of patients are at the center of this enterprise. Results of this research are cited by people debating health policy and making decisions in health care organizations. Increasingly, doctors use such findings to decide how to treat a person with a given medical condition, as they weigh risks to the patient against benefits for particular courses of treatment.

With this diverse field as backdrop, the selections chosen for *The Social Medicine Reader* represent many disciplines, methods, voices, and levels of inquiry. The various writers explore health and illness from the perspectives of patients, health care providers, the medical care system, and society. They address basic but critical questions: What transformations occur as a person becomes a patient? How are illness and disability experienced? What causes disease, and how do we think critically about categories of risk? What does medicine do? Can we even speak of "medicine" as an active force apart from its practice by individuals? What are doctor-patient relationships about—what are the roles and responsibilities of each party? What forces shape the current and future organization and financing of health care?

In addressing these questions, the authors represented in this reader explore the relationships between those who suffer and those who heal, between individuals and cultures, and the medical care system and society at large. Patients' ideas of illness and of treatment are considered alongside those of physicians. We see doctors in the context of the medical culture that shapes them and their work; we see the ethical dilemmas that doctors and patients must face together, and the changing role of physicians within an evolving organization, financing, and delivery system. The social context of ethical debates between patients and doctors emerges from these readings, which present current national debates about social justice, including the ethical underpinnings of a fair distribution of medical care, technology, and opportunities for health and well-being.

The Social Medicine Reader challenges standard ways of thinking about medical categories of disease, social categories of risk, and types of moral reasoning, on which much of the field of bioethics is based. Its many voices reflect both insider and outsider perspectives of the profession, settings, and practice of medicine. They include individual narratives of illness experiences, commentaries by physicians, arguments about complex medical cases, and interpretative as well as data-based material by scholars in the social sciences and the humanities. These are readings with the literary and scholarly power to convey the complicated relationships between medicine and society. They do not resolve the most vexing issues we face today, but illuminate them.

Medicine's impact on society is well documented. Biomedical technology and practice have profoundly affected our institutions and our social relations. Those who create and dispense scientific medicine have gained formidable status and power, both within and outside the world of doctoring. Furthermore, medicine has affected how we think about the most fundamental, enduring human experiences—conception, birth, maturation, sickness, suffering, healing, aging, and death—and it has shaped the metaphors we use to express our deepest concerns. Medical practices and our responses to them have helped to redefine the meaning of age, race, and gender. Through technological advances, medicine has produced new, sometimes terrifying, ethical dilemmas—dilemmas that we are often unprepared to address, and whose terms are expressed in the new vocabularies of science and economics, as well as the more familiar ones of morality and human relations.

Less well documented but equally important are the effects of society on medicine. It is impossible to take account of medicine without paying attention to the place and time of its practice and the social and cultural landscape of which it is a part. Medicine and society are not separate, independent forces, one determining the other; they are interdependent, and shape each other. Giving form and voice to the multiple dimensions of this reciprocal relationship between medicine and society is the principal goal of this volume.

Social influences on medicine are apparent in several ways. First, modern science presumes that the pursuit of knowledge can and should be conducted with minimal bias. Yet medical knowledge and practice, like all knowledge and practice, are shaped by political, cultural, and economic forces, within which doctors' ideas about disease—in fact their very definitions of disease—depend on the role science plays in particular cultures, as well as on the culture of science. Medicine tends to reduce the world to a vocabulary of its own, one that seems immune to the vagaries and vicissitudes of culture. But diseases are not immutable; they are shaped by person, time, and place, and are identified and endowed with significance only within social and cultural contexts.

It is also impossible to give a full account of medicine without considering social class and environment. Despite the power of the biomedical model of disease and the increasing specificity of molecular and genetic knowledge, social factors have always influenced the occurrence and course of most diseases. The classic public health model of disease is a triumvirate of agent, host, and environment, and it is the interaction of host with environment that makes the critical difference. People who are poorly nourished, inadequately housed, or exposed to polluted air and water, and violence and other unpredictable, traumatic events are more susceptible to injury and disease.

Once disease has occurred, the power of medicine to alter its course is constrained by the larger social and economic context. Some diseases have such costly treatments that many patients cannot afford the care or travel to obtain them. For other diseases, difficult changes in behavior that the doctor recommends may simply not fit with the world views of the individual or community.

Beyond these problems, many medical interventions are, themselves, of contested or unclear value. Spending on health care in the United States has long outstripped that of other industrialized nations, but that spending has not resulted in a healthier population. Babies still die at far too high a rate, and cancer, heart disease, and stroke still cause too many adults to suffer premature disability or death. What does our medicine produce? Who benefits from these enormous expenditures of resources?

Nothing better exemplifies society's resistance to medical expansionism than the development of informed consent as the guiding principle for doctor-patient (and researcher-subject) interactions. We Americans cherish personal autonomy and, as a result, the rules of informed consent recognize that the interests of patients can be very different from physicians' judgments of what is best for patients. Contemporary bioethics began by using the language of philosophy to respond to the language of medicine. Now it also draws on literary language and other disciplines to emphasize the multiplicity of persons, interests, and values that come together in medical-moral problems.

At this juncture, it is fair, and indeed advisable to ask, "So what?" So what if medicine is demonstrably social and the social is demonstrably colonized by medicine? This is not news! Perhaps not—but the sociality of medical practice has never been so richly illustrated, so abundantly documented as at present. The cumulative body of literature and scholarly work goes well beyond just recognizing medicine as something other than science and truth. The answer to the "so whats" of this moment is that by critically analyzing the issues, we can open up possibilities, change what seems inevitable, and practice medical education and doctoring in a more self-critical way. The goal now is to ignite and to fuel the inner voices of social, human, and moral analysis among health care professionals—to provoke the conversations from within. The time to begin those conversations and to learn the vocabulary is, along with anatomy and pathology, when the culturing of individuals into medicine is in process. The answer to "So what?" then, will come in the way physicians and health care professionals practice in the coming decades, in clinics, conference rooms, and operating theaters.

The readings that comprise this volume are divided into five parts, each illuminating a different aspect of medicine in society and society in medicine. The first part, "Culture, Experiences of Illness, and Deviance and Disability" addresses topics from the perspectives of medical anthropology. The second, "The Influence of Social Factors on Health and Illness," draws material from the fields of medical sociology and epidemiology. Part III, "The Culture of Medicine and Medical Practice," is based principally on self-reflections of physicians, and on the sociology of medicine and professions. The fourth part, "Health Care Ethics and the Provider's Role," draws from bioethics; the fifth, "Medical Care Financing, Rationing, and Managed Care," brings together critical analyses from medical economics, ethics, and clinical medicine.

Despite differences in method, perspective, and vocabulary, one of the most important characteristics of *The Social Medicine Reader* is that themes reappear from one part to the next. None of the parts deals exclusively, for example, with doctor-patient relationships; each raises issues that are relevant to this theme, based on its particular concerns and perspectives. Similarly, some selections present patients and their loved ones in personal narratives, with all the texture and flavor of emotions; later we consider how race, gender, and class may influence such sentiments and responses. Social justice is another key theme. The selections pose in various ways questions about who gets (or does not get) what kind of care from whom, and why—and with what results. Another recurrent theme is the political economy of health care, and how resources are distributed and controlled at the national and individual level. Not surprisingly, birth and death appear often in the readings. After all, medicine is about witnessing, about accompanying others as they enter, endure, and exit life's entanglements. We are concerned throughout with the artful expression of the anguish, recovery, longing, rage, and ecstasy that accompany illness and healing. Repeatedly, these readings make clear that much of what we encounter in science, in society, and in everyday and extraordinary lives is indeterminate, ambiguous, contradictory, and complex. And because of this inherent ambigu-

ity, the interwoven selections focus directly on conflict—conflict about power and authority, autonomy and choice, and risk and security.

Each part is prefaced by an introductory essay that provides background for the readings—reviewing the theoretical and conceptual issues, academic debates, and perspectives that the selections are intended to illustrate. The parts are also divided into sections, each of which opens with an explanation of the significance of the readings and the rationale for their selection. A bibliography at the end of the volume includes the works cited in these introductory materials.

Every anthology is open to challenge about what has been included and left out, and this reader will be no exception. The study of medicine and society is dynamic, with large bodies of ever-expanding, new literatures from which to draw. We did not include some readings considered "classic" in various fields. In many cases these classics are dated, or are too narrowly focused on disciplinary debates beyond the scope of physicians in training. We have summarized these debates in the introductory essays to each part, so that we could include a wider range of materials more suited to students training as health care providers or researchers.

We have selected readings that worked well in the classroom, provoking discussion and engaging the readers' imaginations. The materials invite self-conscious, multi-level, critical examination. This is inherently difficult and challenging, but educationally rewarding. We learn about ourselves when we study medicine. When physicians turn a critical gaze on their own endeavors, they not only enrich the practice of medicine, but also challenge all of us to reassess our assumptions about medicine's fundamental work. Healing is the enduring task of physicians. It can best be accomplished through an informed joining of the medical and social worlds.

PART I

A Cultural Perspective

of Experiences of Illness, Disability,

and Deviance

Why begin a reader in social medicine with a cultural perspective? We do so because culture is that common fund of ideas, images, beliefs, and behaviors that inform our lives—including our definitions of health and illness, how we respond to disease and injury, and how we experience pain, discomfort, and disfigurement. Cultural practices and meanings that may be taken for granted are the context within which Western biomedicine is produced, learned, and practiced. Culture is the stage, script, lighting, and direction for the drama of illness and treatment—it is influential, but not definitive.

As Clifford Geertz has said, "Anthropology is a science whose progress is marked less by the development of consensus than by refinement of the debate. What gets better is the precision with which we vex each other" (1973, 29). Despite ongoing debate, most contemporary anthropologists view culture as an evolving, collective product, a negotiable and negotiated template for leading and making sense of daily life. They agree, more or less, that (1) culture includes the values, rules, prohibitions, preferences, symbols, meanings, language, and practices that guide how everyday life is lived and how events that fall outside everyday experience are understood; (2) culture is shared among a group of people, despite variations among them in interpretation of principles or in practices; (3) culture endures at a fundamental level, but also changes over time, particularly in expressive modes such as music or dress; (4) cultural form and content are produced and reproduced by those who learn the rules and practice or apply them in daily living.

Culture is not a set of rigid rules or practices that everyone in a particular group follows (see Wright et al. 1993). Taking such a view can lead to stereotyping, or a cookie-cutter view of culture—that it stamps out identical people with identical beliefs. It may be helpful to think of culture as agreed-upon-enough to create recognizably patterned responses to disease, disability, or death.

To examine the nature and meaning of illness and healing, *The Social Medicine Reader* takes a multidimensional perspective that draws on frameworks and findings from a variety of academic disciplines. The most prominent of these are sociocultural and medical anthropology, sociology, social history, and the history of medicine and science. We draw also on fictional and nonfictional accounts from inside and outside the domains of illness and treatment. These vivid narratives of managing illness in daily life and disablement in a lifetime contribute to a textured, biographical understanding of the individuals whose experiences with illness and disability are the center of attention in this section.

The readings that follow identify and work primarily with culture close to home. Differences across cultures in how illness is treated and defined and in what the outcomes of illness are signal that sickness is social as well as biological (Kleinman 1986). We wish to emphasize here that culture works also in what may seem to us the commonplace, unexotic, largely Western settings where biomedicine dominates—and that many of us call home.

Demographers predict that within the next fifty years, white people of European descent in the United States will become a numerical minority again for the first time since the colonization of the North American continent. The social and cultural world of the twenty-first-century United States, its language, music, food, and political figures and forces, will probably be profoundly different from what they were just half a century ago, when the dominant, white, Anglo-Saxon tradition was accepted by many as "American culture," a culture both desirable and superior to others. Members of a dominant culture are inclined to view their own ways as logical and natural, to see culture as something that others have. In this case, *we* have values or principles, *they* have beliefs and customs; *we* have science and knowledge, *they* have traditions and myths. Yet Western history, the social history of science and medicine, and the cultural study of health and illness challenge these dichotomies and show them to be artificial.

The United States has always been a culturally diverse society, home to Anglo-Saxon, African, Native American, and Mediterranean groups (among others) with clear linguistic and cultural boundaries. Ethnicity and cultural diversity are now center stage in the politics, economy, social life, and health care of the late-twentieth-century United States. Rayna Rapp (1993) demonstrates, for example, how the ethnic diversity of both the producers and receivers of biomedical information influences their responses to it. She uses the example of amniocentesis, but the clinicians, scientists, and patients she studies practice many cultures, and this fact makes it impossible to take a simple-minded view of culture as an infallible predictor of responses to and interpretation of medical information. As this multicultural, ethnically diverse society moves into a new century, it is crucial that we understand health, illness, and medical practice as both product and producer of larger social and cultural domains.

As much as we anticipate change, each age and

era develops a sense of inevitability about itself, about its ways and ideas. And so we have about ours, particularly in the realms of science and medicine. Yet, illness categories, both lay and scientific, are, at base, cultural categories, and as such change over time. The historian Michael MacDonald (1989) describes, for example, how in sixteenth- and early-seventeenth-century England suicide was changed from a "heinous crime . . . a kind of murder committed at the instigation of the devil" to a secularized and medical condition. He argues that physicians had little to do with the evolution of concepts of suicide; rather, philosophers, laymen, and particularly coroners' juries lead the way. Suicide was medicalized and reconstrued at first as an abnormality of affect, but not because physicians of the time were developing clinical views of depression or mental disorder. The reason that suicide was classified as an illness was that the family of a person convicted of "self-murder" had to forfeit the property of the deceased, because the person who committed suicide was posthumously convicted of a felony. Heirs protested this double loss of a loved one and material resources, and coroners' juries increasingly helped families avoid this penalty by not ordering inquisitions into questionable deaths, which they might then have been forced to declare suicides. Instead, they returned an increasing number of verdicts of death brought on by insanity, or *non compos mentis*. All this took place within a context of increasing secularization in other social realms.

A social-historical perspective applied to suicide, or to other maladies such as eating disorders (Brumberg 1989), lays bare some of the mechanisms that operate in the continual social construction and reconstruction of ideas about disease and illness. Political, legal, and economic forces often eclipse the influence of medical practice and ideology in these processes, and analyses that take a social-historical view balance unidimensional views that see disease as something defined by medical or biomedical experts.

One has only to catalogue the widely varied conceptions and representations of AIDS in the past decade to recognize how cultural forces can alter the face of a disease. HIV has sparked a mixture of moral, spiritual, virological, neurological, and social explanations. Paul Farmer's (1992) study of understandings of AIDS in Haiti shows how blame and accusation (constituting the "third epidemic"—worse than the disease) dominate American and Haitian views. Accusations of sorcery arise in a Haitian village to account for the disease. The American public fears that the virus was introduced here by "infected" Haitian immigrants. Haitians counter with conspiratorial ideas about U.S. motivations to weaken or defame impoverished black immigrants who will carry the affliction home. Fears of contagion and pollution by outsiders or malevolent others are shared by Americans and Haitians alike. AIDS now infects more women and children of color in the United States than persons who are homosexual, yet AIDS bears the stigma of sinfulness because its first victims in the United States were gay men. In Africa, AIDS has always been a "heterosexual" disease, but because of its spread by and among prostitutes, it attracted a different kind of moral approbation. Ominous diseases like AIDS provide both a window and a mirror into deeply held values, ideas about order, about pollution, and about good and bad.

The reciprocal influence of cultural conceptions, social sentiment and policy, and medical practice is also well demonstrated by remarkable changes during the past three decades in the care and treatment of persons with severe physical and mental disabilities. Institutions for mentally retarded and mentally ill persons have been all but emptied, and even the most seriously impaired individuals now live and receive treatment in community settings. These changes took place because of a confluence of forces: the development of effective drugs and treatments; civil rights litigation that led to the right to "least restrictive" treatments; the desire of public mental health authorities to save money; and the advocacy efforts of severely disabled persons and their families to change the status quo. People with disabilities now have a larger presence in the media, the workplace, and in the overall consciousness of society at large. As importantly, clinical practice and the medical assessment of their abilities have changed dramatically as a result of changes brought about in part by social forces. Had these individuals remained confined in institutions, their ability to work or to navigate public transportation systems, for example, might have remained undiscovered.

Advocates for people with psychiatric disorders take a variety of approaches, each one working a different cultural territory. Some persons with psychiatric diagnoses emphasize civil rights and define themselves as a minority group that is subject to discrimination, for example, in the workplace. Others—like the activist relatives of individuals with schizophrenia—work to redefine these disorders as a kind of disease, that is, to medicalize them by promoting the view that they are malfunctions of the brain. Promotional materials declare schizophrenia to be a "no-fault brain disease," and there are public and professional pressures to replace the term "mental illness" with "neurobiological disorder" or NBD. Indeed, these advocates succeeded recently in what for them was a vital symbolic move—the National Institutes of Mental Health were administratively joined with the National Institutes of Health. Recent public opinion research reveals that most Americans now view depression and schizophrenia as biologically based diseases, though there is much confusion about what kind of disease they might be and what mechanisms are at work.

The approach of this interdisciplinary reader is that the biological and cultural realms are intertwined. That is not to say that culture includes everything. But nearly every part of biological and social life is culturally influenced; life is "cultured." In any locale, for example, the plants that are used for healing, the kind of crops that are grown, and the climate help to shape local customs and beliefs. These customs and beliefs, in turn, interpret or give symbolic meaning to the weather or to medicines or to food. Social hierarchies then often determine how resources are distributed within a group—who gets what and how much and when—which may then influence patterns of disease.

Biology and culture do not stand in opposition, the one fixed and the other malleable. Instead, there is an interplay of biological and cultural forces and factors. Illness is sensate. It is felt in the body through pain, discomfort, and loss or change of function. Illness and injury are embodied—seen, displayed, apparent to self and to others. How we feel, what we feel, what we identify as pain and discomfort and disfigurement are all learned and shaped in cultural contexts. The bodies we expect—and hope—to have are imagined within cultural parameters. The availability of new technologies for replacing knees and hips, for example, in part creates the expectation, not just the possibility, of playing tennis or skiing downhill at age seventy. Cosmetic surgery to rid the face of wrinkles or the body of fat, and expensive new-tech dental implants instead of dentures become the means to as well as the reasons for evolving ideas about bodily shape and function over a lifetime. This interplay between medical technology and bodily expectations is an important example of the mutual molding of culture and medicine.

Prozac, the popular antidepressant medication, presents a similar example of the relationship between evolving technology and expectations—in this case applied to emotional states and intellectual functioning. Prozac offers people the chance to feel more optimistic or happier, when they may not have a diagnosable disease. The possibilities for enhancing the senses of well-being and happiness, courtesy of Prozac, are changing how we view moods and the presence or meaning of sadness and melancholy as part of daily living. Familiar emotions, the blues, and distress are being redefined as diseases to "treat" them with this and other drugs. On the flip side, the argument could be made that if Prozac or other drugs enhance well-being or functioning, this is proof of the presence of an underlying pathology. The debate about Prozac (and other legal and extralegal means of enhancing mood) reflects ongoing disagreement about the definition of will and personal "responsibility" and their roles in preventing dysfunction or maintaining health. Will and responsibility are in turn rooted deeply in Western ideology about independence, individualism, and mastery over nature. The specific cultural questions raised by Prozac are about what sort of sentiments and experiences are accepted as part of life or are subject to removal or reduction via outside intervention or medical treatment.

Social scientists have found it useful to make a distinction between "disease" as a pathological process and biological condition, and "illness" as the personal, socially and culturally influenced experience of impairment or pathology (Fabrega 1974, Kleinman et al. 1978). The distinction between these concepts calls attention to personal experience and pathophysiology as concurrent and legitimate processes, but it also may reinforce an unnecessary separation of biology from culture and of body from person (Taussig 1980). Margaret Lock's (1994) work on aging and menopause in Japan and North America illustrates the intimate interactions between biology and culture. Lock finds that Japanese women physically experience menopause differently from American women. They do not report the "hot flashes" and emotional changeability that Americans do. Rather, their primary sensations

include aching joints and other bodily pains. Likewise, Japanese and American physicians differ widely in how they approach menopause and in their proclivities for prescribing estrogen replacement therapy. Their relationships with patients are embedded in cultural contexts with differing ideas about gender, authority, female biology, and aging. How can it be that Japanese women experiencing menopause actually *feel* differently from American women? Their aching shoulders are as culturally influenced *and* as real as American and Canadian hot flashes, but all the women are going through the same biological process. Or are they?

Culture, then, is deeply implicated in the recognition, experience, and treatment of illness. Illness is also situated in and defined by the roles that individuals are expected to play in society. The most enduring articulation of this perspective is Talcott Parsons's (1951) idea of the "sick role." Parsons, a sociologist, described expectations for people who are ill that are based on American values of responsibility, independence, and productivity. First, based on how severe the illness is, a person is excused from normal social role responsibilities. People are allowed to stay home from school or work if they are ill, for example. Being exempt from responsibilities because of illness is, however, hotly contested in the case of mental illness. In the realm of criminal law, "diminished capacity" and "not guilty by reason of insanity" are legal concepts that express our culture's practice of exempting people of full responsibility if they are sick. Yet recent U.S. history is filled with instances when claiming the exemption caused public outcry, from John Hinckley to Jeffrey Dahmer and John Salvi. These cases demonstrate clearly the social and cultural influences on this intersection of medical and legal concepts.

The second component of the sick role is that a person who is ill deserves to be taken care of, by either family or social institutions, in order to get well. Third, people who are infirm are expected to consider illness as undesirable and are obligated to try to get well—to seek treatment, to change diet, quit smoking, or follow a doctor's orders. Those who violate this expectation—refusing treatment for drug addiction, for example—may lose their deserving-of-help status. In 1994, federal legislation was passed that strictly limited disability income support for people with substance abuse disorders and revoked the benefit for those who did not comply with treatment. In 1995, persons with substance abuse disorders were excluded from eligibility for disability benefits altogether. Even though addiction had clearly been defined as a medical condition, falling within biomedical practice, it did not influence public sentiment or policy regarding the moral status of addicted persons. Cultural ideas about responsibility and will overrode the medical mantle of deservedness via disease.

How people who are sick and those around them respond to illness is part of a cultural code that is learned, often without noticing. Other cultural groups may have different definitions of the sick role, but no matter what kind of healing system prevails, there are well understood codes of conduct for "illness behaviors," another useful concept (Mechanic 1962). Illness behaviors are those practices that accompany disease and dysfunction—from eating chicken soup to chanting all night to appease an offended spirit. Illness behaviors are learned, and although they change over time, American illness behaviors still reflect ancient medical principles of balance among the "humors," or elements of the body, of hot and cold, and wet and dry. Thus many Americans explain the onset of an upper respiratory infection with a story of getting overtired, getting wet and cold, not eating enough of certain foods—not keeping the balance—even though they understand the viral nature of most colds. It is important to remember that while the reach of biomedicine is global, only a minority of the world's population rely solely or even primarily on biomedical care or adhere to humoral beliefs about disease. Ayurvedic, traditional Chinese, and spiritist medical traditions—to name only the most prominent—are also used along with biomedicine by a large proportion of the world population.

Within the United States' diverse society, there are observable differences in how people define illness and behave when they are ill and how they are responded to by others (see Lang 1989). The concept of an "explanatory model" of illness was introduced by physician-anthropologist Arthur Kleinman (1980) as a way of understanding individual patients' illness ideas and practices. In eliciting an illness account or explanatory model, the investigator asks individuals about their terminology for a disease or their pain; their ideas about its etiology; their ideas about how a particular illness works; how long they think it will last; their expectations for the outcome of treatment; their account of the severity of the problem and its impact on their daily lives. These stories of sickness convey what a particular injury or impairment means to individuals and to their loved ones (Brody 1987, Kleinman 1988). Few individuals have consistent, well-developed "models" of their physical or psychological problems, so the explanatory model concept may be most useful as a way to invite individuals to give an account or narrative of their illness.

The interactions of culture, health, illness, and biomedicine are illustrated in the selections that follow. They have been chosen for their depth and richness in conveying the experience of illness, treatment, and disability in cultural context.

Sue E. Estroff

Culture,

Health, and Illness

The readings for this section on culture, health, and illness convey some of the diversity and richness of cultural analyses of health, illness, and biomedical knowledge and practice. Together the readings illustrate different findings and methods and analytic strategies for investigating how cultural context, disease, and biomedicine intertwine. It is fitting that we begin with a clinician's sympathetic inventory of what constitutes a person. Cassell gives us a profoundly cultural rendering of what we in the West recognize as our selves. His rich description of the nature and components of personhood identifies the focal point for illness, suffering, and medical treatment in our society. What makes a person, and how do they suffer? A person has a past, secrets, hopes for the future, and needs for intimacy. Cassell entreats physicians to recognize and reduce suffering by recognizing the persons who have become their patients. In the cultural analyses and illness narratives that follow in this and the next sections, Cassell's leads and cues about the nature of selves that are profoundly Western are illustrated repeatedly and with the added force of individual voices.

Martha Balshem takes an ethnographic and qualitative approach to investigating higher than expected rates of cancer in a working-class neighborhood. Her role is not typical of anthro-

pological work, however, because she was employed as a health educator and the people she interviewed in the neighborhood identified her with the biomedical point of view. Balshem's task was to elicit and analyze the informants' ideas about the nature and causes of cancer in order to more effectively communicate a prevention program. Her article discusses their images of cancer and heart disease and what they thought could be done about it, along with their attitudes toward "scientific knowledge." Like good scientists, the neighborhood residents see the exceptions to medical dogma—the smoker who never gets cancer, the person who eats sausages with no apparent ill effects. Balshem interprets their skeptical reception of the prevention program as a resistance to medical authority, as an assertion of the validity of local knowledge and experience. The residents know that the air pollution from a nearby industry is as likely a culprit as their dietary indulgences in causing cancer, yet they also know they need jobs. Their choices and attitudes cast health education and preventive medicine in a different light. How far can and should such programs go in evaluating or seeking to change people's lifestyles and preferences?

Holly Mathews and her colleagues also investigated the meaning of cancer for their informants, African American women living in eastern North Carolina who were in the advanced stages of breast cancer. As part of a multidisciplinary team, Mathews used interviews to gather data about why these women came for treatment so late in the course of their illnesses. The women's narratives of their experience with breast cancer reveal cultural metaphors and ideas about the body that in turn influence their responses to diagnosis and treatment. Their ideas about good and bad blood and their concerns that tumors will spread when they come in contact with air during surgery differ greatly from the ideas of Balshem's informants. The accounts reported here are not linear or necessarily consistent, but they are richly personal and cultural—and as importantly, often had a determining influence on whether the women remained in treatment. When these views were challenged baldly or ignored by clinicians, some of the women refused further treatment of their illness. This selection raises questions about how such findings might be applied in clinical practice.

The Nature of Suffering
and the Goals of Medicine
Eric J. Cassell

■

The obligation of physicians to relieve human suffering stretches back into antiquity. Despite this fact, little attention is explicitly given to the problem of suffering in medical education, research, or practice. I will begin by focusing on a modern paradox: Even in the best settings and with the best physicians, it is not uncommon for suffering to occur not only during the course of a disease but also as a result of its treatment. To understand this paradox and its resolution requires an understanding of what suffering is and how it relates to medical care.

Consider this case: A 35-year-old sculptor with metastatic disease of the breast was treated by competent physicians employing advanced knowledge and technology and acting out of kindness and true concern. At every stage, the treatment as well as the disease was a source of suffering to her. She was uncertain and frightened about her future, but she could get little information from her physicians, and what she was told was not always the truth. She had been unaware, for example, that the irradiated breast would be so disfigured. After an oophorectomy and a regimen of medications, she became hirsute, obese, and devoid of libido. With tumor in the supraclavicular fossa, she lost strength in the hand that she had used in sculpturing, and she became profoundly depressed. She had a pathologic fracture of the femur, and treatment was delayed while her physicians openly disagreed about pinning her hip.

Each time her disease responded to therapy and her hope was rekindled, a new manifestation would appear. Thus, when a new course of chemotherapy was started, she was torn between a desire to live and the fear that allowing hope to emerge again would merely expose her to misery if the treatment failed. The nausea and vomiting from the chemotherapy were distressing, but no more so than the anticipation of hair loss. She feared the future. Each tomorrow was seen as heralding increased sickness, pain, or disability, never as the beginning of better times. She felt isolated because she was no longer like other people and could not do what other people did. She feared that her friends would stop visiting her. She was sure that she would die.

This young woman had severe pain and other physical symptoms that caused her suffering. But she also suffered from some threats that were social and from others that were personal and private. She suffered from the effects of the disease and its treatment on her appearance and abilities. She also suffered unremittingly from her perception of the future.

What can this case tell us about the ends of medicine and the relief of suffering? Three facts stand out: The first is that this woman's suffering was not confined to her physical symptoms. The second is that she suffered not only from her disease but also from its treatment. The third is that one could not anticipate what she would describe as a source of suffering; like other patients, she had to be asked. Some features of her condition she would call painful, upsetting, uncomfortable, and distressing, but not a source of suffering. In these characteristics her case was ordinary.

In discussing the matter of suffering with lay persons, I learned that they were shocked to discover that the problem of suffering was not directly addressed in medical education. My colleagues of a contemplative nature were surprised at how little they knew of the problem and how little thought they had given it, whereas medical students tended to be unsure of the relevance of the issue to their work.

The relief of suffering, it would appear, is considered one of the primary ends of medicine by patients and lay persons, but not by the medical profession. As in the case of the dying, patients and their friends and families do not make a distinction between physical and nonphysical sources of suffering in the same way that doctors do.[1]

A search of the medical and social-science literature did not help me in understanding what suffering is; the word "suffering" was most often coupled with the word "pain," as in "pain and suffering." (The data bases used were *Psychological Abstracts,* the *Citation Index,* and the *Index Medicus.*)

This phenomenon reflects a historically constrained and currently inadequate view of the ends of medicine. Medicine's traditional concern primarily for the body and for physical disease is well known, as are the widespread effects of the mind-body dichotomy on medical theory and practice. I believe that this dichotomy itself is a source of the paradoxical situation in which doctors cause suffering in their care of the sick. Today, as ideas about the separation of mind and body are called into question, physicians are concerning themselves with new aspects of the human condition. The profession of medicine is being pushed and pulled into new areas, both by its technology and by the demands of its patients. Attempting to understand what suffering is and how physicians might truly be devoted to its relief will require that medicine and its critics overcome the dichotomy between mind and body and the associated dichotomies between subjective and objective and between person and object.

In the remainder of this essay I am going to make three points. The first is that suffering is experienced by persons. In the separation between mind and body, the concept of the person, or personhood, has been associated with that of mind, spirit, and the subjective. However, as I will show, a person is not merely mind, merely spiritual, or only subjectively knowable. Personhood has many facets, and it is ignorance of them that actively contributes to patients' suffering. The understanding of the place of the person in human illness requires a rejection of the historical dualism of mind and body.

The second point derives from my interpretation of clinical observations: Suffering occurs when an impending destruction of the person is perceived; it continues until the threat of disintegration has passed or until the integrity of the person can be restored in some other manner. It follows, then, that although suffering often occurs in the presence of acute pain, shortness of breath, or other bodily symptoms, suffering extends beyond the physical. Most generally, suffering can be defined as the state of severe distress associated with events that threaten the intactness of the person.

The third point is that suffering can occur in relation to any aspect of the person, whether it is in the realm of social roles, group identification, the relation with self, body, or family, or the relation with a transpersonal, transcendent source of meaning. Below is a simplified description or "topology" of the constituents of personhood.

"Person" Is Not "Mind"

The split between mind and body that has so deeply influenced our approach to medical care was proposed by Descartes to resolve certain philosophical issues. Moreover, Cartesian dualism made it possible for science to escape the control of the church by assigning the noncorporeal, spiritual realm to the church, leaving the physical world as the domain of science. In that religious age, "person," synonymous with "mind," was necessarily off limits to science.

Changes in the meaning of concepts like that of personhood occur with changes in society, while the word for the concept remains the same. This fact tends to obscure the depth of the transformations that have occurred between the 17th century and today. People simply *are* "persons" in this time, as in past times, and they have difficulty imagining that the term described something quite different in an earlier period when the concept was more constrained.

If the mind–body dichotomy results in assigning the body to medicine, and the person is not in that category, then the only remaining place for the person is in the category of mind. Where the mind is problematic (not identifiable in objective terms), its very reality diminishes for science, and so, too, does that of the person. Therefore, so long as the mind–body dichotomy is accepted, suffering is either subjective and thus not truly "real"—not within medicine's domain—or identified exclusively with bodily pain. Not only is such an identification misleading and distorting, for it depersonalizes the sick patient, but it is itself a source of suffering. It is not possible to treat sickness as something that happens solely to the body without thereby risking damage to the person. An anachronistic division of the human condition into what is medical (having to do with the body) and what is nonmedical (the remainder) has given medicine too narrow a notion of its calling. Because of this division, physicians may, in concentrating on the cure of bodily disease, do things that cause the patient as a person to suffer.

An Impending Destruction of Person

Suffering is ultimately a personal matter. Patients sometimes report suffering when one does not expect it, or do not report suffering when one does expect it. Furthermore, a person can suffer enormously at the distress of another, especially a loved one.

In some theologies, suffering has been seen as bringing one closer to God. This "function" of suffering is at once its glorification and its relief. If, through great pain or deprivation, someone is brought closer to a cherished goal, that person may have no sense of having suffered but may instead feel enormous triumph. To an observer, however, only the deprivation may be apparent. This cautionary note is important because people are often said to have suffered greatly, in a religious context, when they are known only to have been injured, tortured, or in pain, not to have suffered.

Although pain and suffering are closely identified in the medical literature, they are phenomenologically distinct.[2] The difficulty of understanding pain and the problems of physicians in providing adequate relief of physical pain are well known.[3–5]

The greater the pain, the more it is believed to cause suffering. However, some pain, like that of childbirth, can be extremely severe and yet considered rewarding. The perceived meaning of pain influences the amount of medication that will be required to control it. For example, a patient reported that when she believed the pain in her leg was sciatica, she could control it with small doses of codeine, but when she discovered that it was due to the spread of malignant disease, much greater amounts of medication were required for relief. Patients can writhe in pain from kidney stones and by their own admission not be suffering, because they "know what it is"; they may also report considerable suffering from apparently minor discomfort when they do not know its source. Suffering in close relation to the intensity of pain is reported when the pain is virtually overwhelming, such as that associated with a dissecting aortic aneurysm. Suffering is also reported when the patient does not believe

that the pain can be controlled. The suffering of patients with terminal cancer can often be relieved by demonstrating that their pain truly can be controlled; they will then often tolerate the same pain without any medication, preferring the pain to the side effects of their analgesics. Another type of pain that can be a source of suffering is pain that is not overwhelming but continues for a very long time.

In summary, people in pain frequently report suffering from the pain when they feel out of control, when the pain is overwhelming, when the source of the pain is unknown, when the meaning of the pain is dire, or when the pain is chronic.

In all these situations, persons perceive pain as a threat to their continued existence—not merely to their lives, but to their integrity as persons. That this is the relation of pain to suffering is strongly suggested by the fact that suffering can be relieved, in the presence of continued pain, by making the source of the pain known, changing its meaning, and demonstrating that it can be controlled and that an end is in sight.

It follows, then, that suffering has a temporal element. In order for a situation to be a source of suffering, it must influence the person's perception of future events. ("If the pain continues like this, I *will be* overwhelmed"; "If the pain comes from cancer, I *will* die"; "If the pain cannot be controlled, I *will not* be able to take it.") At the moment when the patient is saying, "If the pain continues like this, I will be overwhelmed," he or she is not overwhelmed. Fear itself always involves the future. In the case with which I opened this essay, the patient could not give up her fears of her sense of future, despite the agony they caused her. As suffering is discussed in the other dimensions of personhood, note how it would not exist if the future were not a major concern.

Two other aspects of the relation between pain and suffering should be mentioned. Suffering can occur when physicians do not validate the patient's pain. In the absence of disease, physicians may suggest that the pain is "psychological" (in the sense of not being real) or that the patient is "faking." Similarly, patients with chronic pain may believe after a time that they can no longer talk to others about their distress. In the former case the person is caused to distrust his or her perceptions of reality, and in both instances social isolation adds to the person's suffering.

Another aspect essential to an understanding of the suffering of sick persons is the relation of meaning to the way in which illness is experienced. The word "meaning" is used here in two senses. In the first, to mean is to signify, to imply. Pain in the chest may imply heart disease. We also say that we know what something means when we know how important it is. The importance of things is always personal and individual, even though meaning in this sense may be shared by others or by society as a whole. What something signifies and how important it is relative to the whole array of a person's concerns contribute to its personal meaning. "Belief" is another word for that aspect of meaning concerned with implications, and "value" concerns the degree of importance to a particular person.

The personal meaning of things does not consist exclusively of values and beliefs that are held intellectually; it includes other dimensions. For the same word, a person may simultaneously have a cognitive meaning, an affective or emotional meaning, a bodily meaning, and a transcendent or spiritual meaning. And there may be contradictions in the different levels of meaning. The nuances of personal meaning are complex, and when I speak of personal meanings I am implying this complexity in all its depth—known and unknown. Personal meaning is a fundamental dimension of personhood, and there can be no understanding of human illness or suffering without taking it into account.

A Simplified Description of the Person

A simple topology of a person may be useful in understanding the relation between suffering and the goals of medicine. The features discussed below point the way to further study and to the possibility of specific action by individual physicians.

Persons have personality and character. Personality traits appear within the first few weeks of life and are remarkably durable over time. Some personalities handle some illnesses better than others. Individual persons vary in character as well. During the heyday of psychoanalysis in the 1950s, all behavior was attributed to unconscious determinants: No one was bad or good; they were merely sick or well. Fortunately, that simplistic view of human character is now out of favor. Some people do in fact have stronger characters and bear adversity better. Some are good and kind under the stress of terminal illness, whereas others become mean and offensive when even mildly ill.

A person has a past. The experiences gathered during one's life are a part of today as well as yesterday. Memory exists in the nostrils and the hands, not only in the mind. A fragrance drifts by, and a memory is evoked. My feet have not forgotten how to roller-skate, and my hands remember skills that I was hardly aware I had learned. When these past experiences involve sickness and medical care, they can influence present illness and medical care. They stimulate fear, confidence, physical symptoms, and anguish. It damages people to rob them of their past and deny their memories, or to mock their fears and worries. A person without a past is incomplete.

Life experiences—previous illness, experiences with doctors, hospitals, and medications, deformities and disabilities, pleasures and successes, miseries and failures—all form the nexus for illness. The personal meaning of the disease and its treatment arises from the past as well as the present. If cancer occurs in a patient with self-confidence from past achievements, it may give rise to optimism and a resurgence of strength. Even if it is fatal, the disease may not produce the destruction of the person but, rather, reaffirm his or her indomitability. The outcome would be different in a person for whom life had been a series of failures.

The intensity of ties to the family cannot be overemphasized; people frequently behave as though they were physical extensions of their parents. Events that might cause suffering in others may be borne without complaint by someone who believes that the disease is part of his or her family identity and hence inevitable. Even diseases for which no heritable basis is known may be borne easily by a person because others in the family have been similarly afflicted. Just as the person's past experiences give meaning to present events, so do the past experiences of his or her family. Those meanings are part of the person.

A person has a cultural background. Just as a person is part of a culture and a society, these elements are part of the person. Culture defines what is meant by masculinity or femininity, what attire is acceptable, attitudes toward the dying and sick, mating behavior, the height of chairs and steps, degrees of tolerance for odors and excreta, and how the aged and the disabled are treated. Cultural definitions have an enormous impact on the sick and can be a source of untold suffering. They influence the behavior of others toward the sick person and that of the sick toward themselves. Cultural norms and social rules regulate whether someone can be among others or will be isolated, whether the sick will be considered foul or acceptable, and whether they are to be pitied or censured.

Returning to the sculptor described earlier, we know why that young woman suffered. She was housebound and bedbound, her face was changed by steroids, she was masculinized by her treatment, one breast was scarred, and she had almost no hair. The degree of importance attached to these losses—that aspect of their personal meaning—is determined to a great degree by cultural priorities.

With this in mind, we can also realize how much someone devoid of physical pain, even devoid of "symptoms," may suffer. People suffer from what they have lost of themselves in relation to the world of objects, events, and relationships. We realize, too, that although medical care can reduce the impact of sickness, inattentive care can increase the disruption caused by illness.

A person has roles. I am a husband, a father, a physician, a teacher, a brother, an orphaned son, and an uncle. People are their roles, and each role has rules. Together, the rules that guide the performance of roles make up a complex set of entitlements and limitations of responsibility and privilege. By middle age, the roles may be so firmly set that disease can lead to the virtual destruction of a person by making the performance of his or her roles impossible. Whether the patient is a doctor who cannot doctor or a mother who cannot mother, he or she is diminished by the loss of function.

No person exists without others; there is no consciousness without a consciousness of others, no speaker without a hearer, and no act, object, or thought that does not somehow encompass others.[6] All behavior is or will be involved with others, even if only in memory or reverie. Take away others, remove sight or hearing, and the person is diminished. Everyone dreads becoming blind or deaf, but these are only the most obvious injuries to human interaction. There are many ways in which human beings can be cut off from others and then suffer the loss.

It is in relationships with others that the full range of human emotions finds expression. It is this dimension of the person that may be injured when illness disrupts the ability to express emotion. Furthermore, the extent and nature of a sick person's relationships influence the degree of suffering from a disease. There is a vast difference between going home to an empty apartment and going home to a network of friends and family after hospitalization. Illness may occur in one partner of a long and strongly bound marriage or in a union that is falling apart. Suffering from the loss of sexual function associated with some diseases will depend not only on the importance of sexual performance itself but also on its importance in the sick person's relationships.

A person is a political being. A person is in this sense equal to other persons, with rights and obligations and the ability to redress injury by others and the state. Sickness can interfere, producing the feeling of political powerlessness and lack of representation. Persons who are permanently handicapped may suffer from a feeling of exclusion from participation in the political realm.

Persons do things. They act, create, make, take apart, put together, wind, unwind, cause to be, and cause to vanish. They know themselves, and are known, by these acts. When illness restricts the range of activity of persons, they are not themselves.

Persons are often unaware of much that happens within them and why. Thus, there are things in the mind that cannot be brought to awareness by ordinary reflection. The structure of the unconscious is pictured quite differently by different scholars, but most students of human behavior accept the assertion that such an interior world exists. People can behave in ways that seem inexplicable and strange even to themselves, and the sense of powerlessness that the person may feel in the presence of such behavior can be a source of great distress.

Persons have regular behaviors. In health, we take for granted the details of our day-to-day behavior. Persons know themselves to be well as much by whether they behave as usual as by any other set of facts. Patients decide that they are ill because they cannot perform as usual, and they may suffer the loss of their routine. If they cannot do the things that they identify with the fact of their being, they are not whole.

Every person has a body. The relation with one's body may vary from identification with it to admiration, loathing, or constant fear. The body may even be perceived as a representation of a parent, so that when something happens to the person's body it is as though a parent were injured. Disease can so alter the relation that the body is no longer seen as a friend but, rather, as an untrustworthy enemy. This is intensified if the illness comes on without warning, and as illness persists, the person may feel increasingly vulnerable. Just as many people have an expanded sense of self as a result of changes in their bodies from exercise, the potential exists for a contraction of this sense through injury to the body.

Everyone has a secret life. Sometimes it takes the form of fantasies and dreams of glory; sometimes it has a real existence known to only a few. Within the secret life are fears, desires, love affairs of the past and present, hopes, and fantasies. Disease may destroy not only the public or the private person but the secret person as well. A secret beloved friend may be lost to a sick person because he or she has no legitimate place by the sickbed. When that happens, the patient may have lost the part of life that made tolerable an otherwise embittered existence. Or the loss may be only of a dream, but one that might have come true. Such loss can be a source of great distress and intensely private pain.

Everyone has a perceived future. Events that one expects to come to pass vary from expectations for one's children to a belief in one's creative ability. Intense unhappiness results from a loss of the future—the future of the individual person, of children, and of other loved ones.

Hope dwells in this dimension of existence, and great suffering attends the loss of hope.

Everyone has a transcendent dimension, a life of the spirit. This is most directly expressed in religion and the mystic traditions, but the frequency with which people have intense feelings of bonding with groups, ideals, or anything larger and more enduring than the person is evidence of the universality of the transcendent dimension. The quality of being greater and more lasting than an individual life gives this aspect of the person its timeless dimension. The profession of medicine appears to ignore the human spirit. When I see patients in nursing homes who have become only bodies, I wonder whether it is not their transcendent dimension that they have lost.

The Nature of Suffering

For purposes of explanation, I have outlined various parts that make up a person. However, persons cannot be reduced to their parts in order to be better understood. Reductionist scientific methods, so successful in human biology, do not help us to comprehend whole persons. My intent was rather to suggest the complexity of the person and the potential for injury and suffering that exists in everyone. With this in mind, any suggestion of mechanical simplicity should disappear from my definition of suffering. All the aspects of personhood—the lived past, the family's lived past, culture and society, roles, the instrumental dimension, associations and relationships, the body, the unconscious mind, the political being, the secret life, the perceived future, and the transcendent dimension—are susceptible to damage and loss.

Injuries to the integrity of the person may be expressed by sadness, anger, loneliness, depression, grief, unhappiness, melancholy, rage, withdrawal, or yearning. We acknowledge the person's right to have and express such feelings. But we often forget that the affect is merely the outward expression of the injury, not the injury itself. We know little about the nature of the injuries themselves, and what we know has been learned largely from literature, not medicine.

If the injury is sufficient, the person suffers. The only way to learn what damage is sufficient to cause suffering, or whether suffering is present, is to ask the sufferer. We all recognize certain injuries that almost invariably cause suffering: the death or distress of loved ones, powerlessness, helplessness, hopelessness, torture, the loss of a life's work, betrayal, physical agony, isolation, homelessness, memory failure, and fear. Each is both universal and individual. Each touches features common to all of us, yet each contains features that must be defined in terms of a specific person at a specific time. With the relief of suffering in mind, however, we should reflect on how remarkably little is known of these injuries.

The Amelioration of Suffering

One might inquire why everyone is not suffering all the time. In a busy life, almost no day passes in which one's intactness goes unchallenged. Obviously, not every challenge is a threat. Yet I suspect that there is more suffering than is known. Just as people with chronic pain learn to keep it to themselves because others lose interest, so may those with chronic suffering.

There is another reason why every injury may not cause suffering. Persons are able to enlarge themselves in response to damage, so that instead of being reduced, they may indeed grow. This response to suffering has encouraged the belief that suffering is good for people. To some degree, and in some persons, this may be so. If a leg is injured so that an athlete cannot run again, the athlete may compensate for the loss by learning another sport or mode of expression. So it is with the loss of relationships, loves, roles, physical strength, dreams, and power. The human body may lack the capacity to gain a new part when one is lost, but the person has it.

The ability to recover from loss without succumbing to suffering is sometimes called resilience, as though nothing but elastic rebound were involved, but it is more as though an inner force were withdrawn from one manifestation of a person and redirected to another. If a child dies and the parent makes a successful recovery, the person is said to have "rebuilt" his or her life. The term suggests that the parts of the person are structured in a new manner, allowing expression in different dimensions. If a previously active person is confined to a wheelchair, intellectual pursuits may occupy more time.

Recovery from suffering often involves help, as though people who have lost parts of themselves can be sustained by the personhood of others until their own recovers. This is one of the latent functions of physicians: to lend strength. A group, too, may lend strength: Consider the success of groups of the similarly afflicted in easing the burden of illness (e.g., women with mastectomies, people with ostomies, and even the parents or family members of the diseased).

Meaning and transcendence offer two additional ways by which the suffering associated with destruction of a part of personhood is ameliorated. Assigning a meaning to the injurious condition often reduces or even resolves the suffering associated with it. Most often, a cause for the condition is sought within past behaviors or beliefs. Thus, the pain or threat that causes suffering is seen as not destroying a part of the person, because it is part of the person by virtue of its origin within the self. In our culture, taking the blame for harm that comes to oneself because of the unconscious mind serves the same purpose as the concept of karma in Eastern theolo-

gies; suffering is reduced when it can be located within a coherent set of meanings. Physicians are familiar with the question from the sick, "Did I do something that made this happen?" It is more tolerable for a terrible thing to happen because of something that one has done than it is to be at the mercy of chance.

Transcendence is probably the most powerful way in which one is restored to wholeness after an injury to personhood. When experienced, transcendence locates the person in a far larger landscape. The sufferer is not isolated by pain but is brought closer to a transpersonal source of meaning and to the human community that shares those meanings. Such an experience need not involve religion in any formal sense; however, in its transpersonal dimension, it is deeply spiritual. For example, patriotism can be a secular expression of transcendence.

When Suffering Continues

But what happens when suffering is not relieved? If suffering occurs when there is a threat to one's integrity or a loss of a part of a person, then suffering will continue if the person cannot be made whole again. Little is known about this aspect of suffering. Is much of what we call depression merely unrelieved suffering? Considering that depression commonly follows the loss of loved ones, business reversals, prolonged illness, profound injuries to self-esteem, and other damages to personhood, the possibility is real. In many chronic or serious diseases, persons who "recover" or who seem to be successfully treated do not return to normal function. They may never again be employed, recover sexual function, pursue career goals, reestablish family relationships, or reenter the social world, despite a physical cure. Such patients may not have recovered from the nonphysical changes occurring with serious illness. Consider the dimensions of personhood described above, and note that each is threatened or damaged in profound illness. It should come as no surprise, then, that chronic suffering frequently follows in the wake of disease.

The paradox with which this paper began—that suffering is often caused by the treatment of the sick—no longer seems so puzzling. How could it be otherwise, when medicine has concerned itself so little with the nature and causes of suffering? This lack is not a failure of good intentions. None are more concerned about pain or loss of function than physicians. Instead, it is a failure of knowledge and understanding. We lack knowledge, because in working from a dichotomy contrived within a historical context far from our own, we have artificially circumscribed our task in caring for the sick.

Attempts to understand all the known dimensions of personhood and their relations to illness and suffering present problems of staggering complexity. The problems are no greater, however, than those initially posed by the question of how the body works—a question that we have managed to answer in extraordinary detail. If the ends of medicine are to be directed toward the relief of human suffering, the need is clear.

Notes

I am indebted to Rabbi Jack Bemporad, to Drs. Joan Cassell, Peter Dineen, Nancy McKenzie, and Richard Zaner, to Ms. Dawn McGuire, to the members of the Research Group on Death, Suffering, and Well-Being of The Hastings Center for their advice and assistance, and to the Arthur Vining Davis Foundations for support of the research group.

1. Cassell, E. Being and becoming dead. Soc Res. 1972; 39: 528–42.
2. Bakan, D. Disease, pain and sacrifice: toward a psychology of suffering. Chicago: Beacon Press, 1971.
3. Marks, R.M., Sachar, E.J. Undertreatment of medical inpatients with narcotic analgesics. Ann Intern Med. 1973; 78:173–81.
4. Kanner, R.M., Foley, K.M. Patterns of narcotic drug use in a cancer pain clinic. Ann NY Acad Sci. 1981; 362:161–72.
5. Goodwin, J.S., Goodwin, J.M., Vogel, A.V. Knowledge and use of placebos by house officers and nurses. Ann Intern Med. 1979; 91:106–10.
6. Zaner, R. The context of self: a phenomenological inquiry using medicine as a clue. Athens, Ohio: Ohio University Press, 1981.

Cancer, Control, and Causality:

Talking about Cancer

in a Working-Class

Community

Martha Balshem

■

In the early 1980s, research based on records of cancer mortality for the city of Philadelphia indicated that two Philadelphia communities were experiencing higher than expected rates of cancer mortality (Dayal, Chiu, Sharrar, Mangan, Rosenwaike, Shapiro, Henley, Goldberg-Alberts, and Kinman 1984). In the parlance of the local tabloids, which quickly reported the findings, these communities were "cancer hot spots." In 1983, a cancer education project was initiated in one of the communities, a white working-class area in the inner city. Project plans called for a baseline survey followed by three years of intensive, community-based educational intervention. The project was to be modeled after several successful community-based projects focused on the prevention of heart disease (Farquhar, Maccoby, Wood, Alexander, Breitrose, Brown, Haskell, McAlister, Meyer, Nash, and Stern 1977; Puska, Koskela, Pakarinen, Puuma-Iainen, Soininen, and Tuomilehto 1976).

To set the context for application of the heart disease project model, the baseline survey for the cancer project included a series of questions on knowledge, attitudes, and practices related to heart disease, along with a set of nearly identical questions on cancer. Results indicated that attitudes toward cancer were significantly and consistently more negative (Amsel, Grover, Bal-

shem, and Gillespie 1984). This raised questions about the applicability of the heart disease project model and left project planners with a conundrum, as quantitative data so often do: it was clear what the survey results said, but not what they meant.

The cancer education project was fielded, nonetheless, and given the name "Project CAN-DO." The name of the project reflected its philosophy: that with regard to cancer prevention, we should focus on factors within our personal control. Residents of the "cancer hot spot" were advised to adopt lifestyle changes—to quit smoking, change their diets, and go for regular cancer screenings—to reduce their risk of cancer. Not long into the project, it became clear that community resistance to program messages was profound, with residents insisting to project health educators that cancer was impossible to prevent and that fate dictated whether or not one would be stricken by the disease.

My own involvement began one year into the program. My duties were to develop and deliver educational programs and to conduct an ethnographic substudy on community attitudes toward cancer. Before describing the investigation that resulted, I will review the theoretical issues that inform my analysis. This review will argue against a literal reading of community statements of belief. Such a reading, typical of the behavioral science perspectives that underlie health education practice, leads only toward a descriptive glossing of community beliefs as "fatalistic." My own reading will recast community statements of belief as purposeful acts in a discourse of resistance.

Working-Class "Fatalism"

Working-class populations in industrial societies are commonly described as fatalistic, often by educators and policy makers who confront working-class resistance to their recommendations. For instance, health educators often call for the reduction of health risks through changes in lifestyle. A standard reference work on cancer prevention states that 75 to 85 percent of all cancer in the United States might be avoided through changes in lifestyle factors such as smoking, diet, and compliance with screening recommendations (Doll and Peto 1981:1205). But working-class people often refuse to change their lifestyles, stating to educators that disease is tied to the activity of fate. They are then labeled "fatalistic" and "hard to reach."

Although health promotion researchers have called for an increasing awareness of the wider context of this "working-class fatalism" (Calnan 1984; Hochbaum 1981; Minkler and Pasick 1986; Pill and Stott 1982, 1985, 1987; Sciandra 1983), the presumption remains that combating fatalism is a basic mission of health education practice. The goal remains the discovery of the shortest path to compliance with the recommendations of scientific medicine. In adopting this goal, health educators define their practice as one that supports and enforces the unequal power dynamic that characterizes the medical encounter.[1] Embedded in the notion of compliance is the basic social relation of clinical medicine, in which the prerogative of defining health status, health risk, and appropriate treatment or action is reserved for the medical scientist or surrogate thereof. Thus, health educators adapt their world view to that of medical science (cf. Trostle 1988).

The inequalities inherent in clinical medical practice have been much investigated in medical anthropology. Power dynamics in the medical encounter have been examined from a variety of viewpoints—including those of sociolinguistics (Fisher and Todd 1983), the explanatory models approach (Kleinman, Eisenberg, and Good 1978), and political economy and social history (Brown 1979; Doyal 1979; Starr 1982). Researchers in health promotion have contrib-

uted their share (Greene, Adelman, Charon, and Hoffman 1986; also see above). A body of widely known, explicitly critical work relates the experience of domination in the medical system to wider processes of social control (Foucault 1975; Freidson 1970; Illich 1976; Taussig 1980; Young 1980; Zola 1972). Recent work on the control of biological reproduction has been particularly clear both on unequal power relationships in the clinical dyad and on how this extends into the realm of public policy decision making (see, for instance, Irwin and Jordan 1987; Martin 1987; Rapp 1988).

Particularly relevant to the issue of working-class fatalism and noncompliance is Taussig's discussion of the "disputes of power" that center on the loss of autonomy to medical professionals. Central to such disputes is the issue of who has the power to define illness and to define appropriate responses to it. In Taussig's analysis, which proceeds from the experience of a hospital patient, the ceding of power to medical authority is uneasy, entailing contradictions that are at least periodically felt to be such by the patient.

In health education practice in working-class communities, we see the same dispute in a different context. The health educator, as surrogate medical scientist, tacitly claims the power to define public health issues and to assign value to different lifestyles. But the context of this practice is very different from that of the clinic: the audience is not, by and large, composed of sick patients, who, in their vulnerable state, are especially inclined to cede power to medical authority. The site of community health education practice is usually a community's home ground— a seniors' center, a church social, a neighborhood shopping center. In this context, we might expect to see a community emboldened to speak its mind.

The conflict between Project CAN-DO educators and residents of their study community is to be understood, then, in terms of issues of authority and resistance. On the surface, their discourse involves disagreements concerning scientific beliefs about cancer, a community critique of the world view of science. But discourse is also practice. Following Herzfeld's (1982) discussion of the uses of rhetoric about fate in Greek discourse, I will explore the ways in which attributions to fate constitute a form of practice in themselves, with a meaning rooted in a still wider social context (cf. Herzfeld 1982:657; also see Herzfeld 1987). Specifically, I will assert that in this community, talking about fate and cancer is a form of everyday resistance (Scott 1985) and an important mechanism in the construction and maintenance of the value ascribed to local tradition.

The Study Community

The Project CAN-DO study community is a very old inner-city area, with small rowhouses and light industry interspersed. At its northern boundary is an important concentration of chemical industry, consisting of two major employers of community residents. The population of the area, numbering about 100,000, is 99 percent white, with large numbers of Polish, Irish, German, and Italian families. Levels of formal education are modest; median annual income was only $13,000 at the time of the 1980 census; and employment is heavily blue collar, with high unemployment rates (Bureau of the Census 1983; Philadelphia City Planning Commission 1982a, 1982b).

It is common for area families to have roots in their neighborhood that go back three or four generations. Many residents seldom leave their neighborhoods, and have limited experience with outside agencies. The social lives of most residents revolve around family, neighborhood, and church. The area is heavily Catholic, with both geographic and ethnic parishes, and most neighborhood children attend Catholic schools.

The tall spires of the various Catholic churches are visible everywhere, and they serve to orient resident and visitor alike. The neighborhoods feel self-contained: streets are narrow and well worn, everyone knows the same people, and few come in or leave without being noticed.

As mentioned above, the neighborhoods also experience high rates of cancer mortality and are known throughout the metropolitan area as a "cancer hot spot." Dayal et al. (1984) present an ecologic analysis of cancer mortality, socioeconomic status, and air pollution levels, suggesting that smoking and occupational exposure—risk factors that correlate with socioeconomic status—explain the high community cancer rates. They carefully acknowledge the limitations of the ecologic approach and point to the possibility of a more complex, perhaps synergistic, role for air pollution. In contrast, popular wisdom connects the high cancer rates to industrial pollution, especially air pollution from the chemical plants. Near those plants, this pollution leaves constant reminders: a white film on the windowsills; a distinctive odor, almost always present; and billowing smokestacks on the weekends, when the local Environmental Protection Agency office closes.

Cancer is an important issue in the neighborhoods, and the Dayal study is fairly well known. Community interpretation of the study downplays the careful caveats of the researchers and defines the study as a scientific denial of the link between cancer and air pollution. The Project CAN-DO focus on lifestyle factors is seen in the same light. Community residents have reason to feel cynical. Despite suggestions that air pollution may reduce the body's ability to fight the spread of cancer cells (see the discussion in Richters 1988), definitive epidemiological research on the link between cancer and air pollution has been defined as prohibitively complex and expensive, and polluters can state that there is no research that clearly shows such a link.

The Public Discourse:
Health Education Practice

In my study of this community, I participated in both public and private discourses about cancer. The public discourse was conducted during my two years of work in the community as a health educator, much of which involved presentations to community groups. These presentations offered an interesting window onto the community.

The reader is asked to imagine a large meeting hall in a Catholic church basement. The floor is linoleum and the walls are yellowish green, with grates over high, small windows. There are 50 or 60 people there, mostly women, for the monthly meeting of the Home and School Association. The people all know one another, and they laugh and joke about recent shared events. Seven or eight women are crammed into a kitchen designed for two, all busily helping to get the coffee on. Ten trays of donuts, cakes, and cookies await the end of the formal meeting. Several sisters from the teaching order are present, including the principal of the church school, who is accorded great respect. The pastor is also present, delighting his parishioners with an energetic display of informality and folksy humor.

The Project CAN-DO team, consisting of myself and a colleague, arrives, carrying a slide/tape projector and assorted paraphernalia. We find the Home and School Association president, who beams at me. "Oh," she says, "you're the cancer lady. Well, let's get you settled in!" The projector is set up on an old piano bench, propped up by a stack of books. Like as not, the slides will be shown on a wall, lending a yellowish green tint to the entire production.

The meeting begins. Business is first, consisting of the treasurer's report on a recent car wash, which earned enough to buy a computer for the eighth graders. A woman from a nearby parish is introduced; carefully coiffed and tailored, she is there to recruit women to clean downtown office buildings at night. The pastor then addresses the audience, gently urging them to support the upcoming holy communion celebration. The meeting has lasted about 20 minutes, and the mood is friendly. The Home and School Association president then announces "the lady from the CAN-DO," who will address the audience on the high-fiber, low-fat diet.

I talk a few minutes, guide the audience through a written questionnaire, and give a slide show. After the slides, I ask if there are any questions. I look out at a sea of faces, all of which look silently back. Some hard work on my part brings out a few comments, mostly brief testimonials from women who already use chicken hot dogs, who have already switched to skim milk, who have done this and more because it is good for their hearts. After these few comments, the silence returns. I bring out a rubber model of five pounds of body fat, which engenders much joking and laughing. I raffle off a hot air popcorn maker, to the delight of all concerned. I then ask if there are any more questions, and the silence immediately returns. I smile and thank the audience, and the meeting adjourns to coffee and cake.

Over coffee and cake, subterranean matters surface. "My sister had cancer," confides one woman, "and the doctors couldn't do nothing for her." "I have a neighbor who eats the old food, and she is 93 years old. Would you like to meet her?" says another, in a joking but pointed spirit. "You mean your husband will eat that stuff? Mine won't," says a third. "You'll never convince most of these people," says the last. "They like their kielbasa too much." "Come by the next church dinner for some really good eating," she adds.

Then, the social climax: I am offered a piece of cake. The offerer, and a goodly number of onlookers, can barely restrain their hilarity. Time stops. Then I accept the cake. There is a burst of teasing and laughter, the conversation becomes easier, and the moment passes. We eat, pack our equipment, and leave.

The general mood of these meetings is friendly, but the health education messages are met with silence. According to one interview respondent, there is social pressure not to speak.

The Private Discourse:
Interviews and Focus Groups

Transcripts of 25 interviews and three focus group discussions document a more private discourse, one with a very different feel. In these settings, talk was easy, and respondents were eager and opinionated. The interview and focus group respondents were all women, recruited both through informal contacts and from a list of respondents to a previous survey. Judging from informal community experience and from one focus group and one formal interview with male respondents, men in the community express views similar to those of the women. However, a systematic exploration of this lies beyond the limits of my data.

The interview sample was representative of community women with regard to the occupation of the household's primary wage-earner and the years of formal education completed by the respondent. All respondents were mothers of school-aged children, and most were in their twenties or thirties. Reflecting the community pattern, half were employed outside the home. Interviews ranged from 45 minutes to two hours, with almost all lasting more than an hour. The three focus groups involved a total of about 18 women and were held at local community centers. Most participants were in their fifties or sixties.

Because of the biases that may be introduced into focus group interviews through the processes of group interaction, all quantitative analyses presented here were conducted both with and without the focus group material. This made no difference in the general trends seen. In the following presentation, I quote from 17 of the 25 interview respondents, and from two of the three focus groups. The quotations selected are representative in both tone and substance, and have not been edited to conform to standard English usage.

Heart Disease and Cancer:
Lifestyle and Environment

As stated above, the Project CAN-DO baseline survey had suggested a sharp contrast between community attitudes toward heart disease and those toward cancer. Finding this contrast interesting—although my purpose was not to focus on the contrast per se—I decided to begin my interviews with a set of questions about heart disease, followed by identical questions about cancer. After this, the interviews were almost entirely unstructured, except for a set of questions at the end concerning dietary habits.

Table 1 presents a list of factors mentioned by interview and focus group respondents in regard to the prevention or causation of cancer, heart disease, or both. Following Pill and Stott (1985), I have classified these as environmental (extrapersonal) or lifestyle factors. As the table shows, environmental factors (172 mentions) were mentioned more often than lifestyle factors (84 mentions) in regard to the prevention and causation of cancer. The opposite pattern was seen for heart disease, with 43 mentions of lifestyle factors and only 12 mentions of environmental factors.

A respondent-by-respondent analysis of the interviews, excluding the focus groups, shows the same pattern. With regard to cancer, environmental factors came more readily to mind than lifestyle factors. Every interview respondent mentioned at least one environmental factor that she considered related to cancer prevention or causation, with an average of three such factors per respondent; in contrast, only 16 respondents mentioned lifestyle factors as causing or preventing cancer. Seven more respondents mentioned lifestyle factors—notably smoking

Table 1. Factors Mentioned as Preventing or
Causing Cancer and Heart Disease

Lifestyle Factors	Cancer	Heart Disease
Diet	35	22
Smoking	16	7
Attitude	7	—
Proper exercise	5	7
Exposure to sun	5	—
Alcohol	4	3
Regular checkups	4	2
Taking care of self	4	—
Caffeine	—	2
Other lifestyle factors	4	—
Total mentions	84	43

Environmental (Extrapersonal) Factors		
Environmental pollution	64	1
Heredity	34	8
Fate/God's will	17	—
Food additives	14	—
Cannot prevent	12	—
Causes not known	9	—
Occupational exposure	7	—
Stress	6	3
Everything causes	5	—
Germs	2	—
Other environmental factors	2	—
Total mentions	172	12

and diet—only to negate or express doubt about their link to cancer (these mentions are not included in Table 1). In contrast, with regard to heart disease, the respondent-by-respondent analysis shows, again, an emphasis on lifestyle factors. Of the 17 respondents who mentioned lifestyle or environmental factors as causes of heart disease, 14 mentioned lifestyle only, three mentioned environment only, and four mentioned both. Although my questions and probes about heart disease and cancer were identical, respondents talked at greater length about cancer. This is reflected in the greater absolute numbers of factors listed in Table 1 under cancer.

Respondent discussions of cancer and heart disease were very different in emotional tone. Each interview respondent was asked, first for heart disease and then for cancer, the following question: "When I say [heart disease/cancer], what does it make you think of?" The following is a representative set of answers, from one respondent, for heart disease and cancer, respectively:

[Heart Disease] The disease, you know, affects the blood stream. The vessels. I mean, it just taxes the heart, which is a muscle, and it just gets weak. You know. And it can't perform the job that it's supposed to do. As good as it's supposed to do it.

[Cancer] Oh, God, I have this terrible thought of cancer—it's like this great big thing that's eating up your whole insides. This big black thing. I just think of it as black. This big black thing that just goes along like a pacman gobbling up your insides. . . . The movie *The Blob,* remember the blob would eat stuff and kept getting bigger and bigger. Well, that's kind of how I think of cancer. This great big blob of stuff that keeps increasing.

To this respondent, as to 14 others, heart disease was a matter of mechanics gone wrong. Respondents sometimes said that they themselves did not know how heart disease worked, but they saw it as a matter of finite knowledge. Heart disease prevention, too, was seen in straightforward terms:

Heart disease . . . say, you're okay, you're smoking, right? First of all, that takes away the oxygen, right? Then you've got the obesity with the cholesterol. That's going to clog your arteries. That's going to cause, you know, damage to the heart, little by little by little.

I never really read up on it. . . . I would just say the heart isn't as strong as yours or mine are. And because of the problem that the heart has, it's working harder and—and at times the heart just can't be working hard all the time. That's how I would put it.

Respondents expressed an easy acceptance of what they perceived as standard scientific knowledge about heart disease. The use of a mechanical model reflected their faith in the ability of modern medical science to understand heart disease fully. Regarding heart disease prevention and causation, 15 respondents made value-neutral statements describing bodily mechanics—high blood pressure, clogged arteries, bad valves, and the like.

The use of the mechanical model, and the faith in medical science that it implies, was not seen in the discussion of cancer. No respondent made straightforward mechanical model statements regarding causation and prevention of cancer. A typical answer to the question "Cancer—what does it make you think of?" was: "Death. Because most of the time when you have cancer you wind up dead, you know. I know there's treatment and all, but in my opinion I think of death." Questions about cancer, unlike questions about heart disease, evoked answers that touched on universal mysteries. In this particular case, as was typical, the respondent lowered her voice as she started to speak about cancer, and came without hesitation to the topic of death.

Fate was another topic often linked to cancer. One respondent spoke of fate in relation to cancer and death:

> If that person dies, it was—you know—that was—it was meant to be that that person would die with that disease. Where you—say you get two people maybe with the same kind where one will pull through, the other one won't.

Another respondent spoke in similar fashion to the general issue of fate and disease control:

This area, that's pretty much the way people are brought up, you know, that you can try to cheat death but it's going to happen sooner or later, so—if it's your day to die and you don't get died one way you're gonna walk in front of a car and get hit and killed anyway.

Statements about fate were usually expressed with conviction, as counterpoints to my presumed advocacy of lifestyle theories of cancer etiology. It was perceived, quite accurately, that such views were in opposition to scientific views of cancer causation, in which lifestyle is awarded center stage. However, respondents did not express a simplistic rejection of the relevance of lifestyle. They usually spoke of fate as one factor in a multifactor etiology, and as one that was simply more powerful than lifestyle:

> I think it's everything you eat and you do and a little bit from up there. . . . If you probably weigh everything out—I don't think you'll ever beat it. I do believe your time is when it is, too.

> But no, I really in my heart think that everything that, they're doing, we're learning, we're saying through education, whatever, is fine. Really. And you should follow, you should try to follow it. Okay? But I still feel that if you're gonna, you know, there's nothing you can do about it. I think it's God's will, that's all. I really do.

Talking about cancer carried us into issues of control over health in ways that talking about heart disease did not. Respondents stressed lifestyle factors when discussing heart disease causation, but stressed environmental forces when speaking of cancer. In discussing cancer, respondents spoke freely and at length of death and fate; discussions of heart disease were more mundane, often touching on mechanical models that indicated faith in the medical establishment's knowledge of the disease. Both the content and the emotional tone of the discourse reflected a more negative underlying attitude toward cancer:

> I just think it's God's will, to tell you the truth, that's my personal opinion because, as I said, this is being a cancerous area and there's people living here and you know, and just their daily life, I guess, you know, their routine, but one might eat good and one might eat bad, one might smoke, one might not smoke, and it's still comin' up, you get it or you don't get it.

> It's probably a lot easier with heart disease because like if you got maybe scar tissue on the heart—okay, they can remove that. Or in the vein—they could cut that part out and they could connect something else. Um— [silence]—you know, with cancer—I mean, that's so—[silence]—totally like the end of everything.

> At least with your heart, if you take care of yourself and do what you're supposed to do, you'll be all right, but cancer—there's no control for it. No matter what you do, it's still there. . . . It's just—you bide your time—until, until—you know, until you die.

Science and Authority

Clearly, talking about cancer brought out feelings of resistance to scientific authority. In the interview and focus group transcripts, there are 34 direct denials of the scientific view of cancer prevention, with 16 mentions of smoking and 11 mentions of diet as factors *not* associated with cancer. In contrast, not a single respondent questioned standard knowledge concerning heart disease. The following illustrate the common skepticism about the link between cancer and lifestyle:

> I don't think cigarettes really gives you cancer—I haven't heard of a lot of people who got cancer from smoking, because people who don't smoke gets cancer of the throat. So you know, you can't say it's smokers that's going to get it when nonsmokers also get it. So it can't just come from that.

> But then how about the people that don't smoke? Like my mother, like I told you, never smoked a day in her life. Why did she die of lung cancer? [Well, why do you think she did?] Beats me. I have no idea, no idea. Wish I knew.

This may be read as a simple contradiction of a scientific message: that smoking and other lifestyle factors cause cancer. But also involved is a rejection of a perceived metamessage: that scientists know definitively what causes cancer. Associated with this is a critique of scientific authority for wrongly discounting the activity of powers beyond its ken.

Respondents expressed anger, frustration, and even disdain in reaction to the perceived arrogance of the scientist. On one hand, went their discourse, science tells us that everything in our environment causes cancer; on the other, it tells us that we can prevent cancer through changes in our lifestyle:

> Every time you turn, like, no matter what you listen to—TV, radio, what have you, all right—this causes cancer, that causes cancer—you know what I mean? So, like, you know, like, all right, I opened my eyes this morning, I just breathed in 29 gallons of cancer. You know what I mean? So, like, just opening your eyes, you're saying, "Hello, cancer."

> Or fluorocarbons in hairspray. Right? You got fluorocarbons in hairspray—you're gonna kick the bucket! Well, for 18 years I was breathing in fluorocarbons; I must be ready to go at any time now. You know? Then they finally took it out. Or, "Hair dye will give you cancer." Well, then, I must have it. I mean

definitely I'm a goner. I don't know when, but I must be a goner because of all these things that they had in there and nobody never told you they weren't any good.

The sarcastic tone, commonly heard, only thinly veils the message—that scientists do not really know what causes cancer. Other respondents delivered this message straightforwardly, with a lively sense of challenge to the interviewer: "Over the last two decades everything has been 'this causes cancer and that'—and people are to the point now where they think everything you eat causes cancer and nobody really knows what causes cancer."

This anger fed into a wider stream of distrust. Expressed by four interview respondents, for instance, was the view that a cure for cancer was being withheld. As one respondent put it: "If you want my honest opinion, I think there is a cure for cancer. I believe deep down there is a cure, but it's the almighty buck again." In this view, the public is victimized by the medical establishment and the government, who conspire to maintain a profitably high level of cancer morbidity.

Talking about cancer drew us into images of victimization. For three interview respondents and for participants in two of the four focus groups, nuclear holocaust was an appropriate image for a victimized world (cf. Sontag 1977). The following quotations are drawn from two of the focus groups:

> [First respondent] You know, it's really a contradiction. Life today. You know? It really is. . . . Everybody's out to scare you. I think that's why people, you know, maybe take the negative attitude, because they think, "God, everybody's just out to," you know. [Second respondent] Everybody's out to get you, no matter what you do, so just enjoy what you do and how you do it. [Why do you think everyone's out to get you? What is it, what is it about the way things are?] [First respondent] I think the world in gen-

eral. The peace and the war and this one fighting that one. When we grew up, we—we had the—the raids—the air raid tests where we would hide under the desks. . . . Now you've got nuclear—where—forget it! You ain't gonna be there!

> No matter whether every person in the United States pickets against the nuclear bomb, if these people in Washington want it, they're gonna do it. You know, and if they want to push the button, they're gonna push it. So you feel like you don't have the control. . . . [What do you have control over in your life?] I think you have control over your family. That part. I don't think you'll ever have control over your government or your health, you know, and anything like that.

And this, from an interview respondent, weaves many issues together:

> It's the same way with the world and world peace and everything. We try, we pray, we talk, we sit down, but there's still that fear in everyone's heart that somebody's gonna push the button. . . . So who controls everything, you know. No matter what we do . . . if you don't eat the proper diet, if you do smoke, if you do drink, and . . . you run your body to the ground, it's gonna catch up with you a lot *sooner* than maybe the person who does everything, that eats all the right things and exercises and doesn't smoke and gets out, you know—but the ironic thing about it, he's the one who drops dead before the guy that's abusing everything! . . . I don't think you control it. And if you're raised and . . . born to the faith that we are, you don't control it. Okay? He might let us think we do, but we don't. Why do babies die? Why are there crib deaths? . . . Why anything? It's just the way it is. You're not gonna change it.

Control, fate, and victimization—these were issues into which talking about cancer led us. Central was a resentment of the authority of science. In many instances, respondent statements about this issue carried such emotional force that they effectively brought my questioning to a halt.

Cancer: A Minion of Fate

From respondent discourse, one may glean an integrated structure of belief about the essential nature of cancer. This view of the nature of the disease is fundamentally different from that propounded by scientific medicine. According to this view, cancer is at the same time "within us all" and "all around us." We are all born with it, and it can be activated by nearly anything—from a serious trauma, such as a major accident, to the most incidental of life events, such as a bump on the breast. It can also be activated by stress, which can mean the wearing effect of everyday living or of an especially difficult period of time. Substances present in the air, earth, and water can also activate it. The causes of cancer are everywhere. Once activated, cancer is invariably fatal:

> Everything to me is cancerous, because it seems like every time you turn around, it causes cancer. I mean, you hear on TV, I mean, you touch somethin' and it might cause cancer.

> I think we're all born with cancer cells, and I think certain things, maybe diseases or the environment, bring them out.

Respondent descriptions of the cancer disease process suggested purposefulness and motivation. Cancer does more than simply grow: it takes over, hits your brain, burns you up, kills you from the inside out. The dominant metaphor (used by ten of the 25 interview respondents) was that cancer eats away at your body. It was spoken of as active, powerful, and impossible to stop:

> Literally, the cancer is eating away the rest of the body—the rest of the cells in the body.

> It just eats you up, I guess. It just starts and it doesn't stop, you know. . . . You always hear of it startin' and that they—it doesn't help, you know. some you hear on TV, they get cured but . . . it just goes and it doesn't stop.

Cancer was described as a "sneaky disease," suggesting that the activity of the disease is capricious:

> Like one day you could be fine and then turn around and you have cancer and it eats away at you.

> It's a sneaky disease. . . . Because it doesn't show itself. . . . There's cancer cells in everybody's body. Somewhere.

It was also described as "the devil's disease," suggesting that cruelty and evil are part of its nature. The following is an excerpt from a memorial article in a community newspaper:

> She was stricken by the devil's disease, cancer, and for 4 years she fought the disease till she had no more strength to fight, she died peacefully only after she was assured we could accept her death. [Betcher and Betcher 1986][2]

As with most minions of fate, cancer may punish those who notice or defy it. To think about cancer, to try to prevent it, is to tempt fate. Cancer testing is "looking for trouble." Respondents seemed hesitant to speak the word "cancer" out loud, and they often referred to cancer as "the big C." Cancer patients are often isolated because people are reluctant to be near them or to speak to them about their disease. Sometimes the word will not even be spoken within the extended family circle of a dying patient. One respondent said of her mother's death: "I don't know if she knew she had cancer. We never talked about it, we never did. But she wasn't stupid—she watched TV, she worked with people. I'm sure, you know, trying to protect us that she didn't discuss it." Another respondent on reactions of a neighbor to news of her husband's illness with cancer: "Oh, they asked me, when they found out—my neighbor—she said, 'What are you going to tell the neighbors?' I said, 'It's not a sin. It's nobody's fault.' "

Many community residents, then, spoke of cancer as a purposeful entity that is capricious, cruel, and evil. The workings of cancer are workings of fate, and fate explains why one person rather than another falls ill. Cancer is a bad fate, in the face of which our bodies are permeable, affording us no protection in the physical and moral world. Because of cancer, our bodies contain and are tied to a force wider than the individual body, and not subject to individual control. The fear of cancer is the fear of annihilation, the fear of death.

Challenging fate is a risky business. Cancer inspires not challenge but taboo: "[Cancer is] taboo. Don't talk about it. If I don't talk about it, you know, or hear about it, I might not get it. You know?"

Cancer Prevention and Defiance

These beliefs support a theory of cancer prevention very different from that taught by scientific medicine. For one thing, everyone is vulnerable, regardless of personal habits. This vulnerability is so complete that making lifestyle changes to lower cancer risk is useless:

I figure I can watch what I'm eating, and do this and do that, but yet I can still get cancer any time. Anybody can, no matter what you do you still can get it, 'cause it doesn't matter what you do or whatever, if it's there, it's there.

I don't think you'll meet anyone who isn't—somewhere isn't going along with the new ideas of not—or cutting down smoking or not smoking or changing food habits . . . but I still feel strongly that . . . if you're gonna get it, you're gonna get it. And there's nothing we can do about it.

No matter what you do—if it's there, it's there. People who even have different lifestyles can get the same kind of cancer. So—either way, you know—if you're going to get it, I think you're going to get it, and that's it.

Can cancer, then, be prevented at all? An answer emerged at various places in the discourse, but perhaps most clearly in stories about the defiant ancestor.

The defiant ancestor, a golden age figure of the grandparental or parental generation, was often invoked by community residents during informal discussions following health education programs. The figure was introduced by eight out of 25 interview respondents, and recognized eagerly by others when I myself introduced it. Respondents stated proudly that they themselves had many of the attributes of these ancestors. The defiant ancestor, so goes the story, smoked two packs of cigarettes a day, ate nothing but lard and bread, never went to the doctor, and lived to the age of 93. The natural questions that followed during the interviews were: What do you think these people did right? Why do you think they lived so long?

Above all else, the defiant ancestor was a hard worker. Physical labor, at work and at home, was the backbone of her existence: "That woman ever since I was born worked and worked and worked . . . woke up 4:30 every morning, did some wash, went to work, came home—she just went—and I think a lot of people, that keeps them going." Moreover, the defiant ancestor did not dwell on disease. Keeping a positive attitude is an important part of staying healthy; refusing to acknowledge symptoms is a way of keeping sickness at bay. Working hard and staying active are the best medicines:

> That was on I think television the other day when they were saying that—I think it was a nurse talking and she said that the people that say, "Oh, my God! I'm afraid I might have cancer! I might have cancer!" They—they're the ones that tend to get it, more so than the ones that say, "Whatever's wrong with me, I'm going to fight it and I'm going to be strong!"

> If you're the type of people that just sit around all the time, you're gonna be sick a lot. If you get up and move and go out and do things, they don't seem to be as sick that often. . . . [The old people] get up at five in the morning and go to bed at nine at night and they work all the time.

> If a person thinks—feels that they're going to get sick, they do get sick. And—because they have that in their mind. . . . Myself, I just take one day at a time, and I don't look at what's going to happen tomorrow because tomorrow might not come.

Part of not dwelling on sickness is staying away from the doctor, ignoring medical advice, and refusing medications:

> You've got to stop and think about these people. They're of the old school, I think, and they know how to work hard. . . . They came over—they worked like horses. They were strong, and I think—years ago, people didn't run to a doctor. They had the old remedies.

> My grandmother, she doesn't, she never went to the doctor's until the last couple months; she was in so much pain that she went. She has an ulcer and you know, and they thought maybe she had something like Reagan had. . . . But it took her until she was in *that much* pain to go.

Working hard and toughing it out—it is a point of pride to delay going to the doctor until you are nearly dysfunctional. Hiding sickness is also prized:

> I would feel that even though if I'm going to die, I'd rather do it longer instead of dying sooner, and making myself happy and the people around me happy so it doesn't even think that I'm dying. Just let it just go my normal life and just be happy and just don't even pay attention that I'm going to die, just keep it going as long as I can.

Even when diagnosed with cancer, those who follow the old ways can show themselves to have resources that medical science does not understand. This story, echoed by others, shows an ancestor who was defiant even in the face of death:

> Like my father—he had leukemia, which is cancer of the blood. They told him that he only had two months to live, and he says, "No way—I'm makin' that summer because I'm going to my boat." And the doctors still can't believe to this day that he made four months. . . . And he died at the end of September. So I think outlook has a lot to do with it. If you make up your mind you're going to do something about it, you can. . . . He was a fighter.

Through discourse about the defiant ancestor, respondents expressed a theory of cancer prevention that was consistent with their expressed view of the disease. If cancer is a minion of fate, then escaping the notice of fate is preventive medicine. An expression of evil purpose—one that seeks to victimize us—is warded off by a positive attitude, by which we refuse to allow evil to overwhelm us. Cancer is also capricious and irrational, striking regardless of direct efforts to control it. Are such efforts, then, counterproductive, serving to challenge forces that we hope will ignore us? The image of the defiant ancestor suggests that dwelling on cancer prevention is foolish. This respondent expressed a common ultimate assessment:

> I feel that even if you're healthy and you don't go to the doctor's you still—you know, you still can live, and even if you smoke and all, you still can live until an age. So it doesn't matter what you do, you still die when your time comes. So it doesn't matter if you change your diet, or stop smoking, when your time's up it's up and there ain't nothin' you can do about it. But 'least they lived to be happy and did what they wanted to do. That's the more important thing.

Discussion

In this high-risk community, talking about cancer means talking about fate. This may be seen as a reflection of heartfelt beliefs. But another understanding may be drawn from looking at the wider context of the discourse.

The Health Educator's View

Scientific medicine is a jealous discipline. It dictates, as a central article of faith, that the only valid road to health is paved with its own recommendations. Health behaviors and beliefs are beyond moral criticism only if they remain on this road. Otherwise, they are problematic and are cast as abnormalities through the process of "medicalization" (Illich 1976; Zola 1972). Scheper-Hughes and Lock summarize this concept as one that describes how

> negative social sentiments . . . can be recast as individual pathologies and "symptoms" rather than as socially significant "signs." This funneling of diffuse but real complaints into the idiom of sickness has led to the problem of "medicalization" and to the overproduction of illness in contemporary advanced industrial societies. In this process the role of doctors, social workers, psychia-

trists, and criminologists as agents of social consensus is pivotal. . . . The medical gaze is, then, a controlling gaze, through which active (although furtive) forms of protest are transformed into passive acts of "breakdown." [1987:27]

Adjunct health professionals, health educators among them, are often concerned to gain legitimacy in the eyes of physicians. This means affiliating themselves with the paradigm of scientific medicine on multiple levels. One way to do this is to adopt a clinical gaze. Through such a gaze, the health educator may see those who do not follow scientific medical advice as being essentially sick. The diagnosis in the case described here would be fatalism. This fatalism may be seen as situated within the individual, like an ear infection or a swollen appendix. Like gaze and diagnosis, treatment is aggressive. The magic bullet is the health education message, delivered to the target population through an appropriate strategy, preferably at a teachable moment. In this military language, describing health education's front in the war against cancer, we see the diffusion and elaboration of one of scientific medicine's fundamental metaphors (see Martin 1988).

In the case of working-class fatalism, medicalization is implicit and not officially recognized by either physician or health educator. The process nonetheless functions to recast resistance to health promotion efforts as a diagnosable pathology. Thus, the world view of medical science is reproduced in a new setting. This may serve to make health promotion efforts to "combat fatalism" seem more legitimate to the physicians on whose acceptance the researcher depends.

This medicalization has at least four consequences. First, it blocks the health educator's view. Along with the clinical gaze comes a pair of blinders. If fatalism is a disease, there is no need to look further at an indigenous etiology that is merely a symptom of this disease. Such an etiology may be dismissed as irrational, and the discourse reported here may be understood only in narrow, adversarial terms.

Second, it obviates the need to develop a critical understanding of the beliefs held by health educators. Without such understanding, health educators have no razor, independent of that of medical science, with which to separate legitimate practice from delusion. For instance, the overall rate for cancer mortality, including all cases of any type, is currently 50 percent; in light of this, the health educator's selling of optimism about the curability of cancer must be considered problematic.

Third, it generates a conceptual schema that allows health professionals to ignore the insights and views of entire communities. With a diagnosis of fatalism, health educators provide clinicians, epidemiologists, and laboratory researchers a vocabulary with which to explain and dismiss the fears of working-class persons and groups. Clinical prejudices are rewritten as scientific understanding. Through medicalization of alternative etiologies, medical science remains a closed system.

Finally, medicalization imparts a moralistic tone to health education practice. The script supplied by medical science constructs the role of the health educator very tightly. This is painful to health educators who identify with their audiences and are not inclined to reduce people to their compliance characteristics. Like anthropologists, health educators often desire to serve as advocates for the communities and people they study.

Such desires notwithstanding, it is extremely difficult for health educators to escape from the worldview of medical science. In the official view of health education campaigns such as Project CAN-DO, local cancer etiologies, through a process of medicalization, are seen only as symptoms of fatalism and denials of objective risk. As such, these health beliefs are material for the construction of a negative other and are part of what makes the "hard to reach" population inscrutable (cf. Said 1978).

The Community View

Most community residents express a set of beliefs about cancer causation, and causation in general, different from that propounded by science. The causal universe they describe is one in which God and luck weave mysterious and unpredictable connections, endangering us all in sometimes purposeful ways. Connections such as that between food and general health coexist with more hidden mechanisms. These mechanisms are ever invisible to scientists, who are too arrogant to admit the reality of anything not within reach of their imagined powers of control. Etiologies that reside within this larger model of causality allow for specific diseases or occasions of disease to be seen as more or less tied to the purposes of fate. For cancer, the tie is seen as being generally strong. The path to survival and cancer prevention in an unpredictable universe is to avoid, to focus elsewhere, and to persevere.

Community residents invoke the moral authority of their ancestors and consider that moral authority irrefutable. Behind this stance is more than a logically consistent position regarding the best way to avoid cancer. The defiant ancestor embodies community ways of life, self-reliance, and defiance of scientific medical advice. The ancestors confront us to say that in local health cosmology, science has not yet exorcised the powers of tradition.

Community residents are aware that scientists regard their worldview as a problem, as a view that needs changing. Scientists, in the residents' interpretation, see themselves as possessing the only valid authority, one that dictates a negating of the value of deep-seated wisdoms. The antagonism that the urban working class feels toward scientific authority is tied into a larger antagonism toward powerful forces from the outside that bear down on the community like a juggernaut, causing social, economic, and health problems that are beyond local control. In this context, local traditions are held up, to self and other, as being of higher value than scientific knowledge. For residents of this high cancer risk community, excluding external views about cancer is important (cf. Douglas 1984).

A low degree of control over life circumstances is central in working-class experience,[3] in contrast to the experience of higher-status persons such as scientists, physicians, and health educators. Community residents clearly feel this in regard to the control of knowledge about cancer. They have relatively little connection, or hope of finding a connection, to the systems by which health professionals gain access to, control, and create information that is accorded scientific legitimacy. They are keenly aware that their chances of influencing public policy on health research are very low. They experience their exclusion from power on many levels, from the disregard that is fostered by medicalization of their views to their inability to prevent the pollution of their air, water, and workplaces.

Thus, the community view is tied to strong feelings about access to power in society. Community members are disinclined to accept their assigned position as "targets" of a health education campaign. They have seen themselves labeled sick, and they have turned this around to label their social and material environment sick. They have considered blaming themselves as victims, and they have rejected the notion. Scientific authority, clearly, does not consider their interpretations of experience valid. So they use rhetoric about fate as a shield, and charge the scientists with hubris.

The Anthropologist's View

My own view begins with the dramatic contrast between the public and the private interactions with me. As members of the public audience, community residents were silent, even sullen, while privately, they eagerly invited me into their homes for interviews that radiated with fun and excitement. Do the public and private discourses bear the same message?

To understand that they do, one must remember the different contexts in which they occur. Public forums like health education programs belong to scientific and educational authority. The scientist (health educator) lectures, and the audience listens, with pastor and principal present. In this context, community residents assume the rebellious stance of the disempowered and alienated student. This stance—an expression of what Willis calls the "counter-school culture" (1977:2)—is central and familiar in working-class life (also cf. Freire 1970). In this way, they resist the position they feel they have been put in, through their wider social disenfranchisement, by institutions of authority such as science. In concrete terms, they look bored.

The teasing and sotto voice hinting that go after the presentation challenge the health educator to get down off the stage and listen. This is shown clearly, for instance, by the teasing that I received about eating an offered piece of cake. We know that you eat cake just like we do, the teasing says, and that you only assume that superior role while standing on the stage. Come down, and we will respond to your lecture.

In contrast, the kitchen, the site of most of the interviews, belongs to the community. There, residents were at last emboldened, transformed into respondents with a purpose. In my view, most saw their interview as an opportunity to enact a performance, to assume a rhetorical stance, in front of a representative of science. In a rare happening, a scientist had made an appearance in the community. More rare still, she had signaled a lowering of interpersonal barriers and had asked to come into community homes. This created an opportunity to express a treasured local value—one expressed among themselves quite often, on the front stoop or in front of the television, but seldom in the actual presence of a scientist. Through the interviews, respondents lived the drama of speaking their views to the outside, to the adversary, who, in a delicious reversal of the usual power mechanisms in the medical encounter, was herself in a position of special vulnerability. Yet the interviews did not have an adversarial feel—perhaps because respondents did not consider the agreement of the interviewer important.

Both public and private responses of the community to their health educators may be seen as what Scott has termed everyday forms of resistance. Scott describes such resistance as "the ordinary weapons of relatively powerless groups: foot dragging, dissimulation, false compliance, pilfering, feigned ignorance, slander, arson, sabotage, and so forth" (1985:29). The more opaque of these methods—false compliance, feigned ignorance—have often been read as peasant fatalism and resistance to innovation. Indeed, as Scott tells us, early views of the intellectual life of subordinate classes portrayed these classes as strongly constrained by the process of hegemony. Scott describes Gramsci's view:

> By creating and disseminating a universe of discourse and the concepts to go with it, by defining the standards of what is true, beautiful, moral, fair, and legitimate, [those in power] build a symbolic climate that prevents subordinate classes from thinking their way free. [1985:39][4]

However, Scott's portrait of lived experience in a peasant village, of everyday practice in a subordinate class environment, supports the argument that hegemony is not an omnipotent process. On the contrary, control of the terms of discourse, the definers of value and belief, is the focus of a potent struggle.

Likewise, in the community described here the struggle is a potent one. Maintaining a rebellious consciousness is part of constructing a valued self, valued community, valued life, in a subordinate class environment. Self and community, valuing and supporting each other, process myriad insults, betrayals, and frustrations. Local belief and tradition, it is asserted, are superior, as is local insight into the workings of authority and hegemony. Community residents assert local control of the value ascribed to local tradition. With regard to beliefs about cancer, their assertions are made in the context of powerfully emotional issues surrounding fate, suffering, life, and death. What is being negotiated is authority: the authority to judge local belief and activity concerning cancer, control, and causality.

Resistance, of course, is also not omnipotent (again, see Scott 1985; also see the discussion in Rebel 1989). The negotiation of powerlessness demands that we realize things in certain contexts that we do not realize in others. The data presented here show a critique of the construction of medical knowledge, but one that is specifically expressed—and perhaps specifically realized—through talking about cancer. When these same respondents talk about heart disease, they express a "routine compliance" with dominant medical models (Scott 1985: 278–284).[5] For residents of this community, talking about cancer opens up a specific text, one that contains an overt and elaborate analysis of dominance and control. There are a number of reasons why this is so.

First is the material nature of the disease. As Sontag so eloquently tells us (1977), and as the material here illustrates, the cancer disease process serves as an apt metaphor for loss of control. Beliefs portraying cancer as uncontrollable have been documented in many populations, including middle-class Americans, working-class African Americans, and respondents to surveys in Britain, France, Israel, and Australia (Adonis 1978; American Cancer Society 1980; Antonovsky 1972; Denniston 1981; Dent and Goulston 1982; Michielutte and Diseker 1982; National Cancer Institute 1986; Ragucci 1981; Salzberger

1976; Sontag 1977). Patterson (1987) shows the presence of such beliefs in the United States in the 19th century. Second, loss of control is a central issue for the postindustrial working class. They are not alone in this: it is a central issue for all of us in the postmodern world and, according to Sontag, acts generally to amplify the dread of cancer (Newman 1989; Reich 1987; Sontag 1977). But for traditionally patriotic poor inner-city whites, the issue is highlighted by the current decline of their class and country, the fading of glory days. This puts in context the general tendency in the United States for groups of lower socioeconomic status to exhibit a special resistance to scientific views on and recommendations for cancer control (Balshem, Amsel, Workman, Balshem, and Engstrom 1988; Celentano and Holtzman 1983; Greenwald 1980; Knopf 1976; Minkler 1981; National Cancer Institute 1986; Rimer, Jones, Wilson, Bennett, and Engstrom 1983).

But to fully understand the meaning of cancer in the study community, one must look at local conditions. Living with high cancer mortality, and with smokestacks and waste dumps, fuels a specific penetration of scientific and medical hegemony, one that resonates with the wider political issue of low control. Ironically and tragically, this penetration focuses on the outward attribution of blame and does not translate into self-preserving practice. Medical advice on the prevention, early detection, and treatment of cancer is rejected, and the rebellious discourse may include smoking, eating a high-fat diet, and avoiding recommended screening examinations.[6] This increases the percentage of cases that are incurable by the time they are diagnosed.[7]

In sum, it is generally true, and particularly so from the vantage point of the study community, that if one is thinking about control, cancer is good to think with. And control is the issue on which community thought about cancer has focused. The community situates the assumptions of cancer control science in a wider context of power and social class. This context is difficult for medical science to recognize. Scientific medicine is often described as a closed system, one that cannot easily work with other points of view (see, for instance, Janzen 1978). In an important sense, what scientific medicine is closed to is an admission of the problematic nature of its own power.

The community critique is also concerned with the issue of causality—that is, with the paradigmatic tendency of science to delimit the causal universe to that which it says and sees. The community critique, as detailed above, defines this as hubris and posits an identity of body and spirit that can be expressed and understood only crudely from within the scientific paradigm. It is no coincidence that the community critique of medical science mirrors that of critical studies in medical anthropology. As the authority of scientific medicine is increasingly challenged, similar critiques surface on many fronts, including that of a progressive consciousness in medicine itself (for instance, Hilfiker 1987; White 1988).

But beyond this interpretation of community discourse as critique lies a view of the discourse as a series of acts and thoughts of resistance. Through this resistance, the community turns the subject of the discourse around and defines the meaning of that discourse for itself. They reject being blamed as victims and targeted for education, and respond with a critique of their own. Thus, we must see not only how they are the subjects of our practice, but how we are the subjects of theirs.

Notes

I would like to thank Zili Amsel, Michael Herzfeld, Ivan Karp, and Emily Martin for their generous and invaluable comments and guidance on this project. Paul Jamison, Barbara Rimer, and Stephen Workman provided professional and moral support of the very best kind. The manuscript has been greatly improved by comments from Howard Balshem, Jane Cowan, Elliott Shore, Mary Steedly, Don Brenneis, and the anonymous reviewers for the *American Ethnologist.* I thank Janet Fitchen, Jeanne Simonelli, and Anna Walsh for the opportunity to present this material at the 88th annual meeting of the American Anthropological Association in Washington, DC, on 19 November 1989. This research was supported by Public Health Service Grant #CA34856 and conducted while I was employed by Fox Chase Cancer Center, Philadelphia, Pennsylvania.

1. Many would replace the word "compliance" with other terms, such as "adherence," that imply dialogue and consensus. This shift is positive, but not paradigmatic. The bottom line in either case is that "they" conform to what "we" advise. Taussig discusses a similar shift in clinical practice, in which the "illusion of reciprocity" is created by the "packaging of 'care,' 'trust,' and 'feelings' " (1980:23). As Trostle points out in a discussion of patient manipulation and terminology: "The word 'compliant' has unfortunate connotations, but the underlying concept also needs reworking" (1988:1306).

2. Permission to quote was given by Arthur Betcher, who, with his wife Mary, wrote this memorial for their beloved daughter, Linda M. Goodwin, who died of cancer at the age of 40. Arthur Betcher agreed to quotation of this material in the hope that it would help researchers understand the sorrow felt by families that lose a loved one to cancer.

3. A vast qualitative literature documents this (see Balshem 1988; Belle 1982; Binzen 1970; Garson 1975; Rubin 1976; Sacks and Remy 1984; Shostak 1980; Tepperman 1976; Willis 1977; and reviews in Balshem 1985 and Burawoy 1979). It is also documented in health promotion research, using quantitative variables such as self-efficacy and locus of health control. Peterson and Stunkard (1989) present an important recent statement on the centrality of beliefs about control to the process of health care decision making. They assert the value of understanding social context in this regard.

4. It is perhaps not uninteresting that I myself was unable to "think my way free" to the present analysis until I was no longer working as a health educator.

5. An analysis of community discourse about heart disease is beyond the scope of this article. In general, however, in American society both medical and lay beliefs about heart disease tend to be tied to a stress model. This model describes the individual heart disease process as a material synecdoche for the everyday harshness of modern life, particularly work life (see, for instance,

Eyer 1975; French and Caplan 1970; Haynes, Feinleib, and Kannel 1980; Karasek, Baker, Marxer, Ahlbom, and Theorell 1981; Rosenman, Brand, Jenkins, Friedman, Straus, and Wurm 1975; Scotch 1963). This entails a focus on the individual disease process that may depoliticize perceptions of the social causation of heart disease, but the process is subtle, and there is assonance between lay and scientific rhetoric (cf. Young 1980). Thus, heart disease is not well suited to carry the sentiments of resistance I have described here.

6. Residents sometimes state that they have already changed their health habits (reduced dietary fat or quit smoking) in order to prevent heart disease, but resist advice to make the same or similar changes in order to prevent cancer. This mechanism is discussed by Ben-Sira (1977). Of course, the extent to which residents have actually changed their health habits, for whatever reason, cannot be assessed through my study.

7. Thus, the rebellion entailed in rejection of scientific recommendations for cancer control is in a sense self-destructive. One interview respondent commented on this irony. But the extent to which this may be generally realized is difficult to assess.

References

Adonis, Catherine. 1978. French Cultural Attitudes towards Cancer. Cancer Nursing 1:111–113.

American Cancer Society. 1980. A Study of Black America's Attitude toward Cancer and Cancer Tests. New York: American Cancer Society.

Ansel, Zili, Prakash L. Grover, Andrew Balshem, and Doris Gillespie. 1984. Heightened Awareness among Residents of an Area Experiencing High Cancer Mortality. MS, Department of Behavioral Science, Fox Chase Cancer Center, Philadelphia, PA, and files of the author.

Antonovsky, A. 1972. The Image of Four Diseases Held by the Urban Jewish Population of Israel. Journal of Chronic Diseases 25:375–384.

Balshem, Martha. 1985. Job Stress and Health among Women Clerical Workers. Ph.D. dissertation. Department of Anthropology, Indiana University.

——. 1988. The Clerical Worker's Boss: An Agent of Job Stress. Human Organization 47:361–367.

Balshem, Martha, Zili Amsel, Stephen Workman, Andrew Balshem, and Paul F. Engstrom. 1988. Development of a Nutrition Education Program for a Blue Collar Community. *In* Advances in Cancer Control: Cancer Control Research and the Emergence of the Oncology Product Line. Paul F. Engstrom, Paul N. Anderson, and Lee M. Mortenson, eds. pp. 65–76. New York: Alan R. Liss.

Belle, Deborah, ed. 1982. Lives in Stress: Women and Depression. Beverly Hills, CA: Sage Publications.

Ben-Sira, Zeev. 1977. Involvement with a Disease and Health-Promoting Behavior. Social Science and Medicine 11:165–173.

Betcher, Mary, and Arthur Betcher. 1986. In Memory—Linda M. Goodwin. Bridesburg Bulletin, September 24.

Binzen, Peter. 1970. Whitetown, U.S.A. New York: Random House.

Brown, E. Richard. 1979. Rockefeller Medicine Men: Medicine and Capitalism in America. Berkeley: University of California Press.

Burawoy, Michael. 1979. The Anthropology of Industrial Work. Annual Review of Anthropology 8:231–266.

Bureau of the Census. 1983. 1980 Census of Population and Housing. Census Tracts, Philadelphia, PA-NY SMSA. Washington, DC: Department of Commerce.

Calnan, Michael. 1984. The Health Belief Model and Participation in Programmes for the Early Detection of Breast Cancer: A Comparative Analysis. Social Science and Medicine 19:823–830.

Celentano, D. D., and D. Holtzman. 1983. Breast Self-Examination Competency: An Analysis of Self-Reported Practice and Associated Characteristics. American Journal of Public Health 73:1321–1323.

Dayal, Hari, C. Y. Chiu, Robert Sharrar, John Mangan, Ira Rosenwaike, S. Shapiro, A. J. Henley, Robert Goldberg-Alberts, and Judith Kinman. 1984. Ecological Correlates of Cancer Mortality Patterns in an Industrialized Urban Population. Journal of the National Cancer Institute 73:565–574.

Denniston, R. W. 1981. Cancer Knowledge, Attitudes, and Practices among Black Americans. Progress in Clinical and Biological Research 53:225–235.

Dent, Owen, and Kerry Goulston. 1982. Community Attitudes to Cancer. Journal of Biosocial Science 14:359–372.

Doll, Richard, and Richard Peto. 1981. The Causes of Cancer: Quantitative Estimates of Avoidable Risks of Cancer in the United States Today. New York: Oxford University Press.

Douglas, Mary. 1984. Standard Social Uses of Food: Introduction. In Food in the Social Order: Studies of Food and Festivities in Three American Communities. Mary Douglas, ed. pp. 1–39. New York: Russell Sage Foundation.

Doyal, Lesley. 1979. The Political Economy of Health. Boston: South End Press.

Eyer, Joseph. 1975. Hypertension as a Disease of Modern Society. International Journal of Health Services 5:539–558.

Farquhar, John W., Nathan Maccoby, Peter D. Wood, Janet K. Alexander, Henry Breitrose, Byron W. Brown, Jr., William L. Haskell, Alfred L. McAlister, Anthony J. Meyer, Joyce D. Nash, and Michael P. Stern. 1977. Community Education for Cardiovascular Health. The Lancet 8023:1192–1195.

Fisher, Sue, and Alexandra Dundas Todd, eds. 1983. The Social Organization of Doctor-Patient Communication. Washington, DC: Center for Applied Linguistics.

Foucault, Michel. 1975. The Birth of the Clinic: An Archaeology of Medical Perception. A. M. Sheridan Smith, trans. New York: Vintage Books.

Freidson, Eliot. 1970. Professional Dominance: The Social Structure of Medical Care. New York: Atherton Press.

Freire, Paulo. 1970. Pedagogy of the Oppressed. New York: Herder and Herder.

French, John R. P., Jr., and Robert D. Caplan. 1970. Psychosocial Factors in Coronary Heart Disease. Industrial Medicine and Surgery 39:31–45.

Garson, Barbara. 1975. All the Livelong Day: The Meaning and Demeaning of Routine Work. Garden City, NY: Doubleday.

Greene, Michele G., Ronald Adelman, Rita Charon, and Susie Hoffman. 1986. Ageism in the Medical Encounter: An Exploratory Study of the Doctor-Elderly Patient Relationship. Language and Communication 6(1/2):113–124.

Greenwald, H. P. 1980. Social Problems in Cancer Control. Cambridge, MA: Ballinger Publishing Company.

Haynes, Suzanne G., Manning Feinleib, and W. B. Kannel. 1980. The Relationship of Psychosocial Factors to Coronary Heart Disease in the Framingham Study. III. Eight-Year Incidence of Coronary Heart Disease. American Journal of Epidemiology 111:37–58.

Herzfeld, Michael. 1982. The Etymology of Excuses: Aspects of Rhetorical Performance in Greece. American Ethnologist 9:644–663.

——. 1987. Anthropology through the Looking-Glass. New York: Cambridge University Press.

Hilfiker, D. 1987. Healing the Wounds: A Physician Looks at His Work. New York: Penguin Books.

Hochbaum, Godfrey M. 1981. Strategies and Their Rationale for Changing People's Eating Habits. Journal of Nutrition Education 13(1), supplement 1:59–65.

Illich, Ivan. 1976. Medical Nemesis: The Expropriation of Health. New York: Pantheon Books.

Irwin, Susan, and Brigitte Jordan. 1987. Knowledge, Practice, and Power: Court-Ordered Cesarean Sections. Medical Anthropology Quarterly 1(3):319–334.

Janzen, John M. 1978. The Quest for Therapy: Medical Pluralism in Lower Zaire. Berkeley: University of California Press.

Karasek, Robert A., Dean Baker, Frank Marxer, Anders Ahlbom, and Tores Theorell. 1981. Job Decision Latitude, Job Demands, and Cardiovascular Disease: A Prospective Study of Swedish Men. American Journal of Public Health 71:694–705.

Kleinman, Arthur, Leon Eisenberg, and Byron Good. 1978. Culture, Illness, and Care: Clinical Lessons from Anthropologic and Cross-Cultural Research. Annals of Internal Medicine 88:251–258.

Knopf, Andrea. 1976. Women's Beliefs about the Causes of Cancer. In Public Education about Cancer. J. Wakefield, ed. pp. 52–61. Geneva: International Union Against Cancer.

Martin, Emily. 1987. The Woman in the Body: A Cultural Analysis of Reproduction. Boston: Beacon Press.

———. 1988. The Cultural Construction of Gendered Bodies: Biology and Metaphors of Production and Destruction. Paper presented at the Vega Day Symposium in Honor of Fredrik Barth, Swedish Society for Anthropology and Geography, April, Stockholm.

Michielutte, R., and R. A. Diseker. 1982. Racial Differences in Knowledge of Cancer: A Pilot Study. Social Science and Medicine 16:245–252.

Minkler, Meredith. 1981. Applications of Social Support Theory to Health Education: Implications for Work with the Elderly. Health Education Quarterly 8(2):147–165.

Minkler, Meredith, and R. J. Pasick. 1986. Health Promotion and the Elderly: A Critical Perspective on the Past and Future. In Wellness and Health Promotion for the Elderly. D. Dychwald, ed. pp. 39–54. Rockville, MD: Aspen Systems Corporation.

National Cancer Institute. 1986. Cancer Prevention Awareness Survey: Wave II. Technical Report. Bethesda, MD: Office of Cancer Communications, National Cancer Institute, National Institutes of Health.

Newman, Katherine S. 1989. Falling from Grace: The Experience of Downward Mobility in the American Middle Class. New York: Vintage.

Patterson, James T. 1987. The Dread Disease: Cancer and Modern American Culture. Cambridge, MA: Harvard University Press.

Peterson, Christopher, and Albert J. Stunkard. 1989. Personal Control and Health Promotion. Social Science and Medicine 28:819–828.

Philadelphia City Planning Commission. 1982a. Selected Population and Housing Characteristics for Philadelphia Census Tracts, 1980. Technical Information Paper 82–19, May. Free Library of Philadelphia, Philadelphia PA.

———. 1982b. Economic and Social Indicators for Philadelphia Census Tracts, 1980. Technical Information Paper 82–41, November. Free Library of Philadelphia, Philadelphia, PA.

Pill, Roison M., and Nigel C. H. Stott. 1982. Concepts of Illness Causation and Responsibility: Some Preliminary Data from a Sample of Working Class Mothers. Social Science and Medicine 16:43–52.

———. 1985. Choice or Chance: Further Evidence on Ideas of Illness and Responsibility for Health. Social Science and Medicine 20:981–991.

———. 1987. The Stereotype of "Working-Class Fatalism" and the Challenge for Primary Care Health Promotion. Health Education Research 2:105–114.

Puska, Pekka, Kaj Koskela, Hilkka Pakarinen, Pirjo Puumalainen, Vaino Soininen, and Jaakko Tuomilehto. 1976. The North Karelia Project: A Programme for Community Control of Cardiovascular Disease. Scandinavian Journal of Social Medicine 4:57–60.

Ragucci, A. T. 1981. Italian Americans. In Ethnicity and Medical Care. Alan Harwood, ed. pp. 211–263. Cambridge, MA: Harvard University Press.

Rapp, Rayna. 1988. Chromosomes and Communication: The Discourse of Genetic Counseling. Medical Anthropology Quarterly 2(2):158–171.

Rebel, Hermann. 1989. Cultural Hegemony and Class Experience: A Critical Reading of Recent Ethnological-Historical Approaches. American Ethnologist 16:117–136, 350–365.

Reich, Robert B. 1987. Tales of a New America. New York: Times Books.

Richters, Arnis. 1988. Effects of Nitrogen Dioxide and Ozone on Blood-Borne Cancer Cell Colonization of the Lungs. Journal of Toxicology and Environmental Health 25:383–390.

Rimer, Barbara, Wendy Jones, Christine Wilson, David Bennett, and Paul Engstrom. 1983. Planning a Cancer Control Program for Older Citizens. Gerontologist 23:384–389.

Rosenman, Ray H., Richard J. Brand, C. David Jenkins, Meyer Friedman, Reuben Straus, and Moses Wurm. 1975. Coronary Heart Disease in the Western Collaborative Group Study: Final Follow-up Experience of 8½ Years. JAMA (Journal of the American Medical Association) 233:872–877.

Rubin, Lillian B. 1976. Worlds of Pain: Life in the Working-Class Family. New York: Basic Books.

Sacks, Karen, and D. Remy, eds. 1984. My Troubles Are Going to Have Trouble with Me: Everyday Trials and Triumphs of Women Workers. New Brunswick, NJ: Rutgers University Press.

Said, Edward W. 1978. Orientalism. New York: Vintage Books.

Salzberger, R. C. 1976. Cancer: Assumptions and Reality concerning Delay, Ignorance and Fear. In Social Anthropology and Medicine. J. B. Loudon, ed. pp. 150–189. New York: Academic Press.

Scheper-Hughes, Nancy, and Margaret M. Lock. 1987. The Mindful Body: A Prolegomenon to Future Work in Medical Anthropology. Medical Anthropology Quarterly 1:6–41.

Sciandra, R. 1983. Effective Communications in Cancer Control. In Progress in Cancer Control III: A Regional Approach. C. Mettlin and G. P. Murphy, eds. pp. 109–112. New York: Alan R. Liss.

Scotch, Norman A. 1963. Sociocultural Factors in the Epidemiology of Zulu Hypertension. American Journal of Public Health 53:1205–1213.

Scott, James C. 1985. Weapons of the Weak: Everyday Forms of Peasant Resistance. New Haven, CT: Yale University Press.

Shostak, Arthur B. 1980. Blue-Collar Stress. Reading, MA: Addison-Wesley.

Sontag, Susan. 1977. Illness as Metaphor. New York: Random House.

Starr, Paul. 1982. The Social Transformation of American Medicine. New York: Basic Books.

Taussig, Michael T. 1980. Reification and the Consciousness of the Patient. Social Science and Medicine 14(B):3–13.

Tepperman, Jean. 1976. Not Servants, Not Machines: Office Workers Speak Out! Boston: Beacon Press.

Trostle, James A. 1988. Medical Compliance as an Ideology. Social Science and Medicine 27(12):1299–1308.

White, Kerr L., ed. 1988. The Task of Medicine: Dialogue at Wickenburg. Menlo Park, CA: Henry J. Kaiser Family Foundation.

Willis, Paul E. 1977. Learning to Labour: How Working Class Kids Get Working Class Jobs. Westmead, Farnborough, England: Saxon House.

Young, Allan. 1980. The Discourse on Stress and the Reproduction of Conventional Knowledge. Social Science and Medicine 14(B):133–147.

Zola, Irving K. 1972. Medicine as an Institution of Social Control. Sociological Review 20(4):487–504.

Coming to Terms with Advanced Breast Cancer: Black Women's Narratives from Eastern North Carolina

Holly F. Mathews, Donald R. Lannin, and James P. Mitchell

■

I went to see the doctor because my arm was aching. He gave me a shot [of cortisone], but it kept on hurting. One day, I was chopping in the garden—I love to chop. It all began that night. It [breast] began to hurt. I thought I had jarred it with the hoe. All of a sudden it kept on hurting. That Saturday night I put a hot cloth on it. It began to run. Sunday, I kept putting cloths on it. It had a risen in it. It was running. That Monday I went to the doctor. He sent me to a surgeon doctor. He checked it over, and I went to the hospital . . . They took it off. I did not get scared. I took God with me . . . I don't have any thoughts about what could have caused it. First, it was a risen. It worked out that it was a risen and a cancer. You have to pray and give it to God. He will take care of it. If anybody's cancer is like mine, I would remove it. In three days it had lumps dripping out of it. I would tell others how I went through it. A lump and a tumor is not the same thing as a cancer. That's why I don't know for sure that mine was a cancer (Lydia, age 72 [1]).

"Coming to terms" is an interesting American expression. Technically, it means to 'compromise, arrive at an agreement, arbitrate' [2]; colloquially, it means to arrive at some understanding and acceptance of a problematic event or experience. Frequently, people come to terms with problematic experiences by putting their thoughts and feelings into words. This act of verbalization implies an attempt not only to conceptualize the experience, but also to define it so that the real work of understanding can begin.

In the narratives to be discussed in this paper, black women from eastern North Carolina draw on multiple sources of knowledge in order to come to terms with a diagnosis of advanced breast cancer—a biomedically-defined disease entity that they often refuse to acknowledge or accept. Their narratives represent a debate over whose terms will be used to label and describe a disease which is new to many of them. This struggle for understanding is made more difficult by the lack of natural contexts for discussion about the nature of the disease since cancer, for a majority of these women, is a taboo topic to be concealed from others, even family and friends (see Balshem [3]). By asking these women to tell us their stories about breast cancer, we created a context in which many of them were able, for the first time, to talk openly about a frightening and often bewildering experience.

The narratives these women produced are the subject of this paper. They are very personal accounts of individual experiences of illness. Yet they also include explanatory commentaries which attempt to relate the meanings of these episodes to an indigenous model of health and disease found in many black communities in the South as well as to popular American notions about cancer and particular biomedical conceptions of breast disease and its treatment. As such, they provide us with an important window into the processes involved in adapting personal experience to pre-existent cultural models, in modifying such models in the light of new information, and in coming to terms with shifts in conceptual reality as perceived by the individual actor in a cultural system.

The narratives are part of a larger study investigating the reasons why some women delay seeking treatment for breast cancer. The study is described first to provide background and context for the narratives. A profile of the women interviewed is then presented along with a discussion of methodology. Finally, the results of the narrative analysis are interpreted in light of recent research on the use of narratives by individuals to conceptualize and understand the experience of illness.

Background for the Study

The narratives come from a study begun in 1988 by the Department of Surgery at the East Carolina University School of Medicine to investigate the reasons why women, and particularly black women in the region, tend in greater numbers than reported nationally, to present with advanced stages of disease when first seeking treatment for breast cancer [4]. Presentation with advanced stage disease is a major issue in breast cancer research because early detection and treatment are known to reduce mortality and suffering [5–7]. Moreover, the survival rates after treatment for breast cancer have been significantly lower for black than for white women primarily because black women present more often with advanced disease, a fact that has been well documented in a number of recent studies [8–10] and by the American College of Surgeons (ASC) Breast Cancer Surveys [11–13] and the Cancer Surveillance, Epidemiology, and End Results (SEER) Program [14].

Between 1 July, 1988 and 30 July, 1991, 400 women who sought treatment for breast cancer in eastern North Carolina received an hour-long, structured interview designed to explore a range of demographic, psychosocial and cultural variables hypothesized to be associated with presentation for treatment with advanced stage disease [15]. In addition, all of these women were asked to complete open-ended, in-depth interviews about their own, personal experiences with breast disease, and their medical records were abstracted to record physician assessments of tumor size and stage at time of presentation as well as physician ratings of subsequent compliance with prescribed treatments.

The East Carolina University Medical School was established ten years ago with a mandate to train family physicians for rural practice and to provide, in conjunction with the Pitt County Memorial Hospital, medical services and preventive care to the people living in the 33-county region of eastern North Carolina. Their jointly sponsored breast clinic is the major treatment site in the region for women with breast abnormalities and has a referral base of 1.5 million people, most of whom live in federally-designated rural areas. Approximately one-third of the region's population is black, although the proportional resident concentration of blacks and whites varies by county. About 25% of this population lives below the poverty line, compared to 14.4% nationally [16].

Women patients entered the breast clinic in one of two ways: referral by a private physician or health department or self-referral directly to the breast clinic. The majority of private physicians and health departments in the rural eastern counties do not have the facilities available to provide advanced screening and treatment of breast disease and so rely on referrals to the ECU breast clinic. In the larger towns (all with populations under 50,000) located in close proximity to the medical center, some private physicians are able to provide advanced screening and treatment for their breast cancer patients. Consequently, the study was designed to draw a consecutive sample of all the women who were either physician- or self-referred to the ECU breast clinic over a three-year period while also interviewing a consecutive sample of women who

sought treatment from a random sample of private physicians practicing in the three larger towns in eastern NC, including Greenville, site of the ECU breast clinic [17].

The 400 women interviewed came from 30 eastern NC counties. Of these 400, 133 or 30.4% were black. There were no significant demographic differences found between the patient population interviewed and the entire breast cancer patient population recorded in the Pitt County Hospital Tumor Registry for eastern North Carolina with regard to age, race, stage of disease, tumor size, patient residence or insurance status [18, p. 25]. Preliminary analyses of the structured interview data focused upon categorizing patients by tumor stage at time of presentation and comparing this classification with the different variables measured in the structured interview. All tumors were staged according to the standardized TNM staging system as described in the 1988 version of the Staging Manual of the American Joint Committee on Cancer [19] using data from both physical examinations, mammography and other diagnostic techniques. For this study, *in situ* carcinomas representing Stage 1 tumors are labeled as "Early Stage" presentation; *local* or invasive cancers localized to the breast representing Stage 2 tumors are labeled as "Middle Stage" presentation; while *regional* cancers in the breast with spread to the regional lymph nodes or pectoral muscles representing Stage 3 tumors and *remote* cancers with distant metastases representing Stage 4 tumors are grouped and labeled as "Late Stage" presentation [19, p. 27].

Black women in the study were significantly more likely than white women to present with advanced or *Late Stage* disease (26% of black as opposed to 11% of white patients); or with *Middle Stage* disease (53% of black as opposed to 39% of white patients); while white women were significantly more likely to present with *Early*

Stage disease (50% of white as opposed to 21% of black patients) [19, p. 26]. This strong association between race and late stage presentation persisted even when the group was stratified by income level, educational level, and method of cancer detection (i.e., breast self exam, physician exam or mammography) and is consistent with results reported in other studies [8, 20].

In an effort to account for the specific effects of race on variation in tumor stage at time of presentation, interaction effects between race and the variables measured in the structured interview were assessed. The categories examined included demographic variables (age, education, residence and occupation); access variables (income, physician utilization, insurance status, available transportation and breast cancer knowledge); social support variables (overall size of social networks and perceived attitudes of male supports toward breast cancer); and psychosocial and cultural variables (fatalism, religiosity and indigenous or "folk" medical beliefs). Those found to be most significantly correlated, in conjunction with race, to late stage presentation included, in order of significance: a high degree of fatalism, a strong sense that men were not supportive of women's suffering, a lack of knowledge of risk factors for breast cancer, lower educational levels overall, and a strong belief in the effectiveness of indigenous or folk treatments for breast disease [19, p. 32]. Access variables did not turn out to influence significantly stage at time of presentation which dovetailed with our independent finding that no differences existed among the patients interviewed with regard to race, income, and educational levels in terms of rate of physician utilization with the only significant difference to emerge being one of age. Older women, of both races and all income levels, did utilize physicians significantly more often than younger women [19, p. 30].

In an effort to further understand the meaning of the findings reported from the quantitative data analysis, the in-depth narratives produced by those black women classified as presenting with late-stage disease were examined in the subsequent phase of the larger study.

Profile of the Patient Population and Description of Methodology

Preliminary analysis of the in-depth interviews focused on 26 narratives produced by black women who presented with late-stage, advanced breast tumors (defined as TNM stage 3 or greater) and who were, therefore, assumed to have delayed a significant amount of time before seeking treatment for breast cancer. During the three-year period from 1988–1991, 34 or 26% of 133 black women patients presented for treatment at the breast clinic with advanced stage disease. After each woman completed the structured interview guide, she was asked to spend another 30 min to 1 hr, at a time convenient with her, telling the interviewer about her personal experiences with breast cancer. Of the 34 women contacted, 5 were very ill from breast cancer having been immediately hospitalized after arrival at the breast clinic. Although most of them did the structured interview, none was able to finish in the in-depth portion. Four of the remaining 29 women contacted were unable to complete the in-depth interview because one became too ill, one died, one refused and another dropped out of treatment and could not be located again. Consequently, the final data set consists of 26 completed in-depth interviews with black women with advanced disease.

Of these 26, 14 were completed prior to diagnosis around the time of biopsy, and the remaining 12 were done retrospectively with patients who had either completed treatment for breast cancer, were in the process of undergoing treatment, or who had refused treatment altogether.

When possible, patients interviewed prior to diagnosis were contacted again on subsequent visits to the clinic as treatment progressed. In addition, those pre-biopsy patients who refused treatment were contacted in their homes for follow-up sessions.

The women interviewed ranged in age from 39–83 years with the majority being over the age of 50. There was no significant difference in the age distribution of advanced stage black patients and the rest of the cancer patient population. Although black women in the cancer study population tended overall to have significantly lower incomes than the white women, those grouped in the late stage category exhibited the same range of variation in income levels as the black women presenting with early and medium stage disease. There were also no significant differences in place of residence between the late and early/medium stage groups of black patients with similar proportions in each category coming from rural, small town, and large town locations. The one significant difference between the groups was educational level, with the late stage group having a significantly higher proportion of women with a low educational level (defining as having completed grade school or less) than the women in the early and medium stage categories who were more likely to have completed high school.

A team of trained interviewers, matched to patients by race and sex, asked the women patients to talk about a standard set of topics related to their personal experience of breast cancer. These topics questioned them about when they had first noticed a breast problem and how; what actions they chose to follow and why; what perceptions they had about causes of the problem; how they felt about their experiences in the medical system; and ended by asking them for their suggestions about how patient care and cancer education efforts could be improved. The interviews employed a conversational style, with the standard topics introduced at points appropriate to the conversation, in order to allow women as much latitude as possible for generating their own narrative structures.

Once the interviews began, most women proceeded with little prompting to talk extensively about their thoughts and feelings. The average interview lasted an hour, but many went longer and were frequently very emotional experiences for both participants and interviewers. When possible, the interviews were tape-recorded; when this was not possible or the patients refused, detailed notes were taken and interview summaries written. The recorded interviews were transcribed onto the computer for software-aided analysis.

All of the coding and analysis was done by the anthropologist on the team using a two-fold strategy. An examination of the overall structure of the narratives yielded insights into both the types of topics introduced and the sequencing of them produced by the respondents. This enabled a better sense of understanding about the issues these women found important as well about the goals they wanted to accomplish in the discussion. The subsequent stage of analysis focused on delineating from the discourse the important metaphors and propositions utilized by patients in conceptualizing and understanding breast cancer in order to try and ascertain the broader cultural models of health and disease that gave meaning to their discussions of individual episodes of illness. To assess the validity of these metaphors and propositions, an iterative procedure was employed. During the ongoing analysis, assumptions derived from the study of initial cases were tested on later interviewees. Second, an attempt was made whenever possible to reinterview patients in order to assess the validity of the analysis of the person's initial interview and to glean additional information to answer questions raised in the iterative process. Eventually,

20 of the 26 women included in the sample were interviewed more than once.

Results of the Narrative Analysis

The 26 interviews analyzed, including the one quoted at the beginning of this article, have a coherent narrative structure. They all begin with a discussion of the origin of symptoms and move chronologically to recount events that occurred relevant to the disorder. Interestingly, unlike illness narratives analyzed in other studies [20, 21], these accounts devote relatively little consideration to the cause of the disorder and direct much more attention to arriving at some label and defining set of features for it. Indeed, many of the breast narratives end with a statement about diagnosis. These narratives, moreover, contain very little commentary on the social roles played by others in the illness, most probably because others are excluded as much as possible from knowing about the condition, and individual women seldom use talk about their symptoms with others outside of the medical system as a way to arrive at a diagnostic label.

The accounts given by the breast cancer patients can thus be seen to mix two types of discourse labeled by Linde [23] as narrative and explanation. They have a narrative structure which begins with an orientation to symptoms and builds to a decision about labeling but with much explanatory justification included along the way. In this sense, they resemble in many respects the stories Farmer collected from rural Haitians when they were initially confronted with the new disease of AIDS [24].

For the majority of these women patients, the concept of breast cancer was fairly new. Although they were familiar with much of the popular discussion on breast cancer, many reported not having heard of it until recently and not having known any one who died from it. As one woman stated, "maybe it was around in the old days but no one knew it, or maybe it's just getting stronger now so they say more are getting it." These women were, in many respects, coming to terms with a novel disorder, and all 26 began their stories in much the same way as did the Haitians when AIDS first became a problem—by attempting to relate their symptoms to an indigenous or "folk" theory of disease based on an imbalance in the blood.

Over time, after receiving an official diagnosis of cancer, these women often struggled to evaluate how popular conceptions of the disease (including, for example, the belief that cancer is always ultimately fatal, medical treatment is degrading and hopeless, and that there is nothing a person can do to prevent cancer) disseminated in the media through television and magazine accounts of personal experiences of cancer and reinforced in general conversations with friends and neighbors about cancer experiences, fit with the indigenous or "folk" definition of the disorder. Finally, for those women who did go through the process of conventional medical treatment for the disease, a third layer of specific biomedical information about breast cancer as well as physician ideas about the need for a therapeutic partnership and positive, fighting spirit during the treatment process began to affect their interpretations of the disorder. Yet despite the similar progression of experience for many of these women, they often varied greatly in the ways in which they handled the contradictions that emerged between these three very different ways of conceptualizing breast disease.

Phase One—The Indigenous Blood Paradigm

All 14 of the black women with advanced disease interviewed prior to diagnosis began their narratives by discussing a host of symptoms connected, they believed, to the presence of a condition known as "dirty" or "bad" blood. The theme of blood figured significantly as well in 10 of the 12 narratives recounted retrospectively by patients with advanced disease. Moreover, segments of the blood model could also be found in about half of the narratives recounted by black women categorized as presenting with early and middle stage disease, but were absent from all of the accounts given by white patients, regardless of stage at time of presentation.

The symptoms they identified included knots or lumps that would "come and go" or move around the body; boils on the skin known as "risens" or "whiteheads," said to be impurities in the blood coming up to get out; aches and pains in the arm and side; and general flushed, feverish feelings coupled with weakness and dizzy or "falling out" spells; and occasionally, flashes of light in the head. For example, Sallie, age 53, reported "It all started with a whitehead I had on my breast. But then it disappeared. But it was a sign of that bad blood trying to get out. So it was there all the time. And then it formed a lump that was there too, but it wasn't coming up." Alternately, Frances, age 76, reported "I had this knot on my stomach. And I went to the doctor and told him about it. But he told me not to worry it was nothing. This was oh, about 1974. But then it moved up to my breast and it began to grow. But it wasn't bothering me. Only it was getting bigger and bigger." Finally, Thelma, aged 41, noted, "It was a real bad time. I was hot and flushed one day, and when I was doing the dishes I started seeing these flashes of light in my head. And that night my arm and my side started hurting and I rubbed the ache out and noticed that lump there had gotten larger. But it wasn't bothering me any."

The reference to bad or dirty blood refers directly to a more inclusive system of beliefs about health and disease common to many black Americans in the South and found, in various forms, in widely distributed African and Afro-Caribbean groups [25]. This belief system attributes good health to the maintenance of balance in the blood. Weidman has labeled this theory found among Haitians as the "blood paradigm" [26]. This paradigm, as documented for the Southeast [27] and in other parts of the United States [28], posits different qualities to blood that is out of balance. It can variously be too high or low, too bitter or sweet, too thick or thin, or too dirty. Any of these conditions is itself seen to be a disorder or to cause other folk illnesses related to the different organs of the body. Treatment usually involves the application of opposites. In the discussion of breast knots and lumps, the women presenting with late-stage disease are drawing on a particular notion of bad blood as blood with "impurities" in it. These impurities are believed to circulate throughout the system and are often talked about as something that is "trying to come out" of the body.

Many women draw connections in their narratives between impurities circulating in the blood and lumps and knots in the body. These lumps are said to be triggered by a bump or blow to the body which causes the impurities in the blood to "clump together in one place." Indeed, 16 of the 26 women with advanced disease described their breast lumps as resulting from bumps or blows bruising the body. For example, in two of the less well elaborated accounts, May and Jean respectively give responses that suggest this connection: "I noticed a knot in my breast in 1989, but it didn't hurt. It just came from bumping into the bed so I put it out of my mind"; "I had a sore spot on my breast that came from bumping into the car door with my groceries. A lump came up there but it never bothered me."

The narratives that make the causal links explicit are more detailed. For example, 66-year-old Clara outlines the connection:

I had a pain in my arm for five years. It was the arthritis jumping on me so I paid it no mind. I also had a knot in my breast all that time, but it would come and go. It wasn't nothing. But then I noticed a few months ago that there was a big knot on my right breast where Mr Jones [an alzheimer's patient she sits for] had been hitting me on the side. You know, if you get a hard enough blow, it makes some kind of blood clot, and if it stays there long enough it's going to form something else.

Lucille, age 75, linked the impurities circulating in dirty blood to the knots formed by a blow or bruise:

That knot I had came and went. If you have dirty blood, the impurities have to go somewhere. And once I passed the change, that blood just stayed in me all the time. It was mounting up. When I fell down that day in the garden, they all came up to that bruise and they made a lump. That's what made it so big.

This chain of logic holds that blood can become dirty either because a person has a tendency that way; has engaged in unclean, unsanitary habits or excessive sexual encounters; or has no way for impurities in the blood to leave the system after menopause. These impurities are circulating in the blood and when they become too numerous or "strong," or when the person is weak with low resistance or has an accident of some kind, the impurities may "come up" into swollen areas, skin sores, or lumps formed under the surface.

In and of themselves, lumps are not bad. They are a normal part of the system as evinced by the fact that if left alone, they tend to come and go. As 57-year-old Olivia put it, "I've had lumps all my life. Sometimes they come on you when things happen. But if a lump is not hurting you then it's nothing to bother with. I believe that if a lump ain't bothering you, you shouldn't bother it. It will probably go away."

However, as Clara indicates in her statement

above, sometimes changes occur in these lumps if they stay in one place long enough. This change is usually described in patient narratives as a fundamental alteration in the character of the lump— it goes from being a static, almost non-living entity that causes no bother or pain, to something animated that begins to take on a life of its own, growing rapidly and becoming bothersome. This transition can happen for several reasons—either a blow or bruise can trigger the growth, an ever-increasing number of impurities in the blood with no other outlet can begin to "move up" or "grow out," or it can just be in one place too long and "take root."

The metaphor, either directly stated or implied in the characterization of lumps in 24 of these 26 narratives, is of a living thing, sometimes explicitly equated to a plant, as when patients refer to lumps as: "a *kernel* under my arm," or "a knot *rooted* in my breast" or a "*growth* that has taken hold in my side." In a very real sense, to borrow Clara's phrase, a lump that stays in one place long enough may become "rooted" to the spot and begin to grow taking on a life of its own that may become bothersome to the woman experiencing it.

Lakoff [29] reports that metaphors serve an important mapping function in cognition by introducing information from physical-world source domains into target domains in the non-physical world which, according to Quinn and Holland [30], enables image-schematic thought. By drawing analogies from physical experience, metaphors assist people in conceptualizing non-physical processes in a concrete, visual way that makes these experiences more tangible and thus accessible to mental processing. For example, when women use the metaphor of a plant to characterize a breast lump which they cannot physically see or necessarily feel, they create a set of images and characteristics that can be used to conceptualize their illness experience in a concrete way and to predict likely entailments. Once a seed beings to root and grow, therefore, it can be expected to get larger. A breast lump growing uncontrollably creates a problem for women because it may "burst through the skin," "make the breast bleed," "take over the breast" or interfere with normal functions and cause pain. Just as plants require nourishment to survive, these lumps may also "keep growing and growing, taking more and more out of me." By logical extension, seeds that are dormant, that have not taken root as evinced by beginning to grow, are not a problem. Consequently, lumps that do not noticeably grow or become bothersome are best left alone.

Many aspects of this view coincide with what women hear generally and are sometimes told explicitly by physicians—i.e. that breast lumps that grow uncontrollably are dangerous because they may spread to other parts of the body and that cancer is a disease that eats you up from the inside out. Similarly, they can also understand the logic of surgery to remove the "growth" from the body. However, the notion of surgery presents a problem for many since it also calls up other, more frightening entailments of the plant metaphor.

Surgery was thought by 20 of the women interviewed to be dangerous because, "cutting on a cancer will make it spread," and "once air gets to a lump it will make it grow." The logic relating these statements to the plant metaphor is usually implied in the narrative accounts but is occasionally elaborated in some detail. Marjorie, age 78, said "I believe, I don't care what kind of lump it is, I believe that if they cut it, it spreads. It might take five years or ten, but it will come back more intensified." Alternatively, 63-year-old Pauline stated, "If you feel you haven't gotten the whole root, then it'll spread. That lump will start to grow again bigger." In both cases, the assumption is that if you want to remove a plant, you must take it out by the roots. If you don't get it all, then it will come back. But also entailed in

these examples is a notion of pruning—that if you just cut it back, the lump will come back stronger and bigger than ever. Consequently, surgery or "going under the knife" is seen by these women to be very dangerous. Unless a lump or knot is extremely bothersome, surgery should be avoided. This is reflected in the desire of many patients to be given a pill that will "poison the growth" or even to undergo radiation treatment which some interpret as "using X-rays to burn up the growth."

Again, these ideas are very similar to ones that patients report hearing from physicians about "taking out the whole cancer," "getting it before it starts to spread" and "making sure to remove the whole thing." However, the notion of catching a lump early and removing it at a point before it starts to grow makes no sense to them. As Frances says: "why would you take out a lump that isn't bothering you. If it's not growing, it should be left alone. Fooling around with it might make it start to act up. I don't hold with cutting on things that ain't bothering you." Such an attitude is also implied in Lydia's statement at the beginning of the paper when she says, "If anybody's cancer is like mine [i.e. a large cancer with lumps dripping out of it], I would remove it." She points this out because, by implication, unless it is such an abnormal type, it should not be disturbed.

The notion of air getting to cancer, discussed in 18 of the 26 narratives, is entailed in the image of plants living outdoors and drawing nourishment from the sun, air and water. This logic suggests that lumps that are enclosed in the body have a limited amount of nourishment. But "opening them up" to the air increases the chances for them to grow and spread. Thus, as 47-year-old Mary explains, "I'm afraid to go under the knife because once that lump is opened up to the air, it will just *blossom* and grow. Even if they try and take it out, the part that's left will be stronger and it will spread."

That the concern with air follows from an entailment of the plant metaphor is made obvious when the previous examples are compared to one given in an interview with a 62-year-old, white patient with early-stage disease. One of the items on the structured interview asked her to agree or disagree with the statement that air getting to a cancer will make it spread. The patient agreed that she had heard people say that was true. When asked why she thought it might be, she replied, "I don't really know but I guess, you know, it's like when a wind comes up on a wildfire and it makes it spread out of control." Obviously, this analogy provides a different but plausible mapping of a physical-world image onto the experience of tumor growth and represents a creative attempt to explain something for which the women had no explanation. Yet this analogy was unique and did not appear in any of the other interviews with white or black patients.

As Quinn and Holland determine in their review of recent studies, metaphors are not extended "willy-nilly from any one domain to any other" but rather a small number of classes of metaphors appear to be used in accounting for particular experiences. As they explain it, "The classes from which speakers select metaphors they consider to be appropriate are those that capture aspects of the simplified world and the prototypical events unfolding in this world, constituted by the cultural model" [30, p. 30]. Clearly, the plant metaphor is doubly compelling in the illness domain. The indigenous or "folk" medical beliefs of many of these black patients are heavily plant oriented, with many traditional herbal remedies being called "root medicines."

Secondly, the plant image itself accounts for many aspects of the particular experiences women have with breast lumps and makes possible many logical entailments about how plants live and grow that seem to predictively account for much of the concrete experiences these women have with breast lumps. Conversely, comparing a breast lump to a wildfire may make it possible to explain how air causes it to spread, but it does not extend logically or satisfactorily to predict and account for other aspects of the experience.

The majority, 22 of the 26 black women who presented with late-stage disease, delayed seeking treatment, they said, because the lumps "weren't bothering them," "did not hurt," or "weren't growing." Only when these conditions changed and the lumps began to become bothersome, painful or extremely large did many of them seek medical help. At this point, some suspected that they might receive a diagnosis of cancer. For many of them, "waiting to see" and "finding out it was cancer" was the worst part of the entire illness experience—an event whose meaning had to be understood with reference to both indigenous conceptions of lumps as well as to popular cultural beliefs about cancer in general.

Popular Knowledge About Cancer

Once these patients began to think about the possibility of cancer, they acknowledged a whole host of feelings about the disease common in popular discourse. Much of what they said paralleled Balshem's descriptions of attitudes toward cancer in Philadelphia [3]. Cancer was seen by patients to be the worst of all diseases because it is always fatal and is essentially incurable. Moreover, cancer is an extremely painful and degrading disease that "strips away your dignity." As 71-year-old Carol said:

> Letting in the idea that it might be cancer was the hardest thing in the world for me. People don't get over cancer. It will always kill you. They might do something for you, but eventually the cancer will come back and get you. It's a horrible, degrading disease that eats you up.

Paradoxically, for many of these women, cancer was seen to have no particular cause. It just, "comes on people for no reason." Much as Balshem observed, these patients reported that everything and nothing can cause cancer, and the reasons why one person and not another falls victim to it are unexplainable. Consequently, for many of the women interviewed, cancer in its whimsical aspects, resembled illnesses that did not respond to conventional categories or cures in the indigenous medical system. Thus, by extension, the only likelihood of finding a cure for cancer was "to turn it over to God." As Ethel, age 58, explained it:

> Cancer is a horrible disease. It just eats you up. The only one powerful enough to overcome it is the Lord. You just have to trust in Jesus to do battle for you and save you from this horrible affliction.

Here the battle metaphor is used to portray a struggle between God, as the all powerful force for good, and cancer as consummate evil, or as another woman put it, "that terrible, evil sickness." While Balshem's informants also embraced this view of cancer as evil, they did not seem to emphasize it as strongly as the breast patients interviewed in this study.

Indeed, many of these women proceeded, after the diagnosis of cancer was received from a physician, to redefine the disorder suffered as a supernatural one which was no longer amenable to treatment with "ordinary means," including physician-prescribed treatments. As Clara expressed it:

> When you know you have cancer, then there's nothing for it but to turn it over to God. If you have enough faith, He will heal it and you don't need no operation. Because there is nothing a doctor can do for you—only God has the power.

It follows that because cancer is a powerful and virtually unstoppable disease once it is activated, women need to be careful not to "stir it up." Balshem reports that her Philadelphia informants view cancer as a minion of fate that may

punish those who notice or defy it. She writes of them that "to think about cancer, to try to prevent it, is to tempt fate. Cancer testing is 'looking for trouble'" [3, p. 161]. For her informants, even speaking the word cancer out loud was potentially dangerous as was talking about the disease openly or acknowledging that others had it. The women interviewed in this study had similar views which mapped well onto their more traditional notions about the characteristics of breast lumps. For example, Selma explained:

> If you have a lump and it's not bothering you, leave it alone. You don't want to get it started. That's why I don't hold with this idea of poking around to look for lumps. Why look for trouble? When that doctor wanted me to have the X-ray on my breast, I told him he was crazy. There's no telling what those X-rays might stir up.

Just as not tempting fate by looking for cancer may protect you, so too refusing to name the disease or acknowledge that you have it is seen as protecting you in some way from suffering its full effects. Janine, age 48, explained her feelings after she went through diagnosis:

> When he told me what it was, well I just couldn't hardly even think about it. To have that disease would be the end. So I just decided then and there that I wouldn't worry no more. That I would give it to God, and that I would never speak of it again. I trusted God to heal me and I believe He has. That's all I need to know.

Once having made this decision, Janine refused surgery and abandoned her radiation treatments. Her condition deteriorated, and she was eventually hospitalized for fluid accumulation in the lungs due to the spread of the cancer. Her lungs were drained, and in an interview that day, she stated that she had been suffering from pneumonia but was feeling much better. When she was rehospitalized two weeks later, she maintained just before her death that pneumonia was killing her. She had not mentioned the word cancer since the day that she received the diagnosis.

Phase Three—Encountering Biomedical Notions of Breast Cancer

In a recent study of American oncology, Good *et al.* [31] have documented a major shift in physicians' attitudes since the 1950s when most felt that a diagnosis of cancer should not be revealed to the patient. Today there is virtual unanimity that diagnoses should be revealed. However, physicians vary in their notions about just when and what should be disclosed to patients in part because they perceive their mission to be one of instilling, not dashing, patients' hopes [31, p. 61]. Many oncologists embrace this mission, not because they believe as some Americans do that the mind can really influence disease, but rather because they believe that hope helps patients adopt a positive attitude which makes forging a "partnership" with them in the healing process easier. As Good *et al.* explain:

> The construction of a partnership is understood as a necessary component of treatment, of getting patients to accept chemotherapy or radiation, and of making patients "work" or be "responsible" for eating well, taking their medication, keeping treatment appointments, and participating in a therapeutic endeavor which is often highly toxic [31, p. 75].

The authors also find that disclosure in oncological practice is not primarily about diagnosis, but rather is more focused on prognosis and treatment. This interest in prognosis appears to correlate directly with the desire to instill hope while the focus on treatment is likely due, as Good *et al.* suggest, to oncologists themselves deriving hope from and demonstrating caring through the treatment process. As they write, car-

ing is conveyed "through offering therapeutic options and holding out hope for the development of new treatments on the cutting edge of biology and medicine" [31, p. 74].

Good *et al.*'s research provides illuminating background for understanding the responses of the late-stage patients interviewed in this study to the biomedical perspective. For 23 of the 26 patients interviewed, diagnosis was not a foregone conclusion. Much of what they wanted to do in their sessions with physicians was to discuss this issue. Yet their physicians were more focused on prognosis and treatment and tended, instead, to shift the talk toward outcomes. Consequently, 19 of the 26 patients with late-stage disease reported feeling "rushed to make a decision," and said that their doctors were "too pushy" or too "quick to jump into something." For others, the physicians' coupling of the dramatic diagnosis of cancer with a desire to perform immediate surgery was a complete turn-off. Of the initial 34 black women diagnosed with late-stage disease, 6 walked out of the clinic at that point and never returned. In this sense, these patients differed dramatically from those studied by Lind *et al.* [32] who were more interested in finding out from physicians about prognosis, disease process and treatment side effects and options than they were in obtaining basic information.

On the other hand, those women who did agree to have conventional treatments were constantly encouraged to be "partners in the *fight* against their disease," "to eat well and build up their strength for the coming *battle*," "to *play the game* and stick with the therapy," and "work with the doctors and nurses to *beat* the disease." Insofar as these women bought into the oncology model, they also tended to embrace the metaphors of warfare and sports used by the clinic staff to encourage them to become "part of the *team*" as partners invested in treatment and survival. Similarly, the patients' conversation began to reflect the use of more scientific terminology in reference to breast cancer. From this new vantage point, they often re-evaluated their initial interpretations about the nature of lumps based on indigenous beliefs or popular conceptions of the disease.

For example, once her treatment was over and the mastectomy completed, Sallie began to incorporate this medical attitude into her interpretations of her experience. She reported feeling like she "had just come through a long battle" and switches from a first person singular voice to the first person plural thereby demonstrating her solidarity with the medical team while shifting her references to popular notions to the third person thereby disassociating herself from them.

> When I found out about the tumor—you know that it was cancer, I didn't know what to do. I didn't see much point in doing anything because, you know, they all say cancer will kill you. There ain't no cure for it. But the people here were so good to me and they told me not to give up—that my family would want me to fight to live and that they would help me. So I took my treatments and I stuck with it. And those X-rays evaporated that tumor down to a little small lump that the doctor took out. And now that we won that fight, the cancer is over. The trick was shrinking that lump so that we could get it all. That's what makes the surgery O.K. so that the cancer won't spread. So I guess maybe I'm here to stay for a while longer.

As Sallie undergoes treatment, her perspective shifts. She does begin to enter into a "partnership" with medical personnel and adopts their language of war to describe the treatment she completed. In the process, her view shifts from a fatalistic acceptance of the inevitable outcome of death which led her to yield to God and a spiritual cure, to an active acceptance of the biomedical view of cancer. In embracing the entailments of the warfare metaphor, her self-definition shifts

from someone doomed to die to that of a survivor of the battlefield—a person who, although scarred from the fight, showed the true "fighting" spirit by working hard and sacrificing to win a victory over the enemy. In the process of articulating this shift in self-image, she clarifies how the medical techniques make surgery, seen as not acceptable in the indigenous model, acceptable from another perspective.

Coming to Terms with Conflicting Interpretations of Breast Disease

Despite the similar progression of experience for many of the women in this group, their efforts to come to terms with conflicting views of the disease varied greatly. Six of the twenty-six women interviewed stuck resolutely to initial interpretations and refused to give up their indigenous beliefs, even in the face of new and conflicting information, while four of the twenty-six completely gave them up in favor of the standard medical explanation. The remaining 16 women, however, worked out some type of accommodation along the lines identified by Strauss [33] in her study of Rhode Island working class men's views of success. Strauss discovered that her informants often held conflicting views simultaneously. In her effort to understand how they managed this, she analyzed their extended discourse and discovered three different ways in which different interpretative schemas can be learned and mentally stored. She labeled one "horizontal containment"—the maintenance of two opposing and contradictory schemas in separate, largely noninteracting cognitive compartments with each being used in a different context. She labels "vertical containment" a situation in which one interpretation is learned more as theory and is thus more easily verbalized than another. Both sets of beliefs are also held in separate, largely noninteracting, cognitive compartments and are expressed in different contexts with different voices. Finally, "integration" is characterized by the co-existence of different and sometimes conflicting ideas in a single schema or in a set of closely connected schemas expressed in a single, consistent voice across contexts [33, p. 315].

A brief examination of three more extended excerpts from narratives recorded after patients had been through the diagnosis and treatment phase illustrates how these different efforts at accommodation parallel the forms identified by Strauss. For example, interviews conducted with 69-year-old Leah both before diagnosis and after her chemotherapy treatments had begun illustrate Strauss' notion of "horizontal containment." In her first interview, Leah explained her disease this way:

> I have these lumps in my body—I've had lumps off and on in my life. They don't hurt or bother me. People say you should leave lumps like that alone because if you bother them, they will start to bother you. They say that if you cut on them they will start to spread and maybe they will turn into cancer. So if this lump does turn out to be something, then maybe I shouldn't have the operation.

In this excerpt, Leah describes the indigenous view of breast lumps. Yet the way in which she discusses these beliefs indicates that for her they are not so much part of her active world view as they are examples of received cultural wisdom. Notice that she repeatedly accesses these beliefs by mentioning that "people say" or "they say" and does not discuss them in the first person as part of her own active belief system.

In a later interview, Leah talks about her disease differently:

> I am not scared of dying because when the Lord decides that my time has come, it will come. And I trust Him and know that He will reach out for me and take me out of this life to a brighter glory, thanks be to Jesus. And you know, I believe it was God himself who revealed this cancer to me. That day that I slipped and fell on the ice and bruised my breast—rubbing that bruise caused me to realize that I had this knot in my breast. And I honestly believe that God directed me to find the knot so that I could be cured. So I trust Him for bringing me this far, and I know that He will take care of me. And He sent me to this doctor and directed him to take the evil out of me to set me free. And I am thankful to him, praise Jesus.

In this passage, Leah describes a personal identification with God as manifested in her first person discussion of her beliefs about God's role in the treatment of her disease.

Clearly, Leah embraces two very different interpretations of her illness. Each was voiced in separate interview contexts, and in none of her sessions did she discuss the two together. They appeared to be organized and stored separately in her mind and accessed under different circumstances and seemed, moreover, to be differentially tied to her sense of personal identity, with her views about God being personally important while her indigenous notions of disease, voiced like lessons from childhood, were not integrated into her daily life. As a result, it is likely to suppose that the two have different levels of motivational intensity for Leah.

The initial receipt of a cancer diagnosis and the subsequent discussion of treatment options immediately caused Leah to fall back on the received wisdom of childhood invoking the "cutting on knots will make them spread" schema. However, the parroting of these notions did not influence her to reject biomedical treatment. She chose surgery, and once that choice was made she rationalized it by shifting to the "God as protector and healer" schema, which eventually came to dominate because it was a more active part of her adult identity and everyday practice and perhaps because it was ultimately more compatible with the biomedical model of the disease since the religious schema's emphasis on the "battle" between a righteous God and the evil enemy cancer mapped well onto the similar use of the battle analogy by the clinic staff.

Alternatively, the excerpt from the interview quoted at the beginning of this paper provides an example of vertical containment. In this passage, Lydia talks about two different interpretations. One, the traditional view, is obviously verbalized easily and in a more theoretical and organized fashion than is the medical interpretation. She begins by identifying her problem as having a "risen" caused by bad blood coming to the surface. She elaborates the cause, the actions taken, and her interpretation. In passing, she also voices the religious interpretation but not in a well-worked out way, saying only that you have to pray and give it to God. Her reference to the medical interpretation is given in a less-well verbalized or theoretically organized fashion. She reports what the doctor did, then from that perspective says that she doesn't have any thoughts about what caused it (meaning, the doctor's version of it as cancer), and ends by saying at some point that she suffered from both a risen and a cancer—a point she later contradicts by saying that the two are not the same. So even though she picked up on the medical interpretation, it was not convincing to her and she does not recount it from a theoretical point of view. Rather she makes short statements about what the doctor said and did almost as a meta-commentary on the indigenous view.

Finally, the story of 39-year-old Sharon demonstrates the attempt to come to some kind of integration—a perspective that appears in her final interview. When she first came in for treatment, Sharon reported that she had a knot that had begun to grow and she wanted the doctor to check on it. When she received the diagnosis of cancer she responded:

> I can't believe that this lump could be cancer. It wasn't really bothering me. I just thought that since it was growing larger, I should get it checked. I just can't make a decision about what to do now. You know, I believe that the Lord is watching over me and He will tell me what to do. I just need time to think and pray.

A few weeks later, when she came back to the clinic, Sharon, who is a minister, heard the clinic staff talking about her and calling her "the preacher." She then reported what happened:

> When I went in to see the doctor, I just told him I didn't want the mastectomy—that I was going to put my faith in the Lord and trust God to cure me. And he said to me, "God can't do everything; you've got to do something for yourself." Well, that did it for me. I got up and walked right out that door because he was questioning everything I have built my life on. So I went home and prayed without ceasing. I asked the people in my church to pray for me too, and I testified to them that God had cured me.

But over time, the tumor grew out of her breast and reached the size of a grapefruit. It bled but she put pads in her bra and kept working. Her friend, an aide at the medical center, was worried and repeatedly urged her to go back to the clinic. Finally, she did return and upon her arrival was seen immediately by several physicians and nurses who gave her much support and encouragement. She explained her situation this way:

> One night when I was praying, the Lord spoke to me and told me it was time now to see a doctor. He directed me to go back so that he could work through the doctors to

cure me. He revealed to me that a medical doctor was needed to cure a medical problem, but that He would be directing him and so I should go along with the treatment and let them remove the knot. So I came back and the day I came, all of the people came down. Three doctors came to talk to me and they discussed what to do about my tumor in front of me, and so just like the Lord said, I was part of the healing process—they were talking to me. And the nurse came down and explained it all to me about how they would first do radiation treatments to shrink the tumor and then operate. And the lady who did the radiation said that God would be on my side and would help me be strong. And all that time while I was waiting and praying, God kept my tumor from getting any bigger, and then He sent me back so the doctors could help me. And now I know what He wants me to do. When I get well, my mission is to work with these doctors to help them talk to patients and tell them about what cancer is and to teach them not to be afraid to have the treatments.

Sharon was able to work out an integration of the religious and medical interpretations of her disease, and in the process, redefined her own self identity and role in life. She is now involved in the medical partnership but has extended this notion of partnership to include God as the team leader and herself as the go-between to bring patients and physicians into a better working relationship with God.

Clearly, the women in this study resolved conflicts brought into the open by the experience of breast disease in very different ways. What remains to be understood are the factors that might account for the different types of accommodations they made. Some clues are suggested in the interviews themselves. In Leah's case, personal experience as an ardent church member appeared to dominate her thinking about cancer to such an extent that the traditional views learned in childhood were less persuasive to her. In Lydia's case, social ties played an integral role in the treatment process. She would have continued to avoid medical attention for her breast had not her granddaughter made the appointment and personally escorted her to see a physician. In order to make the granddaughter happy, Lydia says she went to the doctor and followed through with surgery. But she never really "bought in" to the oncologist's model of breast disease perhaps because her own personal allegiance was still bound to the indigenous system. Lydia's ambivalence is reflected in her refusal to agree with the biomedical definition of her disorder.

Sharon, on the other hand, had a combination of pressures acting on her. She had a bad personal experience with the medical staff when she sought treatment because they made fun of the very core concept in her identity—her role as a minister. Consequently, she rejected the medical system and its interpretation of the disease. But later, after repeated urging from a close friend who worked at the medical center, she did return, although on her own terms and guided by God. Fortunately, she received a more positive reception the second time and was made to feel like an important part of the treatment process by the medical staff. She embraced this identity melding it with her own sense of religious purpose to arrive at an integrated explanation for why she delayed as well as for why she finally sought treatment.

Equally complex is the way in which these varying interpretations affected behavior. In some cases, patients made choices consistent with their expressed views of the disease; in others, they did not. A full account of the meaning of these narratives must eventually attempt to relate them to the broader social context in which the patients operate in order to try and untangle the factors involved in their decisions to accept, reject, or accommodate to new sources of knowledge and in order to more fully understand the complex relationships that exist between mental models and social actions.

Conclusion

This preliminary analysis of a small segment of the total interviews completed raises as many questions as it answers. Although anthropologists have written recently about indigenous etiologies of cancer in French-speaking Canada [34] and northern Italy [35], there has been very little work, with the exception of Balshem's recent article, designed to explore the variation in cancer beliefs within the United States. As a result, it is not surprising that popular medical knowledge, as Saillant writes, has virtually no recognition in the clinic or in oncology [34, p. 100]. This analysis focused specifically on the factors that may contribute to the tendency of some black women in eastern North Carolina to delay seeking treatment for breast cancer until they have an advanced stage of the disease. The limited generalizability of this study must be noted since the beliefs and behaviors of women with advanced stage disease are not necessarily relevant to the behaviors of the majority of women with breast cancer. Nonetheless, a major factor consistently implicated in the continuing disparity in mortality rates for breast cancer between black and white women is the fact that significantly more black than white women present for treatment with late stage disease. Any attempt to promote early detection and treatment seeking behavior in this population must be based on a more complete understanding of the reasons accounting for delay if they are to succeed.

Too often in the past we have assumed that patients who delay seeking treatment for cancer or who fail to utilize the screening services available, are either lacking in knowledge, too poor to access services, denying reality or excessively fatalistic. The labeling of patients as fatalistic is, as Balshem writes, particularly pernicious because fatalism in medical circles is seen as being situated within the individual as a diagnosable pathology [3, p. 164]. Thus efforts at combating delay often focus on eradicating fatalism by supplying individuals with appropriate medical knowledge. Such a stance, as Balshem notes, obviates the need for health practitioners to develop a critical understanding of beliefs held by patients. For as she writes, "If fatalism is a disease, there is no need to look further at an indigenous etiology that is merely a symptom of this disease" [3, p. 164]. Consequently, dialog and discussion are stymied, and physicians often resent and usually dismiss the attempts of patients to come to terms with the cancer diagnosis by telling stories that seem to the physician to be at best irrational and at worst adversarial [3, p. 164].

While fatalism and the other attitudinal variables mentioned above may be part of the complex of behaviors leading to presentation with advanced stage disease, we cannot afford to ignore the fact that these patients also have well-worked out ideas about their own health and about disease—ideas that must be considered if oncologists truly hope to forge a therapeutic partnership with them.

Notes

1. Pseudonyms are used in the text to protect informant confidentiality.
2. Laird, C. *Webster's New World Thesaurus,* p. 448. Warner Books, New York, 1974.
3. Balshem, M. Cancer, control and causality: Talking about cancer in a working-class community. *Am. Ethnolog.* 18, 162, 1991.
4. These data were collected as part of a study entitled "Psychosocial Factors Delaying Breast Cancer Presentation," Donald Lannin, with Jim Mitchell and Holly Mathews, and funded by The American Cancer Soci-

ety, Grant No. PBR-37. Special assistance was provided by Frances Swanson as project manager.

5. Feldman, J. *et al.* The effects of patient delay and symptoms other than a lump on survival in breast cancer. *Cancer* 51, 1226, 1983.

6. Elwood, J. M. and Moorehead, W. P. Delay in diagnosis and long-term survival in breast cancer. *Br. Med. J.* 280, 1291, 1980.

7. Sheridan, B., Fleming, J., Atkinson, L., and Scott, G. The effects of delay in treatment on survival rates in carcinoma of the breast. *Med. J. Aust.* 1, 262, 1971.

8. Briel, H. A. *et al.* Results of treatment of stage I–III breast cancer in black Americans: the Cook County Hospital Experience, 1973–1987. *Cancer,* 65, 1062, 1990.

9. Freeman, H. P. and Wasfie, T. J. Cancer of the breast in poor black women. *Cancer* 63, 2562, 1989.

10. Natarajan, N. *et al.* Race-related differences in breast cancer patients. *JNCI* 56, 1704, 1984.

11. Nemoto, T. *et al.* Management and survival of female breast cancer: Results of a national survey by the American College of Surgeons. *Cancer* 45, 2917, 1980.

12. Wilson, R. E. *et al.* The 1982 national survey of carcinoma of the breast in the United States by the American College of Surgeons. *Surg. Gynecol. Obstet.* 159, 309, 1984.

13. Natarajan, N., Nemoto, T., Mettlin, C. and Murphy, G. P. Race-related differences in breast cancer patients: Results of the 1982 national survey of breast cancer by the American College of Surgeons. *Cancer* 56, 1704, 1985.

14. Baquet, C. R. *et al.* Cancer among blacks and other minorities: Statistical profiles. DHHS Publication No. (NIH) 86–2785 (published by NCI, Bethesda, MD), 1, 1986.

15. The first study period ended on 30 June, 1991, but a subsequent renewal grant from American Cancer Society (No. PRB-64532) has enabled ongoing data collection. As of 30 June, 1992, data had been collected on 530 patients from 30 counties. An additional component of the five-year study has been to collect structured interview data with an identical number of female controls without breast disease randomly selected from the region and matched to patients on the basis of age, race and place of residence. Finally, each patient has been asked to name her confidant—the person she has relied upon most for advice during her experience with breast disease. Structured interviews have also been completed with these individuals.

16. Mathews, H. F. Introduction: a regional approach and a multidisciplinary perspective. In *Herbal and Magical Medicine: Traditional Healing Today* (Edited by Kirkland, J. *et al.*), p. 1. Duke University Press, Durham, 1992.

17. This latter component of the sample was included to ensure adequate representation of the patient pool seen by private physicians, the majority of whom are white middle- and upper-income women.

18. Lannin, D. R., Mitchell, J. P. and Mathews, H. F. Progress report on American Cancer Society grant No. PBR-37, pp. 25–46. Department of Surgery, East Carolina University School of Medicine, Greenville, NC, 1990.

19. American Joint Committee on Cancer. *Manual for Staging of Cancer,* 2nd edn, pp. 127–133. J. B.Lippincott, Philadelphia, 1983.

20. Riggs, R. S. and Noland, M. P. Factors related to the health knowledge and health behavior of disadvantaged black youth. *JOSH* 54, 431, 1984.

21. Price, L. Ecuadorian illness stories: cultural knowledge in natural discourse. In *Cultural Models in Language and Thought* (Edited by Holland, D. and Quinn, N.), p. 313. Cambridge University Press, London, 1987.

22. Early, E. A. The logic of well being: therapeutic narratives in Cairo, Egypt. *Soc. Sci. Med.* 16, 1491, 1982.

23. Linde, C. Explanatory systems in oral life stories. In *Cultural Models in Language and Thought* (Edited by Holland, D. and Quinn, N.), p. 343. Cambridge University Press, London, 1987.

24. Farmer, P. Sending sickness: sorcery, politics and changing concepts of AIDS in rural Haiti. *Med. Anthrop. Q.* 4, 6, 1990.

25. See for example, Ingstad, B. The cultural construction of AIDS and its consequences for prevention. *Med. Anthrop. Q.* 4, 28, 1990; Laguerre, M. *Afro-Caribbean Folk Medicine.* Bergin and Garvey, Granby, MA, 1987; Mathews, H. and Hill, C. E. Applying cognitive decision theory to the study of regional patterns of illness treatment choice. *Am. Anthrop.* 92, 155, 1990.

26. Weidman, H. *Miami Health Ecology Project Report: A Statement on Ethnicity and Health.* University of Miami, Miami.

27. Mathews, H. F. Rootwork: Description of an ethnomedical system in the American South. *South. Med. J.* 8, 885, 1987.

28. Snow, L. F. Traditional health beliefs and practices among lower class black Americans. *Western J. Med.* 139, 820, 1983.

29. Lakoff, G. Classifiers as a reflection of mind: a cognitive

model approach to prototype theory. *Berkeley Cognitive Science Report* 19, 10, 1984.

30. Quinn, N. and Holland, D. Culture and cognition. In *Cultural Models in Language and Thought* (Edited by Holland, D. and Quinn, N.), p. 3. Cambridge University Press, London, 1987.

31. Good, M. J. D., Good, B. J., Schaffer, C. and Lind, S. E. American Oncology and the discourse on hope. *Cult. Med. Psychiat.* 14, 59, 1990.

32. Lind, S. E., Good, M. J. D., Seidel, S., Csordas, T. and Good, B. J. Telling the diagnosis of cancer. *J. Clin. Oncol.* 7, 583, 1989.

33. Strauss, C. Who gets ahead? Cognitive responses to heteroglossia in American political culture. *Am. Ethnolog.* 71, 312, 1990.

34. Saillant, F. Discourse, knowledge and experience of cancer: a life story. *Cult. Med. Psychiat.* 14, 81, 1990.

35. Gordon, D. R. Embodying illness, embodying cancer. *Cult. Med. Psychiat.* 14, 275, 1990.

2

Illness Experiences and Illness Narratives

The three readings in this section explore what suffering, illness, and disability mean to individuals and to those with whom they live and work. Narratives of illness are the stories people tell about how and why they got sick, how and why they think they will get better or not, and what they feel when in pain or hope for in recovery. Virginia Woolf (1986) once described being ill as being in an "undiscovered country," drawing a similarity between being confined and drawn inside oneself by illness to exploring unknown or unfamiliar territory. Busy in the flow of work or daily tasks, we may miss the subtle nuances of light, aroma, the passage of time, and the details of our own bodies that are apparent to the person who is slowed with sickness. Telling a story of sickness to someone who really listens is an important means to reduce the loneliness of being in that undiscovered country. The genre of the illness narrative, or what Ann Hunsaker Hawkins calls "pathography" (1993) has grown enormously just in the past decade. It includes famous authors like William Styron (1990), who writes about being clinically depressed, and Reynolds Price (1994), who retells the tale of his progressive paralysis. Many others who are not so famous also speak of and write about their illness-related hopes and fears, experiences in hospitals and operating rooms, and quiet lonely days at home and in despair (Murphy 1987).

The section begins with another reflection on the nature of suffering, perhaps the quintessential quality of illness. Annie Dillard conveys in no uncertain terms that suffering is an altogether routine part of nature, but like Cassell, she argues that suffering is an extraordinary part of the experience of being human. The deer in her essay that will soon be someone's meal does not ask *why,* but Alan MacDonald, the man who is burned twice over most of his body, does. Dillard accepts and "knows" the suffering of the deer, but she reads daily about Alan MacDonald's horror at knowing he is about to be burnt badly again. Dillard's male companions were aghast that she did not try to save the deer or show the distress they expected of her as a woman. They do not, however, question their own inaction. Dillard's sketch of a fragile, beautiful animal struggling in vain for freedom, for life, raises a tension between the desire to intervene and the excruciating experience of witnessing the suffering of another. When and how much should one intervene if a person is suffering futilely, and when is it more humane to accept the naturalness of death and loss? We return to this topic in part IV on ethics. While Dillard ties suffering to the natural, she also suggests that supernatural explanations may be of some help in understanding "why."

Arthur Frank's account of his serious illnesses and treatment presents a very different interpretation of suffering. Frank, a sociologist, describes the "colonization" of his body by physicians and medicine and his struggle to retain an identity apart from being a patient in a body. *Recognition,* not intimacy or even warmth, is what he seeks from those who treat his body. He wants his sensate and psychological experiences and his other identities to be acknowledged by the doctors and nurses. Frank's experiences of being ill and a patient lead him to conclude that physicians "cue"

or signal to patients how they should behave when sick: courageous, optimistic, and cheerful. How ironic, he observes, that sometimes this elicited illness "performance" is then labeled denial!

The final selection is a story of sickness from a different vantage point—that of a family member. Serious illness almost never happens to a person alone—there are always others who participate and who feel the effects. Told from the vantage point of Rosie's sister, "Silver Water" conveys the complexity and penetrance of chronic illness and suffering within a family. The author, psychotherapist Amy Bloom, gives a fictional (but all-too-accurate) account of a family's misadventures with psychiatric treatment for Rosie, who has schizophrenia. It matters little that Rosie's father is a psychiatrist. Rosie and her family search for competent care and find it only once. They are constrained by limitations in their health insurance and must cope with the chaos and immense pathos of Rosie's deteriorating condition. Rosie and her sister take an uncommon path in resolving their mutual but distinct grief. The story's end may be interpreted as an act of heroic love, or of incomprehensible resignation and defeat.

The Deer at Providencia

Annie Dillard

∎

There were four of us North Americans in the jungle, in the Ecuadorian jungle on the banks of the Napo River in the Amazon watershed. The other three North Americans were metropolitan men. We stayed in tents in one riverside village, and visited others. At the village called Providencia we saw a sight which moved us, and which shocked the men.

The first thing we saw when we climbed the riverbank to the village of Providencia was the deer. It was roped to a tree on the grass clearing near the thatch shelter where we would eat lunch.

The deer was small, about the size of a white-tail fawn, but apparently full-grown. It had a rope around its neck and three feet caught in the rope. Someone said that the dogs had caught it that morning and the villagers were going to cook and eat it that night.

This clearing lay at the edge of the little thatched-hut village. We could see the villagers going about their business, scattering feed corn for hens about their houses, and wandering down paths to the river to bathe. The village headman was our host; he stood beside us as we watched the deer struggle. Several village boys were interested in the deer; they formed part of the circle we made around it in the clearing. So also did four businessmen from Quito who were attempting to

guide us around the jungle. Few of the very different people standing in this circle had a common language. We watched the deer, and no one said much.

The deer lay on its side at the rope's very end, so the rope lacked slack to let it rest its head in the dust. It was "pretty," delicate of bone like all deer, and thin-skinned for the tropics. Its skin looked virtually hairless, in fact, and almost translucent, like a membrane. Its neck was no thicker than my wrist; it was rubbed open on the rope, and gashed. Trying to paw itself free of the rope, the deer had scratched its own neck with its hooves. The raw underside of its neck showed red stripes and some bruises bleeding inside the muscles. Now three of its feet were hooked in the rope under its jaw. It could not stand, of course, on one leg, so it could not move to slacken the rope and ease the pull on its throat and enable it to rest its head.

Repeatedly the deer paused, motionless, its eyes veiled, with only its rib cage in motion, and its breaths the only sound. Then, after I would think, "It has given up; now it will die," it would heave. The rope twanged; the tree leaves clattered; the deer's free foot beat the ground. We stepped back and held our breaths. It thrashed, kicking, but only one leg moved; the other three legs tightened inside the rope's loop. Its hip jerked; its spine shook. Its eyes rolled; its tongue, thick with spittle, pushed in and out. Then it would rest again. We watched this for fifteen minutes.

Once three young native boys charged in, released its trapped legs, and jumped back to the circle of people. But instantly the deer scratched up its neck with its hooves and snared its forelegs in the rope again. It was easy to imagine a third and then a fourth leg soon stuck, like Brer Rabbit and the Tar Baby.

We watched the deer from the circle, and then we drifted on to lunch. Our palm-roofed shelter stood on a grassy promontory from which we could see the deer tied to the tree, pigs and hens walking under village houses, and black-and-white cattle standing in the river. There was even a breeze.

Lunch, which was the second and better lunch we had that day, was hot and fried. There was a big fish called *doncella,* a kind of catfish, dipped whole in corn flour and beaten egg, then deep fried. With our fingers we pulled soft fragments of it from its sides to our plates, and ate; it was delicate fish-flesh, fresh and mild. Someone found the roe, and I ate of that too—it was fat and stronger, like egg yolk, naturally enough, and warm.

There was also a stew of meat in shreds with rice and pale brown gravy. I had asked what kind of deer it was tied to the tree; Pepe had answered in Spanish, "*Gama.*" Now they told us this was *gama* too, stewed. I suspect the word means merely game or venison. At any rate, I heard that the village dogs had cornered another deer just yesterday, and it was this deer which we were now eating in full sight of the whole article. It was good. I was surprised at its tenderness. But it is a fact that high levels of lactic acid, which builds up in muscle tissues during exertion, tenderizes.

After the fish and meat we ate bananas fried in chunks and served on a tray; they were sweet and full of flavor. I felt terrific. My shirt was wet and cool from swimming; I had had a night's sleep, two decent walks, three meals, and a swim—everything tasted good. From time to time each one of us, separately, would look beyond our shaded roof to the sunny spot where the deer was still convulsing in the dust. Our meal completed, we walked around the deer and back to the boats.

That night I learned that while we were watching the deer, the others were watching me.

We four North Americans grew close in the jungle in a way that was not the usual artificial intimacy of travelers. We liked each other. We stayed up all that night talking, murmuring, as though we rocked on hammocks slung above time. The others were from big cities: New York, Washington, Boston. They all said that I had no expression on my face when I was watching the deer—or at any rate, not the expression they expected.

They had looked to see how I, the only woman, and the youngest, was taking the sight of the deer's struggles. I looked detached, apparently, or hard, or calm, or focused, still. I don't know. I was thinking. I remember feeling very old and energetic. I could say like Thoreau that I have traveled widely in Roanoke, Virginia. I have thought a great deal about carnivorousness; I eat meat. These things are not issues; they are mysteries.

Gentlemen of the city, what surprises you? That there is suffering here, or that I know it?

We lay in the tent and talked. "If it had been my wife," one man said with special vigor, amazed, "she wouldn't have cared *what* was going on; she would have dropped *everything* right at that moment and gone in the village from here to there to there, she would not have *stopped* until that animal was out of its suffering one way or another. She couldn't *bear* to see a creature in agony like that."

I nodded.

Now I am home. When I wake I comb my hair before the mirror above my dresser. Every morning for the past two years I have seen in that mirror, beside my sleep-softened face, the blackened face of a burnt man. It is a wire-service photograph clipped from a newspaper and taped to my mirror. The caption reads: "Alan McDonald in Miami hospital bed." All you can see in the photograph is a smudged triangle of face from his eyelids to his lower lip; the rest is bandages. You cannot see the expression in his eyes; the bandages shade them.

The story, headed MAN BURNED FOR SECOND TIME, begins:

> "Why does God hate me?" Alan McDonald asked from his hospital bed.
>
> "When the gunpowder went off, I couldn't believe it," he said. "I just couldn't believe it. I said, 'No, God couldn't do this to me again.'"

He was in a burn ward in Miami, in serious condition. I do not even know if he lived. I wrote him a letter at the time, cringing.

He had been burned before, thirteen years previously, by flaming gasoline. For years he had been having his body restored and his face remade in dozens of operations. He had been a boy, and then a burnt boy. He had already been stunned by what could happen, by how life could veer.

Once I read that people who survive bad burns tend to go crazy; they have a very high suicide rate. Medicine cannot ease their pain; drugs just leak away, soaking the sheets, because there is no skin to hold them in. The people just lie there and weep. Later they kill themselves. They had not known, before they were burned, that the world included such suffering, that life could permit them personally such pain.

This time a bowl of gunpowder had exploded on McDonald.

> "I didn't realize what had happened at first," he recounted. "And then I heard that sound from 13 years ago. I was burning. I rolled to put the fire out and I thought, 'Oh God, not again.'"
>
> "If my friend hadn't been there, I would have jumped into a canal with a rock around my neck."

His wife concludes the piece, "Man, it just isn't fair."

I read the whole clipping again every morning. This is the Big Time here, every minute of it. Will someone please explain to Alan McDonald in his dignity, to the deer at Providencia in his dignity, what is going on? And mail me the carbon.

When we walked by the deer at Providencia for the last time, I said to Pepe, with a pitying glance at the deer, "*Pobrecito*"—"poor little thing." But I was trying out Spanish. I knew at the time it was a ridiculous thing to say.

The Cost of Appearances

Arthur Frank

■

Society praises ill persons with words such as *courageous, optimistic,* and *cheerful.* Family and friends speak approvingly of the patient who jokes or just smiles, making them, the visitors, feel good. Everyone around the ill person becomes committed to the idea that recovery is the only outcome worth thinking about. No matter what the actual odds, an attitude of "You're going to be fine" dominates the sickroom. Everyone works to sustain it. But how much work does the ill person have to do to make others feel good?

Two kinds of emotional work are involved in being ill. The kind I have written about in earlier chapters takes place when the ill person, alone or with true caregivers, works with the emotions of fear, frustration, and loss and tries to find some coherence about what it means to be ill. The other kind is the work the ill person does to keep up an appearance. This appearance is the expectation that a society of healthy friends, co-workers, medical staff, and others places on an ill person.

The appearance most praised is "I'd hardly have known she was sick." At home the ill person must appear to be engaged in normal family routines; in the hospital she should appear to be just resting. When the ill person can no longer conceal the effects of illness, she is expected to convince others that being ill isn't that bad. The minimal acceptable behavior is praised, faintly, as "stoical." But the ill person may not feel like acting good-humored and positive; much of the time it takes hard work to hold this appearance in place.

I have never heard an ill person praised for how well she expressed fear or grief or was openly sad. On the contrary, ill persons feel a need to apologize if they show any emotions other than laughter. Occasional tears may be passed off as the ill person's need to "let go"; the tears are categorized as temporary outbursts instead of understood as part of an ongoing emotion. Sustained "negative" emotions are out of place. If a patient shows too much sadness, he must be depressed, and "depression" is a treatable medical disease.

Too few people, whether medical staff, family, or friends, seem willing to accept the possibility that depression may be the ill person's most appropriate response to the situation. I am not recommending depression, but I do want to suggest that at some moments even fairly deep depression must be accepted as part of the experience of illness.

A couple of days before my mother-in-law died, she shared a room with a woman who was also being treated for cancer. My mother-in-law was this woman's second dying roommate, and the woman was seriously ill herself. I have no doubt that her diagnosis of clinical depression was accurate. The issue is how the medical staff responded to her depression. Instead of trying to understand it as a reasonable response to her situation, her doctors treated her with antidepressant drugs. When a hospital psychologist came to visit her, his questions were designed only to evaluate her "mental status." What day is it? Where are you and what floor are you on? Who is Prime Minister? and so forth. His sole interest was whether the dosage of antidepressant drug was too high, upsetting her "cognitive orientation." The hospital needed her to be mentally competent so she would remain a "good patient" requiring little extra care; it did not need her emotions. No one attempted to explore her fears with her. No one asked what it was like to have two roommates die within a couple of days of each other, and how this affected her own fear of death. No one was willing to witness her experience.

What makes me saddest is seeing the work ill persons do to sustain this "cheerful patient" image. A close friend of ours, dying of cancer, seriously wondered how her condition could be getting worse, since she had brought homemade cookies to the treatment center whenever she had chemotherapy. She believed there had to be a causal connection between attitude and physical improvement. From early childhood on we are taught that attitude and effort count. "Good citizenship" is supposed to bring us extra points. The nurses all said what a wonderful woman our friend was. She was the perfectly brave, positive, cheerful cancer patient. To me she was most wonderful at the end, when she grieved her illness openly, dropped her act, and clearly demonstrated her anger. She lived her illness as she chose, and by the time she was acting on her anger and sadness, she was too sick for me to ask her if she wished she had expressed more of those emotions earlier. I can only wonder what it had cost her to sustain her happy image for so long.

When I tried to sustain a cheerful and tidy image, it cost me energy, which was scarce. It also cost me opportunities to express what *was* happening in my life with cancer and to understand that life. Finally, my attempts at a positive image diminished my relationships with others by preventing them from sharing my experience. But this image is all that many of those around an ill person are willing to see.

The other side of sustaining a "positive" image is denying that illness can end in death. Medical staff argue that patients who need to deny dying should be allowed to do so. The sad end of this process comes when the person is dying but has become too sick to express what he might now want to say to his loved ones, about his life and theirs. Then that person and his family are denied a final experience together; not all will choose this moment, but all have a right to it.

The medical staff do not have to be part of the tragedy of living with what was left unsaid. For them a patient who denies is one who is cheerful, makes few demands, and asks fewer questions. Some ill persons may need to deny, for reasons we cannot know. But it is too convenient for treatment providers to assume that the denial comes entirely from the patient, because this allows them not to recognize that they are cueing the patient. Labeling the ill person's behavior as denial describes it as a need of the patient, instead of understanding it as the patient's *response* to his situation. That situation, made up of the cues given by treatment providers and caregivers, is what shapes the ill person's behavior.

To be ill is to be dependent on medical staff, family, and friends. Since all these people value cheerfulness, the ill must summon up their energies to be cheerful. Denial may not be what they want or need, but it is what they perceive those around them wanting and needing. This is not the ill person's own denial, but rather his accommodation to the denial of others. When others around you are denying what is happening to you, denying it yourself can seem like your best deal.

To live among others is to make deals. We have to decide what support we need and what we must give others to get that support. Then we make our "best deal" of behavior to get what we need. This process is rarely a conscious one. It develops over a long time in so many experiences that it becomes the way we are, or what we call our personality. But behind much of what we call personality, deals are being made. In a crisis such as illness the terms of the deal rise to the surface and can be seen more clearly.

One incident can stand for all the deals I made during treatment. During my chemotherapy I had to spend three-day periods as an inpatient, receiving continuous drugs. In the three weeks or so between treatments I was examined weekly in the day-care part of the cancer center. Day care is a large room filled with easy chairs where patients sit while they are given briefer intravenous chemotherapy than mine. There are also beds, closely spaced with curtains between. Everyone can see everyone else and hear most of what is being said. Hospitals, however, depend on a myth of privacy. As soon as a curtain is pulled, that space is defined as private, and the patient is expected to answer all questions, no matter how intimate. The first time we went to day care, a young nurse interviewed Cathie and me to assess our "psychosocial" needs. In the middle of this medical bus station she began asking some reasonable questions. Were we experiencing difficulties at work because of my illness? Were we having any problems with our families? Were we getting support from them? These questions were precisely what a caregiver should ask. The problem was where they were being asked.

Our response to most of these questions was to lie. Without even looking at each other, we both understood that whatever problems we were having, we were not going to talk about them there. Why? To figure out our best deal, we had to assess the kind of support we thought we could get in that setting from that nurse. Nothing she did convinced us that what she could offer was equal to what we would risk by telling her the truth.

Admitting that you have problems makes you vulnerable, but it is also the only way to get help. Throughout my illness Cathie and I constantly weighed our need for help against the risk involved in making ourselves vulnerable. If we did not feel that support was forthcoming, we suppressed our need for expression. If we had expressed our problems and emotions in that very public setting, we would have been extremely vulnerable. If we had then received anything less than total support, it would have been devastating. The nurse showed no awareness or appreciation of how much her questions required us to risk, so we gave only a cheerful "no problems" response. That was all the setting seemed able to support.

Maybe we were wrong. Maybe the staff would have supported us if we had opened up our problems with others' responses to my illness, our stress trying to keep our jobs going, and our fears and doubts about treatment. We certainly were aware that our responses cut off that support. It was double or nothing; we chose safety. Ill persons face such choices constantly. We still believe we were right to keep quiet. If the staff had had real support to offer, they would have offered it in a setting that encouraged our response. When we were alone with nurses in an inpatient room, the questions they asked were those on medical history forms. In the privacy of that room the nurses were vulnerable to the emotions we might have expressed, so they asked no "psychosocial" questions.

It was a lot of work for us to answer the day-care nurse's questions with a smile. Giving her the impression that we felt all right was draining, and illness and its care had drained us both already. But expending our energies this way seemed our best deal.

Anybody who wants to be a caregiver, particularly a professional, must not only have real support to offer but must also learn to convince the ill person that this support is there. My defenses have never been stronger than they were when I was ill. I have never watched others more closely or been more guarded around them. I needed others more than I ever have, and I was also most vulnerable to them. The behavior I worked to let others see was my most conservative estimate of what I thought they would support.

Again I can give no formula, only questions. To the ill person: How much is this best deal costing you in terms of emotional work? What are you compromising of your own expression of illness in order to present those around you with the cheerful appearance they want? What do you fear will happen if you act otherwise? And to those around the ill person: What cues are you giving the ill person that tell her how you want her to act? In what way is her behavior a response to your own? Whose denial, whose needs?

Fear and depression are a part of life. In illness there are no "negative emotions," only experiences that have to be lived through. What is needed in these moments is not denial but recognition. The ill person's suffering should be affirmed, whether or not it can be treated. What I wanted when I was most ill was the response, "Yes, we see your pain; we accept your fear." I needed others to recognize not only that I was suffering, but also that we had this suffering in common. I can accept that doctors and nurses sometimes fail to provide the correct treatment. But I cannot accept it when medical staff, family, and friends fail to recognize that they are equal participants in the process of illness. Their actions shape the behavior of the ill person, and their bodies share the potential of illness.

Those who make cheerfulness and bravery the price they require for support deny their own humanity. They deny that to be human is to be mortal, to become ill and die. Ill persons need others to share in recognizing with them the frailty of the human body. When others join the ill person in this recognition, courage and cheer may be the result, not as an appearance to be worked at, but as a spontaneous expression of a common emotion.

Silver Water

Amy Bloom

■

My sister's voice was like mountain water in a silver pitcher; the clear blue beauty of it cools you and lifts you up beyond your heat, beyond your body. After we went to see *La Traviata*, when she was fourteen and I was twelve, she elbowed me in the parking lot and said, "Check this out." And she opened her mouth unnaturally wide and her voice came out, so crystalline and bright that all the departing operagoers stood frozen by their cars, unable to take out their keys or open their doors until she had finished, and then they cheered like hell.

That's what I like to remember, and that's the story I told to all of her therapists. I wanted them to know her, to know that who they saw was not all there was to see. That before her constant tinkling of commercials and fast-food jingles there had been Puccini and Mozart and hymns so sweet and mighty you expected Jesus to come down off his cross and clap. That before there was a mountain of Thorazined fat, swaying down the halls in nylon maternity tops and sweatpants, there had been the prettiest girl in Arrandale Elementary School, the belle of Landmark Junior High. Maybe there were other pretty girls, but I didn't see them. To me, Rose, my beautiful blond defender, my guide to Tampax and my mother's moods, was perfect.

She had her first psychotic break when she

was fifteen. She had been coming home moody and tearful, then quietly beaming, then she stopped coming home. She would go out into the woods behind our house and not come in until my mother went after her at dusk, and stepped gently into the briars and saplings and pulled her out, blank-faced, her pale blue sweater covered with crumbled leaves, her white jeans smeared with dirt. After three weeks of this, my mother, who is a musician and widely regarded as eccentric, said to my father, who is a psychiatrist and a kind, sad man, "She's going off."

"What is that, your professional opinion?" He picked up the newspaper and put it down again, sighing. "I'm sorry, I didn't mean to snap at you. I know something's bothering her. Have you talked to her?"

"What's there to say? David, she's going crazy. She doesn't need a heart-to-heart talk with Mom, she needs a hospital."

They went back and forth, and my father sat down with Rose for a few hours, and she sat there licking the hairs on her forearm, first one way, then the other. My mother stood in the hallway, dry-eyed and pale, watching the two of them. She had already packed, and when three of my father's friends dropped by to offer free consultations and recommendations, my mother and Rose's suitcase were already in the car. My mother hugged me and told me that they would be back that night, but not with Rose. She also said, divining my worst fear, "It won't happen to you, honey. Some people go crazy and some people never do. You never will." She smiled and stroked my hair. "Not even when you want to."

Rose was in hospitals, great and small, for the next ten years. She had lots of terrible therapists and a few good ones. One place had no pictures on the walls, no windows, and the patients all wore slippers with the hospital crest on them. My mother didn't even bother to go to Admissions. She turned Rose around and the two of them marched out, my father walking behind

them, apologizing to his colleagues. My mother ignored the psychiatrists, the social workers, and the nurses, and played Handel and Bessie Smith for the patients on whatever was available. At some places, she had a Steinway donated by a grateful, or optimistic, family; at others, she banged out "Gimme a Pigfoot and a Bottle of Beer" on an old, scarred box that hadn't been tuned since there'd been English-speaking physicians on the grounds. My father talked in serious, appreciative tones to the administrators and unit chiefs and tried to be friendly with whoever was managing Rose's case. We all hated the family therapists.

The worst family therapist we ever had sat in a pale green room with us, visibly taking stock of my mother's ethereal beauty and her faded blue t-shirt and girl-sized jeans, my father's rumpled suit and stained tie, and my own unreadable seventeen-year-old fashion statement. Rose was beyond fashion that year, in one of her dancing teddybear smocks and extra-extra-large Celtics sweatpants. Mr. Walker read Rose's file in front of us and then watched in alarm as Rose began crooning, beautifully, and slowly massaging her breasts. My mother and I laughed, and even my father started to smile. This was Rose's usual opening salvo for new therapists.

Mr. Walker said, "I wonder why it is that everyone is so entertained by Rose behaving inappropriately."

Rose burped and then we all laughed. This was the seventh family therapist we had seen, and none of them had lasted very long. Mr. Walker, unfortunately, was determined to do right by us.

"What do you think of Rose's behavior, Violet?" They did this sometimes. In their manual it must say, If you think the parents are too weird, try talking to the sister.

"I don't know. Maybe she's trying to get you to stop talking about her in the third person."

"Nicely put," my mother said.

"Indeed," my father said.

"Fuckin' A," Rose said.

"Well, this is something that the whole family agrees upon," Mr. Walker said, trying to act as if he understood or even liked us.

"That was not a successful intervention, Ferret Face." Rose tended to function better when she was angry. He did look like a blond ferret, and we all laughed again. Even my father, who tried to give these people a chance, out of some sense of collegiality, had given it up.

After fourteen minutes, Mr. Walker decided that our time was up and walked out, leaving us grinning at each other. Rose was still nuts, but at least we'd all had a little fun.

The day we met our best family therapist started out almost as badly. We scared off a resident and then scared off her supervisor, who sent us Dr. Thorne. Three hundred pounds of Texas chili, cornbread, and Lone Star beer, finished off with big black cowboy boots and a small string tie around the area of his neck.

"O frabjous day, it's Big Nut." Rose was in heaven and stopped massaging her breasts immediately.

"Hey, Little Nut." You have to understand how big a man would have to be to call my sister "little." He christened us all, right away. "And it's the good Doctor Nut, and Madame Hickory Nut, 'cause they are the hardest damn nuts to crack, and over here in the overalls and not much else is No One's Nut"—a name that summed up both my sanity and my loneliness. We all relaxed.

Dr. Thorne was good for us. Rose moved into a halfway house whose director loved Big Nut so much that she kept Rose even when Rose went through a period of having sex with everyone who passed her door. She was in a fever for a while, trying to still the voices by fucking her brains out.

Big Nut said, "Darlin', I can't. I cannot make love to every beautiful woman I meet, and furthermore, I can't do that and be your therapist too. It's a great shame, but I think you might be able to find a really nice guy, someone who treats you just as sweet and kind as I would if I were lucky enough to be your beau. I don't want you to settle for less." And she stopped propositioning the crack addicts and the alcoholics and the guys at the shelter. We loved Dr. Thorne.

My father went back to seeing rich neurotics and helped out one day a week at Dr. Thorne's Walk-In Clinic. My mother finished a recording of Mozart concerti and played at fund-raisers for Rose's halfway house. I went back to college and found a wonderful linebacker from Texas to sleep with. In the dark, I would make him call me "darlin'." Rose took her meds, lost about fifty pounds, and began singing at the A.M.E. Zion Church, down the street from the halfway house.

At first they didn't know what to do with this big blond lady, dressed funny and hovering wistfully in the doorway during their rehearsals, but she gave them a few bars of "Precious Lord" and the choir director felt God's hand and saw that with the help of His sweet child Rose, the Prospect Street Choir was going all the way to the Gospel Olympics.

Amidst a sea of beige, umber, cinnamon, and espresso faces, there was Rose, bigger, blonder, and pinker than any two white women could be. And Rose and the choir's contralto, Addie Robicheaux, laid out their gold and silver voices and wove them together in strands as fine as silk, as strong as steel. And we wept as Rose and Addie, in their billowing garnet robes, swayed together, clasping hands until the last perfect note floated up to God, and then they smiled down at us.

Rose would still go off from time to time and the voices would tell her to do bad things, but Dr. Thorne or Addie or my mother could usually bring her back. After five good years, Big Nut died. Stuffing his face with a chili dog, sitting in his unair-conditioned office in the middle of July, he had one big, Texas-sized aneurysm and died.

Rose held on tight for seven days; she took her

meds, went to choir practice, and rearranged her room about a hundred times. His funeral was like a Lourdes for the mentally ill. If you were psychotic, borderline, bad-off neurotic, or just very hard to get along with, you were there. People shaking so bad from years of heavy meds that they fell out of the pews. People holding hands, crying, moaning, talking to themselves. The crazy people and the not-so-crazy people were all huddled together, like puppies at the pound.

Rose stopped taking her meds, and the halfway house wouldn't keep her after she pitched another patient down the stairs. My father called the insurance company and found out that Rose's new, improved psychiatric coverage wouldn't begin for forty-five days. I put all of her stuff in a garbage bag, and we walked out of the halfway house, Rose winking at the poor drooling boy on the couch.

"This is going to be difficult—not all bad, but difficult—for the whole family, and I thought we should discuss everybody's expectations. I know I have some concerns." My father had convened a family meeting as soon as Rose finished putting each one of her thirty stuffed bears in its own special place.

"No meds," Rose said, her eyes lowered, her stubby fingers, those fingers that had braided my hair and painted tulips on my cheeks, pulling hard on the hem of her dirty smock.

My father looked in despair at my mother.

"Rosie, do you want to drive the new car?" my mother asked.

Rose's face lit up. "I'd love to drive that car. I'd drive to California, I'd go see the bears at the San Diego Zoo. I would take you, Violet, but you always hated the zoo. Remember how she cried at the Bronx Zoo when she found out that the animals didn't get to go home at closing?" Rose put her damp hand on mine and squeezed it sympathetically. "Poor Vi."

"If you take your medication, after a while you'll be able to drive the car. That's the deal.

Meds, car." My mother sounded accommodating but unenthusiastic, careful not to heat up Rose's paranoia.

"You got yourself a deal, darlin'."

I was living about an hour away then, teaching English during the day, writing poetry at night. I went home every few days for dinner. I called every night.

My father said, quietly, "It's very hard. We're doing all right, I think. Rose has been walking in the mornings with your mother, and she watches a lot of TV. She won't go to the day hospital, and she won't go back to the choir. Her friend Mrs. Robicheaux came by a couple of times. What a sweet woman. Rose wouldn't even talk to her. She just sat there, staring at the wall and humming. We're not doing all that well, actually, but I guess we're getting by. I'm sorry, sweetheart, I don't mean to depress you."

My mother said, emphatically, "We're doing fine. We've got our routine and we stick to it and we're fine. You don't need to come home so often, you know. Wait 'til Sunday, just come for the day. Lead your life, Vi. She's leading hers."

I stayed away all week, afraid to pick up my phone, grateful to my mother for her harsh calm and her reticence, the qualities that had enraged me throughout my childhood.

I came on Sunday, in the early afternoon, to help my father garden, something we had always enjoyed together. We weeded and staked tomatoes and killed aphids while my mother and Rose were down at the lake. I didn't even go into the house until four, when I needed a glass of water.

Someone had broken the piano bench into five neatly stacked pieces and placed them where the piano bench usually was.

"We were having such a nice time, I couldn't bear to bring it up," my father said, standing in the doorway, carefully keeping his gardening boots out of the kitchen.

"What did Mommy say?"

"She said, 'Better the bench than the piano.'

And you sister lay down on the floor and just wept. Then your mother took her down to the lake. This can't go on, Vi. We have twenty-seven days left, your mother gets no sleep because Rose doesn't sleep, and if I could just pay twenty-seven thousand dollars to keep her in the hospital until the insurance takes over, I'd do it."

"All right. Do it. Pay the money and take her back to Hartley-Rees. It was the prettiest place, and she liked the art therapy there."

"I would if I could. The policy states that she must be symptom-free for at least forty-five days before her coverage begins. Symptom-free means no hospitalization."

"Jesus, Daddy, how could you get that kind of policy? She hasn't been symptom-free for forty-five minutes."

"It's the only one I could get for long-term psychiatric." He put his hand over his mouth, to block whatever he was about to say, and went back out to the garden. I couldn't see if he was crying.

He stayed outside and I stayed inside until Rose and my mother came home from the lake. Rose's soggy sweatpants were rolled up to her knees, and she had a bucketful of shells and seaweed, which my mother persuaded her to leave on the back porch. My mother kissed me lightly and told Rose to go up to her room and change out of her wet pants.

Rose's eyes grew very wide. "Never. I will never . . ." She knelt down and began banging her head on the kitchen floor with rhythmic intensity, throwing all her weight behind each attack. My mother put her arms around Rose's waist and tried to hold her back. Rose shook her off, not even looking around to see what was slowing her down. My mother lay up against the refrigerator.

"Violet, please . . ."

I threw myself onto the kitchen floor, becoming the spot that Rose was smacking her head against. She stopped a fraction of an inch short of my stomach.

"Oh, Vi, Mommy, I'm sorry. I'm sorry, don't hate me." She staggered to her feet and ran wailing to her room.

My mother got up and washed her face brusquely, rubbing it dry with a dishcloth. My father heard the wailing and came running in, slipping his long bare feet out of his rubber boots.

"Galen, Galen, let me see." He held her head and looked closely for bruises on her pale, small face. "What happened?" My mother looked at me. "Violet, what happened? Where's Rose?"

"Rose got upset, and when she went running upstairs she pushed Mommy out of the way." I've only told three lies in my life, and that was my second.

"She must feel terrible, pushing you, of all people. It would have to be you, but I know she didn't want it to be." He made my mother a cup of tea, and all the love he had for her, despite her silent rages and her vague stares, came pouring through the teapot, warming her cup, filling her small, long-fingered hands. She rested her head against his hip, and I looked away.

"Let's make dinner, then I'll call her. Or you call her, David, maybe she'd rather see your face first."

Dinner was filled with all of our starts and stops and Rose's desperate efforts to control herself. She could barely eat and hummed the McDonald's theme song over and over again, pausing only to spill her juice down the front of her smock and begin weeping. My father looked at my mother and handed Rose his napkin. She dabbed at herself listlessly, but the tears stopped.

"I want to go to bed. I want to go to bed and be in my head. I want to go to bed and be in my bed and in my head and just wear red. For red is the color that my baby wore and once more, it's true, yes, it is, it's true. Please don't wear red tonight, oh, oh, please don't wear red tonight, for red is the color—"

"Okay, okay, Rose. It's okay. I'll go upstairs with you and you can get ready for bed. Then Mommy will come up and say good night too. It's okay, Rose." My father reached out his hand and Rose grasped it, and they walked out of the dining room together, his long arm around her middle.

My mother sat at the table for a moment, her face in her hands, and then she began clearing the plates. We cleared without talking, my mother humming Schubert's "Schlummerlied," a lullaby about the woods and the river calling to the child to go to sleep. She sang it to us every night when we were small.

My father came into the kitchen and signaled to my mother. They went upstairs and came back down together a few minutes later.

"She's asleep," they said, and we went to sit on the porch and listen to the crickets. I don't remember the rest of the evening, but I remember it as quietly sad, and I remember the rare sight of my parents holding hands, sitting on the picnic table, watching the sunset.

I woke up at three o'clock in the morning, feeling the cool night air through my sheet. I went down the hall for a blanket and looked into Rose's room, for no reason. She wasn't there. I put on my jeans and a sweater and went downstairs. I could feel her absence. I went outside and saw her wide, draggy footprints darkening the wet grass into the woods.

"Rosie," I called, too softly, not wanting to wake my parents, not wanting to startle Rose. "Rosie, it's me. Are you here? Are you all right?"

I almost fell over her. Huge and white in the moonlight, her flowered smock bleached in the light and shadow, her sweatpants now completely wet. Her head was flung back, her white, white neck exposed like a lost Greek column.

"Rosie, Rosie—" Her breathing was very slow, and her lips were not as pink as they usually were. Her eyelids fluttered.

"Closing time," she whispered. I believe that's what she said.

I sat with her, uncovering the bottle of white pills by her hand, and watched the stars fade.

When the stars were invisible and the sun was warming the air, I went back to the house. My mother was standing on the porch, wrapped in a blanket, watching me. Every step I took overwhelmed me; I could picture my mother slapping me, shooting me for letting her favorite die.

"Warrior queens," she said, wrapping her thin strong arms around me. "I raised warrior queens." She kissed me fiercely and went into the woods by herself.

Later in the morning she woke my father, who could not go into the woods, and still later she called the police and the funeral parlor. She hung up the phone, lay down, and didn't get back out of bed until the day of the funeral. My father fed us both and called the people who needed to be called and picked out Rose's coffin by himself.

My mother played the piano and Addie sang her pure gold notes and I closed my eyes and saw my sister, fourteen years old, lion's mane thrown back and eyes tightly closed against the glare of the parking lot lights. That sweet sound held us tight, flowing around us, eddying through our hearts, rising, still rising.

Experiences of Deviance, Chronic Illness, and Disability

Persons with long-term physical and mental disabilities are more numerous, more politically active, and of greater public and health policy concern in Western societies today than at any previous time. Somewhere between 35 and 43 million Americans have disabling conditions that interfere with their lives to varying degrees. In 1990, about 19.4 million people between the ages of eighteen to sixty-four (or 12.8 percent of the U.S. population) reported that their functioning was limited by a chronic condition. Among this group, 6.7 million persons (4.4 percent of the U.S. population) were so limited that they were unable to work (Vladeck et al. 1993). While most of us are relatively healthy and able-bodied, each of us is only temporarily "able"; we each face loss of comfort and function in varying degrees over the life span. Being disabled is a personal experience, an interpersonal and social challenge, a clinical problem, and a health and social policy concern. In this section, disablement is examined as a social and personal process, viewed from experiential, clinical, and sociological perspectives.

People with chronic illness and disability are present in the clinical practice of medicine in large numbers and challenge the usual assumptions, held by both doctors and patients, about clinical encounters—that there will be a quick cure, just as if they had an acute illness. It is helpful to distinguish between the age-appropriate and expected limitations (aches and pains) that afflict people and those that interrupt normal development and functioning and are not expected. Both the meaning of such ailments to the individual and the clinical response may differ.

Since older people tend to have more chronic conditions, and since there are more and more elderly people in the United States, physicians who practice medicine in this country will find themselves treating more and more persons with chronic illness in the next decades. (We return to this topic in part II.)

At the same time, a great many persons under the age of sixty-five also have chronic illnesses such as rheumatoid arthritis or severe disabilities such as spinal cord injuries. An estimated 31 percent of children under the age of eighteen (about 20 million children) were reported to have at least one chronic health condition, and about 2 million had three or more chronic conditions. In 1993, slightly over 723,000 children were recipients of Supplemental Security Income (SSI), a federal income support program for individuals with severe disabilities (NASI 1994).

What individuals with disabilities have in common is the substantial cost of their care, their inability to pay for all or perhaps any of it, and their needs for resources such as housing, transportation, and food in addition to medical care. Approximately 12 percent of national health care expenditures in 1993, or $108 billion, was spent on long-term care, an increase of 13.9 percent from 1992. Long-term care costs are largely borne by public funds, particularly Medicaid. For example, nursing home costs for all ages represented $38 billion in expenditures in 1986, over 40 percent of which was paid for by Medicaid. Nursing home expenditures increased by 17 percent between 1991 and 1992. Private health insurance pays for less than 1 percent of nursing home costs, and less than 2 percent of all elderly have any long-term health insurance protection (Vladeck et al. 1993).

Yet, as noted above, elderly people represent only part of the disabled population. There are, for example, an estimated 2.5 million people under the age of sixty-five with developmental disabilities, including mental retardation, who require lifelong care and support. In 1986, Medicaid expenditures reached $5.2 billion to pay for intermediate care facilities for persons with severe mental retardation. Despite these large sums of public assistance, the remaining half of long-term care costs for disabled persons were paid out of pocket, by families, spouses, and friends who may deplete resources that they need for their own future care or for other family members. Clearly, paying for long-term medical, habilitative, and rehabilitative care poses difficult questions on resource allocation and public policy on the one hand, and very personal dilemmas for families and spouses on the other. (We return to this topic in part V.)

Having a chronic illness or disability in the United States often means that a person becomes impoverished financially. A person with a severe disability who receives SSI gets a maximum of $5,200 per year, and a recipient of Social Security Disability Insurance (SSDI) gets an average of $7,500 per year. Among disabled persons under sixty-five years old, 38 percent live below the poverty level compared to 16 percent among nondisabled persons. Recent studies show that many people who are unable to work because of disabilities, but who do not qualify for SSI or SSDI, rely solely on their families for material support or have no support at all. Yet an investigation of 145 physically disabled individuals found that, compared to nondisabled persons, those with impairments did not rate their lives as less happy or satisfying. The people with disabilities did, however, rate their lives as more difficult and likely to stay that way. Another study of 88 seriously physically restricted persons (Hahn 1988)

posed the question, "If you were given one wish, would you wish that you were no longer disabled?" Only half said they would wish to remove their disability. Most considered their disability a fact of life, an inconvenience, and a source of frustration. It is not accurate to assume that all disabled persons are bitter, angry, or ashamed of themselves. Neither should we expect each of them to become "happy handicapped" people, practicing exceptionalism in every aspect of their lives.

From a social perspective, illness entails "deviance"—that is, discrepancies in behavior and appearance from what is expected or "normal." Being ill also involves a temporary change in identity. We often say, "I don't feel like myself" when ill, and in some important ways, we are not our customary selves. But when a condition or disease is not temporary but lasts for years, even a lifetime, the challenge of illness to identity can be substantial. In his autobiography, Leonard Kriegel (1991, 47) writes as a person with a disability that "people struggle not only to define themselves but to avoid being defined by others. But to be a cripple is to learn that one can be defined from outside. Our complaint against society is not that it ignores our presence but that it ignores our reality, our sense of ourselves as humans brave enough to capture our destinies against odds that are formidable. . . . Our true selves, our own inner lives, have been auctioned off so that we can be palatable rather than real."

In the readings that follow, Irving Zola takes up the topics of identity and chronic illness in his essay on how we talk about disability, and he provides an introduction to the dynamics of medical and social labeling. Gordon Weaver's character, Finch, suffers with a rough-edged anger at being trapped inside of his spastic body. His anguish about who and what he is give life to Zola and Cassell's arguments about identity and disability being intimately entwined. Finch is apart from everyone, sneering all the way. His unpredictable body prevents him from joining the social world he longs for, and he rejects others whose bodies are like his.

The last reading in this section, also by Zola, sets up a counterpoint. In a fictional account, Zola gives a rare view of two individuals with substantial disabilities engaged in the most human of activities, making love. While the efforts and arrangements they have to make may differ from those of able-bodied people, their emotional and romantic concerns are very familiar. Like Weaver, Zola illustrates some slippery ambiguities about how persons with disabilities are viewed by themselves and others. What seem to be vast differences between their lives and ours may be at some times more apparent than real, and then at others so vast as to be incomprehensible.

Self, Identity, and the Naming Question: Reflections on the Language of Disability

Irving Kenneth Zola

■

"When I use the word, it means just what I choose it to mean—neither more nor less."—Humpty Dumpty

I. The Power of Naming

Language . . . has as much to do with the philosophical and political conditioning of a society as geography or climate . . . people do not realize the extent to which their attitudes have been conditioned to ennoble or condemn, augment or detract, glorify or demean. Negative language inflicts the subconscious of most . . . people from the time they first learn to speak. Prejudice is not merely imparted or superimposed. It is metabolized in the bloodstream of society. What is needed is not so much a change in language as an awareness of the power of words to condition attitudes [1].

A step in this awareness is the recognition of how deep is the power of naming in Western culture. According to the Old Testament, God's first act after saying "Let there be light" was to call the light "Day" and the darkness "Night." Moreover, God's first act after the creation of Adam was to bring in every beast of the field so that Adam could give them names; and "whatsoever Adam called every living creature, that was the name thereof" (Genesis 2:20). Thus what one is called tends "to stick" and any unnaming process is not without its difficulties and consequences [2].

While a name has always connoted some aspect of one's status (e.g. job, location, gender, social class, ethnicity, kinship), the mid-twentieth century seems to be a time when the issue of naming has assumed a certain primacy [3, 4]. In the post-World War II era Erik Erikson [5] and Alan Wheelis [6] noted that "Who am I" or the issue of identity had become a major psychological concern of the U.S. population. The writings of C. Wright Mills [7] as well as the Women's Movement [8], however, called attention to the danger of individualizing any issue as only a "personal problem."

The power of naming was thus recognized not only as a personal issue but a political one as well. While social scientists focused more on the general "labelling" process [9–13] and the measurement of attitudes toward people with various chronic diseases and disabilities [14, 15], a number of "liberation" or "rights" movements focused on the practical implications. They claimed that language was one of the mechanisms by which dominant groups kept others "in place" [16, 17]. Thus, as minority groups sought to gain more control over their lives, the issue of naming—what they are called—was one of the first battlegrounds. The resolution of this was not always clear-cut. For some, the original stigmas became the banner: Negroes and coloreds become Blacks. For others, only a completely new designation would suffice—"Ms." has caught on as a form of address but "womyn," "wimmin" have not been so successful in severing the vocabulary connection to "men."

People with disabilities are in the midst of a similar struggle. The struggle is confounded by some special circumstances which mitigate against the easy development of either a disability pride or culture [18, 19]. While most minority group members grow up in a recognized subculture and thus develop certain norms and expectations, people with chronic diseases and disabilities are not similarly prepared. The nature of their experience has been toward isolation. The vast majority of people who are born with or acquire such conditions do so within families who neither have these conditions nor associate with others who do. They are socialized into the world of the "normal" with all its values, prejudices, and vocabulary. As one generally attempts to rise out of one's status, there is always an attempt to put this status in some perspective. The statements that one is more than just a Black or a woman, etc., are commonplace. On the other hand, where chronic illness and disability are concerned, this negation is almost total and is tantamount to denial. Proof of successful integration is embodied in such statements as "I *never* think of myself as handicapped" or the supreme compliment, "I *never* think of you as handicapped."

What then of the institutions where too many spend too much of their time—the long-term hospitals, sanitoria, convalescent and nursing homes? These are aptly labelled "total institutions" [20], but "total" refers to their control over our lives, not to the potential fullness they offer. The subcultures formed within such places are largely defensive and designed to make live viable within the institution. Often this viability is achieved at such a cost that it cannot be transferred to the non-institutional world.

For most of their history, organizations of people with disabilities were not much more successful in their efforts to produce a viable subculture. Their memberships have been small in comparison to the potential disabled population, and they have been regarded more as social groups rather than serious places to gain technical knowledge or emotional support. And though there are some self-help groups which are becoming increasingly visible, militant and independent of medical influence, the movement is still in its infancy [21]. Long ago, Talcott

Parsons articulated the basic dilemma facing such groups:

> The sick role is . . . a mechanism which . . . channels deviance so that the two most dangerous potentialities, namely group formation and successful establishment of the claim of legitimacy, are avoided. The sick are tied up, not with other deviants to form a "subculture" of the sick but each with a group of nonsick, his personal circle, and, above all, physicians. The sick thus become a statistical status and are deprived of the possibility of forming a solidarity collectivity. Furthermore, to be sick is by definition to be in an undesirable state, so that it simply does not "make sense" to assert a claim that the way to deal with the frustrating aspects of the social system is for everyone to get sick [22, p. 477].

A mundane but dramatic way of characterizing this phenomenon can be seen in the rallying cries of current liberation movements. As the "melting pot" theory of America was finally buried, people could once again say, even though they were three generations removed from the immigrants, that they were proud to be Greek, Italian, Hungarian, or Polish. With the rise of black power, a derogatory label became a rallying cry, "Black is beautiful." And when women saw their strength in numbers, they shouted "Sisterhood is powerful." But what about those with a chronic illness or disability? Could they yell, "Long live cancer" "Up with multiple sclerosis" "I'm glad I had polio!" "Don't you wish you were blind?" Thus the traditional reversing of the stigma will not so easily provide a basis for a common positive identity.

2. Some Negative Functions of Labelling

The struggle over labels often follows a pattern. It is far easier to agree on terms that should *not* be used than the designations that should replace them [23–25]. As with the racial, ethnic [26] and gender groups [27, 28] before them, many had begun to note the negative qualities of certain "disability references" [29, 30]. Others created quite useful glossaries [31].

Since, as Phillips [32] notes, the names one calls oneself reflect differing political strategies, we must go beyond a list of "do's" and "don'ts" to an analysis of the functions of such labelling [33–36]. As long ago as 1651, Thomas Hobbes—in setting his own social agenda—saw the importance of such clarifications, "seeing then that truth consists in the right ordering of names in our affirmations, a man that seeks precise truth has need to remember what every name he uses stands for; and to place it accordingly; or else he will find himself entangled in words as a bird in lime twigs; the more he struggles the more belimed" [37, p. 26].

There are at least two separate implications of such naming which have practical and political consequences. The first is connotational and associational. As Kenneth Burke [38, p. 4] wrote "Call a man a villain and you have the choice of either attacking or avenging. Call him mistaken and you invite yourself to attempt to set him right." I would add, "Call a person sick or crazy and all their behavior becomes dismissable." Because someone has been labelled ill, all their activity and beliefs—past, present, and future—become related to and explainable in terms of their illness [20, 39]. Once this occurs, society can deny the validity of anything which they might say, do, or stand for. Being seen as the object of medical treatment evokes the image of many ascribed traits, such as weakness, helplessness, dependency, regressiveness, abnormality of appearance and depreciation of every mode of physical and mental functioning [17, 40, 41]. In the case of a person with a chronic illness and/or a permanent disability, these traits, once perceived to be temporary accompaniments of an illness, become indelible characteristics. "The individual is trapped in a state of suspended animation socially, is perpetually a patient, is chronically viewed as helpless and dependent, in need of cure but incurable" [17, p. 420].

A second function of labelling is its potential for spread, pervasiveness, generalization. An example of such inappropriate generalizing was provided in a study by Conant and Budoff [42]. They found that a group of sighted children and adults interpreted the labels "blind" and "legally blind" as meaning that the person was totally without vision—something which is true for only a small segment of people with that designation. What was problematic became a given. Another example of this process occurs when disability and person are equated. While it is commonplace to hear of doctors referring to people as "the appendicitis in Room 306" or "the amputee down the hall," such labelling is more common in popular culture than one might believe. My own analysis of the crime-mystery genre [43], noted that after an introductory description of characters with a disability, they are often referred to by their disability—e.g. "the dwarf," "the blind man," "the one-armed," "the one-legged." This is usually done by some third person observer or where the person with the disability is the speaker. The disability is emphasized—e.g. "said the blind man." No other physical or social descriptor appears with such frequency.

Perhaps not unexpectedly, such stand-in appellations are most commonly applied to villains. They were commonplace during the heyday of the pulp magazines, where the disability was incorporated into their names—"One-Eyed Joe," "Scarface Kelly"—a tradition enshrined in the Dick Tracy comic strips. It is a tradition that continues, though with more subtlety. Today we may no longer have "Clubfoot the Avenger," a mad German master-criminal who crossed swords for 25 years with the British Secret Service [44–51], but we do have "The Deaf Man,"

the recurring thorn in the side of Ed McBain's long-running (over 30 years) 87th Precinct novels [52–54]. All such instances can reinforce an association between disability, evil, and abnormality [55].

A very old joke illustrates the pervasiveness of such labelling:

A man is changing a flat tyre outside a mental hospital when the bolts from his wheel roll down a nearby sewer. Distraught, he is confronted by a patient watching him who suggests, "Why don't you take one bolt off each of the other wheels, and place it on the spare?" Surprised when it works, the driver says, "How come you of all people would think of that?" Replies the patient, "I may be crazy, but I'm not stupid."

This anecdote demonstrates the flaw in thinking that a person who is mad is therefore stupid or incapable of being insightful. As the social psychological literature has long noted, this is how stigma comes about—from a process of generalizing from a single experience, people are treated categorically rather than individually and are devalued in the process [56–58]. As Longmore so eloquently concludes, a "spoiling process" [59] results whereby "they obscure all other characteristics behind that one and swallow up the social identity of the individual within that restrictive category" [17, p. 419]. Peters puts it most concretely: "The label that's used to describe us is often far more important in shaping our view of ourselves—and the way others view us—than whether we sign, use a cane, sit in a wheelchair, or use a communication board" [23, p. 25].

While many have offered vocabulary suggestions to combat the above problems of connotation and pervasiveness, few have analytically delineated what is at stake in such name changes [17, 60, 61]. The most provocative and historically-rooted analysis is an unpublished paper by Phillips [32], who delineates four distinct strategies which underly the renaming. While she carefully notes that further investigation may change or expand her categorization, the very idea of her schema and the historical data describing the genesis of each "recoding" remain timely.

"Cripple" and "handicapped," as nouns or adjectives, she sees as primarily "names of acquiescence and accommodation," reflecting an acceptance of society's oppressive institutions. Terms such as "physically challenged" by so personalizing the disability run the risk of fostering a "blaming the victim" stance [62]. Such terms, as well as "physically different," "physically inconvenienced," not only may be so euphemistic that they confound the public as to who is being discussed but also contribute strongly to the denial of existing realities [33]. Two other strategies represent a more activist philosophy. "Handicapper" and "differently-abled" are "names of reaction and reflection" whose purpose is to emphasize "the can-do" aspects of having a disability. To the group of Michigan advocates who coined the term [63], a "Handicapper" determines the degree to which one's own physical or mental characteristics direct life's activities. Anger, says Phillips, is basic to "names of renegotiation and inversion" where the context sets the meaning. Perhaps the best examples occur when disability activists, in the privacy of their own circles, "talk dirty," referring to themselves as "blinks," "gimps," or telling "crip" jokes and expounding on the intricacies of "crip" time. More controversy arises however, when people publicly proclaim such terms as a matter of pride. Recently, for example, many have written about the positive aspects of "being deaf" [64, 65] or, even more dramatically of being a "cripple" [66]. Kriegel [60, 61] says that "cripple" describes "an essential reality," a way of keeping what needs to be dealt with socially and politically in full view. Nancy Mairs [67], a prize-winning poet who has

multiple sclerosis, clearly agrees; and in the opening remarks of her essay, "On Being a Cripple," states it most vividly:

> The other day I was thinking of writing an essay on being a cripple. I was thinking hard in one of the stalls of the women's room in my office building, as I was shoving my shirt into my jeans and tugging up my zipper. Preoccupied, I flushed, picked up my book bag, took my cane down from the hook, and unlatched the door. So many movements unbalanced me, and as I pulled the door open, I fell over backwards, landing fully clothed on the toilet seat with legs splayed in front of me: the old beetle-on-its-back routine. Saturday afternoon, the building deserted, I was free to laugh aloud as I wriggled back to my feet, my voice bouncing off the yellowish tiles from all directions. Had anyone been there with me, I'd have been still and faint and hot with chagrin.
>
> I decided that it was high time to write the essay.
>
> First, the matter of semantics. I am a cripple. I choose this word to name me. I choose from among several possibilities, the most common of which are handicapped and disabled. I made the choice a number of years ago, without thinking, unaware of my motives for doing so. Even now, I'm not sure what those motives are, but I recognize that they are complex and not entirely flattering. People—crippled or not—wince at the word cripple, as they do not at handicapped or disabled. Perhaps I want them to wince. I want them to see me as a tough customer, one to whom the fates/gods/viruses have not been kind, but who can face the brutal truth of her existence squarely. As a cripple, I swagger [67, p. 9].

When Phillips' very titles may imply an evaluation of the particular strategies, it is clear from her own caveats that while many may try to impose their terminology as "the correct language," "None feel really right" [23, p. 25].

3. Recontextualizing Names

The ultimate question, of course, is whether any of these renaming procedures, singly and alone, can deal with the connotational and generalization issues discussed previously. I would argue that the context of usage may be every bit as important (as Phillips implies) as the specific terminology. Thus one of the reasons for all the negative associations to many terms is a result of such contexts. Here social scientists, researchers and clinicians are particularly at fault in their medicalizing of disability [55, 68, 69]. In their writings and in the transmission of these writings by the popular press and media, people with varying diseases and disabilities are inevitably referred to as "patients," a term which describes a role, a relationship and a location (i.e. an institution or hospital) from which many connotations, as previously noted, flow. For the 43 million people now designated as having a physical, mental or biological disability, only a tiny proportion are continually resident in and under medical supervision and are thus truly patients. Similarly, the terms "suffering from," "afflicted with" are projections and evaluations of an outside world. No person with a disability is automatically "suffering" or "afflicted" except in specific situations where they do indeed "hurt," are "in pain" or "feel victimized."

I am not arguing, however, for the complete elimination of medical or physical terminology. As DeFelice cautions, "The disabled movement has purchased political visibility at the price of physical invisibility. The crippled and lame had bodies, but the handicapped, or so the social workers say, are just a little late at the starting gate. I don't like that; it's banal. When we speak in metaphorical terms, we deny physical reality. The farther we get from our bodies, the more removed we are from the body politic . . ." [70].

One meaning I derive from his caution is that we must seek a change in the connotations and the pervasiveness of our names without denying the essential reality of our conditions. Thus biology may not determine our destiny; but, as with women, our physical, mental and biological differences are certainly part of that destiny [71, 72].

A way of contextualizing our relationship to our bodies and our disabilities may not be in changing terms but in changing grammars. Our continual use of nouns and adjectives can only perpetuate the equation of the individual equalling the disability. No matter what noun we use, it substitutes one categorical definition for another. An adjective, colors and thus connotes the essential quality of the noun it modifies. Such adjectives as "misshapen," "deformed," "defective," "invalid"—far from connoting a specific quality of the individual—tend to taint the whole person.

The same is true with less charged terms. Thus "a disabled car" is one which has totally broken down. Could "a disabled person" be perceived as anything less? Prepositions, on the other hand, imply both "a relationship to" and "a separation from." At this historical juncture the awkwardness in phrasing that often results may be all to the good, for it makes both user and hearer stop and think about what is meant, as in the phrases "people *of* color" and "persons *with* disabilities."

Distance and relationship are also at the heart of some very common verb usages. The first is between the active and passive tense. Note the two dictionary meanings:

Active—asserting that the person or thing represented by the grammatical subjects performs the action represented by the verb [73, p. 12].

Passive—asserting that the grammatical subject to a verb is subjected to or affected by the action represented by that verb [73, p. 838].

Thus in describing an individual's relationship to an assistive device such as a wheelchair, the difference between "being confined to a wheelchair" and "using" one is a difference not only of terminology but of control. Medical language has long perpetuated this "disabled passivity" by its emphasis on what medicine continually *does* to its "patients" rather than *with* them [74, 75].

Similarly the issues of "connotation" and "pervasiveness" may be perpetuated by the differential use of the verbs "be" and "have." The French language makes careful distinctions between when to use "être" (be) and when to use "avoir" (have). English daily usage is blurry, but another look at Webster's does show the possibilities.

> be = to equal in meaning
>   to have same connotation as
>   to have identity with
>   to constitute the same class as [73, p. 96].
> have = to hold in possession
>   to hold in one's use
>   to consist of
>   to stand in relationship to
>   to be marked or characterized by
>   to experience
>   SYN—to keep, control, retain, or experience [73, p. 526].

Like the issue of nouns vs prepositions, verbs can also code people in terms of categories (e.g. *x* is a redhead) instead of specific attributes (e.g. *x* has red hair), allowing people to feel that the stigmatized persons are fundamentally different and establishing greater psychological and social distance [76]. Thus, as between the active and passive tense, so it is between "I am . . ." Both specify

a difference in distance and control in relation to whatever it is one "is" or "has." And since renaming relates to alternative images of distance and control, grammar, which tends to be normative, concise, shared and long-lasting, may serve us better than sheer name change. Though I personally may have a generic preference (e.g. for "disability" over "handicap"), I am not arguing for any "politically correct" usage but rather examining the political advantages and disadvantages of each [36].

For example, there may be stages in the coping with a particular condition or in the perceived efficacy of a particular "therapy" (e.g. the 12 steps in Alcoholics Anonymous) when "ownership" and thus the use of "I am" is deemed essential. Those old enough to remember President Kennedy's words at the Berlin Wall, "*Ich bin ein Berliner*" (I am a Berliner), will recall the power of its message of kinship. Similarly, when we politically strategize as a minority group [77] and seek a kinship across disease and disability groups [78], the political coming-out may require a personal ownership best conveyed in terms of "I am . . ."

On the other hand, there are times when the political goals involve groups for whom disease and disability is not a permanent or central issue. On my university campus, for a myriad of reasons, people with mobility impairments are virtually non-existent. Yet we are gradually retrofitting old buildings and guaranteeing accessibility in new ones. The alliance here is among women who are or may become pregnant, parents with small children, people with injuries or time-limited diseases, and others who perceive themselves at risk, such as aging staff or faculty. They rarely see themselves as disabled but often admit to having a temporary disability or sharing a part of "the disabled experience" (e.g. "Now I know what it's like to try to climb all those stairs"). Thus where coalition politics is needed, the concept of "having" vs "being" may be a more effective way of acknowledging multiple identities and kinship, as in our use of hyphenated personal and social lineages—e.g. Afro-American.

4. A Final Caveat

One of the sad findings in Phillips' study [32] is how divisive this struggle over names has become. People thus begin to chastize "non true-believers" and emphasize to others "politically correct" usage. In so doing, we may not only damage the unity so necessary to the cause of disability rights but also fail to see the forest for the trees. Our struggle is necessary because we live in a society which devalues, discriminates against and disparages people with disabilities [77, 79]. It is not our task to prove that we are worthy of the full resources and integration of our society. The fault is not in us, not in our diseases and disabilities [41, 62, 80, 81] but in mythical denials, social arrangements, political priorities and prejudices [82].

Here too, a renaming can be of service not of us but of our oppressors [83]. As Hughes and Hughes [84] note, when we turn the tables and create epithets for our oppressors, this may be a sign of a beginning cohesiveness. Thus the growing popularity of terms like TAB's and MAB's (temporarily or momentarily able-bodied) to describe the general population breaks down the separateness of "us" and "them" and emphasizes the continuity and inevitability of "the disability experience." Thus, too, those who have created the terms "handicappism" [85] and "healthism" [68, 86, 87] equate these with all the structural "-isms" in a society which operates to continue segregation and discrimination. To return finally to the issue of naming, the words of Philip Dunne reflect well the choices and consequences of language:

If we hope to survive in this terrifying age, we must choose our words as we choose our actions. We should think how what we say might sound to other ears as well as to our own. Above all, we should strive for clarity . . .
. . . if clarity [is] the essence of style, it is also the heart and soul of truth, and it is for want of truth that human freedom could perish [88, p. 14].

Notes

1. Saturday Review, Editorial, April 8, 1967.
2. LeGuin, U. K. She unnames them. *New Yorker,* January 21, p. 27, 1985.
3. Friedrich, O. What's in a Name? *Time,* August 18, p. 16, 1986.
4. Vickery, H. Finding the right name for brand X. *Insight,* pp. 54–55, January 27, 1986.
5. Erikson, H. *Childhood and Society.* Norton, New York, 1950.
6. Wheelis, A. *The Quest for Identity.* Norton, New York, 1958.
7. Mills, C. W. *The Sociological Imagination.* Oxford University Press, Oxford, 1959.
8. Boston Women's Health Book Collective. *Women and Our Bodies* (In later revised versions, *Our Bodies Ourselves*). New England Free Press, Boston, 1970.
9. Becker, H. *Outsiders.* The Free Press, Glencoe, IL, 1963.
10. Becker, H. (Ed.) *The Other Side—Perspectives on Deviance.* The Free Press, Glencoe, IL, 1964.
11. Erikson, K. Notes on the sociology of deviance. *Soc. Problems* 9, 307–314, 1962.
12. Erikson, K. *Wayward Puritans: A Study in the Sociology of Deviance.* Wiley, New York, 1966.
13. Schur, E. *Crimes Without Victims.* Prentice-Hall, Englewood Cliffs, NJ, 1965.
14. Siller, J. The measurement of attitudes toward physically disabled persons. In *Physical Appearance, Stigma, and Social Behavior: The Ontario Symposium* (Edited by Herman, P. C., Zanna, M. P., and Higgins, E. T.). Vol. 3, pp. 245–288. Lawrence Erlbaum Associates, Hillsdale, NJ, 1986.
15. Yuker, H., Block, J. Z., and Young, J. H. *The Measurement of Attitudes Toward Disabled Persons.* Human Resources Center, Albertson, NY, 1966.
16. Gumperz, J. J. (Ed.) *Language and Social Identity.* Cambridge University Press, Cambridge, 1982.
17. Longmore, P. K. A note on language and the social iden-

tity of disabled people. *Am. Behav. Scient.* 28, (3), 419–423, 1985.

18. Johnson, M. Emotion and pride: the search for a disability culture. *Disability Rag,* January/February, p. 1, 4–10, 1987.

19. Zola, I. K. "Whose voice is this anyway? A commentary on recent collections about the experience of disability." *Med. Human Rev.* 2, (1), 6–15, 1988.

20. Goffman, E. *Asylums.* Anchor, New York, 1961.

21. Crewe, N., and Zola, I. K. *et al. Independent Living for Physically Disabled People.* Jossey-Bass, San Francisco, 1983.

22. Parsons, T. *The Social System.* The Free Press, Glencoe, 1951.

23. Peters, A. Developing a language. *Disability Rag,* March–April, p. 25, 1986.

24. Peters, A. The problem with "Gimp." *Disability Rag,* July/August, p. 22, 1986.

25. Peters, A. Do we have to be named? *Disability Rag,* November/December, p. 31, 35, 1986.

26. Moore, R. B. *Racism in the English Language—A Lesson Plan and Study Essay.* The Council of Interracial Books for Children, New York, 1976.

27. Shear, M. Equal writes. *Women's Rev. Book* 1, (11), 12–13, 1984.

28. Shear, M. Solving the great pronoun debate. *Ms,* pp. 106, 108–109, 1985.

29. Biklen, D., and Bogdan, R. Disabled—yes; handicapped—no: the language of disability, p. 5, insert in "Media Portrayals of Disabled People: A Study in Stereotypes." *Interracial Books Children Bull.* 8, (3, 6 & 7), 4–9, 1977.

30. Corcoran, P. J. Pejorative terms and attitudinal barriers—editorial. *Arch Phys. Med. Rehabil.* 58, 500, 1977.

31. Shear, M. No more supercrip. *New Directions for Women,* p. 10, November–December, 1986.

32. Phillips, M. J. What we call ourselves: self-referential naming among the disabled. *Seventh Annual Ethnography in Research Forum.* University of Pennsylvania, Philadelphia, 4–6 April 1986.

33. Chaffee, N. L. Disabled . . . handicapped . . . and in the image of God?—Our language reflects societal attitudes and influences theological perception. Unpublished paper, 1987.

34. Gill, C. J. The disability name game. *New World for Persons with Disabilities,* 13, (8), 2, 1987.

35. Gillett, P. The power of words—can they make you feel better or worse? *Accent on Living,* pp. 38–39, 1987.

36. Lindsey, K. The pitfalls of politically correct language. *Sojourner,* p. 16, 1985.

37. Hobbes, T. *Leviathan.* Dutton, New York, 1950.

38. Burke, K. *Attitudes Toward History,* revised edn. Hermes, Oakland, CA, 1959.

39. Link, B. G., Cullen, F. T., Frank, J., and Wozniak, J. F. The social rejection of former mental patients: understanding why labels matter. *Am. J. Sociol.* 1987, 92, (6), 1461–1500, 1987.

40. Goodwin, D. Language: perpetualizing the myths. *Impact, Inc.* (Newsletter of Center for Independent Living, Alton, IL), Vol. 1, No. 2, pp. 1–2, 1986.

41. Zola, I. K. *Missing Pieces: A Chronicle of Living with a Disability.* Temple University Press, Philadelphia, 1982.

42. Conant, S., and Budoff, M. The development of sighted people's understanding of blindness. *J. Vis. Impairment Blindness* 76, 86–96, 1982.

43. Zola, I. K. Any distinguishing features: portrayal of disability in the crime-mystery genre. *Policy Stud. J.* 15, (3), 485–513, 1987.

44. Williams, V. *The Man with the Clubfoot.* Jenkins, London, 1918.

45. Williams, V. *The Secret Hand.* Jenkins, London, 1918.

46. Williams, V. *Return of Clubfoot.* Jenkins, London, 1923.

47. Williams, V. *Clubfoot the Avenger.* Jenkins, London, 1924.

48. Williams, V. *The Crouching Beast.* Hodder & Stoughton, London, 1928.

49. Williams, V. *The Gold Comfit Box.* Hodder & Stoughton, London, 1932.

50. Williams, V. *The Spider's Touch.* Hodder & Stoughton, London, 1936.

51. Williams, V. *Courier to Marrakesh.* Hodder & Stoughton, London, 1944.

52. McBain, E. *Fuzz.* Doubleday, New York, 1968.

53. McBain, E. *Let's Hear It for the Deaf Man.* Random House, New York, 1973.

54. McBain, E. *Eight Black Horses.* Avon, New York, 1985.

55. Conrad, P., and Schneider, J. W. *Deviance and Medicalization: From Badness to Sickness.* C. V. Mosby, St. Louis, 1980.

56. Ainlay, S. C., Becker, G., and Coleman, L. M. (Eds.) *The Dilemma of Difference: A Multidisciplinary View of Stigma.* Plenum, New York, 1986.

57. Jones, E. E., Farina, A., Hastorf, A. H., Markus, H., Miller, D., and Scott, R. *Social Stigma: The Psychology of Marked Relationships.* W. H. Freeman, New York, 1984.

58. Katz, I. *Stigma: A Social Psychological Analysis.* Lawrence Erlbaum Associates, Hillsdale, NJ, 1981.

59. Goffman, E. *Stigma: Notes on the Management of*

Spoiled Identity. Prentice-Hall, Englewood Cliffs, NJ, 1963.

60. Kriegel, L. Uncle Tom and Tiny Tim: reflections on the cripple as Negro. *Am. Scholar* 38, 412–430, 1969.

61. Kriegel, L. Coming through manhood, disease and the authentic self. In: *Rudely Stamp'd: Imaginal Disability and Prejudice* (Edited by Bicklen, D., and Bailey, L.), pp. 49–63. University Press of America, Washington, DC, 1981.

62. Ryan, W. *Blaming the Victim*. Pantheon, New York, 1970.

63. Gentile, E., and Taylor, J. K. Images, words and identity. Handicapper Programs. Michigan State University, East Lansing, MI, 1976.

64. *Disability Rag*. Cochlear implants: the final put-down. March/April, pp. 1, 4–8, 1987.

65. Innerst, C. A will to preserve deaf culture. *Insight*, November 24, pp. 50–51, 1986.

66. Milam, L. *The Crippled Liberation Front Marching Band Blues*. MHO and MHO Works, San Diego, CA, 1984.

67. Mairs, N. On being a cripple. In *Plaintext: Essays*, pp. 9–20. University of Arizona Press, Tucson, AZ, 1986.

68. Zola, I. K. Medicine as an institution of social control. *Sociol. Rev.* 20, 487–504, 1972.

69. Illich, I. *Medical Nemesis: The Expropriation of Health*. Calder & Boyars, London, 1975.

70. DeFelice, R. J. A crippled child grows up. *Newsweek*, November 3, p. 13, 1986.

71. Fine, M., and Asch, A. Disabled women: sexism without the pedestal. *J. Sociol. Soc. Welfare* 8, (2), 233–248, 1981.

72. Fine, M., and Asch, A. (Eds.) *Women with Disabilities—Essays in Psychology, Culture, and Politics*. Temple University Press, Philadelphia, 1988.

73. *Webster's New Collegiate Dictionary*. Merriam, Springfield, MA, 1973.

74. Edelman, M. The political language of the helping professions. In *Political Language*, pp. 59–68. Academic, New York, 1977.

75. Szasz, T. S., and Hollender, M. H. A contribution to the philosophy of medicine: the basic models of the doctor-patient relationship. *AMA Arch Internal Med.* 97, 585–592, 1956.

76. Crocker, J., and Lutsky, N. Stigma and the dynamics of social cognition. In *The Dilemma of Difference: A Multidisciplinary View of Stigma* (Edited by Ainlay, S. C.), pp. 95–121. Plenum, New York, 1986.

77. Hahn, H. Disability policy and the problem of discrimination. *Am. Behav. Scient.* 28, 293–318, 1985.

78. Harris, L. *et al. Disabled Americans' Self Perceptions: Bringing Disabled Americans into the Mainstream*. Study No. 854009. International Center for the Disabled, New York, 1986.

79. Scotch, R. K. *From Goodwill to Civil Rights: Transforming Federal Disability Policy*. Temple University Press, Philadelphia, 1984.

80. Crawford, R. You are dangerous to your health: the ideology of politics of victim blaming. *Int. J. Hlth Services* 7, 663–680, 1977.

81. Crawford, R. Individual responsibility and health politics. In *Health Care in America: Essays in Social History* (Edited by Reverby, S., and Rosner, D.), pp. 247–268. Temple University Press, Philadelphia, 1979.

82. Gleidman, J. and Roth, W. *The Unexpected Minority: Handicapped Children in America*. Harcourt, Brace, Jovanovich, New York, 1980.

83. Saxton, M. A peer counseling training program for disabled women. *J. Sociol. Soc. Welfare* 8, 334–346, 1981.

84. Hughes, E., and Hughes, H. M. "What's in a name." In *Where People Meet—Racial and Ethnic Frontiers*, p. 130–144. The Free Press, Glencoe, IL, 1952.

85. Bogdan, R., and Biklen, D. "Handicappism." *Soc. Policy*, pp. 14–19, March/April, 1977.

86. Crawford, R. Healthism and the medicalization of everyday life. *Int. J. Hlth Services*, 10, 365–388, 1980.

87. Zola, I. K. Healthism and disabling medicalization. In *Disabling Professions* (Edited by Illich, I., Zola, I. K., McKnight, J., Caplan, J., and Shaiken H.), pp. 41–69. Marion Boyars, London, 1977.

88. Dunne, P. Faith, hope, and clarity. *Harvard Mag.* 88, (4), 10–14, 1986.

Finch the Spastic

Speaks

Gordon Weaver

■

The doctor's achievements with problems like mine are famous; his connection with the university—research and occasional lectures—accounts for my choice of this state, city, school. I had, of course, my pick of institutions. He is, I think, basically kind, but too great a scientist to obscure his ministrations with mercy or pity, and for this I am grateful. Though we have met each month for the past five years, we have no . . . what you would call *rapport.*

Answer a leading question: what is Finch? Is he the body, the badly made bundle of nerve ends and motor responses? Or is he the mind, the intelligence, the scholarships and fellowships, the heap of plaques, medallions, scrolls, given in testimony to his brilliance? Or is he something even more than these, a total greater than the sum of his parts? I ask you, does not Finch . . . feel?

Ah, you mock! Finch, you say, Finch of all people! Finch? Poor, pathetic Finch, with his tested and recorded intelligence quotient of two hundred and thirty-three, locked forever in his prison of chaotic muscles. Poor Finch, who falls as easily over a curbstone as an infant toddler over a toy. Unfortunate Finch, whose large, staring eyes often roll wildly behind his thick glasses. Tragic Finch, who must choke and strain like some strangling madman if he is to ask for so much as a drink of water.

You underestimate me.

Stripped to shorts and undershirt, I sit on the edge of the doctor's examination table, legs dangling. With an ordinary tape measure, he checks my calves, thighs, forearms, biceps, to see if any disparity has developed. Kneeling, he exerts pressure on each foot as I pull up against him, testing for any distinction in muscular strength. "Okey doke," he says, pausing to jot conclusions in the thick folder bearing my name that will doubtless one day yield monographs, to his ever-spreading renown. "Ready?" he says, handing pen and folder to the attentive nurse. I do not speak needlessly.

He stands near me, raises his hands, spreads his fingers like a wrestler coming to close with an opponent in the center of the ring. And I see it just that way, a contest, for my amusement. I am very strong.

Relaxation is the secret. I half-close my eyes to concentrate, bombarding my shoulders, arms, hands, fingers, with commands: relax! Gradually, the fingers twitch, release the edge of the table, and slowly my arms rise, fingers open to meet his. He meets me halfway, interlocks his fingers with mine, and we push, face to face. I watch his skin flush, eyes protrude ever so slightly, teeth clench. We push, as earnest as two fraternity boys arm wrestling for a pitcher of beer. I am very strong.

He grunts without meaning to, catches himself, pushes again, then gives up, exhales loudly. "Okay," he says. I smell the aroma of some candied lozenge on his breath. Is there a trace of sweat on his tanned brow? "Okay," he says, "okay now." To save time, the nurse helps him unlace our fingers.

There was an impressive formal reception when I came to the university, five years ago. Not for me alone, of course. Invited were perhaps a hundred new students with some claim to distinction: merit scholars, recipients of industrial science fellowships, national prize-winning essayists, valedictorians in great number. But, except for a small covey of timid and meticulous Negro boys and girls, to whom all the dignitaries paid solemn if perfunctory court, I was easily the center of attention.

Imagine Finch, the spastic, dressed for the occasion. (The habitual fraternity jacket was not to come until my sophomore year, when Delta Sigma Kappa, campus jocks, coming to know me from my work at the gymnasium, adopted me as something of a mascot, perhaps their social service project for the year—the jacket was free, as are the passes to football and basketball games. I could, if I cared to, sit on the players' bench.) I wear a dark suit with vest, and the dormitory housemother has tied a neat, hard little knot in my tie for me. I stand near the refreshment table, as erect as my balance will permit. My left arm is locked into place, palm up, whereon I place a napkin, a saucer, and a clear glass cup of red punch which I have no interest in tasting. With utmost care, I have tenderly grasped the cup's handle between thumb and forefinger, and there I stand, listening, questioning, answering, discussing (I speak extraordinarily well this day!) with a crowd of deans, departmental chairmen, senior professors, polite faculty wives, the president of the student body, and a handful of upperclass and graduate honor students. From time to time a few wander away to make a ritual obeisance to the Negroes, but they return.

Finch, Finch is the main attraction! Finch, with his certified intelligence quotient of two hundred and thirty-three, Finch who probes and reveals yawning gaps in the reading of graduate students ten years his senior, Finch who speaks with authority of science, literature, and contemporary politics, Finch who dares to contradict the holder of the endowed chair in history! Oh, there is glory in this! Finch, who cannot tie a shoelace, cannot safely strike a match, has trouble inserting dimes in vending machine slots—Finch is master here!

The other new students stand on the fringe of my audience, bewildered, or stroll off to stare dumbly at the obligatory portraits of past university presidents and trustees that dot the walls. I grow weary, but the tremor of my head can pass for judicious nodding, the tick in my cheek for chewing gum. The punch in my cup rocks a little. Who is the free man here?

Is it the scholar-professor who must think hard to recall specific points in his dissertation if he is to answer me? Is it the hatchet-faced, balding Dean of Letters and Science who carefully defends the university against its out-of-state rival, which also sought Finch? Is it the beautiful girl who won a regional science fair, but stands here, open-mouthed and silent as Finch explicates the relationship between set theory and symbolic logic? Is it the faculty wife with bleached hair, calculating her sitter's wages, who dares not depart for fear of offending Finch? Or is it Finch, whose brain roars with commands of discipline to his muscles, achieved only with the excruciating tenuous force of his will?

What you might think a disaster was actually the climax of my triumph. I had almost no warning. I felt the spasm that plunged my chin down against my chest, felt a stiffening come over my arms and hands, but no more. As nicely as if I wished it, I tossed my cup of punch up and back over my shoulder, while the saucer snapped in two in my left hand, giving me a rather nasty cut across the palm. There was a fine spray of punch in the air, the cup shattering harmlessly against the wainscotted wall behind me. Only the beautiful winner of the regional science fair forgot herself so far as to shriek as if she had been goosed.

I allowed no time for tension or embarrassment. I spoke quickly, clear as a bell, "Please excuse me," and reached up with the napkin to wipe punch from my forehead and hair. I asked for a chair, was seated, and the conversation continued as before while my hand was bandaged.

Which of you, I ask, would dare such a thing outside your dreams? When I smiled they laughed. And the winner of the science fair blushed, mortified by her outburst, as I related other such experiences in my past for their entertainment.

Above all, do not underestimate me.

The doctor breathes heavily. At my sides, my hands still hold their clawlike, grappling shape. A small victory, I am stronger than he; something to savor for a short time each month. He writes again, says, "I trust you're keeping up with the schedule." I nod, or what passes for a nod. The nurse helps me into my shirt and trousers.

"I can't emphasize that enough, James," the doctor said. He has called me by my first name since I met him; I was, after all, only seventeen when my parents arranged the first consultation.

"I don't want to alarm you," he said, "but there is evidence of unilateral deterioration—" I know the jargon as well as he—"your right side's progressing fairly rapidly. I want you to stay with the schedule, and don't miss the medication. I'm going to write your folks . . ."

I have always kept the schedule. Ever since I can remember, there has been a schedule, exercises, work with weights, isometrics, special breathing and relaxation drills. At home, in my dormitory room, in classes, on regular visits to the gymnasium, I have faithfully kept the schedule. And medication. Pills, occasional injections as new serums and theories prevail. My wristwatch is equipped with a small but persistent buzzer to keep me precisely on the schedule.

"You know the literature on progression yourself . . ." he is saying. The nurse is fastening the buckles on my shoes; I once counted it a great breakthrough to go from snaps to buckles. I looked forward to laces, but no longer care about such matters. The nurse brings my fraternity jacket.

"You do understand the import of what I'm saying, James?" the doctor said. I realized he

wanted more than a nod or flutter of eyelids. I must speak.

I did not forget the beautiful winner of the regional science fair. I saw her now and again during my first quarter at the university. We passed in corridors, joined the same lines in the cafeteria and bookstore, and once, sat in the same aisle in the auditorium to watch a foreign film. Whether she seemed to notice me or not (how, I ask, does one *not notice* Finch?), I never forgot her face as I saw it when my hand was being bandaged at the reception, flushed with distress for her unmannerly and callous shriek at my misfortune with the punch cup. I understood she was emotionally in my debt until I should release her.

As these weeks passed, I began to pay attention, to sometimes go out of my way to meet her as she left a class or walked one of the narrow paths crossing the wide, green campus on her way to or from her dormitory. I found stations, fixed and concealed points, from which to observe her at length. It was not until the first long vacation, however, that I recognized how affected I was by her beauty. Her name was Ellen.

Picture Finch: his father or mother drives him to the public library for a day's work, and he burrows into his books and three-by-five notecards with a determination the envy of any serious scholar. A librarian helps him carry books to a far, quiet corner near a window, where the sun's warm rays belie the frozen, cold stillness of the snow-covered streets and buildings outside. He begins, reads, writes, outlines, and time passes without his knowing it, or caring. But a dingy cloud throws him into shade, or the day has already faded to that dark, chill cast that is a deep winter afternoon. He lifts his trembling head, closes his eyes, sore with strain, and suddenly sees nothing, thinks of nothing, but the beautiful Ellen. History or political science or biology evaporate, and his reality consists only of her pale blond hair, the hazel tint of her bright, large eyes, the unbelievably fresh smoothness of her skin, the light downy hair on her arm, the sparkle of her white, even teeth; to the exclusion of even his lifelong awareness of his insane, spastic body, Finch knows only this beautiful Ellen!

I see, I *feel* the beauty of her movement: her hand glides to gesture, her fingers curl around a pencil, artless as the flow of water, no more self-conscious than the law of gravity; her head tilts, or she throws it to cast her hair back out of her eyes; she sits, crosses one long, sleek leg over the other, and it bobs in time to the animation of her conversation; she arches her back, thrusts out her breasts, and lets her coat slide down her stiffened arms as if they were greased rails; she climbs the steps to her dormitory, her knees churning like pistons, and pauses before the door to stomp snow from her high, black boots; alone on a path (but Finch, hidden, watches!) she holds her books against her stomach, runs, slides like a tightwire walker on a streak of silvery ice.

Ah, thinks Finch, oblivious to his books and the dry, clean smell of the library, *beauty!* She walks and runs, this beautiful Ellen, sits, jumps, with the floating, liquid perfection of some gaudy reptile.

It was Christmas, and I was home with my family, and I had reading and research papers to do, but I—why should I not say it—was in love. Finch was eighteen, and in love for the first time in his life. Yes, *Finch loves!* Or, thought he did. Loved, once.

"Jim?" says a voice outside this absorbing, warming reality—it is his father, or his mother, come at the agreed hour. "Jim, it's time to go, we'll be late for supper." Finch opens his eyes, and it is winter again, cars make slushy noises outside the window, and he must reorder his mind, recall where he left off his research, stack his cards and papers, answer questions, think of real things, when and where and what he is.

It is Christmas Eve night, and my family gathers at the huge tree that dominates our living room. There are special things to eat, and I am allowed a little whiskey for the occasion. My mother is happy in her Christmas way, tears in her eyes as she hands me many expensive gifts, elaborately wrapped—a new fountain pen, made in Germany, with a thick barrel, so much easier for the fingers to circle; a cowhide briefcase with a manacle fitted to the handle so I can lock it to my wrist (this will require new feats of balance, but, to please her, I say nothing of it); an astrakhan hat, in vogue among students this year—she will not have me lack what others have!

I appear to enjoy this annual ceremony as much as they. I give, and get, an enthusiastic hug and kiss as I open each gift, being careful not to too badly smash or tear the fluffy bows and ribbons and bright paper as I unwrap each package, labeled, as always, *To Jim from Santa.* I faithfully follow my father's direction as he films all this, stooped behind his camera and tripod, his words just a bit thick with too much whiskey. I pose, seated on the floor between my younger brother and sister (they are both perfectly ordinary), put my arms around their necks, do my best to smile so that I will not look drunk or half-witted in the movie.

But I go to bed early, pleading fatigue, the ritual splash of whiskey, the research to be done even on Christmas day. I leave them, to seek Ellen, to be alone in my bed and nourish this thrilling, weakening sensation of love that for the first time in my life lets me, makes me, forget myself. My taut body relaxes in stages, by degrees, while my brain whirls gently with real and imaginary visions of this exquisite Ellen. I still hear music, the rattle of happy, sentimental talk as my parents sit up late, drinking and watching old Christmas films—and for the first time in my life, I am not ashamed of the erection that keeps me from sleep.

The good doctor has just informed me that my future is limited. The paralysis, unknown to me as I labor faithfully at my schedules, as I dose myself to the point of nausea, has been progressing. Subtle as a tiny worm, my malady has eaten away at this comic body, devouring days of my life. The figures noted in my folder already record the shrinkage from atrophy. The ultimate and sure end, if progression is not arrested, will be a spasm of sufficient duration, somewhere vital, the throat, the diaphragm, and I will suffocate in a final paroxysm, no different than if I had swallowed a fishbone. Yet he asks me to speak now, reassure him that I understand and face his diagnosis calmly.

He waits, brows lifted, expectant, needing; the nurse returns my file to the cabinet drawer. I speak, for us both, a lie.

"I'm . . . not . . . alarmed," I say, almost effortlessly. True, my mouth twists in shapes wholly unrelated to the words. My tongue emerges as I finish, and I am in danger of drooling idiotically, but the words, slow-paced, are only a little distorted, like the stridency in the voices of the deaf when they sing.

True, no one could take me for normal, but that I speak at all is a minor wonder.

"Good," the doctor said, "good," washing his hands. The nurse has left the room.

I have said, does not Finch feel? But feeling brings on paralysis, interrupts the constant stream of impulses from brain to muscle—feeling means stasis, immobility. I must be alone if I am to allow myself grief or wonder. Solitude waits only on my tortured passage through the waiting room, a perilous descent of the stairs, a short ride on my bicycle to the dormitory.

Back at the university, I determined to call her. Though I might have known she would not refuse me, I shook as if I suffered Saint Vitus' dance, telephone receiver in hand, until she said yes, she would accompany me to a movie. "Will we be walking, Jimmy?" she asked. I faltered, choked, not having thought to the point of specific arrangements. Finch, pride of the history department, flustered like any juvenile! *No,* I managed to stammer: even the closest theater

was a trek across the campus, far enough to be humiliating. I cringed, imagining us, arm in arm perhaps, floundering and swaying on the icy paths. "Oh," Ellen said, and waited for me to speak. I rocked fitfully on the small seat in the booth in the empty dormitory corridor. It might have sounded, in her ear, like the wild and frantic banging of someone prematurely buried.

I nearly mentioned my bicycle, but this was unsafe in winter for me alone—with her, perched on the handlebars, it would have been macabre. "I have a car, Jimmy," she said sweetly. And so we went in her car.

I do not remember what film we saw, for through most of the feature I sat rigid, inching my hand closer and closer to hers. Something happened in the film, something loud, action with bombastic musical accompaniment, and damning myself eternally a coward if I failed to act, at last, with a short, convulsive, clutching thrust, I slipped my hand over hers. She was kind enough to turn her head to me, and smile. We sat that way until the house lights came up, my sweaty palm covering the back of her smooth, cool hand. Surreptitiously, I breathed her delicious perfume, and from the corner of my eye, exulted in the delicate turn of her ear, her nostril, the way her blond hair swept upward on the back of her neck, the soft line of her throat, the faint heaving of her bosom.

We parked at the dormitory complex. It was very cold, and the other cars raised thick, steady clouds of exhaust. Their occupants, clasped in long, intense embraces, moved as shadows behind the frosted windows, all about us. Every few minutes, an engine died, a door opened, and a couple emerged to walk to one or another of the buildings. In the doorway lights we saw clearly their final kissing and fondling.

Ellen left the motor running, and we sat, silent. She wore a heavy coat, open, with a hood, a ring of snowy rabbit fur framing her face. We sat, quiet, while my brain raced, wondering what I should, or would, or could do. I did not want, at first, to touch her, but felt I must. I could feel the tick in my cheek grow worse, knew my limbs were frozen, hands balled in fists in my lap.

"Do you want me to walk with you to your dorm, Jimmy?" she said, and quickly, she leaned toward me, perhaps to open the door for me, I do not know. Somehow it terrified me, and I lurched, as if I had been given an electrical shock, and I spoke.

"No!" I said. I did not mean to touch her, not at first.

My left arm came up, swiftly enough to have given her a jarring slap, but stopped short, and I caressed her cheek and chin. She seemed to lean further toward me. I willed my right hand to take her shoulder and turn her fully toward me. I think she wanted me to kiss her, or thought I wanted to—I looked into her face, and she was, again, smiling, as she had in the theater. Her mouth was open slightly, her eyelids fluttering.

It was then I decided to kiss her, and let myself feel fully the love I had not permitted myself before, ever. I think I may have begun to cry.

I was not in love, I understand now, not in love with this beautiful Ellen, this precocious student of science, with her skin like milk, her grace of movement so inherent and unconscious as to put a dancer or an animal to shame. I did not love her, I say. I felt, then, as I moved my head closer to hers, the welling up of my response to all the love showered on me before, by my family, doctors, nurses, therapists, teachers.

Should not Finch, like you, feel?

I was, surely, crying, making a grotesque sound like the growling of a beast. I was moved by the collective force of all that love—my weepy mother, standing at the end of the parallel handrails, holding back her tears, whispering, *step Jimmy, step, one more step to mother, Jimmy;* my father, carrying me high on his shoulders in the teeth of a biting wind at a football game, cheering, *look at him go, Jimmy!,* suddenly letting me

drop into his arms, hugging me to his chest, saying, *it's okay, Jim, it's okay,* because he thought I felt hurt, unable ever to run like that anonymous halfback; my teachers, *see, James knows, you're all so smart aleck, but James always has the right answer;* my sister, *Jimmy, are you the smartest person in the world?;* an auditorium filled with parents, the state superintendent of education saying, *I cannot say enough in praise of James Finch,* rolls of applause as I move, like some crippled insect, to the podium, everyone's eyes wet . . . I draw Ellen's face close to mine, my hand tightening on her shoulder. Stupidly, I try to speak.

Kiss me, I want to say, with all the force muted by all the tenderness of my need. And I am betrayed once more by my odious body. Ellen's mouth is closed to meet mine, and I gargle some ugly distortion of my intention: *Kwaryoup,* I say, and her eyes pop open in horror. I hold her tightly, feel her resistance, try again—*Keeeebryumbeel* erupts from my throat. She tries to release herself. *Sochavadeebow,* I am saying, trying to reassure her.

"Jimmy!" she says, and pulls at my wrists. "Let go, Jimmy!" I want to comply, but my left hand, nerves along my arm seeming to explode like a string of firecrackers, raises, comes down on her breast. "Jimmy!" she shrieks, and is crying now. "Get away from me, Jimmy, let go of me! Get your hands off me, you're hurting me, Jimmy!"

And it is over, mercifully. The door is open, I crawl or fall out, scramble through the snow on my hands and knees, slobbering, falling, thrashing. Behind me, I hear Ellen's nearly hysterical sobbing.

Ah, Finch, to think you might love! I no longer need to remember this, but when I do, am amused, recalling fairy tales of frogs and princesses, recited, sometimes hour after hour, in an effort to relax me for sleep, by my patient mother. A student of history, I remind myself, should have known better.

No matter. Before the following year was out, I had ceased avoiding her. When we meet now, we can even smile, though we do not speak.

As I leave, other patients in the waiting room pretend not to see me. An old woman with a cane and a platform shoe covers her eyes with a magazine. A palsied man, no more than forty, looks down at his shuddering hands. Another woman, younger, with a perfectly healthy looking child on her lap, suddenly becomes interested in her son's hair, like a grooming, lice- and salt-seeking primate. Yet another woman, her face set in a lopsided grimace, one shoulder permanently higher than the other, merely yawns, closes her eyes, pinches the bridge of her nose between two fingers until I am beyond her, as if she cannot bear her affliction so long as I am before her to remind her of it.

I walk to the door. I stagger like an old wino, head whipping from side to side with the thrust of each leg, as if I keep time to some raucous, private music. My arms are cocked, ready to catch me if I slip. My feet point inward, and my torso tips forward to provide the continuity of momentum, my broad shoulders thrown back to maintain a risky balance.

It is a gait to embarrass, to make children laugh, a clumsy cantering locomotion that results from only the most exacting and determined attention to control. Inside my rolling head, behind my shocked, magnified eyeballs, my brain orders, with utmost precision, each awkward jerk of thigh, leg, foot. Just as I reach the door to the stairs, a voice greets me cheerfully.

"Hello, Jimmy," sings out in a lilting feminine rush of genuine delight. I bang loudly against the door as I stop, gripping the knob with both hands for support. My head nearly hits the panel of thick, opaque glass. I turn with difficulty. "Hello, Jimmy," she says again.

I know her, but not well. She is a disgusting thing to see, a fellow-student. Fat of face and body, her legs are little more than pale pink, waxy skin stretched over bone, her feet strapped to the steel platform of her wheelchair. One arm is horribly withered, the thin, useless fingers held curled in her broad lap. The other is braced for strength to allow her to work the levers that steer her chair. Beneath her seat squats a large, black battery, her source of power. Her neck angles slightly to one side. Someone has recently given her jet black hair a hideous pixie cut.

I know her. She is one of the small, cohesive platoon of handicapped, crippled, maimed university students. They have an association of sorts, advised by a conscientious faculty member who lost an eye in Korea. The university provides a specially equipped Volkswagen van to take them about campus. They have keys to operate freight elevators, and the buildings have ramps to accommodate them. When I came to the university I was invited, by the one-eyed professor, to join their ranks. I even attended one meeting— mostly polio victims and amputees. The agenda was devoted to a discussion of whether or not to extend membership to an albino girl whose eyesight was so bad she could not read mimeographed class handouts. I declined to join, of course, but still receive their randomly published newsletter. We have nothing in common.

She smiles now, lipstick and powder, rouge and eyebrow pencil making a theater mask of her face. "I've never seen you up here before, Jimmy, have you just started coming?" I am struck, suddenly with the awareness that she has an . . . an *interest* in me! I grope frantically to open the door.

I must, and do, speak, but badly, without thinking, so shaken am I with my understanding. *Haroyoup* comes groaning from my lips, like the creaking of a heavy casket lid. Startled and embarrassed, she smiles all the harder, and I push open the door to begin the slow descent of the steep stairs leading to the street where my bicycle waits. Mad Finch, who dared to think he might feel!

At the top of the stairs I turn around, for I must descend backwards. I take the rail with both hands, regulate my breathing, concentrate, then step back, into the air, with one foot . . . I have a special sense of freedom, for I can never know if the foot will find the stair just below, or if I will step backward into space, find nothing, and fall. I am, for an instant, like a blindfolded highdiver who steps off the springboard, uncertain if there is water below.

I am able, momentarily at least, to forget my self-pity in this kind of freedom only I know.

I must not despair! Though Finch wields the chalk no better than a child does a crayon, he cuts surely as a surgeon to the heart of the problem on the blackboard. Though his pronunciation is atrocious, his syntax is exact, his structure flawless, vocabulary well beyond his years. Though his eyes, enlarged behind thick lenses, stare, sometimes roll up in his head, no one reads more or faster, and for amusement he will commit a paragraph or a page to memory in record time.

It is Finch who is free to traverse the lines of caste and class in our community. Finch is the locker room pet of brainless athletes. They challenge him to feats of strength, and lose good-naturedly. From the heights of their chickenwire and toilet paper float thrones, Junoesque sorority queens wave to Finch in the crowd, call him by name. Filthy and morose, the bearded politicals and bohemians, who lurk in the basement of the student union, will take time to read Finch their latest throwaway or poem. Serious students, praying for futures in government or academia, consult Finch before submitting seminar reports.

Oh, I am not lonely!

So, with an effort of will, informed by the discipline of my regimen in physical therapy, weight-lifting, my schedules, I heave, lifting my center of balance upward with an exaggerated shrug of my broad, strong shoulders; then, at the exact moment, a second divided into several parts for pre-cision, I lean to the right, forcing all my weight onto my right leg, onto the raised pedal of my bicycle. There is no continuity, no fluid evolving process of motion, but my timing is correct—my mind has once more concentrated this fool's body into a preconceived pattern—the pedal depresses, the bike rolls forward.

There is an instant when disaster is possible—I am thrown forward with the bike, but my locked left hand grips the handlebar, stops me short of an ignominious and bruising tumble to the pavement. I remember to pull with my right arm, to isolate the individual muscles that will steer out, away from the curb, past the hulk of a parked florist's truck.

I move. Out now, near the center line, I assert the series of stiff, dramatic thrusts of hip and leg that pump me along, past the campus shops, the bus stop.

Students throng the sidewalk, and they call to me. The frat boys, the unmercifully attractive girls, golden and creamy in their expensive clothes, jocks in their letter sweaters and wind-breakers, malcontents in old military jackets. They call: "Ho Finch!" "Jimbo!" "Hi Jimmy!" They grin, wave. "Baby Jim boy!" "Hi Jim," they call.

With careful, paced breathing, I multiply the complexity of my ordeal. Almost one by one, I unlock my fingers from the handlebar. With the strained deliberation of a weight-lifter, I raise it above my head, steering and balance both entrusted to my left arm. Aloft, the tingling spasms are sufficient to produce a casual wave. Like a swimmer shaking water from his inner ear, I rock my head, once, twice, three times, until I face them. Opening my jaw is enough to pull my lips back over my teeth: a smile.

In this instant I am helpless. Were a car to swerve into my path, a pedestrian dart in front of me, all would end in an absurd, theatrical collision—perhaps serious injury. But I prevail.

Now, the breeze in my ears, my glasses vibrating on the bridge of my nose, threatening to fall across my mouth, I speak. My tongue bucks and floats, the stiff planes of my throat shiver, and I respond.

"Jimmy!" they cry. "How you doing, Jimbo!"

Hyaroul explodes my voice, and I can almost see their delight, the fullness of quick and easy tears of sentimental pity form in their eyes. *Hyarouffa!* I say, already plotting how I will lower my right hand, face the road again. *Haluff!* I make an unexpelled breath, not knowing if it is my cry of joy at being alive, known, loved, or a curse far more terrible than any profane cliché they will ever know—because . . . I suspect . . . simply because I cannot answer my own questions, cannot know what is, or is not, Finch.

Tell Me, Tell Me

Irving Kenneth Zola

■

Now I was the one who was nervous. Here we were alone in her room thousands of miles from my home.

"Well, my personal care attendant is gone, so it will all be up to you," she said sort of puckishly, "Don't look so worried! I'll tell you what to do."

This was a real turn-about. It was usually me who reassured my partner. Me who, after putting aside my cane, and removing all the clothes that masked my brace, my corset, my scars, my thinness, my body. Me who'd say, "Well, now you see 'the real me.'" How often I'd said that, I thought to myself. Saying it in a way that hid my basic fear—that this real me might not be so nice to look at . . . might not be up to 'the task' before me.

She must have seen something on my face, for she continued to reassure me, "Don't be afraid." And as she turned her wheelchair toward me she smiled at me that smile that first hooked me a few hours before. "Well," she continued, "first we have to empty my bag." And with that brief introduction we approached the bathroom.

Anger quickly replaced fear as I realized she could get her wheelchair into the doorway but not through it.

"Okay, take one of those cans," she said pointing to an empty Sprite, "and empty my bag into it."

Though I'd done that many times before it

wasn't so easy this time. I quite simply couldn't reach her leg from a sitting position on the toilet and she couldn't raise her foot toward me. So down to the floor I lowered myself and sat at her feet. Rolling up her trouser leg I fumbled awkwardly with the clip sealing the tube. I looked up at her and she laughed, "It won't break and neither will I."

I got it open and her urine poured into the can. Suddenly I felt a quiver in my stomach. The smell was more overpowering than I'd expected. But I was too embarrassed to say anything. Emptying the contents into the toilet I turned to her again as she backed out. "What should I do with the can?" I asked.

"Wash it out," she answered as if it were a silly question. "We try to recycle everything around here."

Proud of our first accomplishment we headed back into the room. "Now comes the fun part . . . getting me into the bed." For a few minutes we looked for the essential piece of equipment—the transfer board. I laughed silently to myself. I seemed to always be misplacing my cane—that constant reminder of my own physical dependency. Maybe for her it was the transfer board.

When we found it leaning against the radiator I reached down to pick it up and almost toppled over from its weight. Hell of a way to start, I thought to myself. If I can't lift this, how am I going to deal with her? More carefully this time, I reached down and swung it onto the bed.

She parallel parked her wheelchair next to the bed, grinned, and pointed to the side arm. I'd been this route before, so I leaned over and dismantled it. Then with her patient instructions I began to shift her. The board had to be placed with the wider part on the bed and the narrower section slipped under her. This would eventually allow me to slip her across. But I could do little without losing my own balance. So I laid down on the mattress and shoved the transfer board under her. First one foot and then the other

I lifted toward me till she was at about a 45 degree angle in her wheelchair. I was huffing but she sat in a sort of bemused silence. Then came the scary part. Planting myself as firmly as I could behind her, I leaned forward, slipped my arms under hers and around her chest and then with one heave hefted her onto the bed. She landed safely with her head on the pillow, and I joined her wearily for a moment's rest. For this I should have gone into training, I smiled silently. And again, she must have understood as she opened her eyes even wider to look at me. What beautiful eyes she has, I thought, a brightness heightened by her very dark thick eyebrows.

"You're blushing again," she said.

"How can you tell that it's not from exhaustion?" I countered.

"By your eyes . . . because they're twinkling."

I leaned over and kissed her again. But more mutual appreciation would have to wait, there was still work to be done.

The immediate task was to plug her wheelchair into the portable recharger. This would have been an easy task for anyone except the technical idiot that I am.

"Be careful," she said. "If you attach the wrong cables you might shock yourself."

I laughed. A shock from this battery would be small compared to what I've already been through.

But even this attaching was not so easy. I couldn't read the instructions clearly, so down to the floor I sank once more.

After several tentative explorations, I could see the gauge registering a positive charge. I let out a little cheer.

She turned her head toward me and looked down as I lay stretched out momentarily on the floor, "Now the real fun part," she teased. "You have to undress me."

"Ah, but for this," I said in my most rakish tones, "we'll have to get closer together." My graceful quip was, however, not matched by any graceful motion. For I had to crawl on the floor until I could find a chair onto which I could hold and push myself to a standing position.

As I finally climbed onto the bed, I said, "Is this trip really necessary?" I don't know what I intended by that remark but we both laughed. And as we did and came closer, we kissed, first gently and then with increasing force until we said almost simultaneously, "We'd better get undressed."

"Where should I start?" I asked.

My own question struck me as funny. It was still another reversal. It was something I'd never asked a woman. But on those rare occasions on which I'd let someone undress me, it was often their first question.

"Wherever you like," she said in what seemed like a coquettish tone.

I thought it would be best to do the toughest first, so I began with her shoes and socks. These were easy enough but not so her slacks. Since she could not raise herself, I alternated between pulling, tugging, and occasionally lifting. Slowly over her hips, I was able to slip her slacks down from her waist. By now I was sweating as much from anxiety as exertion. I was concerned I'd be too rough and maybe hurt her but most of all I was afraid that I might inadvertently pull out her catheter. At least in this anxiety I was not alone. But with her encouragement we again persevered. Slacks, underpants, corset all came off in not so rapid succession.

At this point a different kind of awkwardness struck me. There was something about my being fully clothed and her not that bothered me. I was her lover, not her personal care attendant. And so I asked if she minded if I took off my clothes before continuing.

I explained in a half-truth that it would make it easier for me to get around now 'without all my equipment.' "Fine with me," she answered and again we touched, kissed and lay for a moment in each other's arms.

Pushing myself to a sitting position I removed my own shirt, trousers, shoes, brace, corset, bandages, undershorts until I was comfortably nude. The comfort lasted but a moment. Now I was embarrassed. I realized that she was in a position to look upon my not so beautiful body. My usual defensive sarcasm about 'the real me' began somewhere back in my brain but this time it never reached my lips. "Now what?" was the best I could come up with.

"Now my top . . . and quickly. I'm roasting in all these clothes."

I didn't know if she was serious or just kidding but quickness was not in the cards. With little room at the head of the bed, I simply could not pull them off as I had the rest of her clothes.

"Can you sit up?" I asked.

"Not without help."

"What about once you're up?"

"Not then either . . . not unless I lean on you."

This time I felt ingenious. I locked my legs around the corner of the bed and then grabbing both her arms I yanked her to a sitting position. She made it but I didn't. And I found her sort of on top of me, such a tangle of bodies we could only laugh. Finally, I managed to push her and myself upright. I placed her arms around my neck. And then, after the usual tangles of hair, earrings and protestations that I was trying to smother her, I managed to pull both her sweater and blouse over her head. By now I was no longer being neat, and with an apology threw her garments toward the nearest chair. Naturally I missed . . . but neither of us seemed to care. The bra was the final piece to go and with the last unhooking we both plopped once more to the mattress.

For a moment we just lay there but as I reached across to touch her, she pulled her head back mockingly, "We're not through yet."

"You must be kidding!" I said, hoping that my tone was not as harsh as it sounded.

"I still need my booties and my night bag."

"What are they for?" I asked out of genuine curiosity.

"Well my booties—those big rubber things on the table—keep my heels from rubbing and getting irritated and the night bag . . . well that's so we won't have to worry about my urinating during the night."

The booties I easily affixed, the night bag was another matter. Again it was more my awkwardness than the complexity of the task. First, I removed the day bag, now emptied, but still strapped around her leg and replaced it with the bigger night one. Careful not to dislodge the catheter I had to find a place lower than the bed to attach it so gravity would do the rest. Finally, the formal work was done. The words of my own thoughts bothered me for I realized that there was part of me that feared what "work" might still be ahead.

She was not the first disabled woman I'd ever slept with but she was, as she had said earlier, "more physically dependent than I look." And she was. As I prepared to settle down beside her, I recalled watching her earlier in the evening over dinner. Except for the fact that she needed her steak cut and her cigarette lit, I wasn't particularly conscious of any dependence. In fact quite the contrary, for I'd been attracted in the first place to her liveliness, her movements, her way of tilting her head and raising her eyebrows. But now it was different. This long process of undressing reinforced her physical dependency.

But before I lay down again, she interrupted my associations. "You'll have to move me. I don't feel centered." And as I reached over to move her legs, I let myself fully absorb her nakedness. Lying there she somehow seemed bigger. Maybe it was the lack of muscle-tone if that's the word— but her body seemed somehow flattened out. Her thighs and legs and her breasts, the latter no longer firmly held by her bra, flapped to her side. I felt guilty a moment for even letting myself feel

anything. I was as anxious as hell but with no wish to flee. I'm sure my face told it all. For with her eyes she reached out to me and with her words gently reassured me once again, "Don't be afraid."

And so as I lay beside her we began our loving. I was awkward at first, I didn't know what to do with my hands. And so I asked. In a way it was no different than with any other woman. In recent years, I often find myself asking where and how they like to be touched. To my questions she replied, "My neck . . . my face . . . especially my ears. . . ." And as I drew close she swung her arms around my neck and clasped me in a surprisingly strong grip.

"Tighter, tighter, hold me tighter," she laughed again. "I'm not fragile. . . . I won't break."

And so I did. And as we moved I found myself naturally touching other parts of her body. When I realized this I pulled back quickly, "I don't know what you can feel."

"Nothing really in the rest of my body."

"What about your breasts," I asked rather uncomfortably.

"Not much . . . though I can feel your hands there when you press."

And so I did. And all went well until she told me to bite and squeeze harder, then I began to shake. Feeling the quiver in my arm, she again reassured me. So slowly and haltingly where she led, I followed.

I don't know how long we continued kissing and fondling, but as I lay buried in her neck, I felt the heels of her hands digging into my back and her voice whispering, "tell me . . . tell me."

Suddenly I got scared again. Tell her what? Do I have to say that I love her . . . ? Oh my God. And I pretended for a moment not to hear.

"Tell me . . . tell me," she said again as she pulled me tighter. With a deep breath, I meekly answered, "Tell you what?"

"Tell me what you're doing," she said softly, "so I can visualize it." With her reply I breathed a sign of relief. And a narrative voyage over her body began; I kissed, fondled, caressed every part I could reach. Once I looked up and I saw her with her head relaxed, eyes closed, smiling.

It was only when we stopped that I realized I was unerect. In a way my penis was echoing my own thoughts. I had no need to thrust, to fuck, to quite simply go where I couldn't be felt.

She again intercepted my own thoughts— "Move up, please put my hands on you," and as I did I felt a rush through my body. She drew me toward her again until her lips were on my chest and gently she began to suckle me as I had her a few minutes before. And so the hours passed, ears, mouths, eyes, tongues inside one another.

And every once in a while she would quiver in a way which seemed orgasmic. As I thrust my tongue as deep as I could in her ear, her head would begin to shake, her neck would stretch out and then her whole upper body would release with a sigh.

Finally, at some time well past one we looked exhaustedly at one another. "Time for sleep," she yawned, "but there is one more task—an easy one. I'm cold and dry so I need some hot water."

"Hot water!" I said rather incredulously.

"Yup, I drink it straight. It's my one vice."

And as she sipped the drink through a long straw, I closed my eyes and curled myself around the pillow. My drifting off was quickly stopped as she asked rather archly, "You mean you're going to wrap yourself around that rather than me?"

I was about to explain that I rarely slept curled around anyone and certainly not vice-versa but I thought better of it, saying only, "Well, I might not be able to last this way all night."

"Neither might I," she countered. "My arm might also get tired."

We pretended to look at each other angrily but it didn't work. So we came closer again, hugged and curled up as closely as we could, with my head cradled in her arm and my leg draped across her.

And much to my surprise I fell quickly asleep— unafraid, unsmothered, and more importantly rested, cared for, and loved.

PART II

The Influence of Social Factors

on Health and Illness

The cultural perspectives that underlie the discussion and readings in part I focused attention on the individual and the individual's experience of illness. This was the right place to begin the inquiry. It is individuals, after all, who experience illness, and it is individuals who enter into relationships with physicians and other health care providers. In part II, we turn from the individual to the group, in a discussion of the relationship between the major categories of social group membership—social class, race/ethnicity, gender, and age—and differential risk of illness and mortality. In contrast to part I, the focus in this part is on the risk of disease, as it relates to group membership. While social group membership does affect how we as individuals experience and understand disease, the factors that define our social group can affect us also by directly increasing our chances of suffering illness or early death.

There are different ways to explore the causes and consequences of different rates of illness. Many research studies in epidemiology, medical sociology, and other health-related social sciences have been conducted to define the nature of these differences, and to elucidate their causes. Some of the readings that follow make reference to such studies, but they also include essays and stories that take us beyond the facts and figures, to explore the impact of social roles and social position upon disease and health. They illustrate how people, as individuals who also are members of particular groups, recognize and interpret risk of illness and death. Finally, they challenge us to examine the meanings of risk categories such as race/ethnicity and social class. As in part I, readings are drawn from a variety of sources, from literature, journalism, health policy, and anthropology. For those who wish to complement these perspectives with the more standard approach of social epidemiology, the reference list at the end of the volume includes some of the most cogent and comprehensive review articles.

Over the past century in Western societies, ideas about the causes of disease have changed a great deal. Religion, culture, politics, and scientific discoveries have all contributed to changing definitions of what disease is and why some people suffer from it while others do not (Rosenberg 1962, Brandt 1985). Furthermore, over time, different disciplines have taken different approaches to defining and examining these questions. Epidemiologists describe the frequency and distribution of disease in a population, and focus on immediate risk factors that predict disease. The logic of this perspective is that the more closely related a risk factor is to the biological mechanism of disease, the more likely it will account for the occurrence of that disease, and the more useful it will be in developing an effective intervention. Classic causal pairs include mosquito bites and malaria, walking barefoot in snail-infested waters and schistosomiasis, and living in close quarters with TB-infected people and tuberculosis. While the rise of chronic conditions has required a more complex "web" of explanatory factors than do acute diseases (Kreiger 1995), epidemiology nevertheless continues to emphasize the immediate determinants of disease.

In contrast, sociologists (and others) focus on the structure and social processes of societies, and find that rates of disease can be predicted by knowing the characteristics of a society's class structure (Townsend and Davidson 1982, Navarro 1990), its rate of social change (Durkheim 1951, Cassel 1976), and group characteristics within a society, such as race/ethnicity, gender, and age (Dressler 1993, Kreiger and Bassett 1986, Kreiger et al. 1993, Verbrugge 1989, Waldron 1990, Estes and Binney 1989). In this view, one's position in society determines one's exposure to biological risks, as do the overall social and economic characteristics of that society. As early as 1910, a local government board in England pronounced, "No fact is better established than that the death rate, and especially the death rate among children, is high in inverse proportion to the social status of the population" (cited in Antonovosky and Bernstein 1977, 453). There have been numerous studies since then that confirm this proposition (McKeown 1976, Marmot et al. 1987, Kitagawa and Hauser 1973, Pappas et al. 1993). Thus, in contrast to the view from epidemiology, researchers in this tradition have emphasized the underlying (or co-occurring) social structural causes of disease rather than the factors that are closest to disease when it strikes.

The combination of these two perspectives, including both biological and social factors, produces a more complete model of disease causation (Mosely and Chen 1984). The difficult part is identifying the steps along the way from general social variables, such as level of education, to discrete biological changes. In a common approach to this problem, broad social factors are hypothesized to work through intermediate or "proximate" pathways, such as specific behaviors, to ultimately affect the distribution of the biological factors. The most sophisticated studies involve multilevel models of analysis that include data about the community, family/household, and individual to predict the occurrence of disease. They are appealing because they seem to represent more accurate versions of the way the world works. However, these complex analyses present researchers and readers with many technical and conceptual challenges.

Research on the determinants of heart disease provides an excellent example of the current studies linking biological and social variables in the prediction of disease. The occurrence of coronary heart disease has been consistently shown to be strongly related to economic factors. In societies with little industrial development, heart disease is found mostly in the upper classes, who have greater access to high-fat diets and live long enough to suffer the consequences. In industrialized societies, heart disease is more common among the lower classes. It is also more common among men than women, and in the United States, more common among African Americans than whites (Lasker et al. 1994).

We know which intermediate factors are linked to this higher rate of heart disease in these individuals. They include behaviors such as smoking, eating a high-fat diet, and having a sedentary lifestyle; personality characteristics, especially the hard-driving "type A" personality; stress, involving both major life events and chronic stressors; and the lack of strong social ties. Many of these intermediate characteristics are more common among groups that exhibit greater prevalence of CHD. Smoking, chronic stress, and poor diet are more common among the poor than the rich, for example. Yet, it is also true that "differences among groups and changes within a group over time cannot be completely explained by the cumulative effect of individual behavioral differences" (Lasker et al. 1994, 55). In attempting to account for unexplained differences, Judith Lasker and her colleagues (1994) hypothesized that in addition to the force of individual risk factors, rapid social change seemed to create an increased vulnerability to disease. In their follow-up study of Roseto, an Italian working-class town in Pennsylvania that had un-

usually low heart disease rates until the mid-1960s, they demonstrated that rapid change in marriage patterns, community activities, interaction with the outside world, and social class characteristics were all correlated with a sharp rise in the number of deaths due to heart disease in the decade following 1965.

In another study of differences in death rates, Mac Otten and his colleagues (1990) attempted to explain the consistently higher mortality rate of African Americans compared to whites in the United States for all causes of death. In their study, mortality rates for adults age thirty-five to fifty-four were predicted using six "well established risk factors . . . plus family income." These included smoking, systolic blood pressure, cholesterol level, body-mass index, alcohol intake, and diabetes. The authors found that 31 percent of excess mortality (deaths that exceeded the normal rates for individuals in that age range) of black adults was explained by the six risk factors, and 38 percent by differences in family income. Thirty-one percent of the excess mortality was explained neither by these individual risk factors nor by family income. They suggested that their model might have omitted important individual risk factors (such as exercise), and they also noted that differences in access to health care and in community characteristics, such as the differing social or physical environments of African Americans and whites, might all contribute to the unexplained deaths. Certainly, other research on black-white differences in mortality and morbidity supports these hypotheses (Dressler 1993, Wenneker and Epstein 1989). Genetic explanations, once quite common, have been shown to explain little if any of the difference in death rates between blacks and whites.

Some authors have suggested that these black-white differences in the United States simply show that it is harder to stay healthy if you belong to the lower social classes. Despite recent social change, there continues to be a high correlation between race/ethnicity and the indicators that are frequently used to measure social class: income, education, and occupation—particularly for black Americans. (See section 1 for further discussion of the definition of social class.) In fact, William Dressler (1993) has argued that race—as defined by skin color—has until very recently determined or defined one's social position or class in America. Since most data on health (mortality rate, infant mortality rate, disease prevalence and incidence) continue to be collected by race/ethnicity rather than by these traditional measures of social class, many medical researchers have developed the habit of using race as a shorthand term or proxy for social class.

The attempt to explain away the black-white differences in health by pointing to social class is persuasive, but incomplete. If social class explained these differences, why was the Otten study unable to account for one-third of the excess mortality, when family income was included in their model? In fact, even if one looks within the same education and income groups, at people with similar behavior and genetic risk factors, there are still significant health differences between African Americans and whites (Kreiger et al. 1993, Wise et al. 1985, Wise 1993, James 1994). Race/ethnicity is measuring something else, in addition to the health disadvantage accounted for by social class. Some authors (Dressler 1993) conclude that it is the impact of persistent and institutionalized discrimination in American society. Blacks do not typically have as easy access to medical care as whites do, and even when they are admitted for care, what they get is often inadequate (Wenneker and Epstein 1989). Blacks also could be more subject to long-term stress, which increases a person's susceptibility to disease (James 1994).

While these debates may seem academic, there are real political consequences to them. When differences in individual behavior are used to explain higher risks for morbidity and mortality,

the tendency is to conclude that people have or get the health they deserve. But when research takes a broader approach, focusing on the structure of society and the health risks of living in poverty and of being black in America (including greater exposures to toxic work and living environments, inadequate food and education, and limited access to medical care), health is no longer solely the result of a person's individual initiative or failure. Rather, it is a product of society, and society's economic and cultural forces. This is a complex debate, with no easy resolution. Social class and race/ethnicity may account for a variety of factors that are related to poorer health; yet there are many different pathways, both individual and societal, working together to create greater risk for disease. (See Haan et al. 1989 for an excellent review of this topic.)

To introduce these issues, the readings in section 1, on social class and race/ethnicity offer a combination of stories, cases, and data-based articles. The three readings in this section present statistics on social class and racial/ethnic differences in health and combine them with writings that examine the lived experience of poverty and of being in a minority group. All three readings challenge us to critically evaluate what is being measured by these "variables." While we have chosen to focus on the black-white comparison, it is important to note that there is a substantial and growing body of literature that critically assesses health outcomes of other racial/ethnic sub-groups, particularly Asian and Hispanic Americans. For example, the literature on Hispanic Americans describes a heterogeneous population that generally resembles African Americans in terms of social class, but resembles whites in terms of health status. This "epidemiologic paradox" further challenges social class explanations of black-white differences (Zimmerman et al. 1994, Scribner 1996).

In addition to social class and race/ethnicity, part II considers two other social variables commonly associated with differential health outcomes: gender and age. Although women often fare less well than men in developing nations (Okojie 1994, World Bank 1993, Pearson 1995), studies in the United States and other industrialized countries paint a more complex picture. During the past several decades, gender differences have consistently showed up in morbidity and mortality figures: First, women use health care services more frequently, and they report higher levels of illness, even when reproduction-related conditions are excluded; in contrast, men seek health care less frequently, and often at later stages of disease (Gijsbers van Wijk et al. 1992). Second, women live longer than men; and men have higher mortality rates for all major causes of death—heart disease, cancer, infectious and parasitic diseases, and accidents, poisonings, and violence (Waldron 1990, Verbrugge and Wingard 1987, Wingard et al. 1989).

There are many explanations for these gender differences in morbidity, mortality, and use of health care. The explanations include individual and societal factors, and thus mirror the models that associate class and race/ethnicity with health outcomes. Some locate the causes in biology. The earlier onset of heart disease for men, for example, is often simply attributed to the protective effect of estrogen in premenopausal women. Some research concludes that men are physiologically more inclined toward aggression than women, thus putting them at greater risk for a variety of conditions (LeVay 1993, Fausto-Sterling 1985). As with the debates on race/ethnicity, however, research on gender and health has found that strictly biological explanations are outweighed by other, social causes.

There is strong evidence that different mortality and morbidity rates are related to the different roles that men and women play, and the consequent differences in their individual behaviors. This includes variations in rates of smoking, alcohol and drug use, engaging in other risk-taking behaviors, working in stressful jobs, and exposure to occupational hazards (Verbrugge and Wingard 1987, Verbrugge 1989, Waldron 1990). The fact that men and women are "socialized" differently—particularly in the United States, with its "rugged individualist" role model for young men—makes them connect differently to social networks that provide buffers from the effects of illness (Berkman and Syme 1979). From early childhood on, males and females are taught to have different attitudes toward acceptable ways to respond to illness. Going to the doctor may be a sign of weakness for many men, while for women, seeking help is appropriate behavior. Many of these factors combine to affect disease rates. Explanations for gender difference in rates of heart disease, for example, include the fact that men smoke more than women (Waldron 1990); they exhibit more personality traits associated with heart disease and have fewer buffering social ties (Kaplan et al. 1988, Lasker et al. 1994). These factors also affect treatment. For life-threatening heart disease, men and women receive similar treatment, but when men and women are admitted to hospitals with less serious heart disease, women undergo fewer procedures than men. It is unclear whether women receive less appropriate care or whether men are overtreated (Bickel 1992).

A recent report by Sally Macintyre and her colleagues (1996) cautions against oversimplifying the relationship between gender and health. Their article challenges conventional wisdom that women have poorer health than men. Based on data from two British surveys, they demonstrate a complex pattern of illness reports, with the "direction and magnitude of sex differences in health varying according to the particular symptom or condition and the phase in the life cycle. Female excess is only consistently found across the life span for psychological distress, and is far less apparent, or reversed, for a number of physical symptoms and conditions" (Macintyre et al. 1996, 617). Because morbidity reports are by nature subjective, interpretation of these patterns is difficult. Possible explanations include shifting gender roles, changing rates of illness, and differences in health (as in life expectancy) between societies at different stages of development or with different cultural and religious attitudes toward gender roles. The authors assert that in recent years, the "story" about gender differences in health has become oversimplified, and inconsistencies and complexities in patterns have been overlooked. It is interesting to speculate why such stereotypes have persisted, even in the face of contradictory evidence.

Age, like gender, can be thought of as a simple, biological variable. There is no stronger predictor of mortality than age (Shryock 1980, 393). While the average age at death has changed over time, the relationship between age and mortality is remarkably constant. Yet our view of age—and the various joys and risk that each age will bring—is also a product of the historical moment and of shared expectations about the nature of the human life cycle. This is an era in which, in the United States, most babies survive beyond their first year of life, most mothers do not die in childbirth, and life expectancy increases for each succeeding generation. It is an era in which government labor regulations suggest that we exist in age-specific groups: "youth," "working age," and "retired." We think of age as a fixed numerical category.

It may surprise us to learn that in earlier times in Western culture, "most people had little idea of their chronological age. . . . [It] was determined largely by rites of passage, the rituals surrounding birth, marriage, and death. Since retirement had no place in traditional European folk culture, old age as a stage of life was not set apart by specific transition rituals or customs. Plagues,

famines, epidemics, and infectious diseases prevented most people from growing old, giving it much thought, or associating death exclusively with old age" (Cole 1992, 11).

This scenario differs from our contemporary experience of age and aging. Infectious diseases have been replaced as the leading causes of death by heart disease, cancer, and stroke. As sociologist Renée C. Fox has written, today, "[c]hronic rather than acute conditions prevail, [and these diseases] are harbingers of the physical form in which most of us will die our eventual deaths" (Fox 1986, 15). As life expectancy continues to grow, not just one chronic condition—but several—increasingly characterize the complex picture of the final years of life.

If we had unlimited space in this book, the section on age would feature readings that span the contemporary life cycle, describing age as experience, as well as an epidemiological category, and describing the conditions that are currently associated with each stage. It might consider hyperactivity among young boys, anorexia and other eating disorders among adolescent girls, treatments for menopause, and for job-related stresses. However, striking changes take place at the end of the life span, and those changes have clear policy and planning significance for the future; so we have selected readings that reflect upon the experience of old age. That experience must be viewed in the context of two interrelated changes: the growing number of older people, as life expectancy doubles during the twentieth century, and a change in people's attitudes toward aging and old age in the United States coupled with changes in the scientific understanding of age.

Currently much of the demographic literature on age and health is concerned with measuring trends in mortality and morbidity among the elderly. Mortality researchers are engaged in an ongoing debate about the existence of a biological limit to life expectancy (due to the biological process of growing old). Those who believe that we have reached the limit of human longevity predict that efforts to increase life expectancy through disease control will produce a "rectangularization" of the survival curve as more and more people live out their natural biological life span (Fries 1980, Fries 1984). Those who disagree argue that in recent years there has been an *increase* rather than a decrease in variability of age of death, as well as a slow progression toward later average ages of death for all five leading causes of death (Manton 1982, Myers and Manton 1984).

The second major topic in the debate about age centers on the quality of life that people in old age can expect. The question is whether living longer merely extends illness and dependency, or whether medical advances in the treatment of chronic conditions have produced a "compression of morbidity" (Fries 1980), meaning that people live longer *and* healthier lives. The answer, not surprisingly, depends upon how illness and dependency are measured.

Lois Verbrugge (1984) examined morbidity data obtained from the U.S. National Health Interview Survey over a twenty-three year period (1957–80), and found that both middle-aged and older people were reporting increasing rates of all chronic diseases and impairments. While mortality rates dropped for most major conditions, morbidity from cancer, diabetes, heart disease, hypertension, and arteriosclerosis all increased notably. Furthermore, more older people sought treatment for nonfatal conditions, including respiratory, skin, and musculoskeletal conditions. Eileen Crimmins and her colleagues (1989) extended this analysis by investigating reports of different types of morbidity, ranging from being confined to a bed to being limited only in secondary activities. They found that between 1970 and 1980, reports of general activity limitations due to illness did increase, but reported "bed dis-

ability days" did not. (For those over eighty-five, however, bed disability as well as rates of institutionalization did increase.) Thus, if you limit the definition of illness and disability to days spent in bed, for those below age eighty-five, most of the increase in life expectancy is spent in healthy old age; while if you look at how far a person can participate fully in a normal, active adult life, then in extending life expectancy, we have also increased the years of disability.

Both Verbrugge and Crimmins suggest several reasons for these trends. First, while the risks of developing chronic diseases have probably fallen during the past several decades, improved diagnostic techniques for chronic conditions have also increased the chances of discovering disease at an earlier stage. Further, because people know more about health, they probably report disability more than in the past (Crimmins et al. 1989, 254). These observations help explain the seemingly contradictory correlation between falling mortality and rising morbidity. Authors of several recent articles (Macintyre et al. 1996, Johansson 1991, Murray and Chen 1992) emphasize that illness reports are subjective measures, susceptible to cultural, economic, and historical influences. Making comparisons about health issues across cultures, historical time periods, age, and gender groups, it is clear, is a challenging, perhaps impossible task.

The fact that we now live longer but experience more long-term illness as we age has already affected many aspects of the health care system. Physicians are seeing more patients with multiple chronic conditions. Administrators and government officials must confront the issue of Medicare, and its ballooning cost to the government, particularly as estimates of the size of the over-sixty-five population are continually revised upward. And, since ultimately, responsibility for care of increasingly dependent elderly rests with family and friends, caregivers will encounter difficult emotional, financial, and moral dilemmas. The readings on old age attempt to bring together some of these themes.

These changes are salient for policy and planning, but it is also important to recognize that the experience of old age in America at the end of the twentieth century is influenced by the complex and often contradictory attitudes that we carry in our culture. The dominant view is that the aged are a burden to society, and that old age is a medical problem that can be alleviated through the "magic bullets" of medical science (Estes 1993). In *The Journey of Life: A Cultural History of Aging in America,* Thomas Cole writes, "[M]iddle-class American culture since the 1830s has responded to the anxieties of growing old with a psychologically primitive strategy of splitting images of a 'good' old age of health, virtue, self-reliance, and salvation from a 'bad' old age of sickness, sin, dependency, premature death, and damnation. Rooted in the drive for unlimited individual accumulation of health and wealth, this dualism has hindered our culture's ability to sustain morally compelling social practices and existentially vital ideals of aging" (Cole 1992, 230). In his analysis, Cole reminds us that the biomedical ideal of "successful aging" creates unobtainable goals. "By transforming health from a means of living well into an end in itself, 'successful' aging reveals its bankruptcy as an ideal that cannot accommodate the realities of decline and death. To create genuinely satisfying ideals of aging, we will have to transcend our exclusive emphasis on individual health . . . and revive existentially nourishing views of aging that address its paradoxical nature: . . . the tension between infinite ambitions, dreams, and desires on the one hand, and vulnerable, limited, decaying physical existence on the other—the tragic and ineradicable conflict between spirit and body" (Cole 1992, 238–239).

This part of the reader brings together evidence and interpretation. It unites epidemiological and demographic evidence about the relationships between social factors, health, and illness with nuanced interpretations of the meaning of these relationships. We must constantly challenge conventional categories, the labels we stick on social communities and on illness itself. We do this not only to refine our understanding of the inquiry at hand, but, as Cole so eloquently demonstrates, to understand ourselves as well.

Gail E. Henderson

I

The Relationship between

Social Class, Race/Ethnicity,

and Health

This section begins with an article from the *Journal of the American Medical Association* that reviews current knowledge about the relationships between social class, race/ethnicity, health insurance, and health outcomes. The authors wanted to see if universal health insurance would make up for the disadvantage of poverty when it comes to health. Using a variety of sources and data from international studies, they show that insurance alone is unlikely to make much difference. They also show that while the mechanisms (or proximate variables) through which poverty affects health outcomes may have changed over time, the strength of the relationship between poverty and health has not.

The second selection is a story about the Banes family, a multigenerational household struggling to survive in one of Chicago's poorest neighborhoods. The family members have many serious health problems, including diabetes, kidney failure, hypertension, stroke, and alcoholism. Each problem has been exacerbated by inadequate medical care and medical insurance coverage, and the chapter depicts in depressing detail the difficulties confronting poor families as they attempt to "work the system" to get health care. Members of families like the Baneses are debilitated in the prime of life by conditions that many in the United States experience as diseases of old

age. Why? Is it the low-paying jobs? The crowded housing? Lack of education that might have been a route out of the neighborhood? Is it the stress of living with constant worries about money? It is hard to reduce the causes of their many medical problems to one "social factor."

Social class is a concept that incorporates all of these causes. The Baneses' story illustrates clearly the multidimensional nature of a person's location in the social hierarchy. Although researchers will typically select one or more features, such as education, occupation, or income, to represent social class in statistical analyses, it is important to remember that this strategy is at best a shorthand method, an abbreviation that cannot completely represent such a holistic concept. Furthermore, social class is not only—or even mainly—a set of individual characteristics. Social class defines people within their communities; it is linked to how much access they have to resources, information, and influence (Mechanic 1989, 10).

The Baneses' story raises many questions. How does this family get medical care? What are the barriers to getting care for them, in contrast to a typical middle-class American family with employment-based medical insurance? How are they treated by health professionals? What problems are generated by having to deal with the chronic illnesses experienced by several family members? What are the causes of these illnesses?

Their story also touches on some of the material discussed in Lawrence Wright's article from the *New Yorker*, "One Drop of Blood," which describes the history of racial classification in the United States. Recent challenges to the use of race in medical and public health research (Osborne and Feit 1992, LaVeist 1994) echo Wright's claim that racial categories are social and political constructs. Yet no one would argue that race, as a social designation in a divided society, should be ignored. "Race" still matters; the question is, what is it measuring?

In the case of the Banes family, it seems simplistic to ask whether the key issue for their family is being African American or of lower-class status. Rather, those two identities create a third, different identity: poor black, different from poor, different from black, and also different from poor white or impoverished Hispanic. This kind of critique suggests a need for more thoughtful examination of *what* is measured when researchers use these labels in an attempt to explain differences in health outcomes, and *how* it is being measured.

Socioeconomic Inequalities

in Health: No Easy Solution

Nancy E. Adler, W. Thomas Boyce,

Margaret A. Chesney, Susan Folkman,

S. Leonard Syme

◼

Socioeconomic status (SES) is a strong and consistent predictor of morbidity and premature mortality. Individuals lower in the SES hierarchy suffer disproportionately from almost every disease and show higher rates of mortality than those above them.[1,2] This association is found with each of the key components of SES: income, education, and occupational status. Various approaches have been taken to explain this association. Empirical research has mostly focused on the impact of poverty and its correlates such as poor housing and inadequate nutrition; however, the poverty-related factors have not adequately explained the SES-health association.[3–5] Policy debate has focused relatively more attention on insurance coverage as a remedy to SES-related inequalities in health; some, like Friedman,[6] argue that "although coverage is not the sole determinant of health status it is a key factor in improved health. . . ."

Each of these approaches has limited our understanding of SES influences on health. The focus on health insurance as a means to improve health may deflect attention from other factors that contribute to social inequalities in health status. In this article we argue that insurance coverage alone will have a minor impact on SES-related inequalities in health. A full understanding of health inequalities requires that we consider other factors distributed along the SES hierarchy that are likely to contribute to undue health burdens and that such factors be explored not only among the impoverished, but at all levels of the social class and health gradient.

The Relationship of SES and Health

Differences in mortality by social class and occupation have been documented since the 19th century. For example, in the 1860s, only the more affluent paid taxes. The crude death rate in Providence, RI, in 1865 was 10.8 per 1000 people among the relatively small group of taxpayers vs 24.8 per 1000 people among the large population of non-taxpayers.[7] During the first half of the 20th century, the difference in life expectancy between the highest and lowest SES groups in cities in the United States, England, and Wales was about 7 years.[1]

Socioeconomic status has been associated with mortality measured both at the aggregate level (ie, areas characterized by lower-SES indicators have higher mortality rates) and at the individual level. At the aggregate level, significant differences in mortality rates within census tracts have been associated with the median monthly rents of homes, median family income, and poverty level of the census tract.[8-11] At the individual level, SES is inversely related to all-cause mortality and to the incidence of and mortality from specific diseases including cardiovascular disease, cancer, and respiratory disease.[12-18]

Although associations between SES and health are found over time and in different countries, the mediating variables may not be identical. In earlier times (and currently in developing countries), health advantages of higher SES were likely to be associated with one's ability to avoid infection. For example, the Great Plague of London in 1665 caused a disproportionate number of deaths among the poor who were more suscepti-

ble to disease because of poor nutrition and sanitation and who, unlike the wealthy, could not flee the cities when the disease became epidemic.[18] However, in circumstances where mortality is due primarily to chronic diseases, different mechanisms must be identified. In developed countries, the majority of deaths result from chronic degenerative diseases related to lifestyle behaviors rather than from infection and famine.[19,20] In the remainder of this article, we examine potential pathways by which SES may now be exerting its influence on health and discuss the implications of these pathways for clinical practice and policy choices.

Linear Relationship vs. Threshold Effect

If SES effects are due to poverty and its correlates, one would expect to find a threshold effect above which SES would show little or no association with health outcomes. Studies at both the individual and aggregate levels challenge this expectation. An association of SES and mortality occurs throughout the SES hierarchy. While many studies have only compared those at the bottom of the SES hierarchy with those above, a number of studies that have made more finegrained comparisons report associations of health and SES at every level of the SES hierarchy.[3-5,10,14,21] For example, using 1971 British census data, Adelstein[21] found increasing mortality as occupational status decreased (Fig 1). In a US sample, Kitagawa and Hauser[10] demonstrated a linear association between years of school and mortality ratios (the ratio of observed to expected deaths, Fig 2) and between median family incomes within neighborhoods and mortality ratios of the neighborhoods.

The association of SES and health differs by age and race. Socioeconomic status differences in health are greatest in middle age and early old age compared with both earlier and later in life. There are marked SES differences in infant mor-

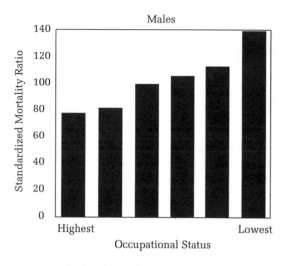

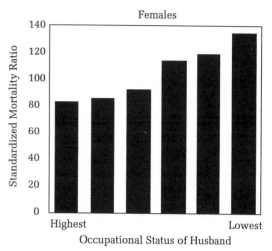

Fig 1. Standardized mortality ratio by occupational status (data from Adelstein[21]).

tality and in the early neonatal period.[22,23] For those who survive, SES differences are comparatively small until much later in life.[22-24] The effects of SES across racial and ethnic groups are more complex, particularly for blacks vs whites. Because blacks are disproportionately represented in lower-SES groups, race and SES are often confounded. Race is more commonly assessed than is SES, and attributions made to racial differences in health outcomes may actually be due, at least in part, to SES.

Studies examining SES and race have come to varying conclusions about their relative impact. For example, when income was taken into account, a 30% higher mortality for blacks vs whites in the Alameda County (California) Study became statistically nonsignificant.[25,26] Similarly, Dayal et al[13] found that racial differences in incidence of and survival from cancer became nonsignificant when SES was controlled for. However, other studies have found that controlling for SES reduces but does not eliminate racial differences in disease and mortality.[17,27,28] The relationships among SES, race, and health may vary depending on the disease or condition. In addition, SES may interact with race. Kessler

and Neighbors[29] reanalyzed eight epidemiologic surveys on psychological distress and found that the effects of race depended on SES level; racial differences in psychological distress were much greater among individuals with lower SES than among those with higher SES. Studies of racial differences in blood pressure have also shown different patterns of association by SES among blacks vs whites.[14,30,31]

Access to Health Care and the SES-Health Gradient

One explanation for the SES-health gradient is that individuals lower in the SES hierarchy have less access to medical care. This explanation supports the belief that universal health insurance could reduce SES differences in health in the United States. However, three sets of findings suggest that while universal health insurance may be a necessary condition, it is not likely to be sufficient to reduce substantially social inequalities in health.

First, countries that have universal health insurance show the same SES-health gradient as that found in the United States—where such in-

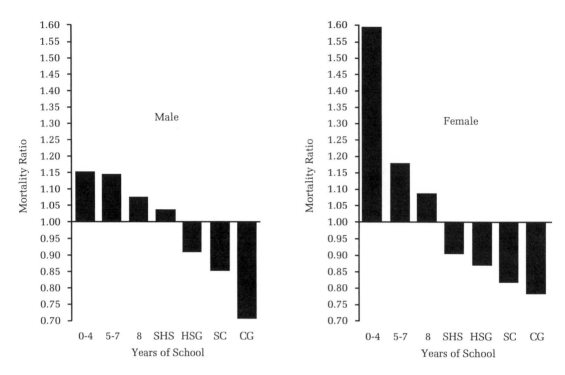

Fig 2. Mortality ratio (observed to expected deaths) by education (data from Kitagawa and Hauser[10]). SHS indicates some high school; HSG, high school graduate; SC, some college; and CG, college graduate.

surance is not provided. In England, Townsend and Davidson[32] concluded that the establishment of the National Health Service was not followed by a reduction of SES differences in health, and that, in fact, SES differences actually widened after its initiation.[18] This may have been due to changes in social conditions that created greater disparities among individuals at different levels of the SES hierarchy. In Scandinavian countries, the SES-health gradient emerges, but it is weaker than in the United States or England.[33-35] This may reflect the more homogeneous populations in these countries, as well as social policies that have reduced social class differences in income and other social resources, in addition to universal health coverage.

Second, SES differences can be found between levels at the upper range of the SES hierarchy.

At upper levels, individuals are likely to have health insurance, making lack of coverage an unlikely explanation for health effects of SES differences. A clear example of both points comes from the Whitehall studies in England. Whitehall I examined 10-year mortality rates of a group of 17,530 British civil servants first studied in 1967 through 1969.[5] Although the subject population was more homogeneous than the general population in that all were employed by the British Civil Service as well as being covered by the National Health Service, a clear gradient still emerged in 10-year mortality across four levels of employment grade. Compared with the top administrators, the executive and professional class had a relative risk (RR) of mortality of 1.6, the clerical staff had an RR of 2.2, and the unskilled laborers had an RR of 2.7.

Third, SES differences appear in a wide range of diseases, both those that are amenable to treatment and those that are not. Bunker and Gomby[36] noted that to the extent to which mortality from malignant diseases reflects differential access to care, a greater SES effect should be found in cancers most amenable to treatment. However, they concluded that "available data show either no effect, or, in fact, a greater discrepancy across social classes for those malignancies least amenable to treatment." Other evidence comes from research within a single treatment setting in which differences in care are presumably minimal and that finds an association of outcome with SES.[13] In a recent study of patients with acute myocardial infarction, patients with more education were found to have lower in-hospital mortality even when age, race, gender, and baseline severity scores were taken into account.[37] In terms of overall mortality, adequacy of care is estimated to account for about 10% of the outcome, while human biological factors and environmental factors each account for 20% and individual factors account for half.[38]

The above argument does not imply that medical care is unimportant. Rather, medical care is but one input into health status and, in some instances, will play a relatively minor role.[39–42] Further, provision of insurance does not ensure equal or adequate access, especially for primary care.[43,44] In those areas that are underserved, individuals with fewer socioeconomic resources will find it more difficult to gain access.[45] Even among individuals in the same area who technically have equal access, true access may differ for those at different SES levels. Individuals with more education and income, who may be more skilled in dealing with bureaucracies and social systems, may be more efficient in determining who provides the best care and in obtaining care when needed.

Individuals with fewer social and economic resources appear to make less use of preventive health services including screening. To some extent, this may reflect insurance-based differences in care. But Hayward et al[46] found that lower-SES women were less likely to have had Papanicolaou tests, breast examinations by a physician, or mammograms independent of age, health status, or frequency of physician visits. Harlan et al[47] found that women with less than a high school education were relatively less likely than those with more education to have been screened for cervical cancer or to have even heard of a Papanicolaou test. Research in Finland found that low-SES women were relatively less likely than those higher in SES to use cancer screening services.[48] Programs involving outreach to increase access will be more effective in reducing SES differentials. For example, Stamler et al[49] examined 5-year all-cause mortality among 11000 hypertensive patients who were randomly referred to standard care or treatment geared to minimizing barriers to care (stepped care). The stepped-care group showed lower mortality than did the standard-care group. In the whole sample, educational level was inversely related to mortality rates; in the stepped-care group, this relationship was reduced, although it still remained significant.

Because insurance alone does not guarantee equal access to and utilization of medical care, and because medical care itself has a limited association with health differences, we must consider other factors that may contribute to SES differentials in health. These must be addressed if substantial reductions in social inequalities in health outcomes are to occur.

Other Factors in the SES Link

Behaviors such as smoking, diet, and lack of exercise are associated with health status.[28,50–52] Early effects of those behaviors are reflected in risk factors such as cholesterol level, obesity, and blood pressure; longer-term effects can be seen in

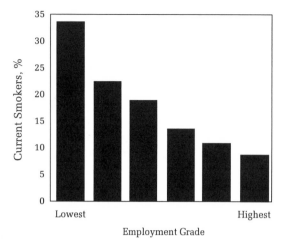

Fig 3. Smoking by employment grade (data from Marmot et al[4]).

disease and premature mortality. Both the behaviors and the risk factors show a linear relationship with SES.

Clear SES differences are shown in rates of smoking. In the Whitehall studies of the British Civil Service, smoking rates in both sexes increased as one went down the employment grade hierarchy. Figure 3 illustrates this association in the sample studied between 1985 and 1988. A significant linear trend by employment grade was also found in prevalence of exercise (the lower the employment grade, the higher the percentage reporting getting no exercise) and diet (the lower the employment grade, the lower the percentage of individuals consuming skimmed milk, wholemeal bread, and fresh fruits and vegetables).[4]

In the United States, similar patterns have been found. For example, in a community sample of 2138 women aged 42 to 50 years studied by Matthews et al,[53] the prevalence of smoking ranged from 45% of those with less than a high school education to 19% of those with advanced degrees. Intermediate rates were found for those with some college (30%) and those with a college degree (23%). Similarly, Winkleby et al[54] found a

strong association of smoking with years of education among both men and women in a community sample of 3349 adults.

Risk factors also increase as SES decreases. In the community sample of women studied by Matthews et al,[53] educational level was significantly associated with cholesterol levels (higher low-density lipoprotein [LDL] and triglyceride levels, lower high-density lipoprotein [HDL], HDL2, and HDL/LDL ratio with less education), systolic blood pressure, glucose tolerance, and body mass index. All risk factors were more adverse the less education the woman had, and the associations persisted when body mass index was taken into account. Kraus et al[14] found a linear gradient between prevalence of hypertension and six levels of SES based on education and occupation among 15,412 white males who were screened for participation in the community-based Multiple Risk Factor Intervention Trial (Fig 4). Smaller numbers of men from other ethnic groups were also studied; the gradient emerged for Hispanics, but not for Asians or blacks. Finally, numerous studies have shown

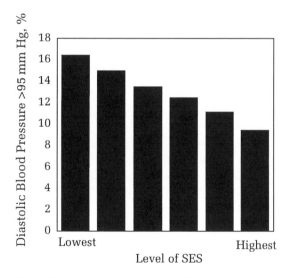

Fig 4. Blood pressure by level of socioeconomic status (SES) (data from Kraus, Borhani, and Franti[14]).

that rates of obesity increase as SES declines, particularly among women.[55-58]

The pattern of health risk behaviors in which those with a higher SES are less likely to smoke and eat high-fat diets and are more likely to exercise has not always been true. Earlier in the 20th century, many of these behaviors (eg, smoking, eating red meat) were not classified as health-risking behaviors but as luxuries. Epidemiological surveys documenting the prevalence of these behaviors are not available for this period. It seems likely that higher-SES individuals were relatively more likely to indulge in these activities. During this time, rates of coronary heart disease were greater in higher-SES groups.[18] However, as health promotion has become more popular, upper-SES groups have been quickest to acquire and act on information regarding health risks. Despite this seeming advantage, a few life-style differences place higher-SES individuals at relatively greater risk for specific diseases. Rates of malignant melanoma are greater in higher-SES groups, which may be due in part to differences in recreational tanning. In addition, rates of breast cancer are greater among higher-SES women, which may reflect differences in child-bearing patterns. However, once breast cancer is diagnosed, survival is positively associated with SES even when stage at diagnosis is taken into account.[13]

Health behaviors represent one pathway by which SES may influence health, but they do not account for all of the association. In the White-hall sample, for example, Marmot et al[5] found that the RR of mortality for lower employment grades was reduced but was still strong when a number of behavioral and risk factors were controlled for.

Other potential pathways by which SES may influence health are through differential exposure to physical and social contexts that are damaging to one's health. The lower an individual is in the SES hierarchy, the more likely he or she is to experience adverse environmental conditions, such as exposure to pathogens and carcinogens at home and at work, and to social conditions, such as crime.[59] As Dutton and Levine[60] note, individuals lower in the social hierarchy experience "more disruption and daily struggle as well as more simple physical hardships."

In addition to the direct health effect of exposure to adverse physical and social conditions, these experiences may trigger psychological processes that affect one's risk of disease. There is increasing evidence that stress plays a role in disease, including heart disease and susceptibility to infection.[61-63] Community studies have demonstrated that the lower one's position in the hierarchy, the greater the reported exposure to stressful life events and the greater the impact of these events on emotional adjustment.[64-66] In a study of 2320 men following a myocardial infarction, Ruberman and colleagues[67] found a strong negative association between years of education and degree of life stress and social isolation; these two variables, in turn, were strongly related to mortality following myocardial infarction. Within groups that were either low on life stress and social isolation or were high on both, education was no longer related to mortality, suggesting that the association of education and mortality was a function of the greater life stress and social isolation of those with less education.

Research on stressful life events has shown that the impact of an event on physical and mental well-being is mediated through the individual's appraisal of the event as stressful; the appraisal is a function of the individual's evaluation of the event and of the resources he or she has to handle it.[68] Appraisal of events as stressful is likely to vary by SES level. Components of SES such as education and income provide resources that can be used to address and resolve threats and may reduce the impact of the event on the body.

Socioeconomic status contributes to the development during childhood of traits and coping resources that may affect risk for disease. Rutter[69] notes that "adverse life events make it more likely that people will act in ways that create threatening situations for themselves." Exposure to greater stress in childhood reduces the likelihood that children will develop "resilience" and increases the chances that they will develop depression and helplessness, characteristics that have been linked to increased risk of disease.[70-71] Placement in the SES hierarchy is also associated with the differential ability of individuals to control their environment. A clear effect is one's ability to avoid risks of disease and injury. For example, safety features in cars (most recently air bags) have been more available in higher-priced cars. There are a myriad of ways in which higher-SES individuals can control their environment, and the experience of control itself has been linked to better health outcomes.[72-73]

Implications for Policy and Clinical Practice

Public health policy is moving toward the provision of health insurance to provide universal access to health care. However, even if this goal is achieved, our review indicates that SES inequalities in health will persist. Differences related to SES in health-damaging behaviors and exposure to adverse physical and psychosocial conditions differentially place those lower in the SES hierarchy at risk of disease and premature mortality. Moreover, successful and effective utilization of care may depend on class-related contextual factors of an individual's daily life. These factors need to be addressed in clinical practice as well as in policy design.

Clinicians and policymakers should be aware that the health effects of social position occur not only at the poverty level—where even conventional wisdom acknowledges disproportionate rates of poor health—but throughout the social class hierarchy. The psychological, behavioral, and biological factors that underlie class-associated vulnerabilities remain incompletely understood, but among those that a physician should attend to involve understanding the patient's health behaviors, exposure to stressful challenges and resources to deal with such challenges, and control over important domains in his or her life that may interfere with modifying health-damaging behaviors and with obtaining adequate care.

Many providers are acutely aware of the possible influences of contextual conditions on patients' health. Yet, they may assume that these become less relevant for patients who are employed, have adequate resources for basic needs, and have access to medical care. Even above the poverty level, however, SES-related factors will affect an individual's ability to engage in health-promoting and disease-preventing behaviors, including effective use of health care services.

In many settings, job status affects the individual's control over the scheduling of his or her work: usually a manager has more flexibility than a foreman, and a foreman has more than a line worker. Control over one's work circumstances affects the individual's ability to not only obtain care, but also to follow through on prescribed regimens. For example, in a recent study of San Francisco, Calif, bus drivers, 60% of drivers with diagnosed hypertension were found to be untreated or uncontrolled despite full and complete access to primary medical care services (unpublished data, Muni Study of Stress and Hypertension, July 1991). Further exploration revealed that many drivers prescribed antihypertensive diuretics were unable to comply with treatment because bathrooms were not accessible during their tightly scheduled bus routes. This example highlights the need for physicians to consider the impact of treatment regimens on individual patient life-styles and the implications of this for their ability to adhere to treatment. In the case of hypertension, physicians may want to consider alternative treatment regimens (eg, nondiuretic antihypertensive medications, dietary changes that accommodate to the variety of foods available to the patient) that balance clinical efficacy with the likelihood that the patient will be able to accommodate the treatment into his or her life.

Our analysis underscores the importance—increasingly recognized within clinical medicine—of a strong program of preventive services accessible to populations of primary care patients. Unfortunately, preventive services may actually be offered in reverse order to the degree of need; those lower in the SES hierarchy, who have the highest rates of health-risking behaviors and risk factors, are least likely to receive information and services. Individuals at the lower ends of the SES hierarchy are more likely to use emergency departments and clinics where continuity of care is not possible and concern about prevention a luxury. Even as one ascends the SES ladder, programs to help with quitting smoking, losing weight, and learning stress management techniques are relatively more available to those at the top. At worksites with preventive health programs, for example, opportunities for exercise, smoking cessation, and stress management are often offered first to the top executives and management. Within physicians' offices, there may be a similar bias toward addressing these issues with better-educated, higher-income patients.

Health promotion programs and physician recommendations are frequently designed with upper-SES individuals in mind. For example, recommendations to increase exercise presume that patients have access to safe environments where they can swim, walk, or jog. Physicians need to recognize not only the importance of discussing risk behavior increases with patients who are lower on the SES ladder, but also that recommendations need to be tailored to the patient's life circumstances. For example, in suggesting exercise, it will be helpful to explore with patients when and where this could be accomplished, both helping them to overcome real or perceived barriers and to identify opportunities of which they may not be aware.

Beyond providing access to care and using clinical practice to reduce social inequalities in health, other inequalities associated with SES will also need to be addressed to reduce substantially the current strong association of SES and health. Vågerö,[34] for example, attributes the fact that class differences in health are smaller in Sweden than in England to differences in income spread rather than to differences in health services. As noted earlier, Sweden's social welfare policies result in a more even distribution of income compared with England's. Other data show that in developed countries, the average life expectancy is associated with how egalitarian the income distribution is; the more egalitarian the distribution, the higher the life expectancy.[74,75] Of developed countries, the United States is among the least egalitarian nations in income distribution.[75] Thus, those concerned with the health of the nation need to be aware of social policies that increase the gap among levels in the SES hierarchy even if we enact policies that provide access to care.

In short, no single strategy will significantly reduce social inequalities in health. The problem needs to be addressed by physicians at multiple levels, from general social policy to the details of clinical practice. Expanded health care coverage and equal access to care may help reduce SES differentials in health, but attention must also be given to SES-related, social, environmental, and psychological resources that influence health risk, the effective utilization of health care, and adherence to prevention and treatment regimens. Physicians have important roles to play in reducing SES inequalities in health. They can increase the likelihood that their recommendations for prevention and treatment will be effective for lower-SES as well as upper-SES patients by providing clinical care that is sensitive to SES-related influences on health and health behaviors. Physicians who are aware of the increased need for outreach to patients as SES declines can also take part in community health initiatives that increase the focus on those lower in the SES hierarchy. Finally, physicians may wish to consider advocacy for social policies to address SES inequalities that have an impact on health.

Notes

Preparation of this essay was supported by the John D. and Catherine T. MacArthur Foundation Network on Determinants and Consequences of Health-Promoting and Disease-Preventing Behavior.

1. Antonovsky, A. Social class, life expectancy and overall mortality. *Milbank Q.* 1967;45:31–73.

2. Syme, S.L., Berkman, L.F. Social class, susceptibility and sickness. *Am J Epidemiol.* 1976;104:1–8.

3. Haan, M.N., Kaplan, G.A., Syme, S.L. Socioeconomic states and health: old observations and new thoughts. In: Bunker, J.P., Gomby, D.S., Kehrer, B.H., eds. *Pathways to Health.* Menlo Park, Calif: The Henry J. Kaiser Family Foundation; 1989:76–135.

4. Marmot, M.G., Smith, G.D., Stansfeld, S. et al. Health inequalities among British civil servants: the Whitehall II study. *Lancet.* 1991;337:1387–1393.

5. Marmot, M.G., Shipley, M.J., Rose, G. Inequalities in death—specific explanations of a general pattern? *Lancet.* 1984;1:1003–1006.

6. Friedman, E. The uninsured: from dilemma to crisis. *JAMA.* 1991;265:2491–2495.

7. Chapin, C.V. Deaths among taxpayers and nontaxpayers, income tax. Providence, 1865. *Am J Public Health.* 1924;14:647–651.

8. Coombs, L.C. Economic differentials in causes of death. *Med Care.* 1941;1:246–255.

9. Haan, M.N., Kaplan, G.A., Camacho, T. Poverty and health: prospective evidence from the Alameda County Study. *Am J Epidemiol.* 1987;125:989–998.

10. Kitagawa, E.M., Hauser, P.M. *Differential Mortality in the United States: A Study of Socioeconomic Epidemiology.* Cambridge, Mass: Harvard University Press; 1973.

11. Patno, M.E. Mortality and economic level in an urban area. *Public Health Rep.* 1960;75:841–851.

12. Berg, J.W., Ross, R., Latourette, H.B. Economic status and survival of cancer patients. *Cancer.* 1977;39:467–477.

13. Dayal, H.H., Power, R.N., Chiu, C. Race and socioeconomic status in survival from breast cancer. *J Chronic Disability.* 1982;35:675–683.

14. Kraus, J.F., Borhani, N.O., Franti, C.E. Socioeconomic status, ethnicity, and risk of coronary heart disease. *Am J Epidemiol.* 1980;111:407–414.

15. Marmot, M.G., Adelstein, A.M., Robinson, N., Rose, G.A. Changing social-class distribution of heart disease. *BMJ.* 1978;2:1109–1112.

16. Marmot, M.G., Rose, G., Shipley, M.J, Hamilton, P.J.S. Employment grade and coronary heart disease in British civil servants. *J Epidemiol Community Health.* 1987;32:244–249.

17. Steinhorn, S.C., Myers, M.H., Hanky, B.H., Pelham, V.F. Factors associated with survival differences between black women and white women with cancer of the uterine corpus. *Am J Epidemiol.* 1986;124:85–93.

18. Susser, M., Watson, W., Hopper, K. *Sociology in Medicine.* 3rd ed. Oxford, England: Oxford University Press; 1985.

19. Caldwell, J.C. *Theory of Fertility Decline.* London, England: Academic Press; 1982.

20. Omran, A.R. The epidemiologic transition: a theory of the epidemiology of population change. *Milbank Q.* 1971;49:509–538.

21. Adelstein, A.M. Life-style in occupational cancer. *J Toxicol Environ Health.* 1980;6:953–962.

22. Gould, J.B., LeRoy, S. Socioeconomic status and low birth weight: a racial comparison. *Pediatrics.* 1988; 82:896–904.

23. Wise, P.H., Meyers, A. Poverty and child health. *Pediatr Clin North Am.* 1988;35:1169–1186.

24. House, J.S., Kessler, R.C., Herzog, A.R. Age, socioeconomic status, and health. *Milbank Q.* 1990;68:383–411.

25. Haan, M.N., Kaplan, G.A. The contribution of socioeconomic position to minority health. In: Heckler, M., ed. *Report of the Secretary's Task Force on Black and Minority Health: Crosscutting Issues in Minority Health.* Washington, DC: US Dept of Health and Human Services; 1985.

26. Kaplan, G.A., Haan, M.N. Socioeconomic position and health: prospective evidence from the Alameda County Study. Presented at the 114th annual meeting of the American Public Health Association; Las Vegas, Nev; September 29, 1986.

27. Devesa, S.S., Diamond, E.L. Association of breast cancer and cervical cancer incidences with income and

education among whites and blacks. *J Natl Cancer Inst.* 1980;6:515–528.

28. Otten, M., Teutsch, S., Williamson, D., Marks, J. The effect of known risk factors on the excess mortality of black adults in the United States. *JAMA.* 1990;263:845–850.

29. Kessler, R.C., Neighbors, H.W. A new perspective on the relationships among race, social class, and psychological distress. *J Health Soc Behav.* 1986;27:107–115.

30. Harburg, E., Erfurt, J.C., Chape, C., Hauenstein, L.S., Schull, W.J., Schork, M.A. Socioecological stressor areas and black-white blood pressure. *J Chronic Dis.* 1973;26:595–611.

31. James, A.J., Strogatz, D.S., Wing, S.B., Ramsey, D.L. Socioeconomic status, John Henryism, and hypertension in blacks and whites. *Am J Epidemiol.* 1987;126:664–673.

32. Townsend, P., Davidson, N. *Inequalities in Health: The Black Report.* Harmondsworth, England: Penguin; 1982.

33. Lundberg, O. Causal explanations for class inequality in health—an empirical analysis. *Soc Sci Med.* 1991;32:385–393.

34. Vågerö, D. Inequality in health—some theoretical and empirical problems. *Soc Sci Med.* 1991;32:367–371.

35. Vågerö, D., Lundberg, O. Health inequalities in Britain and Sweden. *Lancet.* 1989;2:35–36.

36. Bunker, J.P., Gomby, D.S. Preface: socioeconomic states and health: an examination of underlying process. In: Bunker, J.P., Gomby, D.S., Kehrer, B.H., eds. *Pathways to Health.* Menlo Park, Calif: The Henry J. Kaiser Family Foundation; 1989:xv–xxiv.

37. Tofler, G.H., Muller, J.E., Stone, P.H. et al. Comparison of long-term outcome after acute myocardial infarction in patients never graduated from high school with that in more educated patients. *Am J Cardiol.* 1993;71:1031–1035.

38. U.S. Dept. of Health, Education and Welfare. *Healthy People: The Surgeon General's Report on Health Promotion and Disease Prevention.* Washington, D.C.: U.S. Dept of Health, Education and Welfare; 1979.

39. Kim, K., Moody, P. More resources, better health? a cross-national perspective. *Soc Sci Med.* 1992;34:837–842.

40. Doll, R. Health and the environment in the 1990s. *Am J Public Health.* 1992;82:933–941.

41. Winkelstein, W. Jr. Medical care is not health care. *JAMA.* 1993;269:2504.

42. Diehr, P.K., Richardson, W.C., Shortell, S.M., LoGerfo, J.P. Increased access to medical care. *Med Care.* 1991;10:989–999.

43. Dalen, J.E., Santiago, J. Insuring the uninsured is not enough. *Arch Intern Med.* 1991;151:860–862.

44. Haas, J.S., Udvarhelyi, S., Morris, C.N., Epstein, A.M. The effect of providing health coverage to poor uninsured pregnant women in Massachusetts. *JAMA.* 1993;269:87–91.

45. Ginzberg, E., Ostow, M. Beyond universal health insurance to effective health care. *JAMA.* 1991;265:2559–2562.

46. Hayward, R.A., Shapiro, M.F., Freeman, H.E., Corey, C.R. Who gets screened for cervical and breast cancer? results from a new national survey. *Arch Intern Med.* 1988;148:1177–1181.

47. Harlan, L.C., Bernstein, A.B., Kessler, L.G. Cervical cancer screening: who is not screened and why? *Am J Public Health.* 1991;81:885–890.

48. Salonen, J.T. Socioeconomic status and risk of cancer, cerebral stroke, and death due to coronary heart disease and any disease: a longitudinal study in eastern Finland. *J Epidemiol Community Health.* 1982;36:294–297.

49. Stamler, R., Hardy, R.J., Payne, G.H. et al. Educational level and five-year all-cause mortality in the hypertension detection and follow-up program. *Hypertension.* 1987;9:641–646.

50. Paffenbarger, R.S., Hyde, R.T., Wing, A.L., Lee, I.M., Jung, D.L., Kampert, J.B. The association of changes in physical-activity level and other lifestyle characteristics with mortality among men. *N Engl J Med.* 1993;328:538–545.

51. Wilhelmsen, L. Coronary heart disease: epidemiology of smoking and intervention studies of smoking. *Am Heart J.* 1988;115:242–249.

52. Centers for Disease Control. *Smoking, Tobacco and Health: A Fact Book.* Rockville, Md: U.S. Dept of Health and Human Services, Public Health Service, Office on Smoking and Health; 1987.

53. Matthews, K., Kelsey, S., Meilahn, E., Kuller, L., Wing, R. Educational attainment and behavioral and biologic risk factors for coronary heart disease in middle-aged women. *Am J Epidemiol.* 1989;129:1132–1144.

54. Winkleby, M., Fortmann, S., Barrett, D. Social class disparities in risk factors for disease: eight-year prevalence patterns by level of education. *Prev Med.* 1990;19:1–12.

55. Cauley, J.A., Donfield, S.M., LaPorte, R.F., Warhaftig, N.E. Physical activity by SES in two population-based cohorts. *Med Sci Sports Exercise.* 1991;23:343–352.

56. Jeffrey, R.W., French, S.A., Forster, J.L., Spry, V.M. Socioeconomic status differences in health behaviors related to obesity: the Healthy Worker Project. *Int J Obes.* 1991;15:689–696.

57. Kahn, H.S., Williamson, D.F., Stevens, J.A. Race and weight change in U.S. women: the roles of socio-economic and marital status. *Am J Public Health.* 1991;81:319–323.

58. Sobel, J., Stunkard, A.J. Socioeconomic status and obesity: a review of the literature. *Psychol Bull.* 1989; 105:260–271.

59. Stokols, D. Establishing and maintaining health environments. *Am Psychol.* 1992;47:6–22.

60. Dutton, D.B., Levine, S. Overview, methodological critique, and reformulation. In: Bunker, J.P., Gomby, D.S., Kehrer, B.H., eds. *Pathways to Health.* Menlo Park, Calif: The Henry J. Kaiser Family Foundation; 1989: 29–69.

61. Byrne, D.G., Whyte, H.M. Life events and myocardial infarction revisited: the role of measures of individual impact. *Psychosom Med.* 1980;42:1–10.

62. Cohen, S., Tyrrell, D.A.J., Smith, A.P. Psychological stress in humans and susceptibility to the common cold. *N Engl J Med.* 1991;325:606–612.

63. Cohen, S., Tyrrell, D.A.J., Smith, A.P. Negative life events, perceived stress, negative affect, and susceptibility to the common cold. *J Pers Soc Psychol.* 1993; 64:131–140.

64. McLeod, J.D., Kessler, R.C. Socioeconomic status differences in vulnerability to undesirable life events. *J Health Soc Behav.* 1990;31:162–172.

65. Cohen, S., Wills, T.A. Stress, social support and the buffering hypothesis. *Psychol Bull.* 1985;98:310–357.

66. House, J.S., Kessler, R., Herzog, A.R., Mero, R., Kinney, A., Breslow, M. Social stratification, age, and health. In: Scheie, K.W., Blazer, D., House, J.S., eds. *Aging, Health Behaviors, and Health Outcomes.* Hillsdale, NJ: Lawrence Erlbaum; 1991.

67. Ruberman, W., Weinblatt, E., Goldberg, J.D., Chaudhary, B.S. Psychosocial influences on mortality after myocardial infarction. *N Engl J Med.* 1984;34:552–559.

68. Folkman, S., Lazarus, R.S., Gruen, R.J., DeLongis, A. Appraisal, coping, health status, and psychological symptoms. *J Pers Soc Psychol.* 1986;50:571–579.

69. Rutter, M. Psychosocial resilience and protective mechanisms. *Am J Orthopsychiatry.* 1987;57:316–330.

70. Carney, R.M., Rich, M.W., Freedlan, K.E. et al. Major depressive disorder predicts cardiac events in patients with coronary artery disease. *Psychosom Med.* 1988; 50:627–633.

71. Booth-Kewley, S., Friedman, H.S. Psychological predictors of heart disease: a quantitative review. *Psychol Bull.* 1987;101:343–362.

72. Rodin, J., Langer, E. Long-term effects of a control-relevant intervention with the institutionalized aged. *J Pers Soc Psychol.* 1977;35:897–902.

73. Rodin, J. Aging and health: effects of the sense of control. *Science.* 1986;233:1271–1276.

74. Wilkinson, R.G. Income distribution and mortality: a 'natural' experiment. *Sociol Health Illness.* 1990; 12:391–412.

75. Wilkinson, R.G. Income distribution and life expectancy. *BMJ.* 1992;304:165–168.

"Where Crowded Humanity Suffers and Sickens": The Banes Family and Their Neighborhood

Laurie K. Abraham

∎

Robert Banes sat on the edge of his hospital bed, cradling his queasy stomach. A thin cotton gown hung on him like a sack. At five feet, eleven inches, Robert weighs only 137 pounds.

Robert's kidneys stopped functioning when he was twenty-seven. He received a transplant a year later, but his body rejected the new kidney after six years. Since then he has required dialysis treatments three times a week. Dialysis clears his body of the poisonous impurities that healthy people eliminate by urinating, but the treatments cannot completely restore his health, and Robert periodically spends a couple of days in the hospital. This time, he had been admitted to the University of Illinois Hospital because he had been urinating blood for a week, a problem that did not appear terribly serious to doctors but nonetheless had to be checked.

Feeling nauseated, Robert was not paying much attention to the game show that droned from his television. A nurse came in and stuck a thermometer in his mouth. Earlier in the day, Robert had undergone a cystoscopy, a procedure in which doctors put a miniaturized scope into his bladder to look for the source of his bleeding. He had not been told the results of the test, so he asked the nurse when his doctor would be stopping by. He also wanted to know how much longer he would have to stay in the hospital.

"You may have to go to surgery," the nurse said vaguely, flipping through his chart. A cloud passed briefly over Robert's face; the thought of surgery scared him, though he did not admit that to the nurse. Instead, he changed the subject.

"I guess I don't get dinner today," he said.

"You didn't get dinner?" she asked, surprised.

"I need some before I get sick."

"Don't do that," the nurse muttered as she walked out the door.

A minute later Robert hurried to the bathroom. "I was probably throwing up because I didn't have no food to push it down," he said, referring to the missed dinner. Robert returned to his bed and lay down, curling his knees into his stomach and pulling a blanket over his shivering body.

Four years before his kidneys failed, Robert was diagnosed with focal glomerulosclerosis, a progressive scarring of the kidneys that eventually destroys them. Focal glomerulosclerosis can be slowed though not cured, but Robert's disease went at its own destructive pace because he did not get medical treatment until his kidneys had reached the point of no return. None of Robert's low-paying, short-term jobs had provided health insurance, and he could not wriggle into any of the narrow categories of government-sponsored insurance, which are generally reserved for very poor mothers and children, the elderly, and the permanently disabled. In other words, Robert had not been poor-parent enough, old enough, or sick enough to get care.

The game show gave way to the news and a report about a "summer virus" that was infecting children. Robert frowned. He and his wife, Jackie, have two daughters and a son: eleven-year-old Latrice, four-year-old DeMarest, and one-year-old Brianna. "Don't tell me that," he sighed. That is Robert's typical response to bad news: he prefers to avoid it.

At the moment, however, Robert would not have minded a little bad news about his own condition. Since he had been admitted to the hospital on July 5, he had not been urinating as much blood, which frustrated him and Jackie. They felt he almost had to *prove* to doctors that he was sick.

Through his open door, Robert could see his wife arrive for an early evening visit. At five feet, ten inches, Jackie is only one inch shorter than her husband, but she weighs twenty pounds more than he does. When she smiles, her pretty, heart-shaped face gets full and round, captivating her baby daughter, who pokes at her cheeks and giggles, making Jackie giggle, too.

Jackie was not smiling that day, however. When she is in public, Jackie can look impassive, even defiant, though this vanishes when her curiosity gets the better of her. She walked slowly past the nursing station looking straight ahead, moving almost regally, her muscular thighs curving beneath her slacks. Next to her husband's brittle frame, Jackie stood like an oak.

She pulled up a chair next to the hospital bed, and Robert began to relay the sketchy medical update he had heard from the nurse. Jackie listened silently; then she responded in the way she sometimes does when she feels overwhelmed.

"I'm going away for a while," Jackie said coolly. "What are you all going to do without me?"

Robert did not reply. He knew, as she did, that she wasn't going anywhere; she was just letting off steam. Today had been her day to pay the bills, which she does in person since they are usually past due, and she had ridden the bus for hours in 90-degree heat.

Jackie told her husband to call home and tell Latrice to take some drumsticks out of the freezer for dinner. Jackie's invalid grandmother, with whom the family lives in one of Chicago's poorest neighborhoods, answered the phone, so Robert gave her the instructions instead. But a few minutes later Latrice called back because she was not sure her great-grandmother had heard the message correctly. In the way other children

might memorize their parents' work numbers, Latrice had memorized the phone number for the university hospital, as well as for Mount Sinai Hospital Medical Center, where her great-grandmother frequently had been hospitalized. Jackie repeated the dinner instructions and hung up the phone. "I need the bed," she said.

She began to empty the stuffed grocery bag she had carried into the hospital. It contained two new T-shirts, underwear, and socks for Robert, a day-old piece of cake from Brianna's first birthday, which he had missed, a can of Sprite, and a bunch of grapes.

The couple watched part of another game show and talked about a report they had heard about a family found murdered mysteriously on the bottom of a lake. This story came from one of the tabloid news programs, whose bizarre stories the family regularly discusses. Then Jackie called home again to check on the children, who were home with her grandmother. The call was not reassuring: one of them had dropped cake on the rug, the other two had stepped in it, and DeMarest reportedly was taunting his great-grandmother.

"I need you to stay in here over the weekend so I can get things straightened out," Jackie wearily told her husband. When one or the other of her sick family members are hospitalized, Jackie sometimes considers it a chance to regroup, to get things together before she has to start taking care of everyone again.

Before Jackie left, she filled the plastic grocery bag she had emptied earlier. From Robert's belated dinner, she took a wedge of leftover chocolate cake home for DeMarest. She took packets of low-salt French dressing, salt, and sugar that Robert had squirreled away from his meal trays, as well as a roll of medical tape left by a nurse. Jackie carefully folded the foil Brianna's birthday cake had been wrapped in and stashed that in her bag, too.

Then she gave Robert $5.00 to pay for his hospital TV, which cost $3.25 a day. Robert slowly walked Jackie to the elevator, past a dimly lit room where the floor's patients congregated. One of the patients, a man about Robert's age, had earlier informed Robert that he was scheduled for a second transplant the next day. He told Robert that he had rejected his first transplanted kidney because he drank a case of beer in one evening—the kind of story that, true or not, flies back and forth among kidney transplant patients.

"This is my wife, Jackie," Robert said to a middle-aged woman sitting on the edge of the day room, closest to where the couple walked. "Nice to meet you," the woman said. Jackie smiled wanly, heading for the door.

The University of Illinois Hospital is part of what is known as the Illinois Medical Center, a 560-acre area just west of the Loop, Chicago's downtown. The center has the highest concentration of hospital beds in the United States, some 3,000 among its four institutions.[1] In addition to the University of Illinois, there is Cook County Hospital, one of the best-known, last remaining, and, as the ancient edifice continues to crumble, most notorious public hospitals in the country, and Rush-Presbyterian-St. Luke's Medical Center, an institution that caters to those who, unlike Robert and Jackie, are privately insured. The Veterans Administration West Side Medical Center is also located there.

The medical and technological might of the complex contrast dramatically with the area around it. Just past the research buildings and acres of parking lots lie some of the sickest, most medically underserved neighborhoods in the city. Medical wastelands abut abundance in American cities because health care is treated as a commodity available to those who can afford it, rather than a public good, like education. Though public schools invariably are better in prosperous suburbs than in poor city neighborhoods, every state at least provides every child with a school to attend, no matter what her family's income. The country has not even come that

far with health care. Medicaid, the state and federal health insurance program intended for the poor, covers less than half of them, and much of the program is left to the states' discretion, so that a Southerner, for example, generally has to be poorer to receive Medicaid than a Northerner.

Even for those poor who manage to squeeze into Medicaid, the government's commitment to providing health care for them does not approach a commitment to equality. Just as education remains in practice separate and unequal, medical treatment for poor people with Medicaid or even Medicare (the government insurance for the elderly) is, in all but exceptional cases, conducted in a separate, second-rate environment.

The Banes family lives in the shadow of the Illinois Medical Center complex, twenty-five minutes southwest by way of the number 37 bus, which runs along Ogden Avenue. The street cuts diagonally across the city from the gentrified lakefront neighborhoods just north of the Loop to the bungalow enclaves of white ethnic suburbs that border Chicago on the southwest. Jackie and Robert live in between, on the West Side, the city's newest and poorest ghetto.

The streets were still lit by the late afternoon sun when Jackie climbed onto the bus for her trip home. Settling her bag on her lap, she fretted that doctors were going to release Robert before they figured out what was wrong with him. A person can only get so far with a "green card," she said, using the street name for the cards issued to families covered by Medicaid. "You need Palmer Courtland kind of money to get anywhere," she complained. Palmer Courtland is a self-made millionaire on "All My Children," a soap opera Jackie and Robert watch.

In addition to the hospitals and their services, programs in a clutch of other buildings near Ogden attempt to palliate what are often conditions born of poverty. There is the Illinois State Psychiatric Institute, the West Side Center for Disease Control, the Chicago Lighthouse for the Blind, and a bit further southwest, the Cook County Juvenile Court, which handles crimes by children, and those against them by their parents.

These buildings are strung along the Eisenhower Expressway, which zips from the booming Western suburbs into Chicago's downtown, whose dramatic growth in the past two decades has bypassed the West Side. Jackie rarely ventures into the Loop. From her perspective, the eight-lane highway is an escape route for the employees of the various hospitals and social service institutions, for people who do not carry poverty home with them in a plastic bag.

As Ogden turns more sharply to the west, it crosses into Jackie's neighborhood of North Lawndale, a name that carries the same ominous weight in Chicago as the South Bronx or Watts carry nationwide.[2] North Lawndale was the subject of a series in the *Chicago Tribune* in 1985 that examined the lives of the so-called underclass. Many people who work and live in North Lawndale were disturbed by what they thought was a distorted, overly negative picture of their neighborhood; the series' very name, "The American Millstone," is hated because it suggests a neighborhood that is no more than a burden to be cast off.

Jackie had never heard of the *Chicago Tribune* series; she reads the *Chicago Sun-Times,* whose pithy city coverage is preferred by poor Chicago blacks. Yet many of her observations of the neighborhood could have served as grist for the millstone.

"My auntie's building got burnt down," Jackie said matter-of-factly one day, pointing to an empty lot where her Aunt Nancy's apartment building used to stand. "Drug dealers moved in." The narrow lot is two lots away from the stone three-flat where Jackie grew up with her grandmother. The building has survived, though its balcony has disappeared and graffiti circles its porch columns. It is just a half-block away from

where the family lives today. Since she was eight, Jackie has only once moved from this block, and that was a short three miles north to live with Robert at his mother's house. Her dreams of a better life are circumscribed by the neighborhood. She talks about getting out, but out means a strip of stone and brick three-flats about four blocks west. "I've always liked it up in that area," she said. "It looks like the middle-class people lives up in there, especially during the summer. All the trees are green and everyone has grass. And the buildings look well kept. You can just tell it's homeowners." Her assessment is accurate—the homes are better tended—but it is hardly out of the neighborhood. The buildings there may be relative castles, but the moat protecting them from the drugs and violence that pervade North Lawndale is narrow enough to step across.

As the bus hissed and groaned up Ogden, it passed Mount Sinai Hospital, which lives the same hand-to-mouth existence as the poor blacks and Hispanics it serves. More than the University of Illinois, Mount Sinai is the Baneses' hospital. It is where Jackie's grandmother, Cora Jackson, had been repeatedly hospitalized because of complications from diabetes that eventually resulted in the amputation of her right leg. It's where Jackie's father was rushed after he suffered a stroke caused by high blood pressure. And on a happier note, it's where Jackie gave birth to Brianna a year ago.

At one time or another, the Baneses and Cora Jackson have sought (and not sought) health care in every way available to the poor. When uninsured—Robert, when his kidneys were deteriorating, and Jackie, when pregnant with Latrice—they delayed care, then went to Cook County Hospital. Later, when Jackie went on welfare, she and the children became eligible for Medicaid.

Meanwhile, some of Mrs. Jackson's medical bills were paid by Medicare, which covers the elderly and disabled, rich and poor alike. Robert also got Medicare but only after his kidneys stopped working. People with renal failure have special status under the program: they are the only group covered on the basis of their diagnosis and regardless of age or disability. Mrs. Jackson had been sporadically eligible for Medicaid, too, which she needed because Medicare does not pay for such important things as medications. Her Medicaid coverage had been fitful because she was enrolled in what is called the "spend-down" program. She qualified for Medicaid only during the months that her medical expenses were so high they forced her income to drop below a "medically needy" level set by the state. Notably, neither Mrs. Jackson, nor anyone else in the family, had ever been covered by private insurance.

Leaving Mount Sinai, the bus cut through Douglas Park, which spreads to the north and south of Ogden. Douglas and two other West Side parks were designed in 1870 as a system of "pleasure grounds" linked together by grand boulevards. Progressive reformers came to envision them as breathing spaces to provide respite from crowded tenements and other urban ills.[3] In its heyday from 1910 until 1930, when North Lawndale was populated by first- and second-generation Jews, bands gave free concerts on weekends, couples paddled rowboats on the lagoon just to the north of Ogden Avenue, and children swam in what was one of the city's first public swimming pools—which, with its baths, was considered as important for public hygiene as it was for recreation.

Except for the players and fans at soccer and baseball games, the park these days is barely dotted with people, a young Hispanic couple walking on a path on the south side of Ogden—the Hispanic side—or several dozen black children splashing in the lagoon to the north—the African-American side. Ogden is a dividing line between Hispanics and African Americans in North Lawndale, and the race line holds in the park as firmly as it does anywhere else in the neighborhood.

Though the park's glory has faded, it is the last piece of deliberately open land that Jackie passed on the Ogden bus. The rest of it consisted of a series of vacant lots, some of which run together for a block or more and which residents euphemistically call "prairies." As it was summer, some of the lots were covered with reedy grasses and weeds, frilly Queen Anne's lace, and deep brown stands of dock plant. Others were piled high with refuse—in one case, what looked like enough decaying furniture to fill an office. In another lot, a building had fallen in on itself, likely prey to the brick thieves who complete the destruction started when buildings are abandoned by landlords who can't afford their upkeep, then are stripped of sinks, stoves, and fixtures, and then finally picked apart, brick by brick. In still other lots, large fernlike weeds flourished, creating an urban jungle that suggests what a parish priest in a similar neighborhood in New Jersey called "panther beauty, beauty you don't want to mess with."[4]

As for the brick and stone two-flats, or old three-story apartment buildings still standing, it is often difficult to tell whether they are occupied or not. Rusty steel grates are locked across nearly every door, even those of the ubiquitous churches. Signs are hand painted and peeling, and since plywood is used to cover most street-level windows, even establishments that still do business have a boarded-up look.

Worse yet, dozens of storefronts have been reduced to gaping holes, outlined by shards of glass that form jagged frames for dark rooms of rubble. Only the foolhardy, or a drug addict desperate for a place to get high, would step inside.

The shrouded condition of the neighborhood unnerves Jackie. Even the local drugstore, whose windows are blocked with ugly, prehistoric stone, can seem foreboding. "You used to be able to see *in* the drugstore," Jackie complained. "Shoot, now you wonder if you get in somewhere, are you going to make it out safe?"

At one corner along the bus route, Jackie pointed to a currency exchange where several scraggly men clustered. "That's a hangout for IV-drug users," she observed with disgust, going on to tell about a nearby bar that peddled do-it-yourself packets for free-basing cocaine. Jackie had noticed the drug paraphernalia when she once stopped at the bar to change a dollar bill. "When I saw that, I told the man I'd skip the change," Jackie said proudly, comparing herself to Father George Clements, a local African-American priest who mounted a boycott against stores that sold drug-related products.

Currency exchanges, storefront churches, auto parts shops, liquor stores and taverns, hot dog stands, and a beauty shop or two are the only businesses left on Ogden, which used to be one of the city's major commercial streets. The largest establishment in the neighborhood, Lawndale Oldsmobile, closed more than two decades ago. Its windowless, graffitied shell has been a fixture in North Lawndale since Jackie was a child. By the time she and her grandmother moved to Chicago from Tupelo, Mississippi, in the early 1960s, the neighborhood was already in rapid decline. The Eastern European Jews who had settled the area in the early part of the century had virtually vanished by the mid-1950s, replaced by black migrants from the South. Driven by the changing nature of their businesses as well as the deteriorating neighborhood, North Lawndale's major companies fled soon after: Sears Roebuck, International Harvester, and Western Electric either departed or reduced the size of their operations. Today, the bruised and battered buildings along Ogden give sad testimony to North Lawndale's knockout blow: the ravaging riots that fol-

lowed Martin Luther King Jr.'s assassination in 1968. After that, most remaining middle-class blacks fled.

In 1960, Lawndale's population peaked at 125,000; by 1980, it had plummeted to 62,000; by the end of that decade, it fell to 47,000.[5] Statistics describing the economic status of the people who remain are discouraging: almost one of every two people is on welfare; three of every five potential workers are unemployed;[6] and three of every five families are headed by women,[7] whose earning power is, of course, significantly less than that of two-parent families.

Accompanying this kind of poverty is a shocking level of illness and disability that Jackie and her neighbors merely take for granted. Her husband's kidneys failed before he was thirty; her alcoholic father had a stroke because of uncontrolled high blood pressure at forty-eight; her Aunt Nancy, who helped her grandmother raise her, died from kidney failure complicated by cirrhosis when she was forty-three. Diabetes took her grandmother's leg, and blinded her great-aunt Eldora, who lives down the block.

Chicago's poor neighborhoods have always been its sickest. In 1890, a medical writer graphically described the conditions that were contributing to rampant disease among the city's immigrant industrial workers. "[Their] sole recourse usually is to the tenement where, heaped floor above floor, in a tainted atmosphere, or in low fetid hovels, amidst poverty, hunger and dirt, in foulness, want and crime, crowded humanity suffers, and sickens, and perishes; for the landlord here is also the airlord, the lord of sunlight; lord of all the primary conditions of life and living; and these are doled out for a price, failing which the wretched tenant is turned out to seek a habitation still more miserable."[8]

The diseases that killed in the nineteenth century lent themselves to such dramatic prose. They were the great epidemics, smallpox, cholera, and typhoid fever. Such bacteria-borne infectious diseases festered because of a water supply periodically tainted by sewage and were easily spread in the crowded living quarters of poor city neighborhoods. With the coming of better sanitation methods, which included reversing the flow of the Chicago River so that the city's sewage would be sent to southern Illinois and Missouri rather than into Lake Michigan, these epidemics were largely conquered, though other age-old communicable diseases such as tuberculosis, sexually transmitted diseases, and, recently, childhood measles, still disproportionately plague Chicago's poor.

One reason infectious diseases retain their foothold among the poor remains substandard housing, which is bad and getting worse in North Lawndale. A recent survey by an economic development group found that only 8 percent of the neighborhood's 8,937 buildings were in good to very good condition. The rest were abandoned, on the verge of collapse, or in need of repair.[9]

Dr. Arthur Jones has visited many of these decrepit buildings on house calls to patients too sick to make it into his clinic, which is located on Ogden almost directly behind Jackie's apartment. The clinic, Lawndale Christian Health Center, was founded by Dr. Jones and several other urban missionaries in 1984 and has succeeded, by most all accounts, at providing affordable and humane health care.

Dr. Jones told of one woman who was suffering a severe case of hives caused by an allergic reaction to her cat, yet repeatedly refused to get rid of the animal. "I really got kind of angry," Dr. Jones remembered, "and then she told me that if she got rid of the cat, there was nothing to protect her kids against rats." Another woman brought her two-year-old to the clinic with frostbite, so Dr. Jones dispatched his nurse practitioner to visit her home a block away from Jackie's. The nurse discovered icicles in the woman's apartment be-

cause the landlord had stopped providing heat. The stories go on, most involving landlords who cannot afford to keep up their buildings and tenants who cannot afford to leave them.

By these standards, the Baneses' apartment is in good shape. They have to contend with an occasional rat and wage a constant battle against roaches, but the landlord has kept the two-flat in decent repair; his sister lives on the first floor.

For the most part, the diseases that Jackie and her family live with are not characterized by sudden outbreaks but long, slow burns. As deadly infectious diseases have largely been eliminated or are easily cured—with the glaring exceptions of AIDS and now drug-resistant tuberculosis—chronic diseases have stepped into their wake, accounting for much of the death and disability among both rich and poor. The difference is that for affluent whites, diabetes, high blood pressure, heart disease, and the like are diseases of aging, while among poor blacks, they are more accurately called diseases of *middle*-aging.

In poor black neighborhoods on the West Side of Chicago, including North Lawndale, well over half of the population dies before the age of sixty-five, compared to a quarter of the residents of middle-class white Chicago neighborhoods.[10] Though they occur more often on the West Side, the three most common causes of premature mortality in the two areas would correspond—heart disease, diabetes, and high blood pressure—were it not for one fatal condition that increasingly is considered a major public health problem: homicide. It ranks sixth in the white neighborhoods but is the number two killer of West Siders under sixty-five.[11] Alcohol and drugs are the poisons that induce many of the West Side's deaths, whether from homicide or heart attack. Thirteen percent of fatalities in that part of the city are directly attributable to alcohol and drugs, four times the rate in white, middle-class neighborhoods.[12]

These statistics are not, of course, unique to Chicago. A study of premature mortality in Harlem showed that black men there were less likely to reach the age of sixty-five than men in Bangladesh.[13] "When sixty-seven people die in an earthquake in San Francisco, we call it a disaster and the President visits," said Dr. Harold Freeman, one of two Harlem Hospital Center physicians who conducted the study. "But here everyone is ignoring a chronic consistent disaster area, with many more people dying. And there is no question that things are getting worse."[14]

Though genetic differences still are occasionally cited in medical literature in order to explain disproportionate disease among blacks, nearly all health experts put most of the blame on poverty—and the lack of access to care and hardscrabble lifestyles that accompany it. The situation worsened during the mid-1980s when the gap in life expectancy between the two races began to widen for the first time in history. Blacks' life expectancy has been less than whites' for as long as health statistics have been gathered, though since the turn of the century both races have lived a little longer each year. But from 1985 to 1988, blacks' life expectancy declined each year while whites' continued to creep ahead.[15] In 1989, blacks regained some of the time they lost, when their life expectancy rose slightly, but only to the 1984 level of 69.7 years.[16]

The starkest contrast in longevity is between white and black men, largely because of spiraling rates of homicide and AIDS among minorities. DeMarest, who was born in 1985, can be expected to live for sixty-four years and ten months, whereas an average white boy born that year will live eight years longer.[17] Jackie knows her son's chances of living a long life are not good, but she does not spend much time brooding about the dangers that await him. For now, she keeps him close to home and hopes for the best.

When Jackie stepped down from the bus after visiting Robert at the hospital, it was late in the day; the sun was about level with her shoulders. As she waited to cross Ogden, she glanced back toward the city, where the 110-story Sears Tower was silhouetted against the blue sky. The tower had been a beacon to Jackie as a child. "That was one ambition me and my cousin used to have. We wanted to walk to the Sears Tower." They never made it past a local shopping strip.

Jackie proceeded across Ogden toward the back of her own stone and brick two-flat, which, fortunately, is about a half-block removed from the harsh four-lane street. Her second-floor back porch, where her children had been playing earlier, was now empty. They had gone inside, since they are under orders not to venture beyond the fifteen-square-feet of the porch. To help make sure they don't, Jackie locks a metal gate across the steps.

The day before Robert was hospitalized, the family had gathered on the porch to celebrate the Fourth of July. It was a normal holiday, normal at least for a family that resigns itself to sickness in the same way that other families resign themselves to being polite to an unwelcome guest.

Robert slumped in a chair, next to the grill, spatula propped up on his knee. His eyes were glassy and he looked more drained than usual. Suffering the side effects of whatever was causing him to urinate blood, he had not been eating well. The rest of the family welcomed the light breeze that cooled the porch, but Robert was shivering despite his long-sleeved sweatsuit.

While Robert listlessly tended the grill, Jackie tossed a salad in the kitchen, then mounded uncooked chicken, ribs, and hamburgers into a large aluminum roasting pan. She took the meat out to the porch for her husband to grill, but when she saw how tired he looked, she took over.

Jackie has not worked outside of her home since Latrice was little and does almost all of the cooking for the family. This pattern was established long ago, when Jackie was a young teen-ager living alone with her grandmother, whom she calls "Mom," or "Mama." By the time Mrs. Jackson got home from her job cooking and wait-ressing at a truck stop, she wanted no part of the kitchen, so Jackie began making dinner on week nights. "I became sort of like the Hazel in the family. Mom the hubby that go to work; I was the wife."

Jackie said she rather enjoyed being in charge at home, picking up after her grandmother, chid-ing her for tossing her bra and girdle over the shower-curtain rod when she came home from work. But Mrs. Jackson, who left for work at 5 A.M., was not moved by her granddaughter's re-quests to please, please put her clothes in her room. "I lay them where I take them off," Mrs. Jackson would tell Jackie. And that was the end of it.

Mrs. Jackson has never been one to waste words with her family, Jackie said, but as she has grown sicker, she has spoken less and less. The Fourth of July was no exception. While the rest of the family talked and listened to Latrice's porta-ble radio on the back porch, Mrs. Jackson sat qui-etly in her wheelchair in the front room, eating from a plate Jackie had fixed for her.

Mrs. Jackson's right leg was amputated in late April because of an infection. First, half of her foot had been removed in February, which doc-tors had hoped would obviate the need for fur-ther amputation. But after a month and a half of erratic outpatient care, Mrs. Jackson's condition worsened, and her leg had to be amputated, too. Like many diabetics, Mrs. Jackson suffers from peripheral vascular disease, a chronic illness that causes blood vessels to thicken and restricts the flow of blood so that infections cannot heal.

Though she wasn't saying much, Mrs. Jack-son looked fresh and more alert than she had recently. Wearing a red-and-white gingham dress, she sat up almost erect in her wheelchair, and when Brianna scuttled into the room, she watched her quizzically. Mrs. Jackson had to wait for the family's life to parade before her since she refused Jackie's offers to push her to the back porch. Several notes from hospital social workers in Mrs. Jackson's medical chart said the elderly woman worried about being a burden to her granddaughter; and perhaps that was part of the reason she chose to stay inside.

Then, too, getting the wheelchair through the kitchen to the back porch is something of a pro-duction. Jackie has to move the kitchen table and chairs, and even then, Mrs. Jackson's wheelchair barely fits through the narrow hallway connect-ing the living room and kitchen. The five-room apartment does not easily accommodate three children and three adults, especially since Mrs. Jackson began to require extra equipment such as a portable commode, a walker, and, of course, a wheelchair.

Mrs. Jackson's world had shrunk to include her bedroom and the front room that adjoined it. Emblems of her life cluttered her dark wood dresser. There were a dozen or more brown pill bottles, two Bibles, gauze pads and antiseptic spray, an unopened pack of Red Man chewing tobacco (for a habit she had acquired in Mis-sissippi), latex gloves, and a small photo album. A picture of Latrice in first grade was stuck in the dresser's mirror. A black patent leather handbag and two church hats, one a deep red knit with fur trim, the other decorated with large gold sequins, hung on its corner. The hats were getting dusty. Since Mrs. Jackson's leg was amputated, she had not been able to go to the First Baptist Church on Sundays, her favorite activity of the week. The situation was especially sad because she had not been a woman who spent much time at home, according to Jackie. "As long as I know this lady, she's been the get-up-and-go type. She has really been stripped of all her worldly duties." Jackie remembers her grandmother as her conduit to the outside world; she often boasts about Mrs. Jackson's legendary knowledge of bus routes.

"Mama used to show me this way, showed me that way; she got around." Though it is hard to imagine somebody being so stoic, Mrs. Jackson never complained about being homebound, Jackie said, or pined for fresh air and sunshine.

Back on the porch, it was relatively quiet, except when two fire trucks screamed out of the station behind the apartment. No trees or bushes grow on the small patch of dirt and weeds in the back yard the Baneses share with the tenant below, but a tree on the lot behind them provides some shield from the constant traffic on Ogden.

Robert perked up when his twenty-year-old half-sister Lativa and her boyfriend arrived. "See, he looks a lot better," Jackie said ruefully. "He gets tired of the same old faces."

The couple indeed brought a burst of vitality to the porch. Lativa was home on leave from the Army, and brought birthday presents for Brianna, whose first birthday was two days away, and for DeMarest, who would not turn five until after Lativa returned to her base in North Carolina.

After dinner, Jackie allowed Latrice and DeMarest to walk to a nearby liquor store to get snowcones, a favorite in the neighborhood. On sweltering summer days, adults and children drag folding chairs and coolers out to the curb and settle in. They pump red, blue, or green syrups into paper cones filled with scoops of chipped ice and sell them to passers-by. Latrice cherishes the rituals of holidays, including the trip for snowcones, so she made sure she and her brother honored the Fourth with their choices, blue-raspberry and watermelon flavors for Latrice, blue-raspberry and strawberry for DeMarest.

Munching on their snowcones as they walked home, the two children passed a narrow general store that was closed for the holiday. Its owner, Jim Downing, a tough sixty-year-old with the hard body of someone thirty years younger, sells a little bit of everything. Hand-painted signs propped outside his establishment hawk pecans,

extermination service (by Mr. Downing, who went to jail for several weeks for using dangerous, illegal chemicals), roach spray, and $39 burglar gates, one of which the Baneses bought and Mr. Downing mounted across their back door. Jackie does laundry in the two washing machines that are crammed into Mr. Downing's store, and Latrice comes here regularly to buy candy, or pick up soda or a gallon of milk for her mom. Mr. Downing tots up her charges on the back of a brown paper sack, testing Latrice's arithmetic as he goes. If the Baneses are running short of cash, he lets them run a tab.

Dessert and dinner finished, the family waited for darkness to fall, then went to the back yard to set off Roman candles and firecrackers that popped when Latrice or DeMarest flung them to the ground. During the night, Robert continued to urinate blood, and the next morning, he reported to the University of Illinois Hospital.

He went home after three days, on a Friday. Doctors told him to return the next Monday for surgery. The medical tests had revealed that the blood was coming from the stump of his rejected kidney, and they wanted to correct the problem. They called late that afternoon and told him they had changed their minds; they would wait to see if the bleeding cleared up on its own. It did.

Notes

1. Chicago and Cook County Health Care Summit, *Chicago and Cook County Health Care Action Plan: System Analysis and Design* (April 1990), ambulatory care chapter, p. 46.
2. Nicholas Lemann, "The Origins of the Underclass," *Atlantic Monthly,* June 1986, p. 36.
3. Chicago Park District and Chicago Public Library, special collections, *A Breath of Fresh Air: Chicago's Neighborhood Parks of the Progressive Reform Era, 1900–1925* (1989), p. 21.
4. The Rev. Michael Doyle's description of depressed South Camden, New Jersey, was included in an article by Wayne King, "Saving an Urban Wasteland," *New York Times,* 16 August 1991, p. B-2.

5. Chicago Department of Planning, *U.S. Census of Chicago: Race and Latino Statistics for Census Tracts Community Areas and City Wards: 1980, 1990* (February 1991), p. 71.

6. *Chicago Tribune* staff, *The American Millstone* (Chicago: Contemporary Books, 1986), p. 96.

7. Personal communication with Marie Bousfield, demographer for the Chicago Department of Planning, 1991. Figure based on calculations from the 1990 U.S. Census.

8. Thomas Bonner, *Medicine in Chicago 1850–1950* (Urbana: University of Illinois Press, 1991), pp. 20–21.

9. *Chicago Tribune* staff, *The American Millstone,* p. 258.

10. Chicago and Cook County Health Care Summit, Chicago and Cook County Health Care Action Plan, draft appendix, communities in need, pp. 1 and 4.

11. Chicago and Cook County Health Care Summit, Chicago and Cook County Health Care Action Plan, draft appendix, pp. 1 and 4.

12. Chicago Department of Health, *Communities Empowered to Prevent Alcohol and Drug Abuse Citywide Needs Assessment Report,* working draft (December 1991), appendix c, p. 71.

13. Colin McCord and Harold P. Freeman, "Excess Mortality in Harlem," *New England Journal of Medicine* 322, no. 3 (18 January 1990): 173–77.

14. Elisabeth Rosenthal, "Health Problems of Inner City Poor Reach Crisis Point," *New York Times,* 24 December 1990, p. 9.

15. Personal communication with Thomas Dunn, National Center for Health Statistics, vital statistics branch, January 1993.

16. Ibid.

17. Personal communication with Robert Armstrong, actuarial advisor, Division of Vital Statistics, National Center for Health Statistics, March 1993.

One Drop of Blood

Lawrence Wright

■

Washington in the millennial years is a city of warring racial and ethnic groups fighting for recognition, protection, and entitlements. This war has been fought throughout the second half of the twentieth century largely by black Americans. How much this contest has widened, how bitter it has turned, how complex and baffling it is, and how far-reaching its consequences are became evident in a series of congressional hearings that began last year in the obscure House Subcommittee on Census, Statistics, and Postal Personnel, which is chaired by Representative Thomas C. Sawyer, Democrat of Ohio, and concluded in November, 1993.

Although the Sawyer hearings were scarcely reported in the news and were sparsely attended even by other members of the subcommittee, with the exception of Representative Thomas E. Petri, Republican of Wisconsin, they opened what may become the most searching examination of racial questions in this country since the sixties. Related federal agency hearings, and meetings that will be held in Washington and other cities around the country to prepare for the 2000 census, are considering not only modifications of existing racial categories but also the larger question of whether it is proper for the government to classify people according to arbitrary distinctions of skin color and ancestry. This discussion arises at a time when profound de-bates are occurring in minority communities about the rightfulness of group entitlements, some government officials are questioning the usefulness of race data, and scientists are debat-ing whether race exists at all.

Tom Sawyer, forty-eight, a former English teacher and a former mayor of Akron, is now in his fourth term representing the Fourteenth Dis-trict of Ohio. It would be fair to say that neither the House Committee on Post Office and Civil Service nor the subcommittee that Sawyer chairs is the kind of assignment that members of Con-gress would willingly shed blood for. Indeed, the attitude of most elected officials in Washington toward the census is polite loathing, because it is the census, as much as any other force in the country, that determines their political futures. Congressional districts rise and fall with the shifting demography of the country, yet census matters rarely seize the front pages of home-town newspapers, except briefly, once every ten years. Much of the subcommittee's business has to do with addressing the safety concerns of postal workers and overseeing federal statistical mea-surements. The subcommittee has an additional responsibility: it reviews the executive branch's policy about which racial and ethnic groups should be officially recognized by the United States government.

"We are unique in this country in the way we describe and define race and ascribe to it charac-teristics that other cultures view very differ-ently," Sawyer, who is a friendly man with an open, boyish face and graying black hair, says. He points out that the country is in the midst of its most profound demographic shift since the eighteen-nineties—a time that opened "a period of the greatest immigration we have ever seen, whose numbers have not been matched until right now." A deluge of new Americans from every part of the world is overwhelming our tra-ditional racial distinctions, Sawyer believes.

"The categories themselves inevitably reflect the temporal bias of every age," he says. "That be-comes a problem when the nation itself is under-going deep and historic diversification."

Looming over the shoulder of Sawyer's sub-committee is the Office of Management and Bud-get, the federal agency that happens to be respon-sible for determining standard classifications of racial and ethnic data. Since 1977, those catego-ries have been set by O.M.B. Statistical Directive 15, which controls the racial and ethnic stan-dards on all federal forms and statistics. Direc-tive 15 acknowledges four general racial groups in the United States: American Indian or Alaskan Native; Asian or Pacific Islander; Black; and White. Directive 15 also breaks down ethnicity into Hispanic Origin and Not of Hispanic Origin. These categories, or versions of them, are present on enrollment forms for schoolchildren; on ap-plication forms for jobs, scholarships, loans, and mortgages; and, of course, on United States cen-sus forms. The categories ask that every Ameri-can fit himself or herself into one racial and one ethnic box. From this comes the information that is used to monitor and enforce civil-rights legis-lation, most notably the Voting Rights Act of 1965, but also a smorgasbord of set-asides and entitlements and affirmative-action programs. "The numbers drive the dollars," Sawyer ob-serves, repeating a well-worn Washington adage.

The truth of that statement was abundantly ev-ident in the hearings, in which a variety of racial and ethnic groups were bidding to increase their portions of the federal pot. The National Co-alition for an Accurate Count of Asian Pacific Americans lobbied to add Cambodians and Lao to the nine different nationalities already listed on the census forms under the heading of Asian or Pacific Islander. The National Council of La Raza proposed that Hispanics be considered a race, not just an ethnic group. The Arab Ameri-can Institute asked that persons from the Mid-dle East, now counted as white, be given a separate, protected category of their own. Senator Daniel K. Akaka, a Native Hawaiian, urged that his people be moved from the Asian or Pacific Islander box to the American Indian or Alaskan Native box. "There is the misperception that Native Hawaiians, who number well over two hundred thousand, somehow 'immigrated' to the United States like other Asian or Pacific Island groups," the Senator testified. "This leads to the erroneous impression that Native Hawaiians, the original inhabitants of the Hawaiian Islands, no longer exist." In the Senator's opinion, being placed in the same category as other Native Americans would help rectify that situation. (He did not mention that certain American Indian tribes enjoy privileges concerning gambling concessions that Native Hawaiians currently don't enjoy.) The National Congress of American Indians would like the Hawaiians to stay where they are. In every case, issues of money, but also of identity, are at stake.

In this battle over racial turf, a disturbing new contender has appeared. "When I received my 1990 census form, I realized that there was no race category for my children," Susan Graham, who is a white woman married to a black man in Roswell, Georgia, testified. "I called the Census Bureau. After checking with supervisors, the bureau finally gave me their answer: the children should take the race of their mother. When I objected and asked why my children should be classified as their mother's race only, the Census Bureau representative said to me, in a very hushed voice, 'Because, in cases like these, we always know who the mother is and not always the father.'"

Graham went on to say, "I could not make a race choice from the basic categories when I enrolled my son in kindergarten in Georgia. The only choice I had, like most other parents of multiracial children, was to leave race blank. I later found that my child's teacher was instructed to choose for him based on her knowledge and observation of my child. Ironically, my child has been white on the United States census, black at school, and multiracial at home—all at the same time."

Graham and others were asking that a "Multiracial" box be added to the racial categories specified by Directive 15—a proposal that alarmed representatives of the other racial groups for a number of reasons, not the least of which was that multiracialism threatened to undermine the concept of racial classification altogether.

According to various estimates, at least seventy-five to more than ninety per cent of the people who now check the Black box could check Multiracial, because of their mixed genetic heritage. If a certain proportion of those people—say, ten per cent—should elect to identify themselves as Multiracial, legislative districts in many parts of the country might need to be redrawn. The entire civil-rights regulatory program concerning housing, employment, and education would have to be reassessed. School-desegregation plans would be thrown into the air. Of course, it is possible that only a small number of Americans will elect to choose the Multiracial option, if it is offered, with little social effect. Merely placing such an option on the census invites people to consider choosing it, however. When the census listed "Cajun" as one of several examples under the ancestry question, the number of Cajuns jumped nearly two thousand per cent. To remind people of the possibility is to encourage enormous change.

Those who are charged with enforcing civil-rights laws see the Multiracial box as a wrecking ball aimed at affirmative action, and they hold those in the mixed-race movement responsible. "There's no concern on any of these people's part about the effect on policy—it's just a subjective feeling that their identity needs to be stroked," one government analyst said. "What they don't understand is that it's going to cost their own groups"—by losing the advantages that accrue to minorities by way of affirmative-action programs, for instance. Graham contends that the object of her movement is not to create another protected category. In any case, she said, multiracial people know "to check the right box to get the goodies."

Of course, races have been mixing in America since Columbus arrived. Visitors to Colonial America found plantation slaves who were as light-skinned as their masters. Patrick Henry actually proposed, in 1784, that the State of Virginia encourage intermarriage between whites and Indians, through the use of tax incentives and cash stipends. The legacy of this intermingling is that Americans who are descendants of early settlers, of slaves, or of Indians often have ancestors of different races in their family tree.

Thomas Jefferson supervised the original census, in 1790. The population then was broken down into free white males, free white females, other persons (these included free blacks and "taxable Indians," which meant those living in or around white settlements), and slaves. How unsettled this country has always been about its racial categories is evident in the fact that nearly every census since has measured race differently. For most of the nineteenth century, the census reflected an American obsession with miscegenation. The color of slaves was to be specified as "B," for black, and "M," for mulatto. In the 1890 census, gradations of mulattoes were further broken down into quadroons and octoroons. After 1920, however, the Census Bureau gave up on such distinctions, estimating that three-quarters of all blacks in the United States were racially mixed already, and that pure blacks would soon disappear. Henceforth anyone with any black ancestry at all would be counted simply as black.

Actual interracial marriages, however, were historically rare. Multiracial children were often marginalized as illegitimate half-breeds who didn't fit comfortably into any racial community.

This was particularly true of the offspring of black-white unions. "In my family, like many families with African-American ancestry, there is a history of multiracial offspring associated with rape and concubinage," G. Reginald Daniel, who teaches a course in multiracial identity at the University of California at Los Angeles, says. "I was reared in the segregationist South. Both sides of my family have been mixed for at least three generations. I struggled as a child over the question of why I had to exclude my East Indian and Irish and Native American and French ancestry, and could include only African."

Until recently, people like Daniel were identified simply as black because of a peculiarly American institution known informally as "the one-drop rule," which defines as black a person with as little as a single drop of "black blood." This notion derives from a long-discredited belief that each race had its own blood type, which was correlated with physical appearance and social behavior. The antebellum South promoted the rule as a way of enlarging the slave population with the children of slaveholders. By the nineteen-twenties, in Jim Crow America the one-drop rule was well established as the law of the land. It still is, according to a United States Supreme Court decision as late as 1986, which refused to review a lower court's ruling that a Louisiana woman whose great-great-great-great-grandmother had been the mistress of a French planter was black—even though that proportion of her ancestry amounted to no more than three thirty-seconds of her genetic heritage. "We are the only country in the world that applies the one-drop rule, and the only group that the one-drop rule applies to is people of African descent," Daniel observes.

People of mixed black-and-white ancestry were rejected by whites and found acceptance by blacks. Many of the most notable "black" leaders over the last century and a half were "white" to some extent, from Booker T. Washington and

Frederick Douglass (both of whom had white fathers) to W. E. B. Du Bois, Malcolm X, and Martin Luther King, Jr. (who had an Irish grandmother and some American Indian ancestry as well). The fact that Lani Guinier, Louis Farrakhan, and Virginia's former governor Douglas Wilder are defined as black, and define themselves that way, though they have light skin or "European" features, demonstrates how enduring the one-drop rule has proved to be in America, not only among whites but among blacks as well. Daniel sees this as "a double-edged sword." While the one-drop rule encouraged racism, it also galvanized the black community.

"But the one-drop rule is racist," Daniel says. "There's no way you can get away from the fact that it was historically implemented to create as many slaves as possible. No one leaped over to the white community—that was simply the mentality of the nation, and people of African descent internalized it. What this current discourse is about is lifting the lid of racial oppression in our institutions and letting people identify with the totality of their heritage. We have created a nightmare for human dignity. Multiracialism has the potential for undermining the very basis of racism, which is its categories."

But multiracialism introduces nightmares of its own. If people are to be counted as something other than completely black, for instance, how will affirmative-action programs be implemented? Suppose a court orders a city to hire additional black police officers to make up for past discrimination. Will mixed-race officers count? Will they count wholly or partly? Far from solving the problem of fragmented identities, multiracialism could open the door to fractional races, such as we already have in the case of the American Indians. In order to be eligible for certain federal benefits, such as housing-improvement programs, a person must prove that he or she either is a member of a federally recognized Indian tribe or has fifty per cent "In-dian blood." One can envision a situation in which nonwhiteness itself becomes the only valued quality, to be compensated in various ways depending on a person's pedigree.

Kwame Anthony Appiah, of Harvard's Philosophy and Afro-American Studies Departments, says, "What the Multiracial category aims for is not people of mixed ancestry, because a majority of Americans are actually products of mixed ancestry. This category goes after people who have parents who are socially recognized as belonging to different races. That's O.K.—that's an interesting social category. But then you have to ask what happens to their children. Do we want to have more boxes, depending upon whether they marry back into one group or the other? What are the children of these people supposed to say? I think about these things because—look, my mother is English; my father is Ghanaian. My sisters are married to a Nigerian and a Norwegian. I have nephews who range from blond-haired kids to very black kids. They are all first cousins. Now, according to the American scheme of things, they're all black—even the guy with blond hair who skis in Oslo. That's what the one-drop rule says. The Multiracial scheme, which is meant to solve anomalies, simply creates more anomalies of its own, and that's because the fundamental concept—that you should be able to assign every American to one of three or four races reliably—is crazy."

These are sentiments that Representative Sawyer agrees with profoundly. He says of the one-drop rule, "It is so embedded in our perception and policy, but it doesn't allow for the blurring that is the reality of our population. Just look at— What are the numbers?" he said in his congressional office as the leafed through a briefing book. "Thirty-eight per cent of American Japanese females and eighteen per cent of American Japanese males marry outside their traditional ethnic and nationality group. Seventy per cent of American Indians marry outside. I grant you that the enormous growth potential of multiracial marriages starts from a relatively small base, but the truth is it starts from a fiction to begin with; that is, what we think of as black-and-white marriages are not marriages between people who come from anything like a clearly defined ethnic, racial, or genetic base."

The United States Supreme Court struck down the last vestige of anti-miscegenation laws in 1967, in Loving v. Virginia. At that time, interracial marriages were rare; only sixty-five thousand marriages between blacks and whites were recorded in the 1970 census. Marriages between Asians and non-Asian Americans tended to be between soldiers and war brides. Since then, mixed marriages occurring between many racial and ethnic groups have risen to the point where they have eroded the distinctions between such peoples. Among American Indians, people are more likely to marry outside their group than within it, as Representative Sawyer noted. The number of children living in families where one parent is white and the other is black, Asian, or American Indian, to use one measure, has tripled—from fewer than four hundred thousand in 1970 to one and a half million in 1990—and this doesn't count the children of single parents or children whose parents are divorced.

Blacks are conspicuously less likely to marry outside their group, and yet marriages between blacks and whites have tripled in the last thirty years. Matthijs Kalmijn, a Dutch sociologist, analyzed marriage certificates filed in this country's non-Southern states since the Loving decision and found that in the nineteen-eighties the rate at which black men were marrying white women had reached approximately ten per cent. (The rate for black women marrying white men is about half that figure.) In the 1990 census, six per cent of black householders nationwide had non-black spouses—still a small percentage, but a significant one.

Multiracial people, because they are now both

unable and unwilling to be ignored, and because many of them refuse to be confined to traditional racial categories, inevitably undermine the entire concept of race as an irreducible difference between peoples. The continual modulation of racial differences in America is increasing the jumble created by centuries of ethnic intermarriage. The resulting dilemma is a profound one. If we choose to measure the mixing by counting people as Multiracial, we pull the teeth of the civil-rights laws. Are we ready for that? Is it even possible to make changes in the way we count Americans, given the legislative mandates already built into law? "I don't know," Sawyer concedes. "At this point, my purpose is not so much to alter the laws that underlie these kinds of questions as to raise the question of whether or not the way in which we currently define who we are reflects the reality of the nation we are and who we are becoming. If it does not, then the policies underlying the terms of measurement are doomed to be flawed. What you measure is what you get."

Science has put forward many different racial models, the most enduring being the division of humanity into three broad groupings: the Mongoloid, the Negroid, and the Caucasoid. An influential paper by Masatoshi Nei and Arun K. Roychoudhury, entitled "Gene Differences between Caucasian, Negro, and Japanese Populations," which appeared in Science, in 1972, found that the genetic variation among individuals from these racial groups was only slightly greater than the variation within the groups.

In 1965, the anthropologist Stanley Garn proposed hundreds, even thousands, of racial groups, which he saw as gene clusters separated by geography or culture, some with only minor variations between them. The paleontologist Stephen Jay Gould, for one, has proposed doing away with all racial classifications and identifying people by clines—regional divisions that are used to account for the diversity of snails and of songbirds, among many other species. In this Gould follows the anthropologist Ashley Montagu, who waged a lifelong campaign to rid science of the term "race" altogether and never used it except in quotation marks. Montagu would have substituted the term "ethnic group," which he believed carried less odious baggage.

Race, in the common understanding, draws upon differences not only of skin color and physical attributes but also of language, nationality, and religion. At times, we have counted as "races" different national groups, such as Mexicans and Filipinos. Some Asian Indians were counted as members of a "Hindu" race in the censuses from 1920 to 1940; then they became white for three decades. Racial categories are often used as ethnic intensifiers, with the aim of justifying the exploitation of one group by another. One can trace the ominous example of Jews in prewar Germany, who were counted as "Israelites," a religious group, until the Nazis came to power and turned them into a race. Mixtures of first- and second-degree Jewishness were distinguished, much as quadroons and octoroons had been in the United States. In fact, the Nazi experience ultimately caused a widespread reexamination of the idea of race. Canada dropped the race question from its census in 1951 and has so far resisted all attempts to reinstitute it. People who were working in the United States Bureau of the Census in the fifties and early sixties remember that there was speculation that the race question would soon be phased out in America as well. The American Civil Liberties Union tried to get the race question dropped from the census in 1960, and the State of New Jersey stopped entering race information on birth and death certificates in 1962 and 1963. In 1964, however, the architecture of civil-rights laws began to be erected, and many of the new laws—particularly the Voting Rights Act of 1965—required highly detailed information about minority participation which could be gathered only by the decennial census, the nation's supreme instrument for gathering demographic statistics. The expectation that the race question would wither away surrendered to the realization that race data were fundamental to monitoring and enforcing desegregation. The census soon acquired a political importance that it had never had in the past.

Unfortunately, the sloppiness and multiplicity of certain racial and ethnic categories rendered them practically meaningless for statistical purposes. In 1973, Caspar Weinberger, who was then Secretary of Health, Education and Welfare, asked the Federal Interagency Committee on Education (FICE) to develop some standards for classifying race and ethnicity. An ad-hoc committee sprang into being and proposed to create an intellectual grid that would sort all Americans into five racial and ethnic categories. The first category was American Indian or Alaskan Native. Some members of the committee wanted the category to be called Original Peoples of the Western Hemisphere, in order to include Indians of South American origin, but the distinction that this category was seeking was so-called "Federal Indians," who were eligible for government benefits; to include Indians of any other origin, even though they might be genetically quite similar, would confuse the collecting of data. To accommodate the various, highly diverse peoples who originated in the Far East, Southeast Asia, and the Pacific Islands, the committee proposed a category called Asian or Pacific Islander, thus sweeping into one massive basket Chinese, Samoans, Cambodians, Filipinos, and others—peoples who had little or nothing in common, and many of whom were, indeed, traditional enemies. The fact that American Indians and Alaskan Natives originated from the same Mongoloid stock as many of these peoples did not stop the committee from putting them in a separate racial category. Black was defined as "a person having origins in any of the black racial groups of Africa," and White, initially, as "a person having origins in any of the original peoples of Europe, North Africa, the Middle East, or the Indian subcontinent"—everybody else, in other words. Because the Black category contained anyone with any African heritage at all, the range of actual skin colors covered the entire spectrum, as did the White category, which included Arabs and Asian Indians and various other darker-skinned peoples.

The final classification, Hispanic, was the most problematic of all. In the 1960 census, people whose ancestry was Latin-American were counted as white. Then people of Spanish origin became a protected group, requiring the census to gather data in order to monitor their civil rights. But how to define them? People who spoke Spanish? Defining the population that way would have included millions of Americans who spoke the language but had no actual roots in Hispanic culture, and it excluded Brazilians and children of immigrants who were not taught Spanish in their homes. One approach was to count persons with Spanish surnames, but that created a number of difficulties: marriage made some non-Hispanic women into instant minorities, while stripping other women of their Hispanic status. The 1970 census inquired about people from "Central or South America," and more than a million people checked the box who were not Hispanic; they were from Kansas, Alabama, Mississippi—the central and southern United States, in other words.

The greatest dilemma was that there was no conceivable justification for calling Hispanics a race. There were black Hispanics from the Dominican Republic, Argentines who were almost entirely European whites, Mexicans who would have been counted as American Indians if they had been born north of the Rio Grande. The great preponderance of Hispanics are mestizos—a continuum of many different genetic backgrounds. Moreover, the fluid Latin-American concept of race differs from the rigid United States idea of biologically determined and highly distinct human divisions. In most Latin cultures, skin color is an individual variable—not a group marker—so that within the same family one sibling might be considered white and another black. By 1960, the United States census, which counts the population of Puerto Rico, gave up asking the race question on the island, because race did not carry the same distinction there that it did on the mainland. The ad-hoc committee decided to dodge riddles like these by calling Hispanics an ethnic group, not a race.

In 1977, O.M.B. Statistical Directive 15 adopted the FICE suggestions practically verbatim, with one principal exception: Asian Indians were moved to the Asian or Pacific Islander category. Thus, with little political discussion, the identities of Americans were fixed in five broad groupings. Those racial and ethnic categories that were dreamed up almost twenty years ago were not neutral in their effect. By attempting to provide a way for Americans to describe themselves, the categories actually began to shape those identities. The categories became political entities, with their own constituencies, lobbies, and vested interests. What was even more significant, they caused people to think of themselves in new ways—as members of "races" that were little more than statistical devices. In 1974, the year the ad-hoc committee set to work, few people referred to themselves as Hispanic; rather, people who fell into that grouping tended to identify themselves by nationality—Mexican or Dominican, for instance. Such small categories, however, are inconvenient for statistics and politics, and the creation of the meta-concept "Hispanic" has resulted in the formation of a peculiarly American group. "It is a mixture of ethnicity, culture, history, birth, and a presumption of language," Sawyer contends. Largely because of immigration, the Asian or Pacific Islander group is considered the fastest-growing racial group in the

United States, but it is a "racial" category that in all likelihood exists nowhere else in the world. The third-fastest-growing category is Other—made up of the nearly ten million people, most of them Hispanics, who refused to check any of the prescribed racial boxes. American Indian groups are also growing at a rate that far exceeds the growth of the population as a whole: from about half a million people in 1960 to nearly two million in 1990—a two-hundred-and-fifty-nine-per-cent increase, which was demographically impossible. It seemed to be accounted for by improvements in the census-taking procedure and also by the fact that Native Americans had become fashionable, and people now wished to identify with them. To make matters even more confounding, only seventy-four per cent of those who identified themselves as American Indian by race reported having Indian ancestry.

Whatever the word "race" may mean elsewhere in the world, or to the world of science, it is clear that in America the categories are arbitrary, confused, and hopelessly intermingled. In many cases, Americans don't know who they are, racially speaking. A National Center for Health Statistics study found that 5.8 per cent of the people who called themselves Black were seen as White by a census interviewer. Nearly a third of the people identifying themselves as Asian were classified as White or Black by independent observers. That was also true of seventy per cent of people who identified themselves as American Indians. Robert A. Hahn, an epidemiologist at the Centers for Disease Control and Prevention, analyzed deaths of infants born from 1983 through 1985. In an astounding number of cases, the infant had a different race on its death certificate from the one on its birth certificate, and this finding led to staggering increases in the infant-mortality rate for minority populations—46.9 per cent greater for American Indians, 48.8 per cent greater for Japanese-Americans, 78.7 per cent greater for Filipinos—over what had been previously recorded. Such disparities cast doubt on the dependability of race as a criterion for any statistical survey. "It seems to me that we have to go back and reevaluate the whole system," Hahn says. "We have to ask, 'What do these categories mean?' We are not talking about race in the way that geneticists might use the term, because we're not making any kind of biological assessment. It's closer to self-perceived membership in a population—which is essentially what ethnicity is." There are genetic variations in disease patterns, Hahn points out, and he goes on to say, "But these variations don't always correspond to so-called races. What's really important is, essentially, two things. One, people from different ancestral backgrounds have different behaviors—diets, ideas about what to do when you're sick—that lead them to different health statuses. Two, people are discriminated against because of other people's perception of who they are and how they should be treated. There's still a lot of discrimination in the health-care system."

Racial statistics do serve an important purpose in the monitoring and enforcement of civil-rights laws; indeed, that has become the main justification for such data. A routine example is the Home Mortgage Disclosure Act. Because of race questions on loan applications, the federal government has been able to document the continued practice of redlining by financial institutions. The Federal Reserve found that, for conventional mortgages, in 1992 the denial rate for blacks and Hispanics was roughly double the rate for whites. Hiring practices, jury selection, discriminatory housing patterns, apportionment of political power—in all these areas, and more, the government patrols society, armed with little more than statistical information to ensure equal and fair treatment. "We need these categories essentially to get rid of them," Hahn says.

The unwanted corollary of slotting people by race is that such officially sanctioned classifications may actually worsen racial strife. By creating social-welfare programs based on race rather than on need, the government sets citizens against one another precisely because of perceived racial differences. "It is not 'race' but a *practice* of racial classification that bedevils the society," writes Yehudi Webster, a sociologist at California State University, Los Angeles, and the author of "The Racialization of America." The use of racial statistics, he and others have argued, creates a reality of racial divisions, which then require solutions, such as busing, affirmative action, and multicultural education, all of which are bound to fail, because they heighten the racial awareness that leads to contention. Webster believes that adding a Multiracial box would be "another leap into absurdity," because it reinforces the concept of race in the first place. "In a way, it's a continuation of the one-drop principle. Anybody can say, 'I've got one drop of *something*—I must be multiracial.' It may be a good thing. It may finally convince Americans of the absurdity of racial classification."

In 1990, Itabari Njeri, who writes about interethnic relations for the Los Angeles *Times,* organized a symposium for the National Association of Black Journalists. She recounts a presentation given by Charles Stewart, a Democratic Party activist: "If you consider yourself black for political reasons, raise your hand." The vast majority raised their hands. When Stewart then asked how many people present believed they were of pure African descent, without any mixture, no one raised his hand. Stewart commented later, "If you advocate a category that includes people who are multiracial to the detriment of their black identification, you will replicate what you saw—an empty room. We cannot afford to have an empty room."

Njeri maintains that the social and economic gap between light-skinned blacks and dark-skinned blacks is as great as the gap between all blacks and all whites in America. If people of more obviously mixed backgrounds were to mi-grate to a Multiracial box, she says, they would be politically abandoning their former allies and the people who needed their help the most. Instead of draining the established categories of their influence, Njeri and others believe, it would be better to eliminate racial categories altogether.

That possibility is actually being discussed in the corridors of government. "It's quite strange—the original idea of O.M.B. Directive 15 has nothing to do with current efforts to 'define' race," says Sally Katzen, the director of the Office of Information and Regulatory Affairs at O.M.B., who has the onerous responsibility of making the final recommendation on revising the racial categories. "When O.M.B. got into the business of establishing categories, it was purely statistical, not programmatic—purely for the purpose of data gathering, not for defining or protecting different categories. It was certainly never meant to *define* a race." And yet for more than twenty years Directive 15 did exactly that, with relatively little outcry. "Recently, a question has been raised about the increasing number of multiracial children. I personally have received pictures of beautiful children who are part Asian and part black, or part American Indian and part Asian, with these letters saying, 'I don't want to check just one box. I don't want to deny part of my heritage.' It's very compelling."

This year, Katzen convened a new interagency committee to consider how races should be categorized, and even whether racial information should be sought at all. "To me it's *offensive*—because I think of the Holocaust—for someone to say what a Jew is," says Katzen. "I don't think a government agency should be defining racial and ethnic categories—that certainly was not what was ever intended by these standards."

Is it any accident that racial and ethnic categories should come under attack now, when being a member of a minority group brings certain advantages? The white colonizers of North America conquered the indigenous people, imported African slaves, brought in Asians as laborers and then excluded them with prejudicial immigration laws, and appropriated Mexican land and the people who were living on it. In short, the nonwhite population of America has historically been subjugated and treated as second-class citizens by the white majority. It is to redress the social and economic inequalities of our history that we have civil-rights laws and affirmative-action plans in the first place. Advocates of various racial and ethnic groups point out that many of the people now calling for a race-blind society are political conservatives, who may have an interest in undermining the advancement of non-whites in our society. Suddenly, the conservatives have adopted the language of integration, it seems, and the left-leaning racial-identity advocates have adopted the language of separatism. It amounts to a polar reversal of political rhetoric.

Jon Michael Spencer, a professor in the African and Afro-American Studies Curriculum at the University of North Carolina at Chapel Hill, recently wrote an article in *The Black Scholar* lamenting what he calls "the postmodern conspiracy to explode racial identity." The article ignited a passionate debate in the magazine over the nature and the future of race. Spencer believes that race is a useful metaphor for cultural and historical difference, because it permits a level of social cohesion among oppressed classes. "To relinquish the notion of race—even though it's a cruel hoax—at this particular time is to relinquish our fortress against the powers and principalities that still try to undermine us," he says. He sees the Multiracial box as politically damaging to "those who need to galvanize peoples around the racial idea of black."

There are some black cultural nationalists who might welcome the Multiracial category. "In terms of the African-American population, it could be very, very useful, because there is a need to clarify who is in and who is not," Molefi Kete Asante, who is the chairperson of the Department of African-American Studies at Temple University, says. "In fact, I would think they should go further than that—identify those people who are in interracial marriages."

Spencer, however, thinks that it might be better to eliminate racial categories altogether than to create an additional category that empties the others of meaning. "If you had who knows how many thousands or tens of thousands or millions of people claiming to be multiracial, you would lessen the number who are black," Spencer says. "There's no end in sight. There's no limit to which one can go in claiming to be multiracial. For instance, I happen to be very brown in complexion, but when I go to the continent of Africa, blacks and whites there claim that I would be 'colored' rather than black, which means that somewhere in my distant past—probably during the era of slavery—I could have one or more white ancestors. So does that mean that I, too, could check Multiracial? Certainly light-skinned black people might perhaps see this as a way out of being included among a despised racial group. The result could be the creation of another class of people, who are betwixt and between black and white."

Whatever comes out of this discussion, the nation is likely to engage in the most profound debate of racial questions in decades. "We recognize the importance of racial categories in correcting clear injustices under the law," Representative Sawyer says. "The dilemma we face is trying to assure the fundamental guarantees of equality of opportunity while at the same time recognizing that the populations themselves are changing as we seek to categorize them. It reaches the point where it becomes an absurd counting game. Part of the difficulty is that we are dealing with the illusion of precision. We wind up with precise counts of everybody in the country, and they are precisely wrong. They don't reflect who we are as a people. To be effective, the concepts of individual and group identity need to reflect not only who we have been but who we are becoming. The more these categories distort our perception of reality, the less useful they are. We act as if we knew what we're talking about when we talk about race, and we don't."

Gender and Health

The readings on gender and health begin with an article by Claire Horton, "Women Have Headaches, Men Have Backaches," which provides a case study for discussion about the intersection of biology and gender roles. Horton, a German anthropologist, draws a rich portrait of the different ways men and women in a small Appalachian community are expected to live, to get sick, and to recover. Her evidence is based on in-depth, intensive interviews and observations with a relatively small number of residents. This type of research is used to investigate social processes that would be impossible to study with a survey questionnaire. The results tell us a great deal about a case, or a small sample of people, but may not be representative of a larger population. What are we to make of "evidence" from such a study? Horton is making a strong statement about the importance of gender and gender roles for understanding the kinds of health problems that people experience. While her case may be persuasive, not all gender differences in health and illness are so obvious.

A very different view is provided in the excerpt from Bobbie Ann Mason's book, *Spence + Lila,* which describes Lila's experience with surgery for breast cancer. Her apparently unemotional reaction to the news and the surgical procedure is in sharp contrast to that of her grown daughters, who are outspoken in their concern and aggressively protective in their interactions with Lila's health care providers. Several connections to readings from part I can be made—to cancer patients in the Balshem and the Mathews et al. articles, as well as to the woman featured in the Cassell essay. Taken together, these stories illuminate the ways in which gender, social class, and age all affect the way illness is experienced.

The short story by Doris Betts is a fictional account of one woman's experience caring for her husband's disabled brother. Both the Betts story and the excerpt from *Spence + Lila* point to the particular role of women as caregivers. In Mason's story, Lila's daughters engage their mother's physician in a rather combative relationship. In Betts's story, the family is portrayed as a uniquely powerful web of choices, relationship, roles, and memories. The obligation of family members to carry on the care-taking role is a theme in the next section as well.

Women Have Headaches, Men Have Backaches: Patterns of Illness in an Appalachian Community
Claire F. Horton

■

This is a study of psychosocial health phenomena observed in a small town and its adjacent rural households in southern West Virginia. The focus of the study stems from an investigation proposed by the Marshall University School of Medicine, Department of Family and Community Health, in Huntington, West Virginia. The anomalies under study were the presenting complaints of incapacitating backaches among the men and headaches among the women who sought care at a local health clinic. The symptoms of the women with headache did not conform to the more readily understood patterns such as true migraine and psychosomatic presenting problems, and many of the men appeared to have symptoms with few objective signs or clinical evidence of pathology.

The thesis of this paper is that this sexually disparate pain and disability syndrome is psychosocial rather the intrinsically medical. The men have backaches, the women have headaches. How could this be? Some of the answers to the question may be found in economics and in the local values determined by the religious beliefs and morals. There may be many other contributory factors to be traced, and it is certainly possible that analogues of similar phenomena may occur in a variety of other settings.

The town and farm setting under consideration

is classified as "Appalachian." There are many ways of defining the term. This group of Appalachian people has its own ethno-classification and collective self-image. In speaking of themselves, both men and women use descriptions of themselves such as "mountain people" and they say "goodchristianpeople," and "goodchristianwomen." The syllables of the latter are rapidly run together, making three words good and christian and women sound as one word. The evaluation "goodchristianwoman" is heard constantly and is a special term of respect. The "goodchristian" description is not so frequently applied to men. This would suggest a social and sexual differential in many values and behavioral norms. The belief system and its morals relate sickness to good and evil. Suffering may be seen as punishment or as a divine means of character-building. Physical pain and psychological stress are to be endured. Sometimes faith can heal. A social-sexual dichotomy emerges in the general forms, not only of behavioral norms, but also in physical affliction: "Men and women get taken different."

The research method of this essay has not been rigorously controlled. The research has, however, been undertaken in much greater depth than an ordinary reconnaissance or trial pretest. An invitation to participate in the project to do research as an anthropologist resulted in numerous visits with members of the community over the past year. The rural health clinic and the staff personnel were sympathetic to the research undertaking. Certain perplexing, medically atypical cases among the clinic clientele were discussed. All of them included headache or backache complaints. These patients were invited to cooperate by giving interviews and to contribute their time to the study.

Home interviews using open-ended questions were undertaken. Fourteen women and ten men cooperated and gave generously of their time. Interviews lasted four to seven hours each. There were also numerous conversations with husband and wife together. Spousal evaluations of each other were illuminating. In addition, in order to obtain an anthropological overview of the community, special activities were undertaken. These included visits to schools, church services, community activities and interviews with members of the business and professional community.

This general setting is the background for the pursuit of explanations of the sexually dichotomized question: why do men have backaches and women have headaches? Could it be a genetic sex-linked trait? Could it be a diet differential? An economic phenomenon? Conversion hysteria divided by gender? An expression of stress? While the biogenic elements may factor in the dual syndrome, given the physical male-female dimorphism, the social factors appear to be the more probable causation. In Appalachia it is a cultural norm that men should do the work requiring muscular strength, and that women should devote their energies to the care and socialization of the children they produce. One social worker exclaimed ruefully, "The women are *only* breeding housewives." This is how it appears to an outsider. To one who has become an accepted friend, albeit from the outside, the image of the woman becomes one of a realistic, sound, good person. There may be negatives, of course, but the positive attributes of the "goodchristianwoman" are the expectation. Then why the headaches?

The headache is mentioned in muted tones commonly associated with mourning death. If talking with an outsider, women refer to the headache as "migraine." Men refer to the phenomenon as "sick headache." With few exceptions the headache is considered to be a female affliction. THE headache is but one of many tribulations that plagued the 14 women in this study. The goodchristianwomen are expected to endure not only headaches, but all hardships uncomplainingly, inexhaustibly [1]. The husband may be a neglectful "sorry" sort, but must be respected in public. No matter how many undisciplined, noisily demanding children compete for attention, the mothers respond positively. Women maintain a soft voice and pleasant speech. Hardworking, the goodchristianwomen have been socialized to be boundlessly forebearing, endlessly forgiving. Complaint, even the mildest protest when fatigued or when harassed by their families, is not a cultural option [2]. Anger is denied. They tend to turn their resentment inward and blame themselves.

Library research has yielded information about the incidence and prevalence of the headache and backache problems, and has offered some excellent theoretical interpretations of mechanisms and social dynamics involved. The library resources also had useful data about Appalachia in general, and some specific local information about the political and economic history of the area. West Virginia is the only state which is entirely classified politically as Appalachian. Much of the contemporary Appalachian conditions can be traced to historical antecedents.

After the discovery of the Cumberland Gap in 1750, the western lands were first opened to settlement. Scots-Irish and English were among the earliest to populate these heavily forested hills. After 1830, new alternative mountain routes deflected immigration westward. This sealed off these earlier settlers, culturally as well as geographically. The isolated communities maintained a cultural continuum until the turn of the century when the lumbering industry "invaded" the seclusion. The timbermen included diverse ethnic elements. Local communities accepted a few of the newcomers who wished to remain, sometimes to marry and to become part of the resident population. A matrifocal social structure effected the cultural absorption of the newcomers. To a lesser extent this was true when industrial coal mining began in the 1920s [3–6].

The tenacity of many characteristics of the past

century in this area is sometimes surprising. The slowly changing culture is full of residual traits and material relics that evoke a romantic nostalgia in many observers [7]. Contrariwise, there is an equally distorted perception of the culture among outsiders: ignorant, ragged, lazy, filthy, hard-drinking hillbillies. Actually, the population consists of a wide gamut of socioeconomic types and personalities [8–10]. It is safe to generalize and say that they are preponderantly good, solid citizens. Some of their members do indeed break laws. The society, however, condemns lawlessness. The culture heroes continue to be frontiersmen Daniel Boone and Davy Crockett [11]. The daring, adventuring man goes forth, the woman keeps the hearth, nurtures the values and maintains the morals. This makes for conservative cultural bonding.

Pearsall wrote in 1966 "Old values remained, but not the means to achieve them" [12]. During the intervening years since this was written there have been massive world changes. Inevitably, some small changes took place in the town, and fewer occurred in the farming environs where the study was undertaken. Two or three computers have been installed. There have been some changes in social relations. There is no longer a pattern of courtship at home. The adults are deeply concerned about "sinful lust." Most mothers dread the possibility of pregnancy in their nubile daughters, but youngsters are encouraged to date and select their mates. Teen-age marriages continue to be the norm, but this is slowly changing. Some young girls now want more education rather than marrying immediately after graduating from high school. Young married women and adolescents are permitted to take jobs without being censured as "floozies." But there are still only two types of females: goodchristianwomen and floozies.

The bible and conservative protestants are the foundation of morals and norms. The members of the more expressive church groups also have consonant views and standards [13]. It is the church, the collective of beliefs and values of the residents, which sets the expectations of proper behavior, duties, obligations and responsibilities, and which limits the bounds of tolerance [14]. The biblical precept of being a "separate people" is clearly understood. The community is not scripturally "fervent" in welcoming strangers. However, they can be very hospitable when they feel comfortable about receiving outsiders. These are very old, deeply rooted value patterns.

There are some perceptible changes in institutionalized religion and morals. An example of such change is seen in an increasing condemnation of home distilleries because of the rising alcoholism in youth. There seems to be a shift in attitudes which sets apart the conventional fundamentalist churches of established denominations vis-à-vis the Holy Rollers, which include the Pentacostals and Holy Ghost congregations. In past times the religious exhuberance was more compartmentalized in events such as camp meetings and revivals. The old time religion continues to flourish with certain modifications. And the solid values of the belief system extend beyond the church. Under this rubric come patriotism, regional loyalty, and the right for men to provide for their families and perhaps to improve their education and life style.

Despite the technological and economic changes, the social organization is still built around the family. The cohesiveness extends throughout the community. Family poverty is increasing: 20% of the population is on welfare [15]. Social Security is a major factor in the economy. There is a decline in the returns from small farming [16] and small merchandising. Road maintenance and other services have suffered from lack of adequate funding. Appalachia has always known poverty [17], but the general rise in American standards and the heightening of communication has sharpened the awareness of problems. The realization of the contrast between the affluent lives portrayed on television and their own impoverishment has been distressing. In their need, many have resorted to kin for ego support and socio-psychological survival.

From these summary statements it is obvious that the dominant systems in the social structure are family and religion. The family and the belief systems are at the core of the psychosocial factors which may be operative in health care.

People regard headaches as just one more burden to be denied, endured, suppressed or treated by home remedies [18]. But if the sufferer vomits, head pain becomes THE headache. Women can permit themselves to be quiescent, on bedrest, for a day or two. Ordinarily, this would be considered gross self-indulgence since women expect and are expected to be ceaselessly active. However, in local ethnomedical lore, vomiting and/or hospitalization validate women's assumption of a uniquely replete sick role. Their privileges include: passivity—"all that rest," family cosseting—"all that visiting" and lavish provisions—"all that food."

Of the 14 women interviewed concerning their experiences with THE headache, 7 had been hospitalized for surgery on at least three occasions; 3 had experienced 10 operations. Since the age of 30, all the women had undergone a succession of surgeries classified as the "Big Three": thyroidectomy, cholecystectomy and hysterectomy. The cholecystectomy was usually the first of the series of attempts to alleviate "stomach pains" and also to relieve their "nervousness." Since this procedure failed to provide permanent relief, they returned for hospitalization, after a 2–3 year interval, usually for a thyroidectomy. About 2 years later, a hysterectomy was performed. Subsequently, adhesions were detected. Later various lingering stubborn stomach pains required biennial admissions for diagnostic surgical action requiring 2-week hospitalizations.

Although detailed information concerning

their headaches was more difficult to elicit, hospitalization experiences were discussed readily. Rather than a hardship, the patients seemed to regard this painful 2-year surgical cycle as a "vacation from life," "doing nothing but watching color TV," surrounded by children and the large maternal family and even visited by their minister. An elderly informant succinctly summed it up: "bein' fed, in bed, 'nuff said."

Moreover, three of the women were anticipating future periodic "vacations" for exploratory operations, since they had "paid their dues," anatomically speaking and were "entitled" to subsequent hospital stays.

The ill and their families are plentifully provided for with food offerings from wives' devoted kith and kin. Realizing that their family is being cared for, invalids are freed from all responsibilities of the day. They need take no thought for the morrow, because when they emerge from the sickroom, they will find their homes immaculate, their children attended, their larders replenished and dinners prepared for the next 2 days. When Appalachian women care for the sick, they "don't fool around," but do "mean business." The female kin and community members who rally around the "really sick" women are firmly bound together in a reciprocal network [18]. The extensive system involved in the care of chronic illness is not extended to childbirth. They believe that parturition is a family affair, and that giving birth is a short intensive "job" rather than an illness. "Birthing" is regarded as a natural process that satisfies a deep human need and brings the reward of children.

Advent of children prompts strengthening of family ties in the community, and particularly in the church. After the birth of their first child, many teen-age mothers assume a more actively devout role in their fundamentalist churches. Various positive cultural rewards spur their religious involvement, such as enhanced status in both family and community. Re-

ligious observance is a wifely obligation [19], but church attendance provides a benevolent infinitely accommodating support group. Some young women do not appreciate these social benefits until they have been absent from church for a prodigal period. Then they suffer from social isolation caused by the rigid gender segregation in the community. They complain about the paucity of female associational groups, and about the virtual absence of alternative role strategies for women. Finally, these women have the burden of full-time child care for which they are assigned almost total responsibility [20]. If and when these "lost ones" "return to the fold" (church), they will find the goodchristianwomen eager to join in their penitent prayers for spiritual guidance and blessing.

The fundamentalist churches reinforce the socialization process begun in the young mother's parental home, and preachers deliver sermons repeating what mothers teach their daughters by precept and example [21]. They are expected to "give and forgive" and to have no individual goals apart from their spouses' wishes. As goodchristianwomen they are urged to be enduring, submissive and subordinate to their men. By example they are to be so charitable, so forbearing that the most shiftless obdurate husbands will be brought into the christian fold in answer to their wives' prayers and by their pious examples. Observing young womens' struggles to fulfill this mission, the church members sweetly and sturdily champion long-suffering wives whose marriages are turbulent and distressing. But on no account will the goodchristianpeople countenance the dissolution of the family unit. They hold women responsible for family cohesion and continuity. Mothers must be the mortar of their marriage.

The husband is the product of the same family situation that socialized the bride. His own upbringing, however, included hero models of successful young married men who seem to pay very little attention to home and family. The stereotype of the strong silent man is approved. They invariably refer to the fathers as "my daddy." The fathers were the authoritarians in the family, contrasting with mothers who acted, of course, as goodchristianwomen. Men portray sisters as well as mothers as controlled and unthreatening. In keeping with the child-rearing practices prevailing in this area of Appalachia, these men were raised in remarkably permissive homes. Their older brothers, sisters, cousins and the entire extended family lavishly indulged them when they were very young. Neighbors, church members, "ate us up. As young boys we could do pretty much as we liked. At home we had plenty of good healthy food" and "candy was always around."

Looff has described the rich dependency gratification [22]. He concluded that he found while such abundantly indulged children could relate readily to outsiders with warmth and trust, often this warmth was combined with wild, impulsive, aggressive behavior [23]. This seeming anomaly may result from the combination of the indulgence with frequent, severe, arbitrarily administered physical punishment. On the whole, however, the permissiveness is pervasive, and the incidence of the harsh, sometimes cruel words and whippings is brief. For example poor rural parents finding themselves in a public situation where "upper class" people can witness their children misbehaving are likely to issue abrupt commands and demand instant obedience. Some trivial act can precipitate heavy-handed chastisement. An example of this: "Go pick up that peanut shell." Any hesitation in complying with the order may result in a forceful beating. In an observed incident, a stern-faced but impassive father ordered his boy to "get another napkin." The youngster paused, and the father seized him by the arm and struck him repeatedly with resounding force. Onlookers turned away uncomfortably, but without disapproval. One man, about 35, recalled, "Mostly my parents were easy. But if my father used 'that voice,' I didn't know what was wanted, only that I do—something—right now." Parents impose the strictest conformity on their children because they dread community censure. A pervasive sense of inferiority causes parents to switch from the easy atmosphere in the household to an unexpected authoritarianism in public. Consequently the children learn a quick submission to peremptory demands.

Another example of glaring inconsistency was offered by one of the informants interviewed. In his case, the parents provided abundant sweets to him and his siblings. A school teacher called the family's attention to severe dental decay and explained that this was a result of eating excessive amounts of sugars. The father looked at him and fumed, "I told you not to eat all that candy." This man, when he was a child, felt accountable for his parent's permissiveness.

Gratification of a sweet tooth is rewarding and fosters a form of expectation and dependency in boys and girls alike. The parents' teaching makes clear the areas of mutual indulgence and the area of sex difference in behavior and rewards. Fathers carry their sons in their arms a little more than they do their daughters. Obviously the gender of the children is established by clothes. The boy also gets toys and presents which differ from the girl's gifts. The parental voices change when they are talking about or to an infant boy or girl. How soon the baby notices this is debatable. However, from the time he can stand or walk, the male baby is subject to different parental action sets at home. When he starts walking, older male relatives begin to involve him in kinetic models of aggression, making mock threatening gestures toward him and encouraging reciprocal punches. The child is questioned and falsely accused of faults such as being "mean" or "bad." Little boys set their solemn faces toward their accusers and strike back somewhat uncertainly. By contrast, little girls are picked up and hugged more frequently, especially by maternal kin. The boys are taught to protect their "poor little sister."

At the age of 3 a little boy receives a baseball cap from his father or surrogate patrikin. This is their universal symbol of changing status from "baby" to "boy." The cap is a statement that he will become an outdoor type, and will participate in team sports. All his male kin encourage him to "play hard, play rough." The boy also learns that he does not have to perform demeaning household work. This is generally recognized by the age of 5.

By the time they are 7 years old, many young males will have received their first rifles and will be taught to shoot "like Daniel Boone." Squirrels are their earliest targets, as squirrel hunting is an important economic activity in this area. By the age of 9, good marksmanship is obligatory, especially so if they accompany male kin on hunting trips.

An authentic expensive "whittling jacknife" is a ritual birthday gift for 9-year-old boys. This is in preparation for a favorite activity of older, "loafering" male gatherings. By this age, too, most boys have become the "spitting image" of their tobacco-chewing elders. In imitation, the boys assertively spew huge gobs of spit, especially in public places. Spitting symbolizes authority, masculinity and sexual prowess. Even marital intentions are declared by a unique spitting ritual as courting couples stroll together; the future bride conscientiously holds up an empty Coke can for the convenience of her expectorating betrothed. With spitting, technique counts: men who can spit the farthest win prestigious prizes at local county fairs. Championship does not correlate with age. Some youngsters whose voices are still changing make a good showing.

School attendance until the age of 16 is the law. Education for boys has a very low priority [24]. Traditionally children dropped out of school to help out on the farm [25]. At present any work that needs to be done, or a special so-cial activity, or even a child's declaration "he just didn't want to go to school today" is accepted as a reasonable excuse for truancy.

The boys whose voices have begun to change start to show a reluctance to go to church. This is one of the first moves toward breaking away from their mother's authority. Men and women do not sit together during church service [26]. The mother keeps the children with her [27]. Pubescent males shift from their mother's section to merge with a peer group on the men's side of the church. Subsequently, many of these boys cluster about male gatherings in the churchyard [28]. With time, they stop going to church with regularity. Initially, their mothers protest this insurgency, then yield, leaving their sons to the world of men and the "good old boys."

The "good old boys" are the explicitly designated reference group of most country boys. Baseball is the game the males play most. Every male is expected to play with spirit. Non-players should watch and cheer. Successful baseball and football players are considered ideal types to become high school principals. Sports serve as a ladder to opportunity.

While many American youths aspire to drive a sports car by their sixteenth birthday, country boys yearn for a "quarter-ton," which is a pick-up truck. The vehicle, however, is not an ordinary "stock job." It must be customized, equipped with special chrome stripping, painted in loud colors with creative decoration. Another option is special racing tires. The trucks are used to drive to work, to baseball games and to hunting and fishing preserves. The vehicle is more than stylized transportation. The community expects young fellows to be different and allows them full expression of their individuality through the medium of the truck.

The ideal image of the "good old boy" is a good-looking, powerful, athletic, hard-working man. The "good old boy" status is sometimes maintained into the late twenties. The number of young men trying to sustain this role diminishes. They are worn down by hard work, hard living and heavier family responsibilities. A 30-year-old "good old boy" cannot begin to compete with a 17-year-old "good old boy." Fighting is the best way to settle disagreements. The men in the age range of 18–22 years seem to combine the best method of muscle, experience and "streetwise" aggression. They are greatly admired and are called "mean" and "mean as a snake." A "mean old guy" over 30 may even be a recipient of disability compensation and may be able to assert his manhood by starting an argument or starting a fight—assailing his antagonist—only to be pulled away from combat by friends who will then carry on the fight. Mere words are counterproductive, action settles things and gets things done [29, 30].

There is no fighting to speak of on the job. The grim business of earning money to support the family is compartmentalized and is external to "home" milieu. It is in the work place of employment that men develop their crippling "pain in the cupplings" (backaches). They do experience headaches which are described as exceedingly painful, but as "different from the sick headache" which afflicts women. The men's headaches are explained by "that awful air in the mine . . . can't hardly breathe" or by "that terrible noise of the saws and machines—can't hear yourself think." Women's headaches are mysterious and inexplicable.

As the headache is to women, low back pain is to men. All of the men interviewed have low backaches which they claim incapacitate them. All have received disability compensation for a work related injury, incurred during their employment in one of the heavy industries: mining, lumbering or glass. Although their workers' compensation temporary disability benefits have been terminated, these men have refused to enroll in the state-provided vocational training programs that would prepare them for different, less

physically demanding work. In their view, a painful back condition is permanently and totally disabling, rendering them incapable of ever performing any work. Thus, when these claimants refuse all offers of alternative types of work, their behavior is regarded by those in authority as incomprehensible if not intransigent.

These patients have assumed that they *are* disabled. To many observers, their pain appears to be relatively mild. But the impression remains that while these descriptions might be exaggerated, they are usually honest. One reason might be that there is a difference of perception about injury between the general society and in this special cultural pocket. In rural West Virginia, the individual who has injured a hand, foot, eye, or even suffers what, to the larger society, would be considered minor damage, he is viewed as totally and permanently incapacitated. Partializing or compartmentalizing of the body part affected so that the person may proceed with work activities is simply not credible. Nor is vocational rehabilitation considered to be a viable alternative for the victim is no longer expected to be required to work. He has been, so to speak, "honorably discharged" from the labor front.

In this area of Appalachia, disability is not experienced as it would be in the general middle-class United States, as a sharp insulting surprise. Disability is not only inevitable, but it inevitably accompanies age. As one informant explained, that it is not a matter of "if" you'll be crippled, only "when." Human bodies, "poor flesh at best," are not presumed to function well, especially as they grow older. An invading set of ailments— "arthuritis" (arthritis), "sugar" (diabetes), "high-blood" (hypertension) are expected by the age of 40. As with injuries, these unavoidable disorders are judged to be irremediable and irreversible. Even fit, healthy, hard-working young males are resigned to being "past it" by their thirtieth birthday.

This belief concerning this aging health condition is not unique in rural, lower class Appalachia. Rainwater notes the pessimism of the lower class persons in his study who are resigned to an aging process that will leave them functionally impaired by their thirties [32]. Although they are apprehensive of illness, he discovered that the individuals rarely organized their lives around sickness [33]. In contrast, Appalachians in this West Virginia county do. Moreover, they define both disability and the disability role differently [34].

These Appalachians hold that kin, kith, church and community are personally and morally accountable for the maintenance of the sick and disabled [35]. The goodchristian must minister unstintingly to ailing fellow church members and neighbors. Prayers are offered for their recovery at school meetings, public picnics, and at most public gatherings. Even at old country music shows, there will be a pause during the performance to pray for the "sick and the shut-ins."

Goodchristianmembers are also fearful that failure to be supportive will cause the community to perceive them as selfish and "cruelhearted." The community deplores interviewers for the Department of Human Services as gratuitously "cruel." Since Christian responsibility toward the ill is so manifestly clear, the social worker who fails to distribute funds to godfearing recipients is "iniquitous." One woman fumed, "there must be a special place in hell for the likes of spiteful people like them."

There is an unconditional compassion for the disabled. Certain behavior, however, is requisite for the patient to merit the uncritical warm response and respect given to the "deserving." The deserving-disabled will be ranked in terms of a hierarchy of values. The first qualification is to "Be Clean." The person must have a clean body, his family must wear clean clothes, his house must be clean. This validates the claimant's good moral fiber and his right to receive the social benefits of disability.

Second, "Don't be do-less." The patient should "stir about." He is not expected to hold a "paying job," but he must not be idle. There is a semantic hurdle to clear. The word "work" means gainfully employed. What we classify as genuine work which is not remunerative is called "ginning." "Work" entails the futureless, joyless, monotonous, dangerous drudgery that is performed away from home. "Ginning" is the quite industrious "doing things around the house." Ginning includes repairing the car, sawing cordwood, helping with harvesting and barn-raising, planting a garden, travelling long distances over bumpy roads in a pick-up truck to go hunting. Family and neighbors admire the man for enduring his pain bravely. This approval is heightened by use of prostheses. The deserving-disabled worker is not a "sorry" man, he is not "do-less." He is a well-regarded member of the community.

The third requirement is that the man be "nice." Niceness is characterized by being friendly, speaking to everyone, attending church and going to funerals. He should not "cuss," and must not "touch a drop." Drinking is an indication that a man is less than a nice person; worse, he is not a Christian and his soul is in deplorable condition.

Fourth, he must obtain a medical doctor's certification of disability, which validates his disabled role and enables him to claim a compensation award.

Fulfillment of these points ensures his standing in the community. The use of a prosthesis sometimes enhances the sufferer's status to the point of being heroic. The family and community value permanence, consequently the permanent invalid has increased prestige and need not try to find "work" [36, 37].

The injured man's wife vociferously backs up the statements and declarations about his condition and pain. She tells any listener repeatedly that he deserves compensation. She uses her role and function of being the family news-bearer to spread the word throughout the family and church, and to the wider community in general. This behavior is not just moral support. The legitimacy of the claim for compensation is now of major economic importance in family maintenance. The family feels entitled to anything and everything that can be obtained to offset the health breakdown, the injury and the backache.

The interviews with disabled back injured workers provide yet another dimension. Considerable insight into the home situation was obtained by talking together with these men and their wives. Invariably, the wives dominated the discussion stressing her husband's suffering, his inability to work and his right to compensation [38]. In brief, the wives appear to have no doubt of their husband's claim. Although in-laws, neighbors, others in the community may have reservations, she has none. We suggest that in keeping with the Appalachian cultural values, the disbelief concerning her husband's disability may well be denied conscious expression. Maintenance of the stability of the family is a core value in Appalachia [39]. To question a husband's posture is unthinkable, as it could result in diminished family solidarity [40, 41]. Further, in the traditionally Appalachian view, the husband must provide financial support for his family. If a wife suggested that her husband had abdicated his responsibility, it would "cast disrespect on him" as breadwinner. Supporting his claim to disability enables these concepts of family role relations to remain intact. Yet another strong incentive for wives to support their husband's statements is the real need for a family income more reliable than that provided by the disabled husband's sporadic work patterns as unskilled laborers, workers in sawmills or as housepainters, carpenters, etc. Wages were never as dependable or as regular as disability compensation payments. Therefore, these women reinforce their husband's claim to incapacity declaring "he just can't do any work."

The central importance of the wife's role in family maintenance has been observed elsewhere [42]. As mentioned the wife is the spokesperson for the family. Looff has explained these verbal skills are due in part to their remaining in school longer than males [43]. Thus, wives tend to be better educated than their spouses. In addition, women in Appalachian culture are the mediators between the family and the outside community. State and Federal agencies have not utilized these resources effectively, preferring to impose the standard, dominant pattern on this variant subculture. For example, the Department of Human Services, still called "welfare" by most rural West Virginians has insisted that the men, the husbands themselves, initiate applications for financial assistance. But to Appalachians, welfare contacts are the domain of women. In order to resolve the conflict between the governmental and cultural situation, a worker from the Department of Human Services will complete applications with the wife, who must then take the form home for the husband's signature.

It is the wifely support that keeps the man "feeding off the system." Spouse support is one of the most crucial aspects of disability in Appalachia. As one informant expressed it, "If the wife were to put her foot down and tell her husband to go back to work, then he would go back to work." The speaker, however, and all the other women interviewed believed that no wife would be so "hard-hearted" or so impractical. Thus, disability becomes an accepted and acceptable identity likely to be achieved either involuntarily through accident or inevitably by aging.

The socioeconomic factor in male backache syndrome clarifies seeming anomalies. Cultural perception and roles take on a certain logic. The man is socialized for dependence [44, 45]. The pampered rebel, the homesick fighting man, the authoritative, strong silent patriarch has been taught primary dependence on his mother and secondary dependence on his wife, although it is his responsibility to provide for them, and he feels guilty and inadequate if he fails [46, 47]. He also has a dependence on the larger society: the "good old boys," the church, the union. When a man's strength is broken as he fulfills his work obligations, he is released from monotonous and dangerous heavy labor, and can accept an honorable dependence. He can slip into a richly nurturing niche. His personal gains are accompanied by advantages others derive from his disability [48]. Bokan defines these benefits as tertiary gains [49]: his family gains a dependable income, his community gains a full-time non-dependent resident and the health care professional gains a permanent patient. These social factors combine to sustain and maintain the patient's pain behavior. However, some of these benefits are offset by emotional costs. Becoming an "honorable burden" on his family diminishes the patient's stress; accommodating to the patient's increased dependency augments the family's stress.

Many articles on headaches seem to multiply the questions of etiology. Migraines can be caused by diets, allergies and stress. The last item, *stress,* is both inherent in the physical environment and in the psychosocial domain. It is complex and often completely camouflaged. The socially precipitating factors of the "THE headache" among females are more obscure. Many medical doctors believe the onset of headaches result from the inability to escape social pressures. As a local physician observed: "When they become sick of it all, they get sick. They simply 'bail out' for a while." This is a patent example of a well-known stress sequence. Another probable stress response among some of the men is seen in reactions following mine accidents. Experience and memory of extreme pain and the terror of return to work precipitates recognizable conversion disorder.

Similar escape from stress is well known to psychiatrists and physicians. The pattern-

ing here is unfamiliar, and the intensity of the psychosomatic pain is seldom recorded. Joint, tendon and muscle problems are definite and physical and, therefore, generally more comprehensible. The term "migraine" headaches may be more of a classification of a severe headache, whether it is experienced by either males or females, and whether it is felt on only one side of the head or both sides. The precipitating "triggers" of headache are often social or environmental stresses [50, 51]. The genetic patterning of THE headache in some families also shows a genetic factor in its occurrence, and this could be inherited as a histo-incompatibility, an allergy or as vascular sensitivity. Diet and low grade infections are practically homogeneous in this location, but these possible causes of headache should also be considered in searching for possible etiology. The powers of suggestion have been closely observed for centuries but these are likely to be dismissed in our scientific climate as "merely" psychosomatic. Some behavioral scientists and anthropologists, however, have been studying the phenomena of suggestive health concomitants for some years. "It might be that there is a psychogenic stimulus which directly affects hormones and enzymes which consequently is pathologically expressed. Or it may be evident in unexpected remissions. This is comparable to psychogenic sexual arousal" [52]. A current statement along these lines: "Belief kills: Belief heals. . . . The significance of these beliefs in disease causation and cure is the same as that of microorganisms and medicinals. . . . We described these phenomena as ethnomedicogenic" [53]. In the Appalachian region, which is under study, given the religion and social value system this psychosocial factor emerges as a definite possibility in exploring the phenomenon.

Doctors and social scientists continue to search for interactions of culture and illness. Recent concepts have been articulated which may help us develop insights on the types of complaints or disorders, such as the term "somatoform" [55]. This notion postulates that there are difficult problems which are polysymptomatic and pathophysiological processes in which the patient within his given culture has an idea of certain symptoms which become realized in scientifically testable actual pathology. In other words, it would seem that imagination (psychosomatic?) becomes a biochemical and histological reality. This would explain, at least in part, the male backache and female headache in question.

The cultural mind-sets expressed in relation to bodily symptoms are found in other parts of the world. The French, for example, have a tendency to attribute a variety of malaises to the liver. They admonish one another, "*ne faites pas de la mauvaise bile.*" Numerous cultural groups from central Europe, West Africa and South America place great emphasis on constipation and "open bowels." Certain rural areas in our country deny that rheumatism is a disease, "that is only part of old age; just like wrinkles." It may therefore be argued that the backaches and headaches are, in part, a cultural attribution.

Belief may be seen as a pathogen. Many West Virginians strongly believe that men are likely to suffer backaches, that most women have paralyzing headaches. They believe in faith healing and in the inevitability of the loss of health as they age. When more research on rituals, symbols, medical therapy and cultural psychological factors in Appalachian communities is correlated with the puzzling problem of the male backache and female headache, we may hope to reach a clearer understanding of the medical phenomenon.

Notes

The author gratefully acknowledges the contributions of two friends and colleagues: Robert B. Walker, M.D., Director of Rural Health Research, Department of Family and Community Health, Marshall University School of Medicine and Jane Phillips, Ph.D., Professor of Anthropology, Howard University. Also, special acknowledgment must be made for support from the Claude Worthington Benedum Foundation in Pittsburgh, Pennsylvania for support to attend the 1983 Annual Meeting of the Society for Applied Anthropology in San Diego, California at which the first draft of this paper was presented.

1. De Craemer, W. A. A cross-cultural perspective in personhood. *Milbank Meml Fund Q. Hlth Soc.* 61, 19–34, 1983.
2. Katon, W., Kleinman, A., and Rosen, G. Depression and somatization: A review, part 1. *Am. J. Med.* 72, 131, 1982.
3. Belcher, J. C. Population growth and characteristics. In *The Southern Appalachian Region: A Survey* (Edited by Ford, T. R.), pp. 37–53. University of Kentucky Press, Lexington, 1962.
4. Pearsall, M. Communicating with the educationally deprived. *Mount. Life Wk* 42, 8–11, 1966.
5. Ford, T. R. (Ed.) The passing of provincialism. In *The Southern Appalachian Region: A Survey*, pp. 9–34. University of Kentucky Press, Lexington, 1962.
6. Schwartzweller, H. K. *et al. Mountain Families in Transition.* Pennsylvania State University Press, University Park, 1971.
7. Pearsall, M. Cultures of the American south. *Anthrop. Q.* 39, 128–144, 1966.
8. Campbell, J. C. *The Southern Highlander and His Homeland,* p. 14. Russell Sage Foundation, New York, 1921.
9. Whetherford, W. D. and Brewer, D. D. *Life and Religion in Southern Appalachia,* pp. 161–162. Friendship Press, New York, 1962.
10. Coreil, J. and Marshall, P. Locus of illness control: a cross-cultural study. *Hum. Org.* 41, 132, 1982.
11. Botkin, B. A. *A Treasury of Southern Folklore.* Crown, New York, 1949.
12. Pearsall, M. *op cit.,* p. 133.
13. Brewer, E. D. C. Religion and the churches. In *The Southern Appalachian Region: A Survey* (Edited by Ford, T. R.), pp. 201–218. University of Kentucky Press, Lexington, 1962.
14. Ford, T. R. *op. cit.,* pp. 24–25.
15. Eligibility Specialist, West Virginia Department of Human Services, Charleston, WV. Personal Communication.
16. Schwartz, J. L. Rural health problems of isolated Appalachian Counties. In *Rural and Appalachian Health* (Edited by Nolan, R. L. and Schwartz, J. L.), p. 24. Charles C. Thomas, Springfield, 1973.
17. Schwartz, J. L. *Ibid.,* pp. 32–35.

18. Coreil, J. *op. cit.,* pp. 132–133.
19. Hicks, G. L. *Appalachian Valley,* pp. 44–45. Holt, Rinehart & Winston, New York, 1976.
20. Gotts, E. E. Home-based early intervention. In *Rural Psychology* (Edited by Childs, A. W. and Melton, G. B.), p. 341. Plenum Press, New York, 1982.
21. Whetherford, W. D., and Brewer, E. C. D. *Life and Religion in Southern Appalachia,* p. 67. Friendship Press, New York, 1962.
22. Looff, D. H. *Appalachia's Children: The Challenge of Mental Health,* pp. 52–53. University of Kentucky Press, Lexington, 1971.
23. Looff, D. H. *Ibid.,* pp. 55, 117–118.
24. Pearsall, M. *Little Smokey Ridge: The Natural History of a Southern Appalachian Neighborhood,* pp. 141–145.
25. Schwartzweller, H. K. *et al. op. cit.,* pp. 32–33, 35.
26. Hicks, G. L. *op cit.,* p. 46.
27. Reul, M. R. *Territorial Boundaries of Rural Poverty: Profiles of Exploitation,* p. 239, Center for Rural Manpower and Public Affairs, Michigan State University, East Lansing, 1974.
28. Hicks, G. L. *op. cit.,* pp. 46–48.
29. Looff, D. H. *op. cit.,* pp. 117–118.
30. Surface, W. *The Hollow,* pp. 118–123. Coward-McCann & Geoghegan, New York, 1971.
31. Garreau, J. *The Nine Nations of North America,* pp. 68–69. Avon Books, New York, 1981.
32. Rainwater, L. The lower class: health, illness and medical institutions. In *Encounters with the Poor* (Edited by Deutscher, I., and Thompson, E. J.), p. 262. Basic Books, New York, 1968.
33. Rainwater, L. *Ibid.,* pp. 263–265.
34. Rainwater, L. *Ibid.,* p. 265.
35. Hicks, G. L. *op. cit.,* pp. 36–49.
36. Gotts, E. E. Home-based early intervention. In *Rural Psychology* (Edited by Childs, A. E., and Melton, G. B.), p. 341. Plenum Press, New York, 1982.
37. Hicks, G. L. *op. cit.,* pp. 74–75.
38. Looff, D. H. *op. cit.,* pp. 86–88, 1971.
39. Friedl, J. Health Care Services and the Appalachian Migrant. Report for the National Center for Health Services Research, 1978.
40. Thomas, J. *The Blue Ridge Country,* p. 49. Duell, Sloan & Pearce, New York, 1942.
41. Looff, D. H. Rural appalachians and their attitudes toward health. In *Rural and Appalachian Health* (Edited by Nolan, R. L., and Schwartz, J. L.), pp. 22–23. Charles C. Thomas, Springfield, 1973.
42. Reul, M. R. *op. cit.,* p. 185.
43. Looff, D. H. *op. cit.,* p. 87.
44. Weller, J. *Yesterday's People: Life In Contemporary Appalachia,* p. 26. University of Kentucky Press, Lexington, 1966.
45. Reul, M. R. *op. cit.,* p. 185.
46. Reul, M. R. *Ibid.,* p. 185.
47. Sternback, R. A., Wolfe, S. R., Murphy, R. W. *et al.* Traits of pain patients: the lower back "loser." *Psychosomatics* 14, 226–229, 1973.
48. Spengler, D. M. *Low Back Pain: Assessment and Management.* Grune & Stratton, New York, 1982.
49. Bokan, J. A., Ries, R. K., and Katon, W. J. Tertiary gain and chronic pain. *Pain* 10, 331–335, 1981.
50. Eaton, W., Kleinman, A., and Rosen, G. Depression and somatization: a review, part II. *Am. J. Med.* 72, 243, 1982.
51. Hamryk-Gutt, R. and Rees, W. L. Psychological aspects of migraine. *J. Psychosomat. Res.* 17, 141–143, 1973.
52. Philips, J. The elements to consider in ethnomedicine. *Folk Healthways* I, No. 3, 2, 1960.
53. Hahn, R. A., and Kleinman, A. Belief as pathogen; belief as medicine: "voodoo death" and "the placebo phenomenon" in anthropological perspective. *Med. Anthrop. Q* 14, No. 4, 3, 1983.
54. Wolff, B. B., and Langley, S. Cultural factors and the response to pain: a review. *Am. Anthrop.* 70, 494–501, 1968.
55. *Diagnostic and Statistical Manual of Mental Disorders,* 3rd Edition, pp. 241–252. American Psychiatric Association, Washington, DC, 1981.

Spence + Lila

Bobbie Ann Mason

■

One

On the way to the hospital in Paducah, Spence notices the row of signs along the highway: WHERE WILL YOU BE IN ETERNITY? Each word is on a white cross. The message reminds him of the old Burma-Shave signs. His wife, Lila, beside him, has been quiet during the trip, which takes forty minutes in his Rabbit. He didn't take her car because it has a hole in the muffler, but she has complained about his car ever since he cut the seat belts off to deactivate the annoying warning buzzer.

As they pass the Lone Oak shopping center, on the outskirts of Paducah, Lila says fretfully, "I don't know if the girls will get here."

"They're supposed to be here by night," Spence reminds her. Ahead, a gas station marquee advertises a free case of Coke with a tune-up.

Catherine, their younger daughter, has gone to pick up Nancy at the airport in Nashville. Although Lila objected to the trouble and expense, Nancy is flying all the way from Boston. Cat lives nearby, and Nancy will stay with her. Nancy offered to stay with Spence, so he wouldn't be alone, but he insisted he would be all right.

When Cat brought Lila home from the doctor the day before and Lila said, "They think it's cancer," the words ran through him like electricity. She didn't cry all evening, and when he tried to hold her, he couldn't speak. They sat in the living room in their recliner chairs, silent and scared, watching TV just as they usually did. Before she sat down for the evening, she worked busily in the kitchen, freezing vegetables from the garden and cooking food for him to eat during her stay in the hospital. He couldn't eat any supper except a bowl of cereal, and she picked at some ham and green beans.

He knew she had not been feeling well for months; she'd had dizzy spells and she had lost weight. The doctor at the local clinic told her to come back in three months if she kept losing weight, but Cat insisted on taking her mother to Paducah. The doctors were better there, Cat insisted, in that know-it-all manner both his daughters had. Cat, who was careless with money, didn't even think to ask what the specialists would charge. When she brought Lila home, it was late—feeding time. Spence was at the pond feeding the ducks, with Oscar, the dog. When Oscar saw the car turn into the driveway, he tore through the soybean field toward the house, as if he, too, were anxious for a verdict.

They had told Lila that her dizzy spells were tiny strokes. They also found a knot in her right breast. They wanted to take the knot out and do a test on it, and if it was cancer they would take her whole breast off, right then. It was an emergency, Lila explained. They couldn't deal with the strokes until they got the knot out. Spence imagined the knot growing so fast it would eat her breast up if she waited another day or two.

They're crawling through the traffic on the edge of Paducah. When he was younger, Spence used to come and watch the barges on the river. They glided by confidently, like miniature flat-tops putting out to sea. He has wanted to take Lila for a cruise on the *Delta Queen,* the luxury steamboat that paddles all the way to New Orleans, but he hasn't been able to bring himself to do it.

He turns on the radio and a Rod Stewart song blares out.

"Turn that thing off!" Lila yells.

"I thought you needed a little entertainment," he says, turning the sound down.

She rummages in her purse for a cigarette, her third on the trip. "They won't let me have any cigarettes tonight, so I better smoke while I got a chance."

"I'll take them things and throw 'em away," he says.

"You better not."

She cracks the window open at the top to let the smoke out. Her face is the color of cigarette ashes. She looks bad.

"I guess it's really cancer," she says, blowing out smoke. "The X-ray man said it was cancer."

"How would he know? He ain't even a doctor."

"He's seen so many, he would know."

"He ain't paid to draw that conclusion," Spence says. "Why did he want to scare you like that? Didn't the doctor say he'd have to wait till they take the knot out and look at it?"

"Yeah, but—" She fidgets with her purse, wadding her cigarette package back into one of the zipper pockets. "The X-ray man sees those X-rays all day long. He knows more about X-rays than a doctor does."

Spence turns into the hospital parking lot, unsure where to go. The eight-story hospital cuts through the humid, hazy sky, like a stray sprig of milo growing up in a bean field. A car pulls out in front of him. Spence's reactions are slow today, but he hits the brakes in time.

"I think I'll feel safer in the hospital," Lila says.

Walking from the parking lot, he carries the small bag she packed. He suspects there is a carton of cigarettes in it. Cat keeps trying to get Lila to quit, but Lila has no willpower. Once Cat gave her a cassette tape on how to quit smoking, but Lila accidentally ran it through the washing machine. It was in a shirt pocket. "Accidentally on purpose," Cat accused her. Cat even told Lila once that cigarettes caused breast cancer. But Spence believes worry causes it. She worries

about Cat, the way she has been running around with men she hardly knows since her divorce last year. It's a bad example for her two small children, and Lila is afraid the men aren't serious about Cat. Lila keeps saying no one will want to marry a woman with two extra mouths to feed.

Now Lila says, "I want you to supervise that garden. The girls won't know how to take care of it. That corn needs to be froze, and the beans are still coming in."

"Don't worry about your old garden," he says impatiently. "Maybe I'll mow it down."

"Spence!" Lila cries, grabbing his arm tightly. "Don't you go and mow down my garden!"

"You work too hard on it," he says. "We don't need all that grub anymore for just us two."

"The beans is about to begin a second round of blooming," she says. "I want to let most of them make into shellies and save some for seed. And I don't want the corn to get too old."

The huge glass doors of the hospital swing open, and a nurse pushes out an old woman in a wheelchair. The woman is bony and pale, with a cluster of kinfolks in bluejeans around her. Her aged hands, folded in her lap, are spotted like little bird dogs. The air-conditioning blasts Spence and Lila as they enter, and he feels as though they are walking into a meat locker.

Two

She felt that lump weeks ago, but she didn't mention it then. When she and Spence returned from a trip to Florida recently, she told Cat about it, and Cat started pestering her to see a specialist. The knot did feel unusual, like a piece of gristle. The magazines said you would know it was different. Lila never examined her breasts the way they said to do, because her breasts were always full of lumps anyway—from mastitis, which she had several times. Her breasts are so enormous she cannot expect to find a little knot. Spence says her breasts are like cow bags.

He has funny names for them, like the affectionate names he had for his cows when they used to keep milk cows. Names like Daisy and Bossy. Petunia. Primrose. It will be harder on him if she loses one of her breasts than it will be on her. Women can stand so much more than men can.

She makes him leave the hospital early, wanting to be alone so she can smoke a cigarette in peace. After he brought her in, he paced around, then went downstairs for a Coke. Now he leaves to go home, and she watches him from behind as he trudges down the corridor, hugging himself in the cold. Lila is glad she brought her housecoat, but even with it she is afraid she will take pneumonia.

In the lounge, she smokes and plays with a picture puzzle laid out on a card table. Someone has pieced most of the red barn and pasture, and a vast blue sky remains to be done. Lila loves puzzles. When she was little, growing up at her uncle's, she had a puzzle of a lake scene with a castle. She worked that puzzle until the design was almost worn away. The older folks always kidded her, but she kept working the puzzle devotedly. She always loved the satisfying snap of two pieces going together. It was like knowing something for sure.

Her son Lee towers in the doorway of the lounge. She stands up, surprised.

"Did you get off work early?" He works at Ingersoll-Rand.

"No. I just took off an hour, and I have to go back and work till nine. They're working me overtime this month." He has lines on his face and he is only thirty-two.

He hugs her silently. He's so tall her head pokes his armpit, where he has always been ticklish.

"I didn't know you were that sick in Florida," he says. "We shouldn't have dragged you through Disney World."

"I knew something was wrong, but I didn't know what." She explains the details of the X-rays and the operation, then says, "I'm going to lose my breast, Lee."

"You are?" The lines on his face freeze. He needs a shave.

"They won't know till they get in there, but if it's cancer they'll go ahead and take it out."

"Which one?"

"This one," she says, cupping her right breast.

A woman with frizzy red hair hobbles into the lounge, her hospital gown exposing her fat, doughy knees. "I was looking for my husband," she says, "but I reckon he ain't here."

Lila waits for the woman to leave, then laughs. She's still holding her breast. "You don't remember sucking on these, do you, Lee?" She loves to tease her son. "You sucked me dry and I had to put you on a bottle after two months. I couldn't make enough milk to feed you."

With an embarrassed grin, Lee looks out the window. "I believe you're making that up."

Four

Lila says, "They sure don't let you get lonesome here—all the traipsing in and out they do at all hours."

Cat and Nancy are hovering over the bed, staring at her with an unnatural sort of eagerness. "Did you sleep?" Cat asks.

"Off and on," says Lila. She tries to sit up against the pillow, but she feels woozy from this morning's medicine. "That coffee last night made me jumpy, but they give me some pills and a shot."

Nancy says, "That's outrageous! There was no good reason to give you coffee. You should have refused it."

Cat's earrings dangle in Lila's face. Lila's mind feels fuzzy, far away. She is afraid the operating room will be cold.

"Are you scared?" Nancy asks, holding Lila's hand.

"They work you over too much for you to be scared. I haven't had time to think." Lila squeezes Nancy's hand and reaches for Cat's. "You girls are being good to me," she says. "I sure am lucky."

"Well, we care about you," Cat says.

"You're going to be just fine, Mom," says Nancy. "You're tough."

"I guess I better say goodbye to my jug," Lila says, laughing and looking down at herself. "If Spence don't hurry on here, he's going to miss his chance."

Just then Spence appears, still in short sleeves. Yesterday she tried to tell him to wear long sleeves, but he wouldn't listen to her. After giving Nancy a hug, he steps back and eyes her up and down to see how much older she seems.

"You look poor as a snake," he says. "Why didn't you bring Robert?"

"He's going off to camp tomorrow. Jack's taking him up to New Hampshire. It's the same place he went last year, where they go on treks into the mountains."

"Bring him down here. I'll see that he communes with nature." Spence grins at Nancy.

"I'm sure you will. You'll have him out planting soybeans." Nancy twists out of a nurse's way.

"It would be good for him," Lila says sleepily. "Working out in the fields would teach him something."

She closes her eyes, vaguely listening to Spence and the girls talk. If this is her time to go, she should be ready. And she has her family with her, except for Lee, who had to work. She feels she is looking over her whole life, holding it up to see how it has turned out—like a piece of sewing. She can see Cat trying on a dress Lila has made for her, and Lila checks to see whether it needs taking up. She turns up the hem, jerks the top to see how it fits across the shoulders, considers an extra tuck in the waist. In a recurrent

dream she has had for years, she is trying to finish a garment, sewing fast against the clock.

They are still chattering nervously around her when the surgeon appears. He's young, with sensitive hands that look skilled at delicate finger work. Lila always notices people's fingers. Nancy and Cat keep asking questions, but Lila is sleepy and can't follow all that he is saying. Then he moves closer to her and says, "If the biopsy shows a malignancy, I'm going to recommend a modified radical mastectomy. I'll remove the breast tissue and the lymph nodes under the arm. But I'll leave the chest muscles. If you follow the physical therapy, then you'll have full use of your arm and you'll be just fine." He smiles reassuringly. He resembles a cousin of Lila's—Whip Stanton, a little man with a lisp and a wife with palsy.

"How small would the lump have to be for you to recommend a lumpectomy instead?" Nancy asks the doctor.

"Infinitesimal," he says. "It's better to get it all out and be sure. This way is more certain."

"Well, more and more doctors are recommending lumpectomies instead of mastectomies," Nancy argues. "What I'm asking is, what is the dividing line? How large should the lump be for the mastectomy to be preferable?"

Lila sees Spence cringe. Nancy has always asked questions and done things differently, just to be contrary. "Nancy, Nancy, quite contrary," they used to tease her.

The doctor shrugs and leans against the wall. "It depends on a number of factors," he says. "You can't reduce it to a question of size. If it's an aggressive tumor, a fast-growing one, then a smaller lump might be more dangerous than one that has grown slowly over a longer period of time. And my suspicion is that this is an aggressive tumor. You can get a second opinion if you want to, but we've got her prepped, and if the second opinion was in favor of a lumpectomy, then wouldn't you have to go for a third opinion, so you could take two out of three? But in this case, time is of the essence." The doctor grins at Lila. "What do you think, Mrs. Culpepper? You look like a pretty smart lady."

"Why, you're just a little whippersnapper," Lila says. "All the big words make me bumfuzzled. I guess you know your stuff, but I got you beat when it comes to producing pretty daughters." She has heard he is single, and she heard the nurses joking with him. She can't keep her mind on the conversation. It's as though she's floating around the room, dipping in and out of the situation, the way the nurses do.

Eight

Lila feels as though she has been left out in a field for the buzzards. The nurses are in at all hours, making no special effort to be quiet—a nurse who checks dressings, another one who changes dressings, a nurse with blood-thinner shots three times a day, a nurse with breathing-machine treatments, various nurses' aides who check temperature and blood pressure, the cleaning woman, the mail lady, the priest and nuns from the hospital, the girls who fill the water jugs, the woman who brings the meal trays, the candy stripers selling toiletries and candy and magazines from a cart. Lila can't keep track of all the nurses who come to check her drainage tube—squirting the murky fluid out of the plastic collection bottle, measuring the fluid intake and output, writing on charts. The nurses walk her around the entire third floor twice a day, accompanied by her I.V. bag, wheeling on a stand. Spence is nervous, bursting in anxiously, unable to stick around. And the girls are in and out, bringing her little things—a basket of flowers from the gift shop downstairs and some perfume. Lee and Joy brought a rose in a milk-glass bud vase. The church sent pink daisies. The old woman in the other bed has no flowers.

The surgeon told Lila she could live without a breast. "You couldn't live without a head, or a liver, or a heart," he said when he informed her in the recovery room that he had removed her breast. "But you can live without a breast. You'll be surprised."

"It would be like living without balls," Lila replied. "You'd find that surprising too, but you could probably get along without them."

Lila is not sure she said that aloud, and remembering it now, she is embarrassed that she might have, under the influence of the drugs. She's surprised Nancy hasn't said the same thing to the doctor's face.

Lila hears the old woman in the other bed grunting and complaining. "I'll not leave here alive!" she shouted when a nurse gave her a bath. "You're wasting your time fooling with me."

By the second day after her surgery, Lila is no longer hooked to the I.V. She plucks at the hospital gown in front where her bandage itches. The drainage tubes irritate her skin. She feels weak, but restless. "I'm afraid my blood's too thin already," she tells the nurse who comes with the blood-thinner shot.

"No, this is what the doctor wanted," the nurse says.

"I'm getting poked so full of holes I'm like a sifter bottom."

Besides the shots, there are the tests. They have wheeled her into the cold basement three times to run her through their machines. They have scanned her bones, her liver, her whole body, looking for loose cancer cells. Now the cancer doctor comes in to tell Lila the results of the tests: The cancer has spread to two out of the seventeen lymph nodes that were removed. Spence isn't there yet, but Cat and Nancy fire questions at him. Lila's head spins as the doctor explains that once the cancer has reached the lymph nodes, it has gone into the bloodstream, and then it can end up anywhere. The news doesn't quite register.

"I'm recommending chemotherapy," the doctor says.

"Is that cobalt?" Lila asks weakly. The doctor is young and reminds her of the odd-looking preacher who led the revival at church last year. The preacher had a long nose and wore a gold shiny suit.

The doctor says, "No. This will be a combination of three drugs—Cytoxan, methotrexate and 5FU." He explains that she will have a chart showing two weeks of treatments, then a three-week rest period, then two weeks of treatments, and so on. She will get both pills and shots. Like dogs teaming up on a rabbit, Cat and Nancy jump on him about side effects.

"This particular treatment is tolerated very well," he says. "That's not to say there won't be side effects. A little hair loss, a little nausea. Some people react more adversely than others."

Lila can't keep her mind on what he's saying. "I've got plenty of hair," she says, tugging at her curls. "And it's coarse, like horse hair." The last permanent she got didn't take on top.

"You're going to have to lay off the smoking too," the doctor says, consulting his clipboard.

"They won't let me smoke here," Lila says. She bummed a cigarette from a visitor in the lounge the night before, but it burned her lungs and tasted bitter. She couldn't finish it.

The cancer doctor says now, "Cigarettes will interfere with the chemotherapy."

"See!" Nancy says triumphantly. "Doctor's orders. And you wouldn't listen to us."

"These girls snitched my cigarettes," Lila says to the doctor. "Is that any way to treat an old woman that's stove up in the hospital?"

"Best thing for you," the doctor says with a slight grin.

Fourteen

A woman from the mastectomy support group arrives the next afternoon, bringing Lila a temporary pad to stuff in her brassiere until she can be measured for a permanent one. Lila feels embarrassed because both her daughters and Spence are right there. Spence is reading the newspaper noisily, rattling the pages and jerking them out smooth. Lila worries about his nerves.

"It's called a prosthesis," the woman explains. Lila did not catch her name. Cheerful and little, pert as a wren, she stands beside the bed, speaking to Lila like a school-teacher. She presents Lila with the object, which is in a plastic bag.

"Law," says Lila. "That weighs a ton." It reminds her of those sandbags used to hold down temporary signs on the highway.

"I can tell you're surprised," the woman chirps. "We don't realize the weight we're carrying around. You can put a strain on your back if you don't get properly fitted. So don't just stuff your bra with any old thing to make it look right. It's got to feel right and it's got to be the right weight, or you can run into serious problems."

The woman says she has had a mastectomy herself, and presumably she is wearing one of these sandbags in her brassiere. Lila notices Spence squirming. Nancy and Cat don't jump on this woman the way they did on the doctors. Cat is playing solitaire and Nancy is reading a book. Mrs. Wright is asleep.

The woman tells a long tale about her own mastectomy. "I was worried about recurrence," she says. "And I did have a lump to come in the other breast. It was tested and it was benign, but I made the decision to have the second breast removed too. I just didn't want to take the chance of having cancer again. Now that may sound extreme to you, but it was just the way I felt. So I'm free from worry, and the prosthesis works just fine."

The woman's little points are as perky as her personality. If the originals were that small, she probably doesn't miss them, Lila thinks. The woman talks awhile about balance, and then she talks about understanding. She has a packet of materials for Lila to read. "You may get depressed over losing part of your femininity," she says. "And we want you to know we're available to help." Lila listens carefully, but she can't think of anything to say.

"The doctors were skeptical when we started our organization," the woman says, leaning toward Lila and speaking in a confidential half-whisper. "But after we advertised, we had fifty women come to the first meeting. There was a great need for this, and we want you to know that we're there to serve you."

"Would I have to come all the way to Paducah?"

"Yes. That's where we hold our meetings, on the first Monday night of each month."

"Well, I don't get out much at night. And I don't like to drive on that Paducah highway."

"Let me urge you just to try it and see what it does for you. I'll give you the names of some people to contact." She talks on and on, about how the family should be understanding. In the packet are letters to daughters and sons and husbands. Spence and the girls are pretending they aren't there. "The letters say things that you may be uncomfortable saying, things you might be afraid to say, but they will explain your feelings at this delicate time when you need emotional support. All you have to do is send the appropriate letter to your daughters and your husband and to your sons, if you have any. It will be a nice surprise for them if you just send them in the mail. It's a much easier way for you to communicate your feelings."

"My girls have stood by me," Lila says, nodding proudly at Cat and Nancy. "And my boy works long hours and can't come as often, but he does when he can. Nancy flew all the way down here from New York."

"Boston," Nancy says, peering over her reading glasses.

"That's the same thing to us down here," the woman says with an apologetic smile.

"How much will this thing cost?" Lila asks. "If you charge by the pound, it might be high." She laughs at herself. She wonders why the woman didn't replace her breasts with big ones. Small-breasted women were always envious of Lila.

"The important thing is to get the proper fitting. With your fitting, and the bra and the prosthesis, the package comes to about a hundred and fifty dollars."

"Good night!" Lila and Spence cry simultaneously.

"But it's an important investment."

After the woman has gone, Spence says, "Will Medicare cover that?"

"I doubt it," Lila says. "I failed to ask her. Law, I hope I don't have to have false teeth anytime soon! I won't be able to keep track of that much stuff."

"You don't need that thing. We can rig you up something."

"Why, shoot, yes," Lila says. "I ain't spending a hundred and fifty dollars for a falsie."

Nancy laughs. "I read about a woman who stuffed her bra with buckshot, and she got stopped at the airport by the metal detector."

Cat says, "I heard about a woman who had an inflatable bra, and she went up in an airplane, and with the change in air pressure they exploded!"

They're all laughing, and Lila spontaneously tosses the prosthesis to Spence. "Catch!" she cries. Spence snatches it out of the air and flings it to Nancy and Nancy tosses it to Cat. Cat starts to throw it to Lila but stops herself, probably realizing Lila's right arm is weak. Lila is laughing so much her stitches hurt. Cat hands her the little sandbag and Lila says, "Well, it'll make a good pincushion."

They all laugh even harder then because Lila is in the habit of keeping stray straight pins and safety pins fastened to her blouse, and more than once in her life she has accidentally jabbed her breast with a pin.

The Mother-in-Law

Doris Betts

∎

I cross the alley which runs between the back of the neighborhood grocery and the back of *her* house. I believe it is 1932. Now softly to the lighted bedroom window to part the dry spirea twigs and see through the cloudy pane.

Already yellowing, she rests in the high bed and breathes through her mouth. She is barely forty and her heart does not want to stop; it beats against the cancer like a fist on a landslide.

They sit around her bed. Husband, three sons. Another long evening. They talk over the day like any ordinary family.

There is the youngest boy, Philip. Black eyes and silence. In ten more years, he will marry me.

She does not ask them the only question which still concerns her: Will you look after Ross? So they do not answer. If I could slip into the room and make her hear, I would whisper, "Yes, of course"; but she has never heard of me, and never will.

I am a ghost here and my other self is skipping rope in another state.

Snow on the alley. Nathan, the eldest, hangs back. He feels responsible for everything he sees, and started living through a long lens at an early age. Ahead of him, Ross is scraping fingers in the snow, slinging handfuls behind him. My future husband walks sideways, so he can look ahead

and watch Ross at the same time. He lacks Nathan's sense of duty; with him, all is instinct.

They come to the rear of the grocery store, where trucks unload at the ramp and fermenting produce is piled in cans. Since the woolen mill closed, the cans rattle all night. People trot up the alley carrying tow sacks.

With his good arm, Ross makes a snowball spatter on their empty garage. The car has been sold. Nathan tries to decide whether the thump disturbs their mother. My husband throws snow, too, and makes his ball fall short. By instinct.

Nathan stops, points. Above the loading ramp, the grocer has installed two poles with electric lights which will shine directly on the garbage cans. Now the boys must keep their window shades pulled at night to avoid recognizing the fathers of friends.

They turn in the sagging wire gate to their back yard. Under the snow lie *her* crowded iris; the stalks of uncut chrysanthemums rattle when Ross limps through. Nathan reaches out to help him across a drift. Before he can grasp the hand, my future husband has dropped snow down Ross' back; they roll and tussle. Philip gets wetter. A draw—Ross laughs. I am watching the scene with my own hand out; if I were to change this or that?

They walk through my transparent arm and climb the back steps. The pattern is set.

Mr. Felts has asked the grocer not to burn his big lights all night long. "They shine in her window." She sleeps so little now, even with medicine. All night he hears the "sooo—soooo" as she sucks breath through her clenched teeth.

The grocer says the police advised it. His windows, door locks are being broken. Obliquely he blames Mr. Felts for the Depression, because he is an accountant and is still working the town's math when its weaving machines have stopped.

The grocer's son ran a machine. "I better leave them on."

Mr. Felts fastens her window shade with thumbtacks. Still the gold leaks in. The shine frightens her; she knows the back alley has never been bright. If there is a fire, Ross will not be able to get away.

Again Mr. Felts begs the grocer. Those who raid the garbage cans do it hastily now, half blinded, in a clatter. She hears; she sucks air faster. One night a metal lid rolls down the entire alley and spins out with a twang against the corner curb. She—who never missed church until this illness—cries out about Ezekiel's chariot.

Next morning, in full sight of the neighborhood, Mr. Felts heaves bricks at the light until both bulbs are broken. He wants to throw one at the grocer, too, but Nathan stops him.

March. When they come home from the funeral, Ross hurries to the bedroom. He does not understand she will not lie there anymore. Only Nathan was old enough to see inside the box. He takes Ross now onto the back steps and speaks for a long time about death and Heaven. Ross hits him.

In her bedroom, their father pulls outward gently on the shade. One by one, the thumbtacks pop onto the floor like buttons off a fat man. My husband smiles when he sees this; my ghost smiles. How I am going to love him!

Crying at last, Ross slams the back door and screams his name.

"Come here," Philip says. "Help me pick up these tacks."

Ross was born with a bad arm and leg. One eye is fixed and useless; there is slight vision in the other. While there was money, the Felts saw many doctors. Casts and splints were used; his night brace banged the bars of the crib when he dreamed.

His spectacles are plain glass and thick glass, so his brain seems to be bulging out through the magnified eye which strains to see shapes, light,

and shadow. Ross is intelligent and, thanks to *her,* well adjusted. She must have bitten her tongue half off the day he climbed onto the garage roof. How her throat swelled shut the first of the hundred times he fell downstairs. But she was successful. All boys fall, Ross thinks.

Summer evenings there was baseball in the vacant lot by the grocer's. Ross batted like a spider, ran bases like a crab. The boys' laughter sounded to him like comradeship. In the bull pen Nathan made sure it was. Philip told me these things.

Now that I have Philip's children, I know how many bloody noses she iced in the pantry. I go into that pantry and watch her from behind the flour bin. She is thinking about the first lumps which have bent her nipple. I understand why she's sure they are harmless; it is not her *turn* for cancer. At night I tap my foot silently by the green chair while she searches her Bible. I'm not a Bible reader myself. I like the Greek myths. She reads St. Paul.

Staring at the green chair, where in more than a decade my other self will sit, she almost meets my eyes, almost pledges to accept any unbeliever who will care for Ross.

"I'm going to be pretty and red-haired," I say—she doesn't care.

"In bed, Philip and I . . ." She can't be bothered.

She dreams beyond me of how Ross kicked against her womb with a foot that could not have been withered. It was Achilles' foot.

Nathan, the dutiful son, has brought her daisies, which she puts absently into a vase. I beg her: Look at my Philip now. He carries no flowers but his black eyes—does she see? Now she embraces Ross and, over his crooked shoulder, gazes deeply at her other sons. She cannot help it; she has begun to bargain. Will they? Can they? Has she prepared them to?

Harmless as marbles, the fragments of her death shift in her breast and another, smaller, rolls in the womb that sheltered Ross and the others. I, Nathan's wife, their children, ours—we hear the bits roll as she looks through time and our faces.

She lets Ross go; the moment passes, will exist in no one's memory but hers and mine.

In 1942, Nathan becomes an army officer. Philip is in high school, unaware that in another state I am in love with a basketball center who owns his own car. We park in it, too; I evade his long arms. Philip's ghost sits in the back seat. I sense him there. I am uneasy, dimly suspecting he exists, fearing his shade is nothing but my frigidity.

This is the year Mr. Felts has almost finished paying the cost of her futile treatment—X-rays and pills—the headstone. He shrinks as the bills shrink; his flesh seems to drain away toward hers. Philip says, "You rest, I'll read tonight." Ross is a college freshman. They take turns with his texts.

The grocery store has been torn down and a warehouse built. Its lights shine day and night, and light up the place in her yard where the iris roots have reared up to lie on the ground like a tumble of potatoes.

At fifteen, I go away to girls' camp in the Blue Ridge Mountains. My parents can afford it. Across the same lake, their church holds summer retreat. Mr. Felts has brought the two younger boys because he promised her. In the dark, Philip smokes secretly after hours and stares over the black water at the lights of the camp where I am sleeping. I can't see what Mr. Felts is doing.

Once, on my horse, I ride across the place where Philip and Ross have had a picnic; they have just gone; maybe no more than a rhododendron bush keeps us from meeting.

Up the hill as they walk away, Ross is asking, "Isn't it time you got interested in girls?"

Now it's time. I go to college in his town. I am eighteen, so ignorant and idealistic that the qualities overlap and blend. My grades are good. I think I will become a social worker and im-prove the world. I sign up to read for blind students.

(Here I must pause. The ghost of my English teacher protests such melodrama, such coincidence. I, too, protest it. I am a tool of the plot, a flat character rung in on the proper page. I say—with Iphigenia—thanks but no thanks! The blade comes on.)

In no time at all, I move from knowing Ross to knowing Philip. I recognize him. He looks like his mother. While we are falling in love, we take Ross everywhere with us. He can ride a gentle mare, swim an awkward backstroke. In the balcony, we explain movie scenes if the dialogue is vague. He hardly notices when we kiss or touch each other. One night, drunk and tired of trying to work out marriage plans, we let Ross drive down a country road—screaming directions, "Right!" and "Left!"—till all three of us hurt from laughing. I kiss Philip so hard my own teeth bite me.

Secretly, Ross talks to me about wanting girls. I repeat it to Philip, whose black eyes go blacker. Nathan is mailing long letters home about how Ross should save himself for his bride.

In spite of what the basketball center said, I am not frigid. Lost at last under Philip, Philip lost in me. In the silence afterward, the ghost of Ross. We get up and dress and go find him and take him for a long walk. Coming home, we sit with our backs against the warehouse, singing. Soprano, tenor, baritone, under the blazing lights.

We marry and the war ends. Ross has a job running a machine he can pedal with one foot. With his checks he buys radios and phonographs. Every morning, Mr. Felts cooks him Cream of Wheat.

Philip and I live over a beauty shop. The smell of hot hair has got into our linens. Philip finishes college; Nathan comes home and begins.

Saturday nights I go to her house and cook a big pot of spaghetti. I am pregnant with our first. Philip is independent and we have refused to cash my parents' checks, which have grown smaller anyway.

I wash the dishes in her sink. Did she cook spaghetti here? Ross likes it. Yes.

Late in the evening when my back aches, I leave the men talking and lie across her bed. They have painted the window sill, but its frame is neatly pocked where the shade was nailed down. I lie there fearful for my child. I ask her: What were the earliest signs? Did you vomit much? Take vitamins?

But she has slipped into the room where Ross and the others are playing cards.

Our daughter is almost ready for kindergarten. The next one is walking and throwing toys; the third sleeps through the night at last. I have got used to the beauty-shop smell.

The telephone rings. Ross says, "I came in? The coffee wasn't fixed?"

I call to our bedroom, "Philip?"

In my ear the telephone: "I can't find where he's gone."

"I'll come," Philip says.

They find Mr. Felts in the furnace room. The shovel is under the coal, and he has gone down around its handle like a wilted vine. His heart tried to get out; all is stained.

We bring Ross home to our four rooms. Afterward I visit her empty house. Where are you, Mr. Felts? What was it like for you? Why did you never say?

Silence. He was as still as Philip is.

Ross lives with us now. Nathan fills out his income tax. He buys insurance policies for Ross. He never forgets a birthday and they ask Ross to dinner once a month. Nathan's daughters go to orthodontists and reducing salons.

I carry four baskets of laundry up these stairs instead of three. Our children like bread pudding. All four are healthy, make noise, eat a lot. They will have straighter teeth when the second set comes in.

Philip works too hard. Some Saturday nights he sits in the kitchen and drinks whiskey alone until his own limbs seem crippled. I have to help him down the hall. "Something worrying you?"

"What could be worrying me?"

I have stopped asking. What he cannot say, I must not. Mostly we talk over our days like any ordinary family.

Sometimes when our bedspring has stopped squeaking, I can hear Ross's squeak. Do the children hear? What will we do when they are too old to share his room? He never complains of the sweat when the vaporizer steams all night and I come in and out with aspirin. Sometimes he sits up in bed to smoke and wait. I'm afraid he'll set the mattress afire some night when I sleep through the smoke.

"Let me light you a cigarette," he always offers.

I always let him. Philip says Ross needs to give us something back.

Lung cancer? I never say that aloud. Secretly, I flush the butt down the toilet.

"I've got more," Ross always calls pleasantly when I come back into the hall.

Now, while the children sleep and Ross sleeps among them and I sit down at last to wait for Philip to come from his overtime work, somebody rattles my garbage can; somebody breathes on my glass, looking in. Somebody's glance like a blaze of light gets under my shade.

I am mending *his* shirt. I am forty, like *her*.

I say to the black windowpane: Yes, we are. Go away.

She understands and her gaze burns past to where Ross still sleeps in a brace in the crib she bought. I understand her, too. Even on weary nights, I am glad her desire found me, drew me to this room.

He's just fine, I say. He will live a long life.

Then, for one icy moment, the ghost of her envy stares at the ghost of mine.

Old Age

The readings in the final section of part II address the meaning of old age and its relation to health and illness. First, in an excerpt from an article on the aging of the baby boom generation, key concepts are defined, including old age, aging, retirement, mental development, and decline. A section on private and public "transfers," where resources are transferred from one sector to another (in this case, for the support of the elderly), illuminates one of the core dilemmas of old age: Who will provide the social and economic support for the ever-increasing number of older people in the United States? This is salient for each of the other readings in this section, and foreshadows the discussion of rationing and social justice in part V.

Daniel Callahan's essay raises questions about the rights and responsibilities of family members for their aged parents. The demands of caring for an elderly relative on a long-term basis can put severe strains on a family's emotional and financial resources. In recent years, two trends have contributed to this dilemma: the increasing number of Americans who survive to old age and are likely to need care, and the increasing number of households headed by single parents, who are less able to muster the resources to care for additional, ill family members (Preston 1984). This is further complicated by the changing definition of the family and of the roles and responsibilities played by family members (Cherlin 1992, Macklin 1991). Who counts as family, and thus, who is responsible for other family members, is by no means an easy question to answer.

Another view of responsibility and advocacy in old age is provided by doctors. Sharon Kaufman's article presents results of a qualitative investigation of the nature of physician decision making in the case of old people who live in the community. During in-depth interviews with forty physicians, she asked how they perceive dilemmas and difficult decisions in geriatric medicine. The doctors reported that they worry about how and when to intervene in patients' lives, to balance risk reduction and safety with independence. They are concerned about the conflict between being advocates for old people, while at the same time asking them to change their behavior and comply with other requests. They are troubled by the lack of clear guidelines for assessing vulnerability and quality of life when pondering placement decisions. These "everyday" ethical dilemmas are concerned with the ability of the elderly to maintain the highest possible quality of life in the face of mounting disability. The cases that Kaufman describes provide tangible evidence of the difficulty that physicians face in balancing competing role demands with their older patients. We will return to this topic in part IV, when we consider ethics and the health care provider's role. As Kaufman points out, one of the most interesting aspects of these dilemmas is the increasing trend toward labeling elderly who are not yet sick, as "at risk" (for falls, functional decline, acute medical problems, or institutionalization) and thus eligible for or "needing" medical intervention. This may be seen as a positive trend, or an example of intrusive medicalization of nonmedical problems.

The final selection is a short story by Ethan Canin, written from the view of an old man ruminating about his stage of life. Ronald Blythe

(1979) has argued that old age is the last frontier, and that this is the first generation to explore this territory. It sounds exciting, but as the introduction to part II reminds us, the social meaning of old age in America is full of contradictions. One critical aspect is loss. The story "We Are Nighttime Travelers" explores the nature of this territory of aging and its losses and satisfactions. The story reflects the paradoxes embedded in the experience of old age—the dreams and the destruction of dreams, desire and the limitations of a deteriorating physical existence. Is this a different view from that of the physicians described by Kaufman? Does the protagonist in Ethan Canin's story achieve an integration of these two sides of old age?

Trends, Issues, Perspectives,
and Values for the Aging of
the Baby Boom Cohorts
John M. Cornman and
Eric R. Kingson

■

Terminology for a National Conversation on Aging

The Terms of Old Age

The concepts and definitions used in any discourse can become dated and misleading. A national conversation on aging ought to start with language that reflects the current state of knowledge, and which seeks to clarify the facts. A sample of some elusive concepts follows, beginning with "old age" itself.

Old Age. "Old age" is a complex and elusive concept. The concept is complex because it simultaneously raises questions for the individual (how am I going to age?), for families (who is going to take care of whom?), for professions (who will pay me how much to deliver services to "old" people?), and for social and economic policies (how many public dollars should we spend on which older people?). Also, the contexts in which "aging" is defined keep changing.

Even though we know the number of people living longer is increasing dramatically, and even though the idea of growing older is hardly new, the concept is elusive because the scientific, social, political, moral, and individual bases for defining "old age" keep changing. Much as the poet William Yeats suggested, death is a man-invented thing, the concept of old age is a social construct, though unlike death, it is a dynamic concept.

Age 65 has been used for many years as the demarcation for old age in the United States and as an important marker for purposes of old age policies, pensions, research, and even for defining old age in the public mind. Sixty-five is often an appropriate age for receipt of private and public retirement benefits, but it also overlooks much of the variability that surrounds the aging process. Biologist Leonard Hayflick (1994) says a person's biological age is more important than the person's chronological age in determining the health status of the individual.

Categories and language, of course, matter, from setting tones and expectations to justifying perceptions and policies. "Old" can be a positive as well as a negative term (venerated and wise, or dated and worn out), but it is seldom used to describe a healthy and active person. An early exception to language that reinforced the view of the old as a homogeneous group can be found in the work of Bernice Neugarten. She was the first to distinguish between the "young-old"—relatively healthy and financially independent older persons of any age, though usually 55 to 74—and the "old-old"—those, usually over age 75, whose activities are often constricted because of significant functional disabilities. Similarly, Mgr. Charles Fahey of Fordham University and others have developed the concept of the "third age" to denote that stage in life after middle age but before the final stage.

The national conversation on an aging society must recognize the limits and variations implied by the term "old age." Most importantly, the conversation must recognize that just as many persons move into the third age and beyond in sound health and financial status, a great many persons in those age groups have pressing health care and financial needs.

Aging. Aging is a lifelong process, common to all species and most societies. Aging should not be confused with aged or old. China is an old society, dating back centuries, and has an aging population, in that the average age of its population is increasing due to the fact the number of older people is increasing faster than the number of younger people (Conner, 1992). A country with a dramatic drop in its birth rate will have an aging population even if life expectancy is not increased. But the study of aging should not be restricted to persons 65 and over. Aging, as a field of interest, should be concerned with the entire course of life, because outcomes in old age—both for individuals and cohorts—are substantially influenced by investments made earlier in life (Kingson, Hirshorn, & Cornman, 1986).

In exploring public values, a national conversation on aging should address the impacts of the aging population as well as the number of people living into and through the third age.

Retirement. The term "retirement" carries several meanings. As an institution, retirement should be understood as a relatively new, evolving, and malleable institution that serves several functions. Beyond protecting against loss of income in later years and supporting late life leisure, retirement policies have been designed to affect labor markets, move unemployment from younger to older workers, and cut labor costs (Graebner, 1980; Schulz, 1995). For retirement to emerge as a social institution, substantial social and economic changes had to occur. The economy had to be capable of supporting a nonworking population. A substantial portion of the population had to live to old age. Decisions had to be made to allocate resources toward a period of "leisure" at the end of the life course. Support had to exist among influential elites and the wider population for the pension and labor force policies that created and later sustained this institution (Kingson & Berkowitz, 1993). By encouraging older workers to retire in exchange for a pension and thereby creating job opportunities for younger ones, public and private pensions, and later, Social Security, helped "grease" the intergenerational transfer of employment opportunities while simultaneously adding a measure of economic protection for older workers. Today, the protections provided to vested workers in good private pension or public employee pension programs is often considerable, but not so for many others. Thus, proposed changes in the institution need to account for the variability among older populations and for interactions across the entire labor force.

As a decision, "retirement" is often misleadingly defined as a choice between full-time paid work and complete withdrawal from the paid work force. In practice, "retirement," if that is a correct term, embraces a wide range of arrangements, activities and uses (Quinn, Burkhauser, & Myers, 1990). People "retire" for many different reasons: because they could afford to, because they wanted to do something else, because of health, because they lost their job. In "retirement," people work, people pursue education or avocations (for some reason called leisure activities), people volunteer, people provide care to relatives and people focus on families or other leisure activities.

Similarly, and for many of the same reasons, "normal retirement age" is an evolving concept. As the stereotypical point of demarcation between middle age and senior citizen status and as the currently-defined age of first eligibility for full Social Security retired worker benefits, age 65 is often considered the normal retirement age. Yet a substantial majority of retired workers define themselves as "retiring" before age 65 and most receive Social Security and, when available, other employment-related retirement pensions before age 65. Arguably, under Social Security, there is no longer a "normal retirement age," but a range of ages from 62 to 70 in which it is normal to retire. When retirement is defined as leaving a long-held job, a full-time job, or beginning to draw Social Security or pension income,

the 50-year trend has been for workers to retire at increasingly younger ages. Defining retirement as *not contributing* to community or the economy in any way (i.e., not doing volunteer work, not providing significant care), the "age of retirement" may well rise as people increasingly work part-time or pursue other productive activities in their so-called retirement years.

As an evolving concept, the definition, meaning and purposes of "retirement" will be determined by the public values defining the meaning and purposes of the third and fourth ages.

Mental Development and Decline. The negative connotations of "being old" imply an automatic state of mental decline and have driven many of society's views of and responses to aging, as well as many gerontological research agendas. However, recent research has found that changes in the mental abilities of older people vary as much as their physical abilities, and that mental decline is not inevitable, at least across far more of the life span than was previously believed (Goleman, 1994). Obviously, viewing the third age (and beyond) as a time of continued involvement and development depends on understanding and valuing the fact that "old age" and mental decline are not inevitably linked. With new understanding of the potentials of older persons ought to come new public values as to opportunities for and responsibilities of older persons.

Stereotypes and Diversity. The complexity and elusiveness of the concepts of "aging" and "aged" can be summed up in one word: "diversity." Indeed, each of the terms discussed above are inadequate because they do not reflect the diversity of the topics which fall under their umbrellas. "Old" is largely determined by an arbitrary chronological age, not by a person's mental or physical health status. People age at different rates. Retirement means different things to different people. People may well become more different than alike as they grow older.

Yet stereotypes too often continue to frame the public discourse on aging issues. Not too long ago, the operative value driving the politics of aging was "old people need and deserve a lot." More recently, old people are seen as "greedy geezers" (Binstock, 1983). Popular commentary continues to emphasize a so-called dependency ratio, which says everyone between 18 and 64 is productive and everyone over 65 is dependent (not gainfully employed), and implies that population aging will impose an unmanageable burden on future cohorts of workers (see Appendix).

Such stereotypes clearly are incorrect and hamper efforts to develop public values and policies which reflect the potentials and needs of an older population. There are a good many older people with little or no need for additional service and support. And there are a good many older persons and a good many families caring for older persons who need an array of services. A national conversation on aging that designates everyone over a certain age as "dependent" not only ignores the contributions older people can and should make, but could lead to a self-fulfilling prophecy.

The national conversation should begin with an appreciation that "aging" and "old age" are dynamic concepts, with recognition that diversity is the hallmark of older populations, and with respect for the uncertainty that must limit all projections. All of which leads to the baby boomers, a misleading stereotype about a generation which is not a generation.

The Diversity of the Baby Boom

As popularly used, the term "baby boom generation" refers to the 76 million people born between 1946 and 1964, 17 million more than would have been born had fertility rates remained at 1940 levels. But aside from a common time frame, there is little else that persons born in 1946 and 1964 share as members of a "generation." The concept of a generation, even more than the concept of old age, is a social construct too often used to make oversimplified statements. The term "generations" has multiple meanings. It is used variously to mean position of vertical lineage within families (e.g., "grandparents"), people involved (or potentially involved) in a social movement in which age-consciousness is important, people currently in a particular age group (e.g., "the elderly"), and people born in a common birth cohort (Bengtson, Cutler, Mangen, & Marshall, 1985). Here, we are using it in the latter sense.

Arguably, it is the 17 million "additional" births, more than the absolute number of births, which has impacted public policies and programs over the life course of the baby boom cohorts. At each stage of that life course, society has had to adapt to dramatic and sudden increases in demands for services and facilities, from building schools, colleges and housing, to training faculty, to expanding law enforcement capabilities, to creating jobs, to providing social services.

Even absent the demographic "bulge," the number and proportion of people living longer would have continued to increase, as they have since the beginning of the century. The increase would have been more gradual, allowing for more measured responses to the aging of the population. The ultimate results, however, would be the same—a permanent shift in the age structure of the population. Once again, it is the unprecedented rapid jump in the number of older people through the first half of the next century which has created the sense of a demographic or aging crisis.

It should be noted further that many of the questions prompted by the aging of the baby boom cohorts regarding potentials, responsibilities and needs of older persons would have arisen without the demographic bulge, but with somewhat less urgency. Therefore, while what follows focuses on older ages, many of the questions and issues are pertinent for people in age cohorts preceding and following the baby boom cohorts.

Of course, the members of the baby boom cohorts have been and are actors in contextual trends which will affect the public values driving aging policies in their later years. They are in the process of constructing the values and politics which will define their third age and beyond. However, the "they" is a diverse lot, with widely different life experiences affecting the goals, aspirations and needs they will have as they age. That diversity must be part of the national conversation on policy directions for an aging population (Kingson, 1992).

The Role of Private and Public Transfers

A broader understanding of the role of transfers will facilitate public discourse on the implications of population aging. Transfers should be understood as public and private; as cash and "in kind." Public transfers are the most visible transfers. The Old Age Health and Income Security system provides an example. These transfers take principally three forms, namely, social insurance (e.g., Social Security and Medicare), public assistance (e.g., SSI and Medicaid) and tax code provisions (e.g., special age-related deductions and incentives for retirement savings through IRAs). Private transfers in this system take a number of forms as well, including employment-based fringes (e.g., private and public employee pensions, health care benefits), family cash transfers (e.g., life insurance, financial assistance from relatives and inheritances), housing, and caregiving (Kingson & Berkowitz, 1993).

Transfers occur to varying degrees and in varying ways throughout life. Early on, individuals and cohorts are primarily recipients of private transfers in the form of family care, housing, and

basic expenses, and of public transfers in the form of education. In youth and middle age, individuals and cohorts both typically transfer more than they receive in the form of caregiving to the young and sometimes to functionally disabled family members, and in tax payments to support the various functions of government. In old age, especially advanced old age, the flow of transfers generally reverses, when the individual is in receipt of Social Security, Medicare transfers, and often family care, when disabled, although many among the old also transfer care and other resources to others as well (Kingson, Hirshorn, & Cornman, 1986). A time-freeze perspective (i.e., cross-sectional) suggests that it is children and the old who receive transfers, and the young adult and middle-aged who give. Such a perspective is often implicit to claims of inequities between cohorts and age groups with respect to the costs and benefits of Social Security and Medicare. A longitudinal perspective does more to highlight the reciprocity over time. From this perspective, the prior contribution of older family members and older cohorts to the young and to society can be seen as justifying the claims of older cohorts to a reasonable return in the form of retirement, health benefits (National Academy on Aging, 1994), and caregiving.

As the work of Elaine Brody (1990), Marjorie Cantor (1991), and Barbara Silverstone (1989) implies, our vision of transfers must extend to include private exchanges of time and care to family members. Although less recognized as an explicit transfer, family and friends are often the sources of critical nonmonetized, long-term care services, including time spent negotiating the complex array of health and long-term care services, house cleaning, meal preparation, shopping, and assisting with personal care. It is now widely acknowledged that the vast majority of functionally disabled elderly persons living in noninstitutional settings rely on family and friends for most, if not all of their care—an estimated 80% of the long-term care going to elderly persons (Olson, 1994).

Even though informal caregiving is *the* critical component of the nation's long-term care system, more often than not, informal caregiving is an afterthought of public policy discussions on long-term care. Policy planners express concern about caregiver stress and the possibility that new home care services may lead to reductions in familial efforts. Researchers note costs, in the form of lost wages and smaller retirement benefits, for those caregivers who must compromise their employment efforts. But serious attention is rarely given to such concerns, in large measure, because of assumptions about who is expected to give care and in the value assigned to this care. Laura Olson (1994, p. 13) points out that in the context of growing social welfare costs, the United States, like many other nations, is placing greater expectations on the family to provide care. "[N]ot only have more females added care of the superannuated to their productive and reproductive roles, but, in addition, these efforts tend to be both invisible and undervalued." Though not an inconsequential concern for men, in a number of fundamental ways, long-term care could be thought about as an explicit women's issue, rather than as a concern that affects women more than men. A broader view of caregiving as a transfer may serve to elevate the visibility of much informal caregiving, increasing the likelihood that these issues will emerge as explicit public policy concerns.

A broader view of transfers may help to move discussion away from narrow and cataclysmic assessments of the momentary value of Social Security and Medicare to any one cohort toward a broader review of how best to deal with financing and benefit reforms in preparation for the retirement of the baby boom cohorts and those who follow. Such reforms, we suggest, will not be achieved by privatizing or means-testing Social Security benefits. These measures could only serve in the long run to undermine political support for the program, an outcome that would be particularly detrimental to low- and moderate-income elders of the future. Without including the entire population in these programs, it is not possible to sustain the large transfers from higher- to low-income persons that occurs within the context of the program. This redistribution within cohorts occurs through such features as the benefit formula, which provides returns to low-wage workers, which are roughly twice as large (i.e., 57% replacement rate) as those to workers paying taxes consistently at the highest level of Social Security taxation (24% placement rate) and through the tax system, which treats up to 85% of Social Security benefits as taxable income. Ultimately, the quality of Social Security and other reforms will be enhanced if we can agree on the questions we need to ask and the values we want to emphasize in moving toward an "older" society, for it is the selection of questions and values which lends meaning to today's trends and will give direction to tomorrow's possibilities.

Appendix

As the number and proportion of older persons changes during the next 60 years, the number of persons aged 18 through 64, the so-called working age population, is projected to decline as a proportion of the entire population. The ratio of elderly persons (65 and over) to every 100 "working age" persons (18 to 64) has increased from about 15:100 persons in 1955 to roughly 21:100 today and is expected to increase to about 36:100 persons in 2030, when all surviving baby boomers are 65 or older. On the one hand, it could be argued that the old age dependency ratio actually understates the implications of population aging. First, it does not capture the aging of the elderly population. The very old population—the group among the elderly with the highest health care and social support costs—is projected to grow in relative and absolute terms, especially as the baby boom cohorts move through their old age. Consequently, the per capita costs of elder support are likely to increase. Second, if middle series Census Bureau and intermediate Social Security mortality assumptions are substantially lower than actual experience, then the overall costs of elder support may be considerably higher. On the other hand, the old age dependency ratio argument seems to overstate and potentially misframe discussion about the pressures arising from population aging in a number of important ways. Analysis based on the "overall dependency" ratio (also called the "total support" ratio)—which includes children under 18 and the elderly as "dependent" populations—leads to a different conclusion (Crown, 1985). During the next 65 years the overall dependency ratio is not projected to exceed the levels it attained in 1964 (Torrey, n.d.). This is because the proportion of population under 18 is projected to decline. Even from 2030 through 2050, the total dependency ratio is projected to be below (about 78:100) what it was during the 1960s (e.g., 83:100 in 1965) when most of the baby boomers were children. While the composition of governmental and private spending for children and elderly persons is different, analysis that includes the expanded notion of dependency ratios does not lead to the automatic conclusion that changing demographics will overwhelm the nation's ability to respond to the retirement needs of future generations (Crown, 1985; Kingson & Berkowitz, 1993). Neither does it suggest that the nation will necessarily be able to meet these needs, since so much depends on future productivity and on such factors as the composition of the workforce (National Academy on Aging, 1994).

References

Bengtson, V. L., Cutler, N. E., Mangen, D. J., & Marshall, V. W. (1985). Generations, cohorts, and relations between age groups. In R. H. Binstock & E. Shanas (Eds.), *Handbook of aging and the social sciences.* New York: Van Nostrand Reinhold.

Binstock, R. H. (1983). The aged as scapegoat. *The Gerontologist, 23,* 136–143.

Brody, E. (1990). *Women in the middle: Their parent-care years.* New York: Springer Publishing.

Cantor, M. H. (1991). Family and community: Changing roles in an aging society. *The Gerontologist, 31,* 337–346.

Conner, K. A. (1992). *Aging America: Issues facing an aging society.* Englewood Cliffs, NJ: Prentice Hall.

Crown, W. H. (1985). Some thoughts on reformulating the dependency ratio. *The Gerontologist, 25,* 166–171.

Goleman, D. (1994, April 26). Mental decline in aging need not be inevitable. *New York Times.*

Graebner, W. A. (1980). *A history of retirement.* New Haven, CT: Yale University Press.

Hayflick, L. (1994). *How and why we age.* New York: Ballantine Books.

Kingson, E. R. (1992, April). *The diversity of the baby boom generation: Implications for their retirement years.* Washington, DC: American Association of Retired Persons, Forecasting and Environmental Scanning Division.

Kingson, E. R., & Berkowitz, E. D. (1993). *Social Security and Medicare: A policy primer.* Westport, CT: Auburn House.

Kingson, E. R., Hirshorn, B. A., & Cornman, J. M. (1986). *Ties that bind: The interdependence of generations.* Cabin John, MD: Seven Locks Press.

National Academy on Aging. (1994, July). *Old age in the 21st century.* Washington, DC: National Academy on Aging.

Olson, L. K. (1994). *The graying of the world: Who will care for the frail elderly?* New York: Haworth Press.

Quinn, J. F., Burkhauser, R. V., & Myers, D. A. (1990). *Passing the torch: The influence of economic incentives on work and retirement.* Kalamazoo, MI: W. E. Upjohn Institute for Employment Research.

Schulz, J. H. (1995). *The economics of aging.* Belmont, CA: Wadsworth Publishing.

Silverstone, B. (1989). *You and your parent: The modern family's guide to emotional, physical, and financial problems.* New York: Pantheon Books.

Torrey, B. B. (n.d.). Guns vs. canes: The fiscal implications of an aging population. *AEA Papers and Proceedings, 72,* 2.

What Do Children Owe Elderly Parents?

Daniel Callahan

■

In the spring of 1983 the Reagan administration announced that states may under Medicaid legally require children to contribute to the support of their elderly parents. At the time a number of states were considering or enacting just such laws. The administration, one spokesman said, was not proposing anything inherently new. It was simply responding to a state request for clarification of the existing Medicaid law, and wanted only to say that state statutes enforcing family responsibility laws were not in conflict with federal policy.[1]

As it turned out, the administration's initiative was a policy shift whose time had not come. While a number of states flirted for a time with new family responsibility policies, only a few (Virginia, Idaho, and Mississippi, for example) actually adopted them, and even fewer seem to be enforcing them. As pressing as the state Medicaid nursing home burden is, it rapidly became clear that there is little general sentiment to force children to provide financially for their elderly parents.[2]

Nonetheless, Reagan's initiative was an important social and policy event and raises significant moral issues. In one form or another, the idea is likely to arise again. Anything that can be done to raise revenue to reduce the Medicaid burden probably will be done. Three questions are thus worth considering. What kind of a moral obligation do children have toward the welfare of their elderly parents? Can it be said that the changed health, longevity, and social circumstances of the elderly justify a shift in traditional moral obligations? Even if children do have some significant duties to parents, is it still legitimate to ask the state to take over much of the direct burden of care?

The first question is of course an old one. Each generation has had to make its own sense of the biblical injunction that we should honor our fathers and mothers. It neither tells us in what "honor" consists nor how far filial obligation should be carried. As a piece of practical advice, however, it once made considerable sense. In most traditional and agricultural societies, parents had considerable power over the lives of their offspring. Children who did not honor their parents risked not only immediate privation, but also the loss of the one inheritance that would enable them to raise and support their own families—land they could call their own.

The advent of industrialization brought about a radical change. It reduced the direct coercive power of parents over their children, setting into motion a trend toward the independence of both parents and children that has been a mark of contemporary society. Though the affective bond between parents and children has so far endured in the face of industrialization and modernity, the combination of actual attachment and potential independence frames the question of the obligation of children toward their elderly parents.

The moral ideal of the parent-child relationship is that of love, nurture, and the mutual seeking for the good of the other. While the weight of the relationship will ordinarily shift according to the age of children and their parents, mutual respect and reciprocity have been a central part of the moral standard. Yet the reality of human lives can stand in the way of the realization of moral ideals. Just as not all children are lovable, neither do all parents give the welfare of their children their serious attention and highest priority. Many children do not find their parents lovable and feel no special sense of duty toward them. Many parents are not happy with the way their children turn out, or with the kind of lives they live, and do not seek to remain intertwined with them.

To what extent, and under what circumstances, flaws and faults of that kind can be said to alter the mutual obligations is obviously an important question. Yet even when the affectional bonds between parent and child are strong, it is still by no means clear what each morally owes to the other. If parents ought to help their children to grow up and flourish, should they go so far as to seriously jeopardize their own future welfare in doing so? If children should honor their elderly parents, how great a sacrifice ought that to entail?

The Changing Status of the Elderly

The present relationship between children and their elderly parents is shaped in part by the changing status of the elderly in society. A rising number and increasing proportion of our population are the elderly. The "young old" (65–75) appear to be in better health than ever, but as people live longer, there is also an increasing number of the "old old" (75+) who are frail and dependent. Despite a variety of public programs and considerable improvement in recent decades, a significant proportion of the elderly (about 25 percent in 1980) still live in poverty or near-poverty. A large proportion do not have immediate family or relatives to whom they can turn for either financial or emotional assistance, and many—particularly women—live alone or in institutions. Even so, as Victor Fuchs notes in summarizing available data, rising income has "made it possible for an ever higher percentage [of the elderly] to maintain their own households, health permitting."[3]

Independence, however, need not mean an absence of family ties. Gerontologists take great pleasure in demolishing what they tell us are two prevalent myths, that the caring family has disappeared, and that the elderly are isolated from their children. There has indeed been a decline in the number of elderly who live with their children or other relatives, from three-fifths in 1960 to one-third in 1980,[4] and an equally sharp drop—down to 1 percent—in the number of elderly who depend upon their children for financial support.[5] Yet it still seems to be true, as Ethel Shanas has noted, that "most old people live close to at least one of their children and see at least one child often. Most old people see their siblings and relatives often, and old people, whether bedfast or housebound because of ill health, are twice as likely to be living at home as to be residents in an institution. . . ."[6] In addition, it is estimated that 60–80 percent of all disabled or impaired persons receive significant family help.[7]

One important change involves the proportion of young and old who believe that children should be financially responsible for their elderly parents. This has shifted downward (from about 50 percent in the mid-fifties to 10 percent in the mid-seventies),[8] and a simultaneous reduction in financial assistance has occurred. However, this need not be taken as an indication of a diminished sense of filial responsibility. The advent of Social Security, and the increasing financial strength of the elderly for other reasons, all indicate important social variables that have reduced financial pressure on children to support parents.

Other social changes could eventually alter that situation. The increasing number of divorced families, of small families, and of families where both spouses work, have created the possibility of a reduced sense of obligation in the future, though that has yet clearly to materialize.[9] In his 1981 book *New Rules,* the pollster Daniel Yankelovich wrote that "one of the most far-reaching changes in [moral] norms relates to what parents believe they owe their children and what their children owe them. Nowhere are the changes in the unwritten social contract more significant or agonizing. The overall pattern is clear: today's parents expect to make fewer sacrifices for their children than in the past, but they also demand less from their offspring in the form of future obligations than their parents demanded of them. . . . Sixty-seven percent [of Americans surveyed] believe that 'children do not have an obligation to their parents regardless of what their parents have done for them.' "[10]

To what extent this shift (assuming it is real) will lead to a change in the behavior and attitudes noted earlier remains to be seen. According to other available data and most commentators, children and families remain the principal source of emotional support and companionship for the elderly. At the same time, there is a pronounced distaste, on the side of both children and parents, for burdening children with financial obligations toward their parents. It seems widely assumed that contemporary life requires a different moral standard. A brief look at the present legal situation is useful in that respect; it brings out some of the ambivalence that exists and opens the way for a more direct look at the moral issues.

What the Law Says

Some twenty-six states at present have statutes that can require children to provide financial support for needy parents. Though erratically administered, difficult to implement, and of doubtful financial value, they remain as testimony to an effort dating back to the early seventeenth century to shift from the public to the private sphere the care of poverty-stricken elderly. While such laws had no precedent in either common law or medieval law, they came into being in England with the Elizabethan Poor Law of 1601, representing a culmination of at least three centuries of

efforts to cope with the problem of the poor in general. The Poor Law did not concentrate on the children of the elderly, but extended the network of potential support to include the fathers and mothers, and the grandfathers and grandmothers, of the poor. The family, as a unit, was to be responsible for poverty-stricken kinfolk.

When these laws passed over into the American scene, during the seventeenth and eighteenth centuries, the focus was on the responsibility of children toward their elderly parents, though a few states have retained the wider scope.[11] Blackstone's famous *Commentaries* succinctly state the moral basis of such a responsibility: "The duties of children to their parents arise from a principle of natural justice and retribution. For to those who gave us existence we naturally owe subjection and obedience during our minority, and honor and reverence ever after; they who protected the weakness of our infancy are entitled to our protection in the infirmity of their age; they who by sustenance and education have enabled their offspring to prosper ought in return to be supported by that offspring in case they stand in need of assistance."[12]

The American state laws were little invoked during the eighteenth and nineteenth centuries, but they were increasingly turned to during the twentieth century, particularly in the aftermath of the depression and World War II. While there is broad historical agreement that the primary purpose of the laws was to protect the public from the burden of caring for the poor, including the elderly, the laws were buttressed by a variety of moral assumptions.[13]

Martin R. Levy and Sara W. Gross have identified three moral premises that underlie the American laws and developed some cogent criticisms of them. First, "the duty of a child to support his parents is a mirror-image of the parents' responsibility to support a child."[14] They point out the doubtful logic of that position. In procreation parents not only bring a child into the world, but by the same action undertake the moral obligation of sustaining that child, whose existence is entirely dependent upon the parents. As Levy and Gross put it, "In the converse situation of the duty of a child to support a parent, there is no proximate cause, no volitional act, and no rational basis for the demand of support. The child has not acted to bring about the life of the parent. While the father assumes the voluntary status of fatherhood, the child assumes no duty by having been born. His birth is the result of the act of the father and mother, and such a result cannot logically or physically be turned into a proximate cause."[15] While they do not deny that there can be a moral bond of love and affection, "moral duty and gratitude, or lofty ideals, cannot be used as a justification for the taking of property."[16] By focusing on "the taking of property," the authors focus on a relatively narrow point.

The second general moral premise turns on what they call "the relational interest of family status."[17] They mean that the simple fact of a family relationship—creating a special tie between parent and child, both biological and social—may itself engender the basis for a demand made upon children to support their elderly parents. Yet they point out that the relational interests are both too broad and too narrow to serve as a reasonable criterion for determining the duty to provide support. "It is too broad in . . . that not all children love and revere their parents. The status of a child confers no special emotional tie in and of itself."[18] It is too narrow in that, if emotional commitment is the standard, then a child would logically be bound to support everyone to whom he or she is tied by emotional commitment, whether family member or not.[19]

The analogy of a contract provides the third moral premise. Since the child was at one time supported by the parent, does not that create an implicit contract requiring that the child in turn support the parent when that becomes necessary? Levy and Gross point out that no direct contract is negotiated between parent and child

when the child is procreated, and that any analogy must thus be based on an implied or quasi-contract. But the analogy of an implied contract does not work: the two parties necessary to the making of a contract did not exist simultaneously. A common standard in the law, moreover, is that neither the carrying out of a duty, nor the promise of rendering a performance already required by duty, is a sufficient condition of a return promise—an obligation to do likewise.[20]

Parents as "Friends"

Although Levy and Gross effectively dispatch the argument that the benefits bestowed by parents upon children automatically entail a duty of the children in return to aid parents, there is considerably more that needs to be said. Are we to hold that the obligation flows in one direction only, that because children were given no choice about being born, they owe nothing whatever to their parents? That seems too extreme. At the least, it fails to explain why in fact many children feel an obligation toward their parents, nor does it sufficiently plumb the moral depths of the family relationship.

The late Jane English also argued that the language of "owing" is mistakenly applied in the circumstances. Children "owe" parents nothing at all—which is not to say that there are not many things that children ought to do for their parents. Instead, she held that "the duties of grown children are those of friends and result from love between them and their parents, rather than being things owed in repayment for the parents' earlier sacrifices."[21] In situations where one person does a favor for another, there may be an obligation to reciprocate, but parents do not do favors for their children in the same sense that strangers or acquaintances may do them for each other. The bond that should unite parents and children is that of friendship, and "friendship ought to be characterized *by mutuality* rather than reciprocity: friends offer what they can give and accept what they need without regard for the total amount of benefits exchanged. And friends are motivated by love rather than by the prospect of repayment. Hence, talk of 'owing' is singularly out of place in friendship."[22] Thus children ought to do things for their parents, but the "ought" is that which follows from friendship; it resists both quantitative measurement and the stricter language of owing something in return for earlier benefits.

While English's argument has some plausibility, it is ultimately unsatisfying. Friendship can certainly exist between parent and child, but it often does not. Quite apart from those circumstances where parents have neglected their children or otherwise alienated their affection, they may have little in common other than their biological origins. Moreover, the nature of the friendship that exists between parent and child can and usually will be different from the kind that exists between and among those who are unrelated. A child might plausibly say that, while he is not a friend of his parents, he nonetheless feels toward them respect and love. To push the same point further, many children actively dislike their parents, find no pleasure in their company, and yet feel they ought to do things for them despite those feelings. In distinguishing between favors and friendship, English says that "another difference between favors and friendships is that after a friendship ends, the duties of friendship end."[23] That may be true enough in the case of nonfamily relationships, but it then raises all the more forcefully the question of whether friendship, however much it may mark a relationship between parent and child, can catch the fullness of the moral bond.

The origin and nature of the parent-child bond—or whatever other relationship may exist— is unique. By the procreation of children parents create a social unit that otherwise would not and could not exist. If children do not select their parents, neither do parents select their individual children (they choose to have *a* child, not *this* child). Even so, the family relationship is not something one can simply take or leave. It is a fundamental and unavoidable part of our social nature as human beings. That psychotherapists can spend a good deal of time untangling problems between parents and children provides at least a clue to the emotional depth of the biological relationship, whether marked by unhappiness or happiness. We can and do drift away from ordinary friendships, but parents stay in our memory and exert their influence even in the face of distance or active hostility. Whether we like it or not, we are in some sense always one with our parents, both because of the unique circumstances by which we came to know them and because of the long period of nurture when we were utterly dependent upon them. The mutual interaction of parents and children, even when friendships exist, cannot then entirely be reduced to the category of friendship. The emotional and biological bond between parent and child gives the relationship a permanent and central place in our lives, quite apart from whether that relationship turns out well or poorly. That cannot be said of friendship in the usual sense of the term.

Capturing Intimacy in Moral Language

Ferdinand Schoeman catches some of this flavor when he argues that the traditional language of morality, that of rights and obligations, does not seem to fit well in describing the bond among family members: "We *share ourselves* with those with whom we are intimate and are aware that they do the same with us. Traditional moral boundaries, which give rigid shape to the self, are transparent to this kind of sharing. This makes for nonabstract moral relationships in which talk about rights of others, respect for others, and even welfare of others is to a certain extent irrelevant."[24] Perhaps Schoeman takes things a bit far, but he tries to make clear that the intimacy of family relationships forces us into revealing and sharing a self that may not be revealed to others on the public stage. While it is often the case that parents do not really know their own child, just as often they do, even when their perceptions differ from those of the child. Whether they understand their child or not, the fact that they shared considerable intimacy when the child was young gives them access to a self that others may never see. For their part, children have unique access to parents, seeing a side of them that may never be revealed to others.

Another powerful candidate for the source of obligation is that of gratitude on the part of children toward their parents. Gratitude would be due, not simply because parents discharged their obligations toward the children, but because in their manner of doing so they went beyond the demands of mere duty, giving voluntarily of themselves in a way neither required nor ordinarily expected of them. As Jeffrey Blustein notes, "Duties of gratitude are owed only to those who have helped or benefited us freely, without thought of personal gain, simply out of a desire to protect or promote our wellbeing. The givers may hope for some return, but they do not give in expectation of it."[25] A consequence of this line of reasoning, however, is that only those parents who did more than was morally required could be said to have a right to the gratitude of their children. And it is by no means obvious that a "debt of gratitude" carries with it a strict obligation to provide like goods or services, that is, to go beyond what is otherwise required.

I am searching here with some difficulty for a way to characterize the ethical nature of the parent-child relationship, a relationship that appears almost but not quite self-evident in its reciprocal moral claims and yet oddly elusive also. We seem to say too much if we try to reduce the relationship to mutual moral duties, rights, and obligations. That implies a rigor and formalism which distorts the moral bond. We say too little if we try to make it a matter of voluntary affection only. Yet we cannot, I suspect, totally dismiss the language of obligation nor would we want to give up the ideal of mutual affection either. If the procreation and physical rearing of a child does not automatically entail reciprocal duties toward the parents when they are needy and dependent, it is certainly possible to imagine a sense of obligation arising when parents have done far more for children than would morally be required of them. My own parents, for example, did not throw me out on my own when I reached eighteen. They sacrificed a good deal to provide me with a higher education, and in fact provided financial support for my graduate education until I was thirty, topping that off by giving my wife and me a down-payment on our first house. They did it out of affection, rather than duty, but I certainly felt I owed them something in return in their old age. There need not be, then, any necessary incompatibility between feeling both affection and a sense of duty. But we lack a moral phrase that catches both notions in one concept; and neither taken separately is quite right.

The Power of Dependence

Another aspect of the relationship between children and their elderly parents bears reflection. Much as young children will have a special dependence upon parents, as those human beings above all others who have a fateful power over their destinies, so many elderly parents can come in dire circumstances similarly to depend upon their children. In a world of strangers or fleeting casual acquaintants, of distant government agencies and a society beyond their control, elderly parents can see in their children their only hope for someone who ought to care for them. Neither parent nor child may want this kind of emotional dependence, and each might wish that there were an alternative. Nonetheless, parents may be forced to throw themselves upon their children simply because there is no other alternative. Who else is likely to care?

Can that sense of utter need, if not for money then only for affection and caring, in and of itself create a moral obligation? It is surely a difficult question whether, as a general matter, a moral obligation is incurred when one human being is rendered by circumstance wholly dependent upon another—whether, that is, the dependency itself creates the obligation, quite apart from any other features of the relationship. A moral claim of that kind will inevitably be controversial, if only because it is (regretfully) common to rest claims of obligation upon implicit or explicit contracts of one kind or another; or upon features of the relationship that can be subjected to utilitarian calculation. It is difficult in this case plausibly to invoke such norms. Still, the power of sheer dependence—whether of newborn child upon parent or elderly, dependent parent upon child—can be potent in its experienced moral demands. The fate of one or more persons rests in the hands of another. The issue, as it presents itself, may be less one of trying to discover the grounds of obligation that would require a response than one of trying to find grounds for ignoring a demand that so patently assaults the sensibilities. It is not so much "must I?" as it is "how can I not?"

Joel Feinberg, commenting on the moral place of gratitude, moves in a similar direction when he writes, "My benefactor once freely offered me his services when I needed them. . . . But now circumstances have arisen in which he needs help, and I am in a position to help him. Surely, I owe him my services now, and he would be entitled to resent my failure to come through."[26] A qualification is in order here: gratitude is ordinarily thought due only when, as noted above, a benefactor has gone beyond ordinary duties. In some cases, parents may have only done their duty, and in such a minimal way that no gratitude seems due them. We are then brought back to the starkest moral situation—in which the dependency only seeks to establish a claim on us.

In trying to unravel the nature of the possible moral obligations, it may be helpful to speak of some specific claims or demands that might be made. Money is by no means the only, or necessarily the most important, benefit that parents can ask of their children. Children can also contribute their time and physical energy, and provide affection and psychological support. On a scale of moral priorities, it would be difficult to persuasively argue that parents have an obligation to deprive their own dependent children of necessary financial support in order to support their elderly parents. By virtue of procreating those children, the latter have a claim upon them that their parents cannot equal. Of course, where a surplus exists after their own children have been taken care of, the financial support of needy parents might become obligatory, particularly if there were no other available sources of support. Ordinarily, however, their principal economic duties will be toward their own children.

The same cannot necessarily be said of providing either physical help or affection to their parents. While the giving of physical help or affection could readily be merged, I think it is useful to distinguish between them. Physical help—such as assistance in moving, cleaning, shopping, and trips to visit friends or doctors—is a somewhat different contribution to the welfare of the elderly than simply talking with them. Parents of young children may not readily be able to adapt their schedules to such demands upon their time or energy. Yet they may be able to provide affection, either by visits at times they find convenient, or through letters and telephone calls. An inability to provide some kinds of care does not exempt children from providing other forms. In fact, the available evidence suggests that affection is most wanted, and it is not difficult to understand why. The uncertainties of old age, the recognition of growing weakness and helplessness, can above all generate the desire to believe that at least some people in the world care about one's fate, and are willing to empathetically share that burden which few of us would care to bear alone—a recognition that life is gradually coming to an end and that nature is depriving us of our body, our individuality, and our future.[27]

In terms of financial obligations, there is considerable evidence from human experience in general, and from state efforts to impose financial burdens upon children in particular, that enforced legal obligations of children toward parents are mutually destructive. If only from the viewpoint of promoting family unity and affection, the provision of economic and medical care for the elderly by the government makes considerable sense. Ben Wattenberg quotes someone who nicely catches an important point: "We [older folks] don't like to take money from our kids. We don't want to be a burden. They don't like giving us money, either. We all get angry at each other if we do it that way. So we all sign a political contract to deal with what anthropologists would call the 'intergenerational transfer of wealth.' The young people *give* money to the government. I *get* money from the government. That way we can both get mad at the government and keep on loving each other."[28]

If the burden of economic care of the elderly can be difficult even for the affluent, it can be impossible for the poor. Moreover, adults with elderly parents ought not to be put in the position of trying to balance the moral claims of their own children against those of their parents, or jeopardizing their own old age in order to sustain their parents in their old age. Though such conflicts may at times be inescapable, society ought to be structured in a way that minimizes them. The great increase in life expectancy provides a solid reason, if one was ever needed, for arguing that all of us collectively through the state—

rather than the children of the elderly—should supply their basic economic support. Both parents and children legitimately want an appropriate independence, not the kind that sunders their relationship altogether or makes it merely contingent upon active affection. A balance is sought between that independence which enables people to have a sense of controlling their own destinies, and those ties of obligation and affection that render each an indispensable source of solace in the face of a world that has no special reason to care for them.

A minimal duty of any government should be to do nothing to hinder, and if possible do something to protect, the natural moral and filial ties that give families their power to nurture and sustain. To exploit that bond by coercively taxing families is, I believe, to threaten them with great harm. It is an action that presupposes a narrower form of moral obligation of children to parents than can rationally be defended. At the same time it promises to rupture those more delicate moral bonds, as powerful as they are conceptually elusive, that sustain parents and children in their lives together. Such bonds do not necessarily rule out financial incentives for children to care for their aged parents, as some recent legislative proposals suggest.[29] But if such incentives are to receive support, in that case considerable care would be needed to guard against an exploitation of parents by avaricious children. There are, I ruefully note, as many ways to corrupt the parent-child relationship as ways to sustain it.

Notes

1. Statement of James L. Scott, Associate Administrator for Operations, Health Care Financing Administration, before the House Select Committee on Human Services, May 16, 1983.
2. *Cf.* the overwhelmingly negative responses to the Administration initiative at hearings conducted by the Subcommittee on Human Services on "Medicaid and Family Responsibility: Who Pays?" May 16, 1983.

3. Victor R. Fuchs, *How We Live: An Economic Perspective on Americans from Birth to Death* (Cambridge: Harvard University Press, 1983), p. 201.

4. Stephen Crystal, *America's Old Age Crisis* (New York: Basic Books, 1982), p. 40.

5. *Ibid.*, p. 52.

6. Ethel Shanas, "The Family Relations of Old People," *The National Forum* 62 (Fall 1982), p. 10. As for the motivation behind the visits of children to their parents, Victor Fuchs cites a study purporting to show "that the number of visits was positively related to the parents' bequeathable wealth . . . ," in Victor Fuchs, " 'Though Much Is Taken': Reflections on Aging, Health, and Medical Care," *Milbank Memorial Quarterly* 62:2 (Spring 1984), p. 160.

7. James J. Callahan, Jr., *et al.*, "Responsibilities of Families for Their Severely Disabled Elderly," paper prepared by the Brandeis University Health Policy Consortium, July 1979, p. iii.

8. Crystal, *op. cit.*, pp. 56–57.

9. *Cf.* Mary Jo Bane, "Is the Welfare State Replacing the Family?" *The Public Interest* (Winter 1983), pp. 91–101.

10. Daniel Yankelovich, *New Rules: Searching for Self-Fulfillment in a World Turned Upside Down* (New York: Random House, 1981), p. 104.

11. For some pertinent analysis of the present state statutes, see, for example, Paul R. Ober, "Pennsylvania's Family Responsibility Statute—Corruption of Blood and Denial of Equal Protection," *Dickinson Law Review* 77 (1972), pp. 331–351; Gregory G. Sarno, "Constitutionality of Statutory Provision Requiring Reimbursement of Public by Child for Financial Assistance to Aged Parents," *American Law Reports Annotation* 75, 3rd (1977), pp. 1159–1178; W. Walton Garrett, "Filial Responsibility Laws," *Journal of Family Law* 18 (1979–80), pp. 793–818; James L. Lopes, "Filial Support and Family Solidarity," *Pacific Law Journal* 6 (July 1975), 508–535.

12. *Commentaries on the Laws of England*, Vol. 1 (Philadelphia: J. B. Lippincott and Co., 1856) book 1, ch. 16, section 1, cited in Jeffrey Blustein, *Parents and Children: The Ethics of the Family* (New York: Oxford University Press, 1982), p. 181. It is worth noting that the People's Republic of China apparently persists in upholding stringent filial obligations. The Constitution of 1982 states that ". . . children who have come of age have the duty to support and assist their parents"; and the Marriage Law of 1980 says that "When children fail to perform the duty of supporting their parents, parents who have lost the ability to work or have difficulties in providing for themselves have the right to demand that their children pay for their support." Cited in Alice and Sidney Goldstein, "The Challenge of an Aging Population in the People's Republic of China." Paper presented at annual meeting of Population Association of America, May 3–5, 1984, Minneapolis.

13. See especially W. Walton Garrett, *op. cit.*, pp. 793–796.

14. Martin R. Levy and Sara W. Gross, "Constitutional Implications of Parental Support Laws," *University of Richmond Law Review* 13 (1979), p. 523.

15. *Ibid.*, p. 524.

16. *Ibid.*, p. 525.

17. *Ibid.*

18. *Ibid.*, p. 526.

19. *Ibid.*, p. 527.

20. *Ibid.*, pp. 527–528.

21. Jane English, "What Do Grown Children Owe Their Parents?" in Onora O'Neill and William Ruddick, eds., *Having Children: Philosophical and Legal Reflections on Parenthood* (New York: Oxford University Press, 1979), p. 351.

22. *Ibid.*, p. 353.

23. *Ibid.*

24. Ferdinand Schoeman, "Rights of Children, Rights of Parents, and the Moral Basis of the Family," *Ethics* 91 (October 1980), p. 8.

25. Blustein, *op. cit.*, p. 177.

26. Joel Feinberg, "Duties, Rights, and Claims," *American Philosophical Quarterly* 3 (1966), p. 139; cited in Blustein, *Ibid.*, p. 176.

27. For further helpful discussions on the general topic, see Andrew Joseph Christiansen, "Autonomy and Dependence in Old Age," Yale University doctoral dissertation, 1982; Abraham Monk, "Family Supports in Old Age," *Social Work* (November 1979), pp. 533–538; Wilma T. Donahue, "What About Our Responsibility to the Abandoned Elderly?" *The Gerontologist* 18:2 (1978), 102–111; Wayne C. Seelbach, "Correlates of Aged Parents' Filial Responsibility Expectations and Realizations," *The Family Coordinator* (October 1978), pp. 341–350; Stanley J. Brady, *et al.*, "The Family Caring Unit: A Major Consideration in the Long-Term Support System," *The Gerontologist* 18:6 (1978), 16–20; Elizabeth S. Johnson and Barbara J. Bursk, "The Relationship Between the Elderly and Their Adult Children," *The Gerontologist* 17:1 (1977), 90–96; Alvin Schorr, ". . . Thy Father and Thy Mother: A Second Look at Filial Responsibility and Family Policy," U.S. Department of Health and Human Services, SSA Publica-

tion No. 13-11953 (Washington DC: Government Print-ing Office, July 1980); W. Andrew Achenbaum, *Old Age in the New Land* (Baltimore: Johns Hopkins Press, 1978), pp. 75–80; Joanne P. Acford, "Reducing Medic-aid Expenditures Through Family Responsibility: Cri-tique of A Recent Proposal," *American Journal of Law and Medicine* 5:1 (Spring 1979), 59–79; "Relative Re-sponsibility," *The Nursing Home Law Letter* (February 1982), pp. 1–8.

28. Quoted by Irving Kristol in a review of Ben Watten-berg's *The Good News Is the Bad News Is Wrong* (New York: Simon and Schuster, 1984), in *The New Republic* (October 29, 1984), p. 37.

29. Representative Mario Biaggi, for instance, introduced a bill in Congress in 1983, H.R. 76, that proposed "to allow a credit against income tax to individuals for maintaining in a household a member of which is a dependent of the taxpayer who has attained age sixty-five." The bill died in committee.

Decision Making, Responsibility, and Advocacy in Geriatric Medicine: Physician Dilemmas with Elderly in the Community

Sharon R. Kaufman

∎

Notions of authority and responsibility in clini-cal medicine have been in flux since the 1960s, when patients became "health care consumers" and started to demand treatment options, health education, and open communication with their doctors (Cassell, 1986; Kaufman, 1993; White, 1988). In geriatrics particularly, shifting notions of physician authority and responsibility, con-sidered along with emergent ideas of patient au-tonomy, create ambiguity about the physician's role in decision making. Most of the literature about physician uncertainty and dilemmas in the care of elderly patients addresses two broad topics: end-of-life decision making in institu-tional settings (Gillick, 1988; Kayser-Jones, 1990; Hodges & Tolle, 1994; Solomon, 1993), and the problems of maintaining autonomy, dignity, and choice for the older person in the nursing home (Agich, 1993; Lidz, Fischer, & Arnold, 1993; Kane & Caplan, 1990; Miles & Meyers, 1994). While deliberation about life prolongation for the old and frail remains problematic, much of geriatric medicine concerns difficult decisions about topics other than the use of life-supportive technologies. And though questions about the re-tention of agency and identity in the nursing home continue to perplex health providers, most older people do not reside in institutions (Rice, 1989; Suzman, Willis, & Manton, 1993).

In a qualitative investigation of how physicians perceive dilemmas and difficult decisions in geriatrics, I found that decisions regarding end-of-life treatments represent only one area of concern for physicians and only one arena in which they define, through their practices, the nature of medical responsibility in the care of older people. In addition, most physicians I spoke with did not describe dilemmas in decision making once their patients were in institutional settings. Rather, in-depth interviews with 40 physicians revealed that they spend a great deal of time and effort confronting three broad problems: first, how much to intervene in patients' lives in order to balance risk reduction and safety with independence, so that frail and sick old people can continue to direct their own lives in the community; second, how to be the best possible advocate for the old person while making demands for medication compliance and behavior change; and third, how to assess vulnerability and quality of life when pondering placement decisions. The expression and discussion of these dilemmas constituted more than half of the data I collected in open-ended interviews about decision making in geriatrics.

Dilemmas concerning the community-dwelling elderly may be thought of as "everyday ethics" (Kane, 1994; Kane & Caplan, 1990) in geriatric medicine. Problems such as those cited above arise routinely in physicians' practices but are somehow not considered as dramatic, important, or worthy of conscious deliberation in the medical or bioethics literatures as are dilemmas that arise from the press to use high technology biomedical interventions at the very end of life in hospital settings. There have been few empirical studies investigating the range of everyday problems and dilemmas physicians face in providing care to older persons who reside in the community and who are not near death. The way in which physicians conceive, address, and solve problems of risk reduction, independence, ad-

vocacy, and intervention will bear directly on the way health care is delivered to older Americans.

This essay explores ways in which physicians view the nature of clinical decision making in the care of their geriatric outpatients. It presents and interprets some primary care physicians' actual descriptions of decision making. Their accounts reveal: (1) how certain problems in geriatrics are understood; (2) how decisions are formulated, weighed, and implemented; and (3) the deliberative process through which clinical responsibility is assessed and practiced.

Methods

This essay is part of a larger investigation of physician conceptualizations, values, conflicts, and explanations that underlie clinical/ethical decision making in the care of older adults. Data consist of in-depth, open-ended interviews with 40 primary care physicians who treat older patients in the community. The analytic task was to discover physician explanations of dilemmas they face, rather than to investigate preconceived variables. By focusing on physician perspectives, the essay is designed to contribute toward a *phenomenology of clinical medicine:* It explores the definitions and meanings of patient-care dilemmas as physicians both describe and attempt to solve them.

Uses of Narrative and Phenomenology

This project responds to recent calls for expanding the work of gerontology to include critical, phenomenological, and humanistic approaches in definitions of problem and explorations of knowledge, theory, practice, and policy (Gubrium, 1992; Luborsky & Sankar, 1993; Moody, 1988a, 1993). Moody (1988a, 1993) proposes that subjective representations of "lived experience" (Benner, 1994a; Husserl, 1931; Merleau-Ponty, 1962) would broaden and deepen the field of gerontology as well as refocus attention on the aging process, the nature of old age, and the role of theory in knowledge production about those topics. I suggest that the aged themselves are not the only useful "object" of study in gerontology. The phenomenological construct of "lived experience" can be applied also to persons whose attitudes and practices shape old persons' lives.

The Sample

The important inclusion criteria for this study was clinicians' experience with an elderly population. Twenty-three of the 40 physicians treated mainly persons over the age of 65 (60% to 100% of their patients). The other 17 physicians noted that 20% to 50% of their patients were elderly. This was a convenience sample generated by "snowball" techniques. I began by interviewing several internists and family practitioners known to me. At the end of those interviews, I asked for the names of other physicians who treat elderly patients. Those individuals were also asked to recommend colleagues to be interviewed. I made every attempt to solicit physicians from different specialties and a range of practice settings. I also tried to interview a broad age range of doctors as well as doctors from a variety of ethnic groups. Forty-two physicians were asked to participate; two declined, citing overburdened schedules. The snowball approach generated the entire sample and included the following: 14 general internists, 4 cardiologists, 10 family practitioners, and 12 geriatricians. Practice settings included: 16 in private or group practice, 13 in community clinics, 5 in public hospitals, 3 in university hospitals, and 2 in Health Maintenance Organizations. The age range was 32 to 71. There were 18 women and 22 men. In addition, the group included 28 white, 5 Hispanic, 4 African American, and 4 Asian physicians.

Interviews

An open-ended interview guide was constructed to elicit physician perspectives about decision making and responsibility in clinical medicine with elderly patients. The questions were intended to be nondirective so that physicians could describe in their own words dilemmas they face and choices they make. Interviews elicited discussion of the following topics: description of current practice; problems of aging; actual decision-making dilemmas; roles and responsibilities in treating the frail elderly and in the dying process; relationships with family and other health professionals; constraints on practice; and discussions of frailty, advocacy, and the allocation of resources. Each interview was face-to-face and lasted at least one hour. Interviews were audiotaped and the tapes were later transcribed verbatim.

The physicians gave narrative accounts (i.e., told stories) in response to my questions about difficult treatment decisions and the dilemmas they pose. Their stories outlined clinical, psychosocial, and contextual problems of at least one case; most physicians discussed three or more cases with me. They described the patient's condition and their own response, emphasized the decision points and why those were troublesome, and if the case had resolved, told its final outcome. This essay focuses specifically on the clinical narrative portions of the conversations.

The Phenomenological Approach: Access to the Moral/Practical Interface

The aim of the phenomenological approach is to use everyday discourse, in this case physician explanations of difficult decisions, to reveal naturally occurring concerns, meanings, and actions (Benner, 1994b). Narrative accounts of actual dilemma situations are details of "lived experience," examples of how difficult decisions are perceived, understood, and embedded in the day-to-day work of clinicians. Narratives illustrate ways in which the storyteller both remembers and engages the problem and relationship with the older person. The accounts reveal what concerns the storyteller—morally, medically, and practically—and illustrate how those aspects of concern cannot be disentangled. Finally, they show how the (partial) "world" of the practitioner, that is, his or her knowledge, relationships, and practices vis à vis a particular patient, is constituted in the storytelling and enacted in clinical/moral problem solving (Benner, 1994b; Leonard, 1994).

Personal stories from physicians whose interactions with the elderly significantly affect them can tell us more about particular values, actual practices, and modes of clinical reasoning than can answers to questions about beliefs or ideology or generalized information about what doctors typically do in conflict situations. The following narrative accounts show: (1) how authority and responsibility are specifically practiced in the doctor/older patient relationship; and (2) that individual understandings of health and illness in late life cannot be removed from moral and social contexts.

Background: Aging and Its Problems

I asked physicians to describe the range of problems they see in geriatrics and the major difficulties of aging and frailty. They defined the intractable problems of aging in terms of both the illnesses and social conditions that produce dependency. The fact that all 40 physicians included the socioeconomic contexts of their patients' lives in their delineation of "medical" problems was an unexpected finding of this study and weakens the stereotype held by many health consumers and health care analysts that

physicians (with the possible exception of board-certified geriatricians, some family practitioners, and psychiatrists) are trained to see, and thus consider in their treatments, only the physical manifestations of disease. These doctors' more broadly based awareness of what constitutes ill health in the elderly has direct implications for how they view responsibility in medicine and how they construct their role as practitioners.

The following excerpts from interviews are illustrative of ways in which physicians conceptualize the problems of being old. The three examples below are typical of this sample.

(1) I see osteoarthritis. Everybody has it. A lot of vascular disease. Both in terms of strokes and cardiovascular disease. A lot of heart disease. Hypertension, diabetes. So the big three would be osteoarthritis, hypertension, diabetes. And then a dabbling of other things after that: the dementias. A lot of my people are low income, so I see a lot of issues surrounding that; people just trying to make ends meet. Problems of housing, problems with safety. How much of what I recommend for them medically can they pay for? Loneliness is a big issue. Real family problems: kids on crack, grandkids that aren't being properly cared for. Worrying about younger people and not having the resources to be able to do much about that. (*Geriatrician, community clinic.*)

(2) Everybody has arthritis, hypertension. Many have heart disease. A lot of them are just deteriorating. A glaring example is the Alzheimer's patient. I see a lot more Parkinson's patients. Families have disintegrated and it's difficult sometimes to get care outside of institutions. People are living longer and they are deteriorating. The problems are mostly financial. People can't afford to buy their medicines. They can't afford long-term

care. Most of the older people have at least two chronic illnesses that require frequent monitoring and lots of medicines, and the expenses for those are outrageous. A little old lady came in yesterday saying, "I can't pay $110.00 a month for my medicine. I'm living on $600.00 a month." And she has no other resources to get it. This is not uncommon. (*Internist, private practice.*)

(3) The common problems—I think they're universal—seem to be about life: concerns about dying and aging and loss of ability to do things that they used to do. On the psychosocial side the problems are mobility, independence, social isolation, depression, anxiety. On the physical side they are painful arthritic conditions which aren't really curable, hypertension, diabetes, heart disease, cancer, chronic lung disease, and strokes. (*Internist, HMO.*)

All 40 physicians view their role to be multifaceted, beyond the strictly biomedical (Engel, 1977), and to consist of managing disease processes, improving or maintaining functional abilities, providing counseling and education to patients and their families, and working to acquire, integrate, and mobilize a wide array of social supports, formal and informal, so that patients can remain in their homes, functioning to the best of their abilities, for as long as possible. Their work embodies a well-known definition of geriatric medicine published in the *Journal of the American Geriatric Society:* "A comprehensive approach to the problems of the elderly, one which skillfully integrates clinical medicine with a mobilization of an array of social support" (Kane, 1988, p. 467). The actual nature of physician decision making which must underly the "comprehensive approach to the problems of the elderly" has not been adequately explored in gerontology.

Defining Dilemmas and the Nature of Decision Making

While physicians talked about many kinds of dilemmas that arise in the care of their community-based vulnerable elderly patients, this essay limits discussion to the three broad dilemmas they most commonly expressed. They are posed here as questions.

First, how, when, and to what degree does one intervene in the lives of frail old people who want to retain their autonomy and continue to live at home? Who is "at risk," what constitutes risk, and who decides? Physicians raised these questions and commented that they are not answered easily because providers and patients view the nature of risk differently. Dilemmas arise because although physicians see direct relationships among self-care ability, compliance, health, and well-being, some of their patients appear unconcerned about nutrition, cleanliness, safety, or symptom reduction. In many cases, what health providers perceive as risks—for example, poor mobility, poor judgment, inability to prepare meals and problems with self-care and managing finances—some patients view as benign states of being for which no intervention is sought or desired. Physicians were troubled when patients expressed a wish to be left alone, without treatment, rather than have their conditions monitored or functional abilities maintained and enhanced.

Second, how far can and should a physician push a patient to modify his or her behavior so that symptoms are relieved, acute problems are resolved, chronic conditions and disabilities are avoided or stabilized, and overall well-being is enhanced? Physicians noted that they sometimes do not know what is the "correct" or "ethical" thing to do regarding attempts to enforce medication compliance, the reduction of squalor in the home, the cessation of tobacco, alcohol or other nonprescription drug use, or the maintenance of in-home services that the patient refuses to employ.

Third, is placement in a skilled nursing facility or board-and-care home necessary or advisable? Placement decisions sometimes were fraught with uncertainty. Doctors were well aware that risk assessment and the perception of need for placement differed among health providers, patients, and family members, that personal and cultural values determine perspective, and that there is no unequivocally "right" thing to do. They also pondered how vulnerable a patient has to be before recommending, urging, or insisting on placement.

When physicians answered my questions—for example, describe a difficult treatment decision or tell me about a dilemma in decision making—they told stories from personal experience in which dilemmas often merged and compounded one another. They did not always articulate dilemmas in terms of the three discrete categories I present here. I have distinguished and separated them analytically to draw attention to some *dimensions* of decisions physicians describe in their everyday work with outpatients. The fact that dilemmas are frequently multidimensional in physician conceptualizations illustrates the complexity of issues with which they struggle and the difficulty of arriving at neat and satisfactory solutions to the problems they see.

The four narratives which follow enable us to see how physicians view some problematic issues in the lives of their elderly patients and how they view their relationships with patients. They represent the "lived experience" of the doctors engaging particular dilemmas, deliberating possible outcomes, and confronting moral and practical concerns. They illustrate that clinical problems are not conceived or addressed either by isolating their component parts or by invoking abstract principles of bioethical theory such as

"autonomy" or "justice" in order to make sense of or solve them. Rather, they show the irreducible nature of certain complex dilemmas in geriatric care.

Clinical Narratives

Example One

There is a guy who is about 78 or so who clearly has dementia and has had a couple of CVAs and lives with his wife who is probably schizophrenic, psychotic to some degree. Their house is a disaster zone and the wife is housebound and she's just as obnoxious as she can be. This is one of the home care patients. The resident goes into this home and there are clothes everywhere and it smells of urine. There is not a big roach or rat history but there is clutter and it's messy.

The resident, the case manager, and probably even Adult Protective Services are involved in this case. They all want to place this guy in [the county nursing home]. They are all saying, "He's in danger because his wife is so nuts, the house is a mess, and his quality of life is terrible." And I don't think he should be placed. My gut feeling is that they'd probably lived in a messy house even before he became ill. The evidence we have is that while the wife is nuts, she's also very committed to him. She tied a string around his waist, which is not an uncommon thing, it's a folk remedy. There are plenty of other patients who come in with strings around their waists. Probably she doesn't feed him right; that's the other thing.

It brings up the issue of what do you do with people who have dementia but who are very clear, consistently, about their choice? This guy does not want to be admitted to [the nursing home]. And there is a marginal living situation. I have spent hours and hours talking to people about this case. I feel like I really want to argue and advocate for him. It represents a class of problems you see in eldercare: older people who live in what are clearly less than ideal circumstances, who tolerate it fairly well, who aren't a danger to themselves. But it's really uncomfortable for us. You walk into somebody's house and it's disgusting. It's dirty and smelly and you say, "Get them out of there!" So how much do we impose our values? We don't have access to the homes of younger people in the same way that we have access to the homes of the elderly. I suspect there are lots of people who live like this. If you live like this when you are young, why shouldn't you be able to live like this when you're old? It's a very tough one . . . I don't know what will happen. We're trying to reframe the goals. One goal may be to have an agency come in and get the house cleaned up. That might be all that's required. (*Geriatrician, hospital-based.*)

Example Two

An 89-year-old woman came in with a hip fracture. All she cared about was going home. She was mildly demented. Not able to manage her money but coherent in terms of other sorts of decision making. There are examples of people in her category that come up all the time: not quite a hundred percent competent, a little fuzzy around things like judgment and organizing their finances, but not so incompetent as to be diagnosed by a psychiatrist. They're really in a gray area in terms of their ability to care for themselves. Really on the borderline. For these kinds of people, it's hard to get services together. They want their independence. They won't sign over their finances to someone else and they won't or can't pay for caregivers, and that's all they need to maintain their independence.

This particular woman lived up a flight of stairs. But she was very clear that she wanted to go home. The nursing staff said, "You can't send this woman home." And I said, "I sure can. We can worry about her safety, we can advise her, but it's her decision." And she was not worried very much about the stairs; she went home and did it.

These sorts of everyday dilemmas are the most complicated. I am constantly having to think: What are my goals? Are my goals to cure the person? To prolong life? To keep the person comfortable? It's not always clear and it's a dynamic and changing process. (*Geriatrician, community clinic.*)

Example Three

The more frequent dilemmas we face in this population of older, frail, inner-city, difficult-to-manage clients with lots of psychosocial problems are about how hard you should push to get them to do something. . . . In order to get the most routine sorts of things done we have to go through fairly intensive maneuvers. All of it can be time consuming.

I had a patient with a big mass in his stomach that was probably malignant. He had lost lots of weight and wasn't doing well and should have had a biopsy. And he wouldn't do it. The question is: How hard do I lean on him? I talk, I try to explain that if this is cancer, it should be taken care of or it can bump you off or cause lots of problems that will make the rest of your life miserable. I give him a chance to answer all the questions and the answer is no. I can insist and tell him that I'm not going to do things he wants, like get him a wheelchair, or see him as often as I have been.

He had plenty of money. He refused to buy medicines for an ulcer which made him feel better, refused to buy glasses, refused to buy a hearing aid. It's obvious these things can improve his quality of life. How hard do you push someone like that? It's often quite difficult to know. Sometimes you can slowly wear down someone's resistance. Given them support, explain why they need to do this or that. And you can make progress, but only if you have the time available to do all that. And in my experience with managed care systems, most of the time that doesn't happen.

The most laissez-faire approach is, "It's his decision; it's none of your business how he makes decisions. It's your job to inform him of the options. . . . You do what the client wants and you respect his wishes." But that's very difficult if in your value system, the benefit of doing what's recommended so far and so obviously outweighs the risks and costs of not doing it. There is no reason to get huffy when someone chooses something you might not choose. But when it's so clearly beneficial and they don't want to do it because they are crazy or rigid, it gets to be difficult.

In many cases, the client is not a full-fledged negotiating partner. Ideally, you explain why it's necessary to do it your way and then you try and negotiate. Often you can't do that. They cannot or will not explain why they want to do it their way. They can't or won't listen to why you think it's necessary. They can't or won't understand. Sometimes they do agree or sort of agree but don't follow through. Those situations can be very difficult. When the client's wishes are unexpressed or pathological or they don't follow through with recommendations, then it really is not so easy to make decisions and feel like you are acting in the most ethical manner possible. It often isn't clear what the most ethical manner is. (*Internist, community clinic.*)

Example Four

I have a man who is very disabled; he does no self-care. He's incontinent; he's in diapers. He coughs up a lot of awful colored phlegm all the time. It is very unpleasant to be around him. He lives with a son who isn't there a lot; the son does about two to three hours of actual care, but otherwise, doesn't do anything. Wouldn't be available for an emergency. The house is really a disaster, not clean at all. They have a paid caregiver who comes twice a day. The son feeds him in the morning, and then the caregiver comes in at noon and again at the end of the day. In between those times, and late into the evening, the patient is alone. He's currently not ambulatory and he can't speak. He can only grunt and groan because of many brain-stem strokes in the past. He's not a very pleasant person. . . . He had been with this home care program for about 4 years, so there's been a kind of long-term concern.

He developed a severe pneumonia and was hospitalized for a month and when he finally recovered enough to consider what he was going to do, he wasn't very ambulatory. He absolutely insisted on returning home. He's not demented. He can write. But he's hard to adequately evaluate in terms of his cognitive function because of his communication problem. Most people won't spend enough time with him trying to communicate. He absolutely refuses to go to a nursing home. He owns the house and understands that he is in danger when left alone because he can't get out. He's willing to take the risk of being in that situation. From what I know, he just wants to be left alone.

When he was discharged from the hospital, I had a nursing agency go out and I tried my best to explain the entire situation. They were very concerned and called me nearly every day to report that he was alone. A physical therapist and home health aide went out there once and the patient smelled from the incontinence so they wouldn't work with him. Ultimately the agency decided they wouldn't work with him. They thought the situation was unsafe; they had questions about liability. They really disliked the situation because of the incontinence and dirt and his being uncooperative and I can understand that.

I don't really like being this man's doctor but I feel very committed, partly because I know no one else would be, and partly because I'm trying to help him with what he wants in his life. He wants to be at home, and I haven't come to my own solid conclusion that that's not possible. He's not mobile now, so he's not such a fall risk. He doesn't try and ambulate. I think we should support him and see what happens and monitor him.

But there are several dilemmas. First, whether this patient is really able to take the risk and responsibility of being alone most of the time. Is he competent to take that risk, so he won't burn up in a fire, or have a heart attack and not be able to get help? And the door is unlocked. Someone could come in and shoot him although I doubt if anyone would go in there. Second, there is the risk of medical problems because of his immobility, especially skin breakdown and the like. And you know, I'm not able to communicate adequately to know if he's willing to take the risk for every one of these points.

I've been told that with any other doctor, he'd probably be in a nursing home. He would have been told he had to go and would not have been able to fight it. I realize I could do that, but I don't wish to do that. I'm pretty invested in trying to help this guy and it takes a lot of time. I think he deserves an adequate trial with adequate services and monitoring to see if things will improve. It's hard convincing other people. So I'm trying to engage people who will be supportive. (*Internist, hospital-based.*)

Medicine's Cultural Conflict: Risk Reduction versus Autonomy

An important feature of medical decision making is that it is both influenced by and embedded in broader social practices and cultural values (Lindenbaum & Lock, 1993; Wright & Treacher, 1982). While medicine has been an extremely powerful force in shaping knowledge in late 20th century life (Cole, 1992; Estes & Binney, 1989), it has also been shaped, in turn, by the larger culture of which it is part (Lock & Gordon, 1988; Kaufman, 1993). The risk discourse permeating

post-industrial society is an example of a powerful cultural form influencing the practice of clinical medicine, especially geriatrics (Kaufman, 1994a).

While a very real need for help, care, and security exists for older people faced with declining abilities, I wish to emphasize that the conceptualization of the elderly "at risk" for falls, institutionalization, functional decline, and acute medical problems is a recent *cultural* phenomenon. Scholars have noted that risk is on the rise as a cultural category (Douglas, 1992; Douglas & Wildavsky, 1982) and that we live in a "risk society" (Beck, 1992), a world made dangerous by technologies of war and industry that produce pollution. Public consciousness of risk and its reverberations in all areas of life has perhaps never been higher (Nelkin, 1989; Slovic, 1987).

In geriatrics particularly, a language of risk, need, safety, and surveillance has emerged in recent decades as a response to the frailties and chronic conditions of the growing "oldest old" population in the United States (American Medical Association, 1990). Much activity in the medical care of older persons focuses on the "need" (Dill, 1993) to minimize risks that health professionals and families perceive as threats to well-being and safety (Shapiro & Tate, 1988).

The need to reduce risk conflicts with the all-pervasive, yet abstract, value of autonomy, that is, the right to maintain adult agency and make independent choices, including that of being left alone. These two values compete in geriatrics, creating ethical conflict for physicians who attempt to care for frail patients in the community. Ethicists have noted and responded to this cultural conflict by delineating kinds and contexts of autonomy vis à vis the diminished capacities of the elderly (Collopy, 1988; Jecker, 1990; Moody, 1988b) in order to show that sick and frail old people can and should retain some choice and dignity as individuals regardless of health status, residence, and degree of dependence on others. Their attempts to fine-tune the concept of autonomy are creative and admirable. Unfortunately, their elaborations are largely theoretical and do not reflect the actual responsibilities physicians and other providers have of weighing safety against relative freedom in small acts on a daily basis. The tension between safety and supervision on the one hand, and risk and independence on the other, remains a major concern for practicing physicians, many frail elderly, and their family members (Kaufman, 1994a, 1994b).

These four narratives illustrate the practical difficulties of balancing safety and health maintenance with independence so that vulnerable old people can remain in the community. When they attempt to acknowledge and support patient choice at the expense of safety or optimal care, physicians may face pressure and criticism from other health professionals as examples Two and Four illustrate. Support of patients' choices can create ethical dilemmas for physicians when patients' treatable conditions go untended (examples Three and Four). Physicians' solutions to the conflict of intervention and risk reduction versus the desire for autonomy are highly individual, reflecting personal and professional values and experience, attitudes toward patient advocacy, and the structural constraints brought to bear on their work by particular agencies and institutions. Sometimes, as the physician in example Three notes, there are no solutions.

Authority and responsibility in regards to risk reduction are contextual and variable. They are described in these narratives as sometimes negotiable. In examples One, Two, and Four, the physicians negotiated with co-workers, enabling their patients to remain at home, at least temporarily. Responsibility was realized in advocacy for the patient's choice to remain at home despite dementia, acute medical conditions, and absence of adequate support or supervision. In example Three, the physician calls attention to his own inability to deliver optimal care because the patient will not negotiate or comply. In that example, the physician struggles with questions of how much to intervene despite the patient's choice and, what in fact, is "responsible" care.

Dimensions of Advocacy

The overarching clinical problem expressed by the physicians, concerning the *degrees, means, and appropriateness of intervention,* dominates most of the data collected from the doctors in this project. That problem, by no means unique to geriatrics, is rooted in medicine's well-known and often criticized directive—do something rather than nothing. The activist stance is shown here to be troubling for physicians who care for elderly in the community. It is also ironic: physicians want to do what they consider necessary and appropriate to improve health, function, and well-being, yet they also defined their role as advocates for older persons who sometimes desired no intervention. Indeed, uncertainty about the doctor's role as patient advocate emerges to a lesser or greater degree in most dilemmas the physicians described. The seemingly insoluble tension between the roles of active physician and patient advocate has become a matter of profound ethical concern in clinical geriatrics and is underexplored in gerontology.

These narratives reveal advocacy to be a complex cluster of moral and clinical decisions and actions which are situation dependent. The physician in example One describes advocacy as limited intervention, perhaps simply cleaning the house in that case, so the patient can continue to reside there despite the fact that "his quality of life is terrible." The physician in example Two separates her "worry" about the patient from her decision to let the patient return to the "risks" of impaired judgment and a flight of stairs. Advocacy in that instance is leaving the patient alone despite colleagues' concerns about safety and competence. In example Three, the inability or refusal of the patient to rationally negotiate a care plan is described by the physician as a potential limit to advocacy because the physician's own values insist on medical intervention to diagnose disease and improve functional capacity. In that case advocacy competes with another value, thorough medical care, to place the physician in an ethical bind. The physician in example Four draws attention to the constraints on her own advocacy stance when it is not shared by a team of health professionals or the agency with which she works. In that example, the limits to advocacy for the nursing agency seem to be constituted by the combination of incontinence, dirt, and the fact that the patient had no social support.

Advocacy is shown in these examples to be more than empathy, philosophy, or action alone. Physicians struggle to formulate ways in which they can both *embody* and *practice* patient advocacy while (1) balancing a medical and social ethic of care; (2) realizing their own values about quality of life in old age; and (3) satisfying coworkers and institutional regulations.

Conclusion: Phenomenology and Clinical Decision Making

A phenomenological approach to physician explanations of dilemmas in the care of older patients allows us to identify some features of the lived experience of clinical/ethical decision making in geriatric medicine. In the analysis of more than 100 dilemmas that 40 physicians described, at least three dimensions of the phenomenology of geriatric medicine emerge. First, dilemmas are not isolated into component parts for deliberation as physicians attempt to solve everyday problems in patient care. Instead, dilemmas are revealed to be multidimensional questions about doing the right thing. In the case of the community-residing frail elderly, dilemmas

are grounded in cultural tensions between risk reduction and autonomy, uncertainty about both advocacy and an ethic of care, and the structural and political constraints on supporting patients' choices.

Second, clinical knowledge is shown to be inextricably tied to moral knowledge about the patient, who is himself conceived in a sociocultural context. Resolving a problem means weighing what is "good for" the patient (Mattingly, 1993; Smith & Churchill, 1986) against the patient's own desires for intervention, improved function, safety, well-being, and agency. In many of the interviews, doctors admitted to not knowing what is best in the long run.

Third, the clinical/moral dilemmas these physicians formulated—When does one intervene to reduce risk? When and how does one advocate for (or insist on) behavioral change? What are the criteria by which to make placement decisions?—point to the fact that authority and responsibility in medicine are often murky notions. An individual practitioner may have clear-cut treatment goals and know what is right and good for a particular patient as in the third example above, only to have those goals derailed by the patient himself, or as the other narratives suggest, by pressures brought to bear on the physician by other health professionals with whom the physician works. Or, competing ideals may vie for dominance in a specific situation, as in the fourth example: In that case the physician knows that an institution would provide better care than the patient receives at home, yet she chooses, for the time being, to honor the patient's wish.

Physician narratives provide one example of how decisions in geriatrics are formulated and understood. They are meant, in the long run, to be supplemented by other forms of qualitative data such as observation of team conference deliberations and interviews with patients, family members, and other health professionals. Clinical narratives can contribute to our understanding of why some decisions in geriatrics are so difficult to make and how moral/medical decisions in geriatrics actually get made. Moreover, ethnographic and phenomenological studies of clinical narratives point to medical authority and responsibility as complex processes influenced by physician values, local institutional worlds, and widespread cultural forms.

Note

The study on which this essay is based was funded by the National Institute on Aging, grant No. AG11538, to Sharon R. Kaufman, P.I. I am indebted to the physicians who participated in this project. Many thanks to two anonymous reviewers for their suggestions on an earlier draft.

References

Agich, G. A. (1993). *Autonomy and long-term care*. New York: Oxford University Press.

American Medical Association Council on Scientific Affairs. (1990). American Medical Association white paper on elderly health. *Archives of Internal Medicine, 150*, 2459–2472.

Beck, U. (1992). *Risk society*. Beverly Hills, CA: Sage.

Benner, P. (Ed.). (1994a). *Interpretive phenomenology*. Thousand Oaks, CA: Sage.

Benner, P. (1994b). The tradition and skill of interpretive phenomenology in studying health, illness, and caring practices. In P. Benner (Ed.), *Interpretive phenomenology* (pp. 99–127). Thousand Oaks, CA: Sage.

Cassell, E. J. (1986). The changing concept of the ideal physician. *Daedalus, 115*, 185–208.

Cole, T. R. (1992). *The journey of life*. New York: Cambridge University Press.

Collopy, B. J. (1988). Autonomy in long-term care: Some crucial distinctions. *The Gerontologist, 28* (Suppl.), 10–17.

Dill, A. (1993). Defining needs, defining systems: A critical analysis. *The Gerontologist, 33*, 453–460.

Douglas, M. (1992). *Risk and blame*. London: Routledge.

Douglas, M., & Wildavsky, A. (1982). *Risk and culture*. Berkeley: University of California Press.

Estes, C. L., & Binney, E. A. (1989). The biomedicalization of aging: Dangers and dilemmas. *The Gerontologist, 29*, 587–597.

Gillick, M. R. (1988). Limiting medical care: Physicians'

beliefs, physicians' behavior. *Journal of the American Geriatrics Society, 36*, 747–752.

Gubrium, J. F. (1992). Qualitative research comes of age in gerontology. *The Gerontologist, 32*, 581–582.

Hodges, M. O., & Tolle, S. W. (1994). Tube-feeding decisions in the elderly. *Clinics in Geriatric Medicine, 10*, 475–488.

Husserl, E. (1931). *Ideas: General introduction to pure phenomenology*. [Translated by W. R. Boyce Gibson.] New York: MacMillan.

Jecker, N. S. (1990). The role of intimate others in medical decision making. *The Gerontologist, 30*, 65–71.

Kane, R. A. (1994). Ethics and long-term care: Everyday considerations. *Clinics in Geriatric Medicine, 10*, 489–500.

Kane, R. A., & Caplan, A. L. (Eds.). (1990). *Everyday ethics: Resolving dilemmas in nursing home life*. New York: Springer.

Kane, R. L. (1988). Beyond caring: The challenge to geriatrics. *Journal of the American Geriatrics Society, 36*, 467–472.

Kaufman, S. R. (1993). *The healer's tale: Transforming medicine and culture*. Madison, WI: University of Wisconsin Press.

Kaufman, S. R. (1994a). Old age, disease, and the discourse on risk: Geriatric assessment in U.S. health care. *Medical Anthropology Quarterly, 8*, 76–93.

Kaufman, S. R. (1994b). The social construction of frailty: An anthropological perspective. *Journal of Aging Studies, 8*, 45–58.

Kayser-Jones, J. (1990). The use of nasogastric feeding tubes in nursing homes. *The Gerontologist, 30*, 469–479.

Leonard, V. W. (1994). A Heideggerian phenomenological perspective on the concept of the person. In P. Benner (Ed.), *Interpretive phenomenology*. Thousand Oaks, CA: Sage.

Lidz, C. W., Fischer, L., & Arnold, R. M. (1993). *The erosion of autonomy in long-term care*. New York: Oxford University Press.

Lindenbaum, S., & Lock, M. (Eds.). (1993). *Knowledge, power and practice*. Berkeley: University of California Press.

Lock, M., & Gordon, D. (Eds.). (1988). *Biomedicine examined*. Boston: Kluwer.

Luborsky, M. R., & Sankar, A. (1993). Extending the critical gerontology perspective: Cultural dimensions. *The Gerontologist, 33*, 440–444.

Mattingly, C. (1993). *What is "the good" for this patient?* Paper presented at the annual meeting of the American

Anthropological Association. Washington, DC, November 17–21.

Merleau-Ponty, M. (1962). *Phenomenology of perception.* London: Routledge and Kegan Paul.

Miles, S. H., & Meyers, R. (1994). Untying the elderly. *Clinics in Geriatric Medicine, 10,* 513–526.

Moody, H. R. (1988a). Toward a critical gerontology: The contribution of the humanities to theories of aging. In J. E. Birren and V. L. Bengtson (Eds.), *Emergent theories of aging* (pp. 19–40). New York: Springer.

Moody, H. R. (1988b). From informed consent to negotiated consent. *The Gerontologist, 28* (Suppl.), 64–70.

Moody, H. R. (1993). Overview: What is critical gerontology and why is it important? In T. R. Cole, W. A. Achenbaum, P. L. Jakobi, and R. Kastenbaum (Eds.), *Voices and visions of aging* (pp. xv–xli). New York: Springer.

Nelkin, D. (1989). Communicating technological risk: The social construction of risk perception. *American Review of Public Health, 10,* 95–113.

Rice, D. P. (1989). The characteristics and health of the elderly. In C. Eisdorfer, D. A. Kessler, and A. N. Spector (Eds.), *Caring for the elderly* (pp. 3–26). Baltimore: Johns Hopkins University Press.

Shapiro, E., & Tate, R. (1988). Who is really at risk of institutionalization? *The Gerontologist, 28,* 237–245.

Slovic, P. (1987). Perception of risk. *Science, 236,* 280–285.

Smith, H. L., & Churchill, L. R. (1986). *Professional ethics and primary care medicine.* Durham: Duke University Press.

Solomon, M. Z. (1993). How physicians talk about futility. *Journal of Law, Medicine, and Ethics, 21,* 231–237.

Suzman, R. M., Willis, D. P., & Manton, K. G. (1993). *The oldest old.* New York: Oxford University Press.

White, K. L. (1988). *The task of medicine.* Menlo Park, CA: The Henry J. Kaiser Family Foundation.

Wright, P., & Treacher, A. (Eds.). (1982). *The problem of medical knowledge: Examining the social construction of medicine.* Edinburgh: University of Edinburgh Press.

We Are Nighttime Travelers

Ethan Canin

∎

Where are we going? Where, I might write, is this path leading us? Francine is asleep and I am standing downstairs in the kitchen with the door closed and the light on and a stack of mostly blank paper on the counter in front of me. My dentures are in a glass by the sink. I clean them with a tablet that bubbles in the water, and although they were clean already I just cleaned them again because the bubbles are agreeable and I thought their effervescence might excite me to action. By action, I mean I thought they might excite me to write. But words fail me.

This is a love story. However, its roots are tangled and involve a good bit of my life, and when I recall my life my mood turns sour and I am reminded that no man makes truly proper use of his time. We are blind and small-minded. We are dumb as snails and as frightened, full of vanity and misinformed about the importance of things. I'm an average man, without great deeds except maybe one, and that has been to love my wife.

I have been more or less faithful to Francine since I married her. There has been one transgression—leaning up against a closet wall with a red-haired purchasing agent at a sales meeting once in Minneapolis twenty years ago; but she was buying auto upholstery and I was selling it and in the eyes of judgment this may bear a key weight. Since then, though, I have ambled on this narrow path of life bound to one woman. This is a triumph and a regret. In our current state of affairs it is a regret because in life a man is either on the uphill or on the downhill, and if he isn't procreating he is on the downhill. It is a steep downhill indeed. These days I am tumbling, falling headlong among the scrub oaks and boulders, tearing my knees and abrading all the bony parts of the body. I have given myself to gravity.

Francine and I are married now forty-six years, and I would be a bamboozler to say that I have loved her for any more than half of these. Let us say that for the last year I haven't; let us say this for the last ten, even. Time has made torments of our small differences and tolerance of our passions. This is our state of affairs. Now I stand by myself in our kitchen in the middle of the night; now I lead a secret life. We wake at different hours now, sleep in different corners of the bed. We like different foods and different music, keep our clothing in different drawers, and if it can be said that either of us has aspirations, I believe that they are to a different bliss. Also, she is healthy and I am ill. And as for conversation— that feast of reason, that flow of the soul—our house is silent as the bone yard.

Last week we did talk. "Frank," she said one evening at the table, "there is something I must tell you."

The New York game was on the radio, snow was falling outside, and the pot of tea she had brewed was steaming on the table between us. Her medicine and my medicine were in little paper cups at our places.

"Frank," she said, jiggling her cup, "what I must tell you is that someone was around the house last night."

I tilted my pills onto my hand. "Around the house?"

"Someone was at the window."

On my palm the pills were white, blue, beige, pink: Lasix, Diabinese, Slow-K, Lopressor. "What do you mean?"

She rolled her pills onto the tablecloth and fidgeted with them, made them into a line, then into a circle, then into a line again. I don't know her medicine so well. She's healthy, except for little things. "I mean," she said, "there was someone in the yard last night."

"How do you know?"

"Frank, will you really, please?"

"I'm asking how you know."

"I heard him," she said. She looked down. "I was sitting in the front room and I heard him outside the window."

"You heard him?"

"Yes."

"The front window?"

She got up and went to the sink. This is a trick of hers. At that distance I can't see her face.

"The front window is ten feet off the ground," I said.

"What I know is that there was a man out there last night, right outside the glass." She walked out of the kitchen.

"Let's check," I called after her. I walked into the living room, and when I got there she was looking out the window.

"What is it?"

She was peering out at an angle. All I could see was snow, blue-white.

"Footprints," she said.

I built the house we live in with my two hands. That was forty-nine years ago, when, in my foolishness and crude want of learning, everything I didn't know seemed like a promise. I learned to build a house and then I built one. There are copper fixtures on the pipes, sanded edges on the struts and queen posts. Now, a half-century later, the floors are flat as a billiard table but the man who laid them needs two hands to pick up a woodscrew. This is the diabetes. My feet are gone also. I look down at them and see two black shapes when I walk, things I can't feel. Black clubs. No connection with the ground. If I didn't look, I could go to sleep with my shoes on.

Life takes its toll, and soon the body gives up completely. But it gives up the parts first. This sugar in the blood: God says to me: "Frank Manlius—codger, man of prevarication and half-truth—I shall take your life from you, as from all men. But first—" But first! Clouds in the eyeball, a heart that makes noise, feet cold as uncooked roast. And Francine, beauty that she was—now I see not much more than the dark line of her brow and the intersections of her body: mouth and nose, neck and shoulders. Her smells have changed over the years so that I don't know what's her own anymore and what's powder.

We have two children, but they're gone now too, with children of their own. We have a house, some furniture, small savings to speak of. How Francine spends her day I don't know. This is the sad truth, my confession. I am gone past nightfall. She wakes early with me and is awake when I return, but beyond this I know almost nothing of her life.

I myself spend my days at the aquarium. I've told Francine something else, of course, that I'm part of a volunteer service of retired men, that we spend our days setting young businesses afoot: "Immigrants," I told her early on, "newcomers to the land." I said it was difficult work. In the evenings I could invent stories, but I don't, and Francine doesn't ask.

I am home by nine or ten. Ticket stubs from the aquarium fill my coat pocket. Most of the day I watch the big sea animals—porpoises, sharks, a manatee—turn their saltwater loops. I come late morning and move a chair up close. They are waiting to eat then. Their bodies skim the cool glass, full of strange magnifications. I think, if it is possible, that they are beginning to know me: this man—hunched at the shoulder, cataractic of eye, breathing through water himself—this man who sits and watches. I do not pity them. At lunchtime I buy coffee and sit in one of the hotel lobbies or in the cafeteria next door, and I read poems. Browning, Whitman, Eliot. This is my secret. It is night when I return home. Francine is at the table, four feet across from my seat, the width of two dropleaves. Our medicine is in cups. There have been three Presidents since I held her in my arms.

The cafeteria moves the men along, old or young, who come to get away from the cold. A half-hour for a cup, they let me sit. Then the manager is at my table. He is nothing but polite. I buy a pastry then, something small. He knows me—I have seen him nearly every day for months now—and by his slight limp I know he is a man of mercy. But business is business.

"What are you reading?" he asks me as he wipes the table with a wet cloth. He touches the saltshaker, nudges the napkins in their holder. I know what this means.

"I'll take a cranberry roll," I say. He flicks the cloth and turns back to the counter.

This is what:

Shall I say, I have gone at dusk through narrow streets
And watched the smoke that rises from the pipes
Of lonely men in shirt-sleeves, leaning out of windows?

Through the magnifier glass the words come forward, huge, two by two. With spectacles, everything is twice enlarged. Still, though, I am slow to read it. In a half-hour I am finished, could not read more, even if I bought another roll. The boy at the register greets me, smiles when I reach him. "What are you reading today?" he asks, counting out the change.

The books themselves are small and fit in the inside pockets of my coat. I put one in front of each breast, then walk back to see the fish some more. These are the fish I know: the gafftopsail pompano, sixgill shark, the starry flounder with its upturned eyes, queerly migrated. He rests half-submerged in sand. His scales are platey and flat-hued. Of everything upward he is wary, of the silvery seabass and the bluefin tuna that pass above him in the region of light and open water. For a life he lies on the bottom of the tank. I look at him. His eyes are dull. They are ugly and an aberration. Above us the bony fishes wheel at the tank's corners. I lean forward to the glass. "*Platichthys stellatus,*" I say to him. The caudal fin stirs. Sand moves and resettles, and I see the black and yellow stripes. "Flatfish," I whisper, "we are, you and I, observers of this life."

"A man on our lawn," I say a few nights later in bed.
  "Not just that."
  I breathe in, breathe out, look up at the ceiling. "What else?"
  "When you were out last night he came back."
  "He came back."
  "Yes."
  "What did he do?"
  "Looked in at me."
  Later, in the early night, when the lights of cars are still passing and the walked dogs still jingle their collar chains out front, I get up quickly from bed and step into the hall. I move fast because this is still possible in short bursts and with concentration. The bed sinks once, then rises. I am on the landing and then downstairs without Francine waking. I stay close to the staircase joists.
  In the kitchen I take out my almost blank sheets and set them on the counter. I write standing up because I want to take more than an animal's pose. For me this is futile, but I stand anyway. The page will be blank when I finish. This I know. The dreams I compose are the dreams of others, remembered bits of verse. Songs of greater men than I. In months I have written

few more than a hundred words. The pages are stacked, sheets of different sizes.

        If I could

one says.

        It has never seemed

says another. I stand and shift them in and out. They are mostly blank, sheets from months of nights. But this doesn't bother me. What I have is patience.

Francine knows nothing of the poetry. She's a simple girl, toast and butter. I myself am hardly the man for it: forty years selling (anything—steel piping, heater elements, dried bananas). Didn't read a book except one on sales. Think victory, the book said. Think *sale.* It's a young man's bag of apples, though; young men in pants that nip at the waist. Ten years ago I left the Buick in the company lot and walked home, dye in my hair, cotton rectangles in the shoulders of my coat. Francine was in the house that afternoon also, the way she is now. When I retired we bought a camper and went on a trip. A traveling salesman retires, so he goes on a trip. Forty miles out of town the folly appeared to me, big as a balloon. To Francine, too. "Frank," she said in the middle of a bend, a prophet turning to me, the camper pushing sixty and rocking in the wind, trucks to our left and right big as trains—"Frank," she said, "these roads must be familiar to you."
  So we sold the camper at a loss and a man who'd spent forty years at highway speed looked around for something to do before he died. The first poem I read was in a book on a table in a waiting room. My eyeglasses made half-sense of things.

        These
        are the desolate, dark weeks

I read

when nature in its barrenness
equals the stupidity of man.

Gloom, I thought, and nothing more, but then I reread the words, and suddenly there I was, hunched and wheezing, bald as a trout, and tears were in my eye. I don't know where they came from.

In the morning an officer visits. He has muscles, mustache, skin red from the cold. He leans against the door frame.

"Can you describe him?" he says.

"It's always dark," says Francine.

"Anything about him?"

"I'm an old woman. I can see that he wears glasses."

"What kind of glasses?"

"Black."

"Dark glasses?"

"Black glasses."

"At a particular time?"

"Always when Frank is away."

"Your husband has never been here when he's come?"

"Never."

"I see." He looks at me. This look can mean several things, perhaps that he thinks Francine is imagining. "But never at a particular time?"

"No."

"Well," he says. Outside on the porch his partner is stamping his feet. "Well," he says again. "We'll have a look." He turns, replaces his cap, heads out to the snowy steps. The door closes. I hear him say something outside.

"Last night—" Francine says. She speaks in the dark. "Last night I heard him on the side of the house."

We are in bed. Outside, on the sill, snow has been building since morning.

"You heard the wind."

"Frank." She sits up, switches on the lamp, tilts her head toward the window. Through a ceiling and two walls I can hear the ticking of our kitchen clock.

"I heard him climbing," she says. She has wrapped her arms about her own waist. "He was on the house. I heard him. He went up the drainpipe." She shivers as she says this. "There was no wind. He went up the drainpipe and then I heard him on the porch roof."

"Houses make noise."

"I heard him. There's gravel there."

I imagine the sounds, amplified by hollow walls, rubber heels on timber. I don't say anything. There is an arm's length between us, a cold sheet, a space uncrossed since I can remember.

"I have made the mistake in my life of not being interested in enough people," she says then. "If I'd been interested in more people, I wouldn't be alone now."

"Nobody's alone," I say.

"I mean that if I'd made more of an effort with people I would have friends now. I would know the postman and the Giffords and the Kohlers, and we'd be together in this, all of us. We'd sit in each other's living rooms on rainy days and talk about the children. Instead we've kept to ourselves. Now I'm alone."

"You're not alone," I say.

"Yes, I am." She turns the light off and we are in the dark again. "You're alone, too."

My health has gotten worse. It's slow to set in at this age, not the violent shaking grip of death; instead—a slow leak, nothing more. A bicycle tire: rimless, thready, worn treadless already and now losing its fatness. A war of attrition. The tall camels of the spirit steering for the desert. One morning I realized I hadn't been warm in a year.

And there are other things that go, too. For instance, I recall with certainty that it was on the 23rd of April, 1945, that, despite German counteroffensives in the Ardennes, Eisenhower's men reached the Elbe; but I cannot remember whether I have visited the savings and loan this week. Also, I am unable to produce the name of my neighbor, though I greeted him yesterday in the street. And take, for example, this: I am at a loss to explain whole decades of my life. We have children and photographs, and there is an understanding between Francine and me that bears the weight of nothing less than half a century, but when I gather my memories they seem to fill no more than an hour. Where has my life gone?

It has gone partway to shoddy accumulations. In my wallet are credit cards, a license ten years expired, twenty-three dollars in cash. There is a photograph but it depresses me to look at it, and a poem, half-copied and folded into the billfold. The leather is pocked and has taken on the curve of my thigh. The poem is from Walt Whitman. I copy only what I need.

But of all things to do last, poetry is a barren choice. Deciphering other men's riddles while the world is full of procreation and war. A man should go out swinging an axe. Instead, I shall go out in a coffee shop.

But how can any man leave this world with honor? Despite anything he does, it grows corrupt around him. It fills with locks and sirens. A man walks into a store now and the microwaves announce his entry; when he leaves, they make electronic peeks into his coat pockets, his trousers. Who doesn't feel like a thief? I see a policeman now, any policeman, and I feel a fright. And the things I've done wrong in my life haven't been crimes. Crimes of the heart perhaps, but nothing against the state. My soul may turn black but I can wear white trousers at any meeting of men. Have I loved my wife? At one time, yes—in rages and torrents. I've been covered by the pimples of ecstasy and have rooted in the mud of despair; and I've lived for months, for whole

years now, as mindless of Francine as a tree of its mosses.

And this is what kills us, this mindlessness. We sit across the tablecloth now with our medicines between us, little balls and oblongs. We sit, sit. This has become our view of each other, a tableboard apart. We sit.

"Again?" I say.

"Last night."

We are at the table. Francine is making a twisting motion with her fingers. She coughs, brushes her cheek with her forearm, stands suddenly so that the table bumps and my medicines move in the cup.

"Francine," I say.

The half-light of dawn is showing me things outside the window: silhouettes, our maple, the eaves of our neighbor's garage. Francine moves and stands against the glass, hugging her shoulders.

"You're not telling me something," I say.

She sits and makes her pills into a circle again, then into a line. Then she is crying.

I come around the table, but she gets up before I reach her and leaves the kitchen. I stand there. In a moment I hear a drawer open in the living room. She moves things around, then shuts it again. When she returns she sits at the other side of the table. "Sit down," she says. She puts two folded sheets of paper onto the table. "I wasn't hiding them," she says.

"What weren't you hiding?"

"These," she says. "He leaves them."

"He leaves them?"

"They say he loves me."

"Francine."

"They're inside the windows in the morning." She picks one up, unfolds it. Then she reads:

Ah, I remember well (and how can I
But evermore remember well) when first

She pauses, squint-eyed, working her lips. It is a pause of only faint understanding. Then she continues:

Our flame began, when scarce we knew
   what was
The flame we felt.

When she finishes she refolds the paper precisely. "That's it," she says. "That's one of them."

At the aquarium I sit, circled by glass and, behind it, the senseless eyes of fish. I have never written a word of my own poetry but can recite the verse of others. This is the culmination of a life. *Coryphaena hippurus,* says the plaque on the dolphin's tank, words more beautiful than any of my own. The dolphin circles, circles, approaches with alarming speed, but takes no notice of, if he even sees, my hands. I wave them in front of his tank. What must he think has become of the sea? He turns and his slippery proboscis nudges the glass. I am every part sore from life.

Ah, silver shrine, here will I take my rest
After so many hours of toil and quest,
A famished pilgrim—saved by miracle.

There is nothing noble for either of us here, nothing between us, and no miracles. I am better off drinking coffee. Any fluid refills the blood. The counter boy knows me and later at the café he pours the cup, most of a dollar's worth. Refills are free but my heart hurts if I drink more than one. It hurts no different from a bone, bruised or cracked. This amazes me.

Francine is amazed by other things. She is mystified, thrown beam ends by the romance. She reads me the poems now at breakfast, one by one. I sit. I roll my pills. "Another came last night," she says, and I see her eyebrows rise. "Another this morning." She reads them as if every word is a surprise. Her tongue touches

teeth, shows between lips. These lips are dry. She reads:

Kiss me as if you made believe
You were not sure, this eve,
How my face, your flower, had pursed
Its petals up

That night she shows me the windowsill, second story, rimmed with snow, where she finds the poems. We open the glass. We lean into the air. There is ice below us, sheets of it on the trellis, needles hanging from the drainwork.

"Where do you find them?"

"Outside," she says. "Folded, on the lip."

"In the morning?"

"Always in the morning."

"The police should know about this."

"What will they be able to do?"

I step away from the sill. She leans out again, surveying her lands, which are the yard's-width spit of crusted ice along our neighbor's chain link and the three maples out front, now lost their leaves. She peers as if she expects this man to appear. An icy wind comes inside. "Think," she says. "Think. He could come from anywhere."

One night in February, a month after this began, she asks me to stay awake and stand guard until the morning. It is almost spring. The earth has reappeared in patches. During the day, at the borders of yards and driveways, I see glimpses of brown—though I know I could be mistaken. I come home early that night, before dusk, and when darkness falls I move a chair by the window downstairs. I draw apart the outer curtain and raise the shade. Francine brings me a pot of tea. She turns out the light and pauses next to me, and as she does, her hand on the chair's back-brace, I am so struck by the proximity of elements—of the night, of the teapot's heat, of the sounds of water outside—that I consider speaking. I want to ask her what has become of us, what has made our breathed air so sorry now, and loveless. But the timing is wrong and in a moment she turns and climbs the stairs. I look out into the night. Later, I hear the closet shut, then our bed creak.

There is nothing to see outside, nothing to hear. This I know. I let hours pass. Behind the window I imagine fish moving down to greet me: broomtail grouper, surfperch, sturgeon with their prehistoric rows of scutes. It is almost possible to see them. The night is full of shapes and bits of light. In it the moon rises, losing the colors of the horizon, so that by early morning it is high and pale. Frost has made a ring around it.

A ringed moon above, and I am thinking back on things. What have I regretted in my life? Plenty of things, mistakes enough to fill the car showroom, then a good deal of the back lot. I've been a man of gains and losses. What gains? My marriage, certainly, though it has been no knee-buckling windfall but more like a split decision in the end, a stock risen a few points since bought. I've certainly enjoyed certain things about the world, too. These are things gone over and over again by the writers and probably enjoyed by everybody who ever lived. Most of them involve air. Early morning air, air after a rainstorm, air through a car window. Sometimes I think the cerebrum is wasted and all we really need is the lower brain, which I've been told is what makes the lungs breathe and the heart beat and what lets us smell pleasant things. What about the poetry? That's another split decision, maybe going the other way if I really made a tally. It's made me melancholy in old age, sad when if I'd stuck with motor homes and the National League standings I don't think I would have been rooting around in regret and doubt at this point. Nothing wrong with sadness, but this is not the real thing—not the death of a child but the feelings of a college student reading *Don Quixote* on a warm afternoon before going out to the lake.

Now, with Francine upstairs, I wait for a night prowler. He will not appear. This I know, but the window glass is ill-blown and makes moving shadows anyway, shapes that change in the wind's rattle. I look out and despite myself am afraid.

Before me, the night unrolls. Now the tree leaves turn yellow in moonshine. By two or three, Francine sleeps, but I get up anyway and change into my coat and hat. The books weigh against my chest. I don gloves, scarf, galoshes. Then I climb the stairs and go into our bedroom, where she is sleeping. On the far side of the bed I see her white hair and beneath the blankets the uneven heave of her chest. I watch the bedcovers rise. She is probably dreaming at this moment. Though we have shared this bed for most of a lifetime I cannot guess what her dreams are about. I step next to her and touch the sheets where they lie across her neck.

"Wake up," I whisper. I touch her cheek, and her eyes open. I know this though I cannot really see them, just the darkness of their sockets.

"Is he there?"

"No."

"Then what's the matter?"

"Nothing's the matter," I say. "But I'd like to go for a walk."

"You've been outside," she says. "You saw him, didn't you?"

"I've been at the window."

"Did you see him?"

"No. There's no one there."

"Then why do you want to walk?" In a moment she is sitting aside the bed, her feet in slippers. "We don't ever walk," she says.

I am warm in all my clothing. "I know we don't," I answer. I turn my arms out, open my hands toward her. "But I would like to. I would like to walk in air that is so new and cold."

She peers up at me. "I haven't been drinking," I say. I bend at the waist, and though my head spins, I lean forward enough so that the effect is of a bow. "Will you come with me?" I whisper. "Will you be queen of this crystal night?" I recover from my bow, and when I look up again she has risen from the bed, and in another moment she has dressed herself in her wool robe and is walking ahead of me to the stairs.

Outside, the ice is treacherous. Snow has begun to fall and our galoshes squeak and slide, but we stay on the plowed walkway long enough to leave our block and enter a part of the neighborhood where I have never been. Ice hangs from the lamps. We pass unfamiliar houses and unfamiliar trees, street signs I have never seen, and as we walk the night begins to change. It is becoming liquor. The snow is banked on either side of the walk, plowed into hillocks at the corners. My hands are warming from the exertion. They are the hands of a younger man now, someone else's fingers in my gloves. They tingle. We take ten minutes to cover a block but as we move through this neighborhood my ardor mounts. A car approaches and I wave, a boatman's salute, because here we are together on these rare and empty seas. We are nighttime travelers. He flashes his headlamps as he passes, and this fills me to the gullet with celebration and bravery. The night sings to us. I am Bluebeard now, Lindbergh, Genghis Khan.

No, I am not.

I am an old man. My blood is dark from hypoxia, my breaths singsong from disease. It is only the frozen night that is splendid. In it we walk, stepping slowly, bent forward. We take steps the length of table forks. Francine holds my elbow.

I have mean secrets and small dreams, no plans greater than where to buy groceries and what rhymes to read next, and by the time we reach our porch again my foolishness has subsided. My knees and elbows ache. They ache with a mortal ache, tired flesh, the cartilage gone sandy with time. I don't have the heart for dreams. We undress in the hallway, ice in the ends of our hair, our coats stiff from cold. Francine turns down the thermostat. Then we go upstairs and she gets into her side of the bed and I get into mine.

It is dark. We lie there for some time, and then, before dawn, I know she is asleep. It is cold in our bedroom. As I listen to her breathing I know my life is coming to an end. I cannot warm myself. What I would like to tell my wife is this:

> What the
> imagination
> seizes
> as beauty must be truth. What holds you
> to what you see of me is
> that grasp alone.

But I do not say anything. Instead I roll in the bed, reach across, and touch her, and because she is surprised she turns to me.

When I kiss her the lips are dry, cracking against mine, unfamiliar as the ocean floor. But then the lips give. They part. I am inside her mouth, and there, still, hidden from the word, as if ruin had forgotten a part, it is wet—Lord! I have the feeling of a miracle. Her tongue comes forward. I do not know myself then, what man I am, who I lie with in embrace. I can barely remember her beauty. She touches my chest and I bite lightly on her lip, spread moisture to her cheek, and then kiss there. She makes something like a sigh. "Frank," she says. "Frank." We are lost now in seas and deserts. My hand holds her fingers and grips them, bone and tendon, fragile things.

PART III

The Culture of Medicine

and Medical Practice

What is the "culture of medicine," and how is it transmitted in the training process? Professions, like other social groups, have cultures: they have specialized languages and ways of understanding, norms of behavior, unique customs, rites of passage, and codes of conduct. In addition to the organizations, publications, jargon, research, and rewards that characterize a profession, there is a prolonged period of adult training that conveys both knowledge and values to new members. And, just as patients are taught how to be sick, doctors, too, undergo an extensive socialization process. This process is the key to understanding physician norms and behavior.

Medical sociologists have long been fascinated with the social processes that transform medical students into counselors and interveners in issues of life and death. How does a person learn to take on such roles? And how does undertaking contact with the most private aspects of human existence change that person? To answer such questions, social scientists examine the educational and clinical experiences that have been shown to mold the attitudes, behaviors, and expectations physicians bring into medical practice.

Classic works on this subject by sociologists such as Howard S. Becker and his colleagues (1961), Robert Merton (1957), Samuel W. Bloom

(1963), and Renée C. Fox (1988) have demonstrated that some of the most powerful themes in medical education may not be apparent to those enrolled in the process. Many students enter medical school with idealistic views of medicine and its goals, and become more realistic and cynical as they move through the training process. Their medical education also places pressures on them to adopt values and views that are consistent with dominant medical beliefs and practices. For example, students learn to intervene actively in the problems of patients. They come to believe that an individual has power to confront disease and biological decline, a view that may not be shared by patients and families who see themselves as less able to resist what happens to them.

Melvin Konner (1987) demonstrates that fundamental identity and role changes generally take place during medical school. Many medical students find they can no longer offer advice to family or friends without being seen as speaking with a professional voice. Medical students see and participate in major life transitions, such as births, injuries, family crises, and deaths. Because their medical training places them close to such important events in people's lives, and pulls them into intense ethical and spiritual dilemmas, they begin to see and conduct their own lives differently, too.

The less-obvious, latent aspects of the socialization process have also received scholarly attention. Renée Fox (1988), for example, has pointed out that despite the enormous quantity of information presented to medical students, a central task in becoming a physician is learning about the uncertainty rather than the certainty of knowledge. Students must learn how to manage the sense of being overwhelmed by new information, to filter a huge amount of detail, and select the most critical parts to retain in memory. Awareness of uncertainty is heightened when students realize that not all questions have an-

swers and that even the finest faculty mentors may be stumped by clinical decisions. As physicians mature, they learn to cope with the uncertainty that comes from constantly changing information, with the need to formulate a clinical diagnosis or prognosis in the face of incomplete data. Communication about this issue, with patients and with other physicians, remains one of the most troubling areas of medical practice.

The sheer quantity of information that a student has to master is only one of the challenges of medical education. Another is the kind of medical experience students are exposed to, and at what point in their training they encounter it. It makes a difference in a student's school experience and attitude to medical practice whether one starts in the emergency room or the well-child clinic. Curricular innovations have been studied by Renée Fox (1988) and Mary-Jo DelVecchio Good (1995), for their potential to make for more caring and humanistic physicians. Entering medical students are now sometimes given early exposure to patients and clinical care. Some medical schools introduce students early on to "normal" health issues, such as pregnancy or routine childhood health maintenance, before they see more life-threatening or chronic diseases. Experiments in community-based care, in humanistic care, in continuity care, and in team-based interdisciplinary care are a feature of some programs. And some medical schools make a point of grounding their educational philosophy and course formulations in the socialization experience, to develop an ethos of caring and guide career directions among medical graduates (Good 1995).

Several physicians-in-training, including Perri Klass (1988), Melvin Konner (1987), Charles LeBaron (1982), and Phillip Reilly (1987), have reflected critically on the aspects of medical education that shape values and behaviors. Peter Conrad (1988) has examined these first-person accounts of the medical school years and concludes, perhaps surprisingly, that over the past three decades little has actually changed in medical school structures and training. Conrad finds that medical school does a fine job in conveying medical information and developing technological skill; however, he notes, there is little in medical education that promotes humanistic medical care. Long hours, sleep deprivation, overemphasis on high-tech solutions, excessive demands and responsibilities placed on students, and hierarchical relations between students, residents, and specialists all contribute to creating competent, but less than compassionate, physicians.

Another important aspect of medical socialization is the training that medical students receive to avoid emotional entanglements and overidentification with the lives and problems of patients. Speaking of "detached concern," sociologists have examined how interactions with mentors and peers model norms of intimacy, and how such rites of passage as the anatomic dissection of a cadaver implicitly teach students to handle suffering, death, and sexuality with professional distance. Frederick Hafferty (1991) carefully explored how students learn the value of emotional detachment in dealing with death and found that much of the socialization occurs within the peer group of medical students—and that values are transmitted by overt group pressure, discussion, ridicule, and humor.

Other studies have highlighted the personal challenges of medical training, in which individuals find it difficult to maintain their own identity while experiencing the conformity of "lock step" classes, a uniform curriculum, and strongly held norms of behavior espoused by peers and role models. Fitzhugh Mullan (1976), an outspoken medical student of the 1960s, wrote about the tensions he felt between his sense of himself as a person and his gradually emerging medical identity. In his battle with school administrators who were enforcing a ban against beards and

mustaches, Mullan felt he was struggling to protect himself from the external forces intent on molding him into what they thought a doctor should be. Although the manifestations of personal identity (dress, hair, political expression) have changed over the years, medical socialization remains a powerful rite of passage.

Internship and the residency years allow doctors in training to use their medical skills and to continue to develop their professional identity. These years of supervised practice often place the new physician in the responsible position of caring for large numbers of hospitalized patients. Among the challenges are the daily work of dealing with patients' privacy and secrets, making life-and-death decisions in the last days of a patient's life, and communicating across racial or cultural lines. Residency training may find new physicians having to deal with insensitivity in themselves, in their colleagues, or in their supervisors, and having to work extremely long hours and cope with exhaustion and the lack of effective supervision, all of which sometimes results in tragic outcomes for patients. Resident physicians may be seen as struggling to balance personal, family, and career demands, while trying to keep from developing a sense of entitlement or arrogance (Gerber 1983).

The study of medical school socialization and clinical training raises questions of what roles physicians and the profession of medicine are expected to fulfill, and a variety of proper and ideal roles for medicine in society have been proposed (Starr 1982, Cassell 1986). Donald Seldin and Gerald Perkoff, in their contributions to this part of the reader, take opposing positions on what the appropriate boundaries of medicine and the use of medical power should be. Seldin sees medicine as a narrowly defined endeavor in which biological, pharmacological, and surgical interventions are used to deal with pain and disability and to postpone death. From his point of view, medicine cannot alter the social and economic conditions that nurture disease. Perkoff, on the other hand, sees medicine as facing a variety of human ills, across a broad front, in which social, biomedical, cultural, and political forces together mold the profession and its responses. These two understandings, set side by side as they are in this reader, challenge medical practitioners to define where they stand on medicine's social roles and its place in responding to community problems.

The kinds of roles and career paths that physicians take on depend in part on who enters the profession. The demography of the medical profession is changing, and as it does so, it more closely reflects the overall makeup of American society. There are now many more women in the profession, and this change in gender distribution could well have effects on how medicine is practiced. More persons from ethnic minorities are becoming doctors and, while we do not yet know how changes in the racial or ethnic makeup of the medical profession will alter medical practice, we know they will make a difference, just as the increase in women will make a difference. Will medicine become more caring, or will more career options arise, as the demography of medical practitioners changes? How is power allocated within medical education—do demographic changes raise real challenges to "old ways"? The short story "The Doctors of Hoyland," by Sir Arthur Conan Doyle (himself a medical practitioner in the late nineteenth and early twentieth centuries), is a reminder that women in medicine have posed questions about career, family, equity, and power for many years. His surprisingly contemporary story is about the conflict that arises between an established male physician in rural England and a highly skilled female physician who starts a practice in the same community. (The story is reprinted at the end of section 2.)

The last issue raised in this part of the reader concerns how physicians and patients relate to each other. Physicians have specific roles in communities, and with patients, and these roles involve responsibilities, privileges, stresses, and rewards. This is most clearly expressed in the doctor-patient relationship. Ethical aspects of this powerful dyad are defined by the rights and duties of each party. (They are also examined in part IV.) Physicians have different types of relationships with patients—each one with different expectations and responsibilities. The readings pose questions such as, How can patients share in the healing process? What are the limits of physician authority and responsibility? And how can physicians balance their roles as doctors caring for individual patients with their broader responsibilities to the community?

For many, these readings will resonate with their own experiences as health workers or as patients. Controversies surround medical education and practice; the roles, power, and import of medicine are all in flux. Political and health policy changes raise career and personal questions. For practitioners, the context, status, and rewards of medical practice are not something they as individuals have total control over, but are determined by decisions made on a societal level. As the readings in part V demonstrate, people working in medicine increasingly need to participate in government and the public policy process if they are to maintain influence over their careers and practices. The culture of medicine, influenced as it is by geography, economics, gender, ethnicity, and politics, has a tradition of shared values and norms that offers a common ground for physicians and their health professional partners to reorganize health care delivery and medical practice as the world around them changes.

Ronald P. Strauss

The Socialization of Physicians

Each year approximately 17,000 students enter the 142 North American medical schools and begin an intense process of personal change and learning that will result in their becoming physicians. They will be there, at the anatomic dissection of a cadaver, the night in the emergency ward, the death watch at an elderly person's bedside, the first placing of a scalpel to skin, or the bringing into the world of a new baby. The process that takes college graduates and makes them young physicians powerfully influences their attitudes, behaviors, and identities. In the selections that follow we learn what that means on an individual level. Melvin Konner reflects on the rites of passage he experienced as a medical student to illuminate the process of medical education. William Branch and his colleagues share encounters with pain, failure, ethical dilemmas, and death, as reported by students in their clinical years. In these reports we hear the voices of medical students angered, moved, or saddened by their experiences, and knowing what impact their medical decisions have on both their patients and themselves. We also see how important the relationship between the medical student and the clinical teacher is for professionalization and role modeling. The demands of medical school are intimidating. How can stu-

dents develop empathy for patients while coping with the institutional norms and pressures of medical training? What is there in medical education that prepares a medical student to deal with a failed resuscitation attempt, to cope with a patient who refuses cancer care, or to face the suffering on a locked psychiatric ward?

The demanding clinical training of physicians as they move beyond medical school is shown here through the eyes of medical students, residents, and attending faculty. Perri Klass shows a young physician dealing with patient privacy and secrets, learning about the entitlements of medical practice. William Winkenwerder Jr. describes the powerful dilemmas faced by medical residents in the care of critically ill persons. His study shows us how a medical resident learns to think independently and make critical decisions, while respecting the values of fellow residents and the attending physicians. His study shows us residents who witness and participate in decisions that sometimes result in poor or ambiguous outcomes, and sometimes in healing, learning first hand about the uncertainty of medical practice.

Abenaa Brewster, a medical student, reacts to the failure of an attending faculty physician to communicate across ethnic barriers. Her short essay gives us an insight into how race may directly intrude on the doctor-patient interaction.

David Asch and Ruth Parker's report on the tragic death of a young patient in New York reveals the long hours and exhaustion that accompany residency training. They describe what it is to be a largely unsupervised resident, not to have slept in eighteen hours, but still asked to make critical patient care decisions at 2 A.M. in a big city emergency room. The issue of reforming the training system becomes a political one, because the public loses confidence in medicine when preventable, tragic outcomes occur.

These readings on clinical training and residency raise critical questions. Is it necessary to make residents work such long, arduous hours? Does residency training develop insensitive attitudes and behaviors among practitioners? What kind of training might better prepare a physician to help in people's life crises and important life passages?

Basic Clinical Skills:

The First Encounters

Melvin Konner

■

For some students in medical school, the ultimate encounter with the patient is not essentially new. This includes the few students who were previously nurses or physician associates and the larger number who have volunteered extensively to work in hospital or other clinical settings. But for many if not most, this experience is the most keenly anticipated and most anxious moment of life as a medical student.

Almost all medical students are young enough so that the naive energy of youth overcomes any natural timidity. To extend the analogy of the adolescent crush, contact with a patient, like marriage, is easier to get into when you are young and, if not foolish, then at least confident, even headstrong. The older you get the more you know, and after a certain point you know too much; you can envision the pitfalls, and you feel embarrassed by what earlier might have been a rough but effective brash éclat. I noticed in myself a level of concern about how I would handle patients, how they would react to me, what I might do wrong that, if not exactly inappropriate, was also not perfectly adaptive. I wanted to be the sort of person who would simply dive in, as so many did all around me.

For example, in a moving clinical exercise during the preclinical years, we visited a rehabilitation hospital for a lecture on the subject of paraplegia by a specialist who was a paraplegic himself—the result of an injury that had taken place within weeks of his graduation from medical school. As might be expected, he remarked on many aspects of day-to-day care, the sort that most physicians prefer to relegate to nurses, with a sensitivity and sympathy that few other physicians could have had. Between the lecture and the patient presentations, we took a break, and as we filed out into the hall to stretch our legs, I saw that one of the patients to be presented—a new quadriplegic—was lying on a portable bed in the hallway. He could not have been more than twenty-one or twenty-two. He was handsome, healthy-looking—his muscles had not had time to deteriorate—and had, as the cliché goes, his whole life ahead of him. Yet he had just lost, permanently, the use of his body below the shoulders. I was one of about forty medical students milling around, spilling out of the classroom into the hallway, all healthy, ambitious and strong; and here, uncomfortably close to me, was a young man about as broken as one could be.

I could not think of anything to say to him. Surely this was a situation in which the wrong words could do damage, and I was highly conscious of the power of my embryonic medical role. I had not been taught the right words, so I was reluctant to say any. Still, the awkwardness of the situation as it was could not be much better than even the wrong words, and I began to grope for some phrases that might be acceptable, that might break the barrier.

During the few seconds that I was preoccupied with this effort, one of my fellow students—a particularly uninspiring athletic type, I thought—walked up to the stretcher, looked down at the crippled young man, and said, "Pretty tough break."

Ouch, I thought. Just the sort of thing I wanted to avoid. "Yeah," said the patient, his face brightening perceptibly.

"How did it happen?" the medical student asked, and they began a conversation in which all the barriers I had envisioned immediately broke down. The emotional topology of the hallway, which for me had been dominated by tension resulting from the lack of communication between the medical students and the patient, had been utterly changed.

I was reminded of the advice I once got as a boy about talking to a girl at a party: if she wants to talk to you, it doesn't much matter what you say first; and if she doesn't want to, it doesn't matter either. Unlike the girls of my youth, however, patients almost always want to be spoken to by doctors (including medical students), but it is not so easy to say the wrong thing. Thus I learned from one of my less inspiring fellow medical students the first lesson of interacting with patients: the doctor is not entitled to be reluctant. However awkward the situation, however discouraging or confusing or ugly the disease, however apparently withdrawn the patient, the doctor must step across the barrier in interpersonal space that everyone else must properly respect.

And yet it was plain to see that the result of this forthrightness was not always good. Teachers and students alike "dove in" with a brusque, abrupt style that many patients disliked. The laying on of hands was reduced to the carrying out of procedures, and words exchanged with the patient were basically viewed as tools to make those procedures go more smoothly.

At my medical school it was arranged for first-year students to have preliminary clinical experiences in hospital settings. I was assigned to a small group led by an immigrant physician who happened to be a superb if slightly pompous neurologist. He used to say, "Touch the patient." This, he explained, was a categorical imperative. No matter what, find an excuse to touch the patient, however reluctant you are, however reluctant you imagine the patient is. If necessary, pretend to check for a fever by putting your hand on the patient's forehead. Take an unnecessary pulse. His words made an indelible impression on me.

On this occasion we stepped out of the elevator onto one of the highest floors of a just-finished hospital tower, a surgical ward so new it seemed to glitter. As we turned a corner into the main part of the ward, we saw and became part of a white-coated commotion around a stretcher. My clinical tutor, as the neurologist was called, introduced me to a young woman who was a third-year medical student engaged in her surgical clerkship. Moans were emanating from within the crowd of hospital whites. The medical student narrated the scene in a cheery lilting tone with a bright, fresh expression on her face; but I was riveted by the moans, which were now taking the shape of the word "Mama," pathetically repeated over and over again. The patient was an old-looking woman (I would now characterize her, in retrospect, as merely middle-aged) who was described as an alcoholic and evidently not *compos mentis*. She was undergoing the procedure of placement of a central line—the insertion of a large-bore needle in a major vein below the clavicle—needed for the pouring in of great volumes of fluid, as well as nutrients and drugs.

The woman did not stop moaning, "Mama, Mama, Mama." (I still cannot get those moans out of my mind. One sees terrible things in medicine, and this was far from the worst I saw, but it was my very first encounter as a student in a hospital; I remember it with the vividness that seems to be preserved for first encounters.) She was frail and small, with a long tangle of orange hair. Curled in the fetal position in a faded yellow hospital gown, she kept repeating her epithet like an uncalm mantra. She was surrounded by large sturdy young men, all handsome and strong of voice. They unfolded her brusquely and efficiently from the fetal curl. Her moans became louder and pierced their moderate, if spirited, professional exchanges: "Mama, Mama, Mama, Mama." Glancing off these was the voice of the cheery young medical student whose explanatory commentary I found harder and harder to listen to. I had a thought that I was to have innumerable times over the next few years, although the feeling that went with it would wane: *Why doesn't somebody touch her forehead? Why doesn't somebody take her hand? Why doesn't somebody say, "It's all right"?*

After a deftly conducted struggle in which the woman's resistance was treated as an annoyance and her cries were ignored, the central line was placed and the residents congratulated one another, as they often and properly do. After all, they are learning, and they deserve and need the praise that goes with new achievement. Also, the central line was for this patient a lifeline, and they could breathe that sigh of relief that comes when, as in a movie, we see a drowning person finally grab hold of a rope.

The patient's body recurled into the fetal position, as the young men stepped away from the stretcher. I was close enough so that without being obtrusive (and they were through with her anyway) I could satisfy my strong urge to touch her. At no point did she stop repeating the plaintive cry, "Mamma." "It's O.K., dear, it's all right," I said, taking her hand and stroking her hair back away from her forehead. She made no obvious response to these gestures, and I naturally thought they might be useless; but that did not mean I should not be making them. Equally, I didn't know whether the residents' matter-of-fact approach to her entered into her experience in any meaningful sense; in retrospect, with greater knowledge of the neuropsychology of brain damage from alcohol and other causes, I can say with some confidence that they didn't know either.

One could wonder, as I shortly did, whether doctors should not maintain a humane approach to patients not only because of the patients themselves but also because of the students and the residents, always likely to act inhumanely because of the stresses of excessive responsibility, overwork, and sleeplessness; or, for the same reason, because of oneself.

This was before I realized that humane acts not directly affecting "care"—a word meaning neither more nor less than medical and surgical intervention for the purpose of favorably altering the course of an illness—are in short supply in the hospital world; that the patient's mental status is only marginally relevant to the effort at helpful verbal or nonverbal communication; and that far from being embarrassed by brusqueness, residents are more likely to be embarrassed by (and to consider not quite professional) acts and gestures that are other than completely instrumental.

One's shock does not last long, but at that point I was still shocked. When the residents were gone and the nurses had removed the patient with her plaintive cries, I looked to the third-year student for some kind of explanation. "What did you think of that?" I asked her.

"Wasn't that great? You have to see a lot of those before you get a feel for them. I'll probably get to place a couple of central lines myself before the clerkship ends."

"Is it difficult to get used to?"

"Oh, it's great, really. The residents are great to you. As long as you do your scut and keep the patients' labs and everything straight. I love it."

I left with a vision of the brightness in her face and with the lilt of her voice in my ears, but I was deeply disturbed by what I had seen. On the bus on the way home I met a psychiatrist whom I had known before I began medical school. I told her about my experience, and she was moderately sympathetic to my concern. But I was looking for something stronger, some sharing of my "obviously" just and righteous anger. The incident was not a surprise to her, and although she deplored it, she seemed to accept it and to consider my reaction somewhat immature, surprisingly so, given my relatively advanced age.

"That's just the way things are," was about what she had to offer. When I confided that I might decide I couldn't be a part of this, she did not take me very seriously. "You'll get used to it," she said. "You don't have to become like them." She left me with the sensible advice that whatever was going on around you, you could and should be the way you wanted to be. "Light your corner," she said finally and emphatically.

My corner was for a period fairly dark. Some time during my first year a young woman physician in my community committed suicide. She had been in the obstetrics department, and was not only a practitioner but an excellent lecturer and teacher. Her case became a subject of constant discussion centered mainly on feminist issues. I knew these were central—she had been in what was virtually the first substantial cohort of women coming into medicine. She had forgone marriage and motherhood, and her situation must have been professionally oppressive and personally lonely.

But I thought there were more issues at stake than could be effectively subsumed under the feminist banner. She had been highly competent and successful, and she had been in obstetrics, generally considered the most hopeful and cheering of medical subfields. Yet she had judged her life not worth living. I thought that there might be lessons about the nature of modern medicine and the awkwardness of the physician's existential situation. In general, suicide risk is higher for men than for women and much higher for physicians than for the population at large. So the death of this young woman cast a shadow over me, too.

At the end of the first year I sat for Part I of the National Medical Board Examinations, and this experience gave me a considerable jolt. For medical students who elect this route to licensure (generally considered the most difficult one) three examinations are taken, Part I normally after the second year. It consists of two full days of multiple-choice questions covering anatomy, biochemistry, physiology, pathology, microbiology, and behavioral sciences. The questions are not of the straightforward "choose the one best answer" type, but of the more bewildering "Choose A if 1 and 3 are right, B if 2 and 4 are right, C if 1, 2, and 3 are right" type; and there are a thousand of them (about one per minute) over the course of two days. Somewhere between 10 and 15 percent of the students who take this test fail.

I was comfortably above that margin and well above the bottom of my own class's performance—not surprising, since I tended to be just about in the middle of the class on most examinations. But I had found the test extremely stressful and felt chastened by my far-from-impressive score. There were many mitigating factors. I was too old for this sort of thing, I told myself, and during the preclinical years this was made most evident by examinations. I had family responsibilities (my daughter was then two and a half, and I used to take her to a sunny little park in the late afternoons and try to memorize preclinical facts while keeping one eye on her wanderings). I had taken some of the basic courses—notably anatomy and biochemistry—six or seven years earlier. Finally, I was taking the exam at the end of the first instead of the second year, so that I could accelerate into the clinical training part of medical school earlier.

All this helped to explain why I didn't do better—I could tell myself it wasn't stupidity, or sloth—but the lesson of the exam came home to me all the more emphatically: my age, my atypical turn of mind, and my stage of life were showing, and these were not ideal for medical school.

But of course I had made my bed and I was going to lie in it. In at least one sense, the worst of it was over. I still had some preclinical sciences to complete, but I was now empowered to set foot on the hospital floor as a student in Basic Clinical Skills. In my interactions with patients I would now have slightly more than spectator status.

It was also the first setting I experienced in medical school in which the class consisted of a small group of students, and after those lecture theaters, the group was almost oppressively intimate. Yet it was very good to have a group small enough to be intimate at all and to provide the sort of friendship and personal support that is needed for the transition to clinical work. We seemed a rather oddball group: an overweight, slow-moving, pleasant fellow with a wry sense of humor whose father was a psychoanalyst but who wanted himself to be a surgeon; a woman with waist-length straight blond hair, appealing in an anorectic sort of way, who was a marathon runner by avocation as well as by austere personality; a handsome, cheerful, harried jock with a mild speech defect who seemed constantly bemused; a Korean student my own age who was doing pathbreaking research in virology and needed this one course for certification in the United States; and me, a misfit anthropologist who couldn't explain himself even to himself, much less to anyone else. Even if I had wanted to, I could not preserve an alienated stance in this group. We were all going through this together.

We had many good discussions, formal and informal. Our teachers were strongly oriented to clinical work and were concerned about psychological and ethical aspects of the doctor-patient relationship. (I did not grasp at the time how unusual this was, and my appreciation of what I was getting was blunted by the erroneous assumption that it was characteristic of clinical training in general.)

In this setting I learned a lot about myself. For example, in one exercise we were given the following problem. A patient needs a kidney transplant. Family members are immunologically surveyed, and a brother is found who can be a technically successful donor. The brother is confidentially interviewed and refuses. The patient is told that no suitable donor is available, "suitability" being understood to include technical factors as well as willingness to donate. I argued strongly that the patient should have been told that his brother was immunologically eligible and had refused to donate; otherwise seeds of suspicion with respect to the whole family might have been sown in the patient's mind. The brother, I thought, should be made to take the consequences of his refusal.

Later I had second thoughts and decided that I had spoken glibly. Kidney donation is a risky enterprise, and it is not at all clear that one owes such a bodily sacrifice to anyone, even a brother. Also, kidney transplants often do not work, and the potential uselessness of the sacrifice cannot be ignored. I did not change my mind exactly. I simply made the single most important discovery one can make about such problems, confirmed many times since: they have no right answer. My appreciation of that fact increased with further clinical encounters. The proposition has a corollary: *whatever* a doctor does in such a situation, it can be viewed from the outside as having been the wrong choice. It is only by living through the anguish of such choices that we come to appreciate the ethical depths they sound.

I also learned things about myself directly. In one exercise we filled out a form designed to assess our state of health, a form that had proved to be superior to a physician's examination in predicting future medical problems. I filled out the form honestly, and at the end was judged to have a "health age" two years older than my chronological age; all the others in the group had a health age younger than their stated age. Either I was in lousy shape or my fellow students were exceptionally vigorous, and either way I was at a disadvantage—for a medical student, the most ironic disadvantage of all.

We had a number of introductory lectures on clinical topics, and the most important of these concerned various aspects of history-taking and physical examination, in support of the complete histories and physicals we were doing regularly. As I had been before, I was a bit diffident in these encounters, finding it hard to cross the conventional barriers to interpersonal interaction that I had built up over half a lifetime. It was especially difficult for me to ask patients questions about their use of alcohol and about their sex lives, subjects we were expected to probe deeply, skeptically, and efficiently. This was all the more difficult since we were not participating in patient care but were there by sufferance; patients had been (quite properly) asked to give their permission to be interviewed and examined by second-year medical students, for the benefit of our education.

My first encounter was comically awkward. Purely by chance, I was assigned to a woman who told me during the brief interview that she was an actress with a local repertory company, the name of which I recognized. She was twenty-two years old, had long auburn hair and large brown eyes, and, although small, carried herself with considerable bearing. She had presence—despite being in the hospital, on a bed, dressed in a drab hospital gown. She was about to be discharged, but her physicians had failed to find the source of the pain she still had, a moderate fluctuating sharp discomfort in the lower left quadrant of her abdomen.

She was not in pain at that moment, and at its worst the pain was not very great, but her poise was noticeably disturbed by worry. She had been talked into letting a student do this examination, and it was the last thing she had to do before leaving the hospital. My charge was to give her a complete *neurological* examination. This was utterly irrelevant to her problem; but it was deemed a good way for me to begin, being the most methodical and meticulous part of the physical examination and the easiest to relate meaningfully to anatomy and physiology. One proceeded literally from head to toe, testing sensation, muscle tone and strength, reflexes, perceptual discrimination and integration, and finally higher coordination of movement and thought.

As in most neurological examinations, there

was no reason to intrude on any part of the body ordinarily considered intimate, and of course I did not. But I soon found out that any part of the body is intimate in the sense that it is protected by the customary barriers of interpersonal space. There are cultures where these barriers are fewer or lighter than they are for us, and others where they are more numerous or severe. But they are always definite and somehow are known to every person in the culture, if only subconsciously. A violation of these strictures, subtle as they may seem, can dramatically transform the nature of a relationship—resulting in embarrassment, in ostracism, in legal action, or even in homicide. Anthropologists had discovered that diplomatic and business failures—for example, in Japan or in Arab countries—may sometimes be traced to missteps in the frame of personal space.

Yet the physician is supposed to cross these barriers briskly, with confidence and aplomb. And the medical student crossing them for the first time must pretend to the same confidence, ignoring the force and weight of all the previous years of obscure but strict training with regard to personal space. I certainly did try to pretend, and my task was greatly complicated by the fact that I was doing my very first physical examination on a woman who promptly aroused in me unmistakable if fleeting feelings of romantic tenderness and sexual desire. I could not imagine that she was unaware of this, and so another dimension of intersubjectivity was added to an already complex interaction.

I was desperately trying to produce from memory the obsessive protracted sequence of the neurological examination, trying to appear professional, trying to conceal (at all costs!) the fact that I had never examined a patient before (which was probably transparently obvious), and trying to carry forward a stream of small talk, all the while suppressing ridiculous lustful sentiments. The simplest things—looking into her mouth, testing the suppleness of her neck, pushing down on her knee to test the muscle strength in her thighs, checking the mobility of her ankle joint—seemed almost intolerably intrusive. Touching the neck or the knee of a beautiful woman was something one earned with an appropriate investment of time and sentiment: candlelight dinners, walks in the moonlight, that sort of thing (or at least, in this age of marvels, a couple of drinks in a singles bar). But to the patient, I was just one of a long line of men and women who had come around to poke at her in the service of various obscure hospital purposes. She understood perfectly well that the rules of interpersonal space are totally different in a medical encounter; it was I who had trouble with the contrast. Understandably, there were moments when the poor young woman almost burst out laughing.

Later I confided my feelings to the group, with the encouragement of the doctor who was leading that day's discussion. He was a very well-meaning man who was appropriately sensitive—indeed almost too much so. (People who say "share" more than twice in one conversation are always suspect to me, and he exceeded this limit by some measure.) He was trying rather desperately to elicit some valuable confessions about our first experience of the physical examination and not getting very far, so I decided to help him out—having been a teacher, I was alert for those moments when panic is setting in because of student unresponsiveness. I said rather flatly that I had had to examine a woman who was very attractive, and that this made me uncomfortable. There was no response from any of my fellow students, who looked at me strangely. "Thank you for sharing that with us," Dr. Clark finally said, and went on to the next topic. I now knew that this was not to be a forum for discussion about learning to be a doctor, as had been claimed, but yet another setting in which everything about you, even feelings, would be judged. I became accordingly diffident about my feelings.

As the weeks went by I became comfortable

with the ritual of the history and physical. The stethoscope, the penlight, and the reflex hammer still seemed foreign, but I was beginning to learn how to use them. We were getting hands-on individual training with our preceptors. We were practicing everything constantly on each other (with the exception of the two most intimate parts of the physical examination, the rectal and vaginal exams, which we practiced on hired models). Two days each week we spent the afternoon with a patient, then presented the patient to our preceptors, and finally returned to the bedside with them. Some of my patients were pieces of human wreckage on the other shore of life. With them the reluctance to touch was different from what it had been with the actress, but this too I overcame—more readily, in fact.

I realize now that I was absurdly meticulous and lengthy in my approach to those first patients. This is true of most beginning clinical students—the less you know, the less confident you feel about leaving out something that might be pertinent. Since I was not engaged in an aggressive and time-pressured approach to the patients' present illnesses, and since I did not have a large panel of patients to think about at the same time, I was able—in fact I felt required—to treat every health problem as important. Each history and physical took about three hours, and my write-up took even longer, involving me as it did in constant consultation of books for the right word, phrase, or explanation. (In patient write-ups, the order is ritualistic, the phrasing formulaic, and the emphasis and reasoning stringently constrained. If they are not, the already problematic circumstances of medical communication and legal vulnerability become impossible.)

How could this process be reduced to one hour for history and physical and one hour for write-up, which was the standard time spent (at best) by interns in their admission work-ups? Actually, since interns might be required to admit up to eight patients in one day, besides attending lectures and rounds and discharging many other duties, it was easy to see that two hours might not be available. So even as I was making my very first inroads into these basic clinical skills, I began to appreciate how they would have to be compromised.

Some interns and residents I met claimed they could be as thorough in an hour or two as I could in six, and at first I found their arguments convincing. But as I got closer to their stage of training, I could appreciate the corners they were cutting (which I would eventually have to cut as well). They focused more narrowly on the present illness, showed less concern for the patient's or, certainly, the family's general health; paid less attention to behavioral and social factors in the patient's illness; were more abrupt and brusque and less responsive to the patient as a human being. The concept of adequate care was eminently flexible, and the judgment about what was really important to give the patient could become very narrow. Of course, when physicians were constantly beset by demands that they reduce costs, they could not feel encouraged to linger with their patients over details that were not immediately essential. Yet such details could turn out to be life-saving in the near term and highly cost-efficient for the future.

In Basic Clinical Skills I had the luxury (for the last time) of giving each patient the fullest conceivable attention. The patients, almost without exception, seemed grateful, and they provided a very instructive set of experiences. There was a sixty-eight-year-old childless widow who had a forty-five-year history of heavy smoking and was now dying of chronic obstructive pulmonary disease. There was a "morbidly obese"—he weighed 389 pounds—forty-five-year-old man who was hypertensive, diabetic, and suffering from numerous recurring painful abscesses in all the creases of his enormous body. All his illnesses were directly related to obesity. A thirty-two-year-old mother of seven suffered from other problems stemming principally from obesity, although she weighed "only" about two hundred pounds: diabetes resulting in kidney impairment, chronic upper abdominal pain, and hypertension. She also had a thyroid problem and chronic asthma, and she was grieving visibly, although it was years past, over her beloved father's untimely death. Her own children had been fathered by a number of different men, and at the time I met her she said she was living and struggling alone.

Another obese man—he weighed 350 pounds—said, "I'm like an alcoholic on food." In addition he was an alcoholic on alcohol. He was now in the hospital, as he had been many times before, for painful swelling in his feet, and this time also in his testicles. His sleep had been sorely troubled by breathing stoppages that woke him—a common problem in the obese—and left him narcoleptic during the day. This had been cured by the surgical opening of a channel into his trachea. But he had been unable to work for about a year due to depression, and he had begun drinking again.

There was a spry seventy-eight-year-old man with a fine wry sense of humor who had just had his gallbladder removed. He had previously had part of his colon removed because of diverticulosis. There was a thirty-four-year-old admittedly promiscuous homosexual, a musician, with a relapse of hepatitis. There was an eighty-three-year-old obese woman with arthritis, hypertension, and leg swelling who had had a bad fall. She was evidently no longer able to take care of herself at home. There was a thirty-nine-year-old man whose lifelong asthma had been exacerbated severely on the day of his separation from a lover. There were cases of cellulitis, thrombophlebitis, cardiac pain, ulcers, cancer, prostatitis, and much more.

What struck me about these patients, aside from the variety of their illnesses, was that many, perhaps most, were hospitalized because of behavioral problems or predispositions. I was not about to blame them, and I don't believe I ever allowed a hint of disapproval to be communicated to them. They taught me a great deal about illness and its treatment and about how to think and talk and act like a doctor. But treatment for many of them was a Sisyphean task, and for some it was almost a fool's errand. Not only was there often very little that could be done for them; but, even more frustratingly, changes in behavior and other preventive measures could have kept them in excellent health in the first place. It was very unusual for any of them to be referred for psychiatric evaluation or even for social service assistance, so they were trapped in a psychological cycle—smoking, drinking, overeating, accident-prone motorcycling, or risky sex—that had brought them into the hospital again and again. Fortunes were being spent on their care by third-party payers, yet these same payers did not deem it suitable to pay for preventive measures or for behavior modification. They would thus never find out whether such methods might be cost-effective—to say nothing of whether they might be the best thing that could happen to these patients.

I discussed all this with a psychiatrist I knew—he had actually recommended me for medical school—who was now head of the Institute of Medicine. He was involved just then in a program recommending the investment of more resources in behavioral medicine on a grand national scale. My interpretation of my patients was old news to him. This was to be only one of many encounters in which I learned that the opinions of those at or near the top of American medicine bore no relation—or, rather, bore only an ironic relation—to actual practice in the trenches.

At this time I seemed to be what I came to call "medically accident-prone." Amusingly, ironically, and probably not entirely coincidentally, I found myself in life situations where my nascent skills seemed to be called for. The first time was on the airplane on the way back from Edinburgh, where I had spoken at a World Health Organization conference on breast-feeding. The pilot's voice scratched over the public address system asking if there were a medical doctor among the passengers. I held my breath for a while, then asked a stewardess what was up. A middle-aged passenger had collapsed, and they feared a heart attack. I was certainly no doctor, but I was feeling the squeeze of responsibility. If I opened my mouth would it do more harm than good? Fortunately, I did not have to answer the question: there were two physicians aboard.

A week or so later I had been attending an intolerably tedious anthropological lecture in a stuffy lecture hall. I had been on the way home from the hospital and still had my little bag with me—it was the only time during medical school when we actually carried those bags—and I was trying to hide it under my seat. The lecturer droned and ostentatiously turned his pages. The air in the room was so thick it was difficult to breathe. As we filed out, I noticed a commotion and saw that a young woman had fainted. Some people got her to a bench, and I rolled up her coat and put it under her legs. She was soon awake, complaining of a pain in her eye, which I tried to examine gently. "I'm a second-year medical student," I said. "I'm not going to touch your eye, but if you like I can look at it." She said that when she fainted she had scratched her eye on her glasses. The eye was teary but looked intact, except for what seemed to be a scratch on the surface of the sclera—the membrane covering the white. She said that she had an ophthalmologist in town, and I offered to call him. I told her to stay where she was.

He was not terribly excited by my story. He said he would see her at his office in an hour. I tried to get him to tell me how worried I should be, and he tried to be noncommittal. "Take a history," he said. There was no revelant history, as

was obvious from what I had already told him. So I simply stayed with her until she got a ride home with her parents. I had judged that this was not an emergency, and I was right.

The third incident, a week or two after that, involved a "consultation" by the rather reckless twenty-four-year-old son of an old friend of mine. The young man, who in every way still acted like a teenage boy, was using the injectable anesthetic ketamine, not a "conventional" street drug. He wanted me to provide him with information about it. I looked over the package insert, already stunned. What I found out was not at all reassuring. Ketamine had a low therapeutic ratio, which meant that the difference between an effective dose and a lethal dose was not very great. For the dreamlike state and occasional hallucinations that were its incidental side effects, he was risking respiratory depression and potentially fatal cardiac arrhythmias. I warned him strongly about these effects, but he did not seem to take my warning very seriously.

After some thought, I told his father about the episode. The young man was living at home and consistently behaved immaturely. His father was always getting him out of trouble. And he was a close friend. I thought that it was important for him to know.

I discussed all three episodes with my preceptors in Basic Clinical Skills. In their estimation I had done the right thing only once, with the young woman in the lecture hall. On the plane, they said, I should have offered to help in any way I could, introduced myself as a second-year medical student, and described the limitations on my knowledge—ludicrously limited, really. I might have been the closest thing to a doctor on the plane, and I was therefore on the spot. I had to get used to that sense of responsibility.

As for my friend's son, they thought I had taken a serious legal risk. He was an adult and was consulting me about a private medical matter. It was a completely privileged communication. For telling my friend his father about the consultation, he could have sued me, probably successfully.

These events made me understand for the first time that my role in life was going to be permanently changed—no, that it had already been changed. I had to begin to relate to the world as a doctor, because that was the way the world would now be relating to me. That entailed the ready acceptance of heavy responsibility, with all its practical, legal, and social consequences. I was no longer just a passenger, or a member of the audience, or a friend. Within and above all those social roles, I was more and more like a physician.

My first surgical experience made a strong impression on me. I was seeing patients one morning with a general surgeon who was conducting his usual clinic, evaluating patients before surgery or following their progress after it. At around noon he said he had to leave to go to a small hospital on the other side of town where a patient was waiting to have an axillary lymph node biopsy. Since he was coming back afterward, I asked him if he would mind my tagging along, and on the contrary he was pleased. As we rode together he spoke reverentially of the surgeon he had trained under who had inspired him to become a surgeon himself. What had been only a famous name to me now became real, and I felt as if I were in the presence of an authentic, impressive tradition that comprised emotion as well as knowledge and skill.

And ritual. When we arrived at the little hospital, the surgeon—a plump, middle-aged Irishman with no pretensions to the status of his teacher—guided me gently through the procedures of sterile technique. The hand washing was so methodical and repetitive, so exceedingly thorough, that it was like a ritual confirmation of the germ theory, a self-reteaching of that theory, every day. The gowning and gloving were equally ritualistic

but more dramatic, since they involved nurses attending the surgeon—and me, his new assistant—like priestesses who, although subordinated, were responsible for the purity of the ritual and who would pounce mercilessly on a technical blemish. I had to put my hands and arms into the gown without letting my fingers contact any part of the front of it. Then I had to plunge my hands, one at a time, into the tight rubber gloves without missing a finger or touching anything or ending up with the fingers too loose. I did my best, as careful as if walking on eggs, and I did not contaminate anything, but the two nurses' pairs of eyes scrutinized me with an unrelenting critical gaze.

The young man on the table was conscious, and his shaved armpit had been prepared with a local anesthetic. I was content to stand and watch, with my rubber-gloved hands gripping each other awkwardly, staying in the sterile area just in front of my chest. The surgeon showed me the lump in the axilla, made his incision, and began quickly and efficiently to explore the wound with his fingers. Suddenly he turned to me. "Put your fingers in and feel it," he said. His own fingers pried the wound open to ease the way for me. There was no avoiding this even if I had wanted to. The young man turned briefly to look at us, but he was not really concerned. I put two fingers of my right hand in and felt in the area where I had seen the shape made by the lump under the skin surface. Timidly, I began to move them around. Finally I felt it, a lump about one centimeter across, smaller than I had expected. I nodded, holding my breath, eye to eye with the surgeon, and removed my hand.

I watched the surgeon take out the offending node and prepare it for pathological study. But that was anticlimactic. I was more interested in the blood on my fingers, the lingering mystery, the feeling in my hand. It was like the feeling or even the smell of a hand used in making love to a woman; my fingers had been inside another person's body, not just in the mouth or the vagina or the rectum, but beneath the protective surface of the skin, the inviolable film set up by millions of years of evolution, the envelope of ultimate individuality. Taking me along with him had been a matter-of-fact random event for the surgeon, but for me it had been an unforgettable experience.

I did not fully appreciate while I was taking Basic Clinical Skills that I was being exposed to two of the best clinical teachers I would encounter in medical school. One was Ross Weinberger, the internist who was my primary supervisor in most of the patient evaluations. He was a socially awkward man with a beak nose and heavy glasses, and an asthenic, slightly stooped frame. He worked for a community health plan with an excellent reputation and he seemed to have no academic ambitions. His general grasp of internal medicine seemed as good as that of anyone I met before or since, but that was not the point really. He was simply *with* the patients in a way I would rarely see again. He had a penetrating gaze that was medically critical yet full of convincing practical warmth—no "sharing" here. He cared, professionally, about the nonmedical aspects of his patients' problems—their characters, their families, their living situations, their incomes. Ignorant as I was, I made the mistake of taking all this for granted. I assumed I had had some bad breaks in certain teaching encounters during the preclinical years, and that now I was embarked on an apprenticeship journey under the command of real doctors. Little did I realize with what longing I would later look back on Dr. Weinberger's simple human decency.

In pediatrics, my supervisor was Ed Gold, who stood out similarly in basic human competence. Pediatricians in general are known for being better people—it sounds silly, but it's true—than most medical specialists. They have accepted the lowest financial status in medicine in exchange for an opportunity to serve in the most nurturant primary care capacity. Ed's touch with children was unsentimental and smooth, but as good as his surname in its ability to calm and even amuse them while he carried out efficiently the necessary examinations and procedures. His handling of parents—the pediatrician's bread and butter—was equally adept. He had worked for a time at the Centers for Disease Control, and he was strongly oriented to preventive medicine.

As a teacher, he managed to confer confidence. He brought out the best in whatever natural skill with children I had, as well as in my experience doing research with children in Africa and my more recent experience as a father. I felt more comfortable with the patients in his consulting room than I had up to then anywhere else in the hospitals and clinics. Toward the end, there was one afternoon when I was closeted for an hour or two with a pair of unusually active ten-year-old twins who were, to use the common expression, bouncing off the walls. I did all that was necessary in interviewing their mother and in observing and examining each of them in turn. I felt in control of the situation and consequently happy.

Ed told me a story that made me appreciate the rigors of internship in a somewhat new and more ominous way. After a long struggle with a deadly illness, he had lost a small child. The parents were grateful to him for the effort—they frequently are—and invited him to their home. They wanted him to be a part of the process of experiencing, and recovering from, their grief. He was touched and was grateful to be with them. They left him alone with a drink in his hand on their living room couch, for a few minutes, while they attended to the dinner they were preparing. He fell asleep, and they left him to sleep, realizing how desperately he needed it.

What struck me was that this unusually sensitive doctor did not have the physical wherewithal to stay awake at such a moment, to serve the function of psychological healing for which he was then badly needed. This was not a man who, in such a situation, would allow himself to fall asleep lightly, and he had felt guilty about it ever since. How bad could the stress of internship be? Worse, evidently, than I had thought.

The parade of exquisitely healthy, normally growing children that came through Ed's clinic, with their usually minor problems, presented a stark contrast to my memory of Africa. That memory in turn made me fear, as it always did, for the health of my own daughter, and of my son who was then soon to be born. Life in general seemed fragile, but children seemed more fragile than anything, and I knew that their basic expectable health and safety was a historical novelty. Not only in Africa but in Europe and the United States a mere century or two before, half of all children could be expected to die.

Near the end of my semester in Basic Clinical Skills, this issue came up in a discussion at the home of a physician who was an expert on public health. He had held a powerful administrative position in internal medicine, and had also made a reputation for himself doing research. But he had given up all that to take a leadership role in the field of public health. People were puzzled, and I, like many others before, gave voice to that puzzlement.

He was forthright, even adamant. Public health measures, not medical care, were responsible for all the important reductions of morbidity and mortality in modern times, he said. This was not news to me and I had little trouble with it, but the vehemence with which he defended this position was surprising. Another physician who joined in the conversation was the designer and implementer of a program for screening newborn infants for hypothyroidism, which if undetected can easily cause profound mental retardation. The two of them insisted not only that public health measures were much more important than medicine, but that medicine had accomplished nothing at all.

I protested. Coronary artery bypass surgery? Appendectomy? Antibiotics? Nothing I mentioned impressed them in the least. The treatments were overrated, the numbers of people saved were trivial compared with the numbers, past and future, saved by preventive measures. I felt like an idiot. Here I was, taking my first steps in clinical work, defending the whole enterprise of clinical medicine in an argument with two men who had spent decades practicing medicine at its best and who had abandoned it and insisted that it was useless. There was no getting around the irony of this exchange, or its implications for the journey on which I had embarked.

Becoming a Doctor:

Critical-Incident Reports from

Third-Year Medical Students

William Branch, Richard J. Pels,

Robert S. Lawrence, and

Ronald Arky

■

"Critical-incident reports" are short narratives of events judged to be particularly meaningful by participants in the events.[1-3] Our medical students wrote such reports at the beginning, in the middle, and in the latter part of their third year, while participating in a required course on the patient-doctor relationship. The students met weekly with faculty members in small groups.[4-6] Assignments for critical-incident reports were open-ended; students were asked to pick an event they felt was important to their learning and to write a short account of it.

An example is this excerpt from a critical-incident report of a third-year medical student who was with a thoracic surgeon examining a patient:

> I think we were both surprised by what we saw. Mrs. M was an extremely obese woman who appeared to have spent the last few days sleeping on the street—she was poorly dressed and extremely malodorous. She greeted us with hostility, telling us how much she hated and distrusted surgeons, and that she was merely seeing us out of courtesy to her internist, whom she very much respected.
>
> Dr. R was obviously surprised by her hos-

tility and lacking any patience replied that if she felt this way then there was nothing he could offer. He pointed out that he believed she had an easily resectable tumor, but if it was not treated she might very well die from it. He carefully explained the procedure, its risks, and the possible complications. Mrs. M reacted to his bluntness with considerable anger, reiterating her position that she refused an operation. She then got off the exam table and left the room. Dr. R was clearly frustrated by this interaction and reacted with some less than flattering remarks about Mrs. M's personality.

> I was also quite upset by this encounter. Here was a woman who had a potentially curable tumor walking away from help. My impression was that she had probably experienced a great deal of pain at the hands of physicians in the past and was not willing to allow them to hurt her again. I felt that Dr. R in letting her leave the room had failed in his job in the most flagrant manner. Had he been more patient, more understanding of her fears, he might have been able at least to win her trust and allow her to begin to contemplate the possibility of surgery. I also felt that it was quite clear that Dr. R did not like the patient and he implied that she was the type of person that he did not like on his service.

In this report, a medical student struggles to reconcile his values with becoming a doctor. As demonstrated by critical-incident reports written by students during their third-year clerkships, such struggles are at the heart of the transition from student to doctor. After reading and rereading 100 such reports,[7] we found that our students' papers focused on a deep-seated conflict—maintaining empathy for patients while becoming acculturated to medicine—even though the students rated their clerkships positively overall as educational experiences. More than 95 percent of the incidents described fell into one of four variants of the expression of this conflict.

Expressions of Empathy

Sometimes students strongly identified with their patients. Temporarily trapped in the locked psychiatric ward, a student knocked on the window. A patient stared. The student banged on the window. The attendant stood up slowly, peered at her, recognized her, and let her out. She thought of a patient, Sylvia, who could not get out. More commonly, students acknowledged being restrained by empathy. "Just how do you approach a patient who happens to be your own age, who's just been told he has something growing in his brain?" Or students expressed their feelings as they watched, attempted to alleviate, or sometimes inflicted suffering. While drawing blood for gas measurements from a dying non–English-speaking man, a student communicated with him "through the anguish on my face" so that he would know "that I was suffering along with him."

Difficulty in Acculturating

Some students described their inability to identify with the team of physicians to which they had been assigned. A woman, working with all-male house staff, found them "chiefly oohing and aahing at attractive nurses." She "feigned a wry smile, just to show that I was not a stick-in-the-mud." When a patient agreed to surgery after hearing that "this operation is your only chance," another student concluded that the patient was "browbeaten into agreeing to the operation" by a resident who "used the specter of death almost as a threat."

Clinic staff invested considerable time in convincing a homeless woman to sign in voluntarily for psychiatric treatment.

There was a lot of excitement among the people working with her that maybe it might be possible to have a real therapeutic exchange with her—maybe she would accept medication. It was at this point that the team found out that the patient's insurance would not cover hospitalization.

She was given $5 and sent by taxi to a homeless shelter. This student concluded, "The whole incident left me quite confused."

The Struggle Between Empathy and Acculturation

In many cases, students recounted their struggles to maintain empathy with patients while assuming the role of doctor. An indigent woman refused to see a medical student in the walk-in clinic. The attending physician explained that it was "a teaching unit" and the patient "had no choice." The patient stormed out. The student wondered "how this patient, who fit the bill for the type of person I had always seen myself helping, actually saw me aligned with Dr. N against her."

Another student described making rounds with a resident:

Dr. X screamed at Mrs. L, "Breathe!" Dr. X slapped her stethoscope on Mrs. L's back and abruptly pushed Mrs. L's shoulder forward. Then Dr. X laughed, embarrassed at her own rudeness. This was a daily ritual. Dr. X made derisive remarks about each patient when we left their room, laughing at her own jokes, patting herself on the back for her wit. The interns laughed nervously. They are team players after all.

This student concluded, "I still like medicine." She had rejected Dr. X's attitude toward patients.

Sometimes students felt betrayed by patients. One "was immensely pleased with myself as I spoke to Mr. Jones," a psychiatric patient. "He frequently began his answers to my questions with 'You see, Rob, what happens now . . .' as if I were a trusted disciple."

Later, Mr. Jones approached.

"Listen, Rob, I can tell you're a man of intelligence. If you could just get back my privileges." Although part of me immediately became aware of his game, the manipulative splitting of the staff that I'd heard of but not yet experienced, I also felt myself being flattered. Perhaps Mr. Jones sensed that I wasn't going to give him what he demanded, but from that point on he opened up less and less. I couldn't help feeling that if I were just a little bit better—a better doctor, a better conversationalist, more empathic?—I would be able to break through to him. . . . In a sense, I selfishly used Mr. Jones much as he had used me. I consistently looked to him to bolster my fragile confidence in my abilities as a physician and empathic listener.

Students were sometimes aware of withdrawing from intimacy with incontinent or grotesque patients at the moment when these patients needed understanding. A young man who had undergone radical neck dissection

would look at me with appreciation and his eyes would say "I'm okay," but a couple of days later he was coughing terribly and trying to push phlegm out through his tracheostomy by producing a huge breath and a cough. He dripped phlegm on my jacket and my hands as I tried to assist him. I didn't make a big deal out of it and just wiped it off. About four days later I came down with a horrible flu. Later, when the patient deteriorated, he seemed barely human. Could he see the horror in my eyes?

Another student "wandered around looking for someone to explain" after witnessing a failed attempt at cardiopulmonary resuscitation.

I was really not sure what I wanted to ask anyway—not about the medical reasons for what was done. What I wanted to know was how it felt to be invading someone's body when there was so little chance of it being any use. And how to switch quickly from being intensely involved in something so personal as death, to acting business-as-usual.

Blending Empathy with Acculturation

Students maintained, and even used, empathy in vexing situations. One student saw the viewpoint of a patient "who was cold toward me no matter how much warmth I extended." The student said, "I am sure that I will not like every patient. Just because a doctor dislikes a patient does not mean that the patient should receive less." Another student compared communicating with the wife of a patient who had had a devastating stroke with her own experiences when her uncle suffered a fatal stroke. She did for the patient's wife what she wished her uncle's doctors had done for her: she provided support.

A student took a personal interest in T.C., a 39-year-old man with AIDS, whom everyone avoided on rounds. The student became the liaison between the patient and his doctors. He successfully advocated giving T.C. more control over his medications. When T.C.'s cryptococcal meningitis worsened, the student took part in telling him. This student concluded, "I think I had an impact on T.C.'s life; he certainly impacted on mine. If I witness his death, I will add one more image to the many already engraved in my mind. What he taught me will always be with me."

Another student inflicted considerable pain while doing a pelvic examination. She concluded that she did not want to stop feeling remorse, which ensured that she would not lose sensitivity. The same student encountered a comatose young victim of a bicycling accident surrounded by his family. She maintained her distance, but felt sad. She reflected that her own brother, who was 20 years old, could have been involved in a similar accident. She wondered if doctors are like voyeurs, but she concluded that she herself felt genuine grief over the death of the patient and "over my inability to reach out and console his family."

Another student felt that the care of his patient consisted of a lot of tests that failed to relieve suffering. On reflection, he concluded that his anger at his team "for not caring more" reflected his search for a convenient target for his own frustration. He wished he had acknowledged his patient's suffering.

Role models were often helpful. A student's pregnant patient had premature rupture of the membranes. The resident assigned to the case hastily and perhaps arbitrarily declared the discharge "purulent" and initiated labor. "With each contraction, the patient's grief seemed to wrack her body, and with the delivery of her tiny infant, still moving in its sac, her sobbing seemed to come from deep inside." This student found solace after talking with a nurse, who herself had delivered a stillborn child. She wrote that she had learned from the compassion and resilience of the nurse, sufficiently so that she could continue to become a doctor.

Students read their critical-incident papers aloud in the groups. As faculty members, we at times responded by sharing our own descriptions of critical incidents. We discussed questions such as what happened, why, and what alternatives or solutions existed. Above all, we listened closely, attempting not to push students to reveal more than they wished, and we tried to help them to clarify their feelings while seeking to gain perspective on the events themselves. Sometimes we were available after class to talk with them. Our students' papers helped us to understand the importance to them of reconciling empathy with patient care, and we hope this understanding enabled us to become better teachers.

Efforts like these to help students keep alive their best instincts and values—efforts we share with teachers at medical schools across the country—deserve to be at the heart of medical education.

Notes

We are indebted to the students who permitted us to quote from their critical-incident reports.

1. Mezirow, J. How critical reflection triggers transformative learning. In: Mezirow, J., ed. Fostering critical reflection in adulthood: a guide to transformative and emancipatory learning. San Francisco: Jossey-Bass, 1990:1–20.
2. Brookfield, S. Using critical incidents to explore learners' assumptions. In: Mezirow, J., ed. Fostering critical reflections in adulthood: a guide to transformative and emancipatory learning. San Francisco: Jossey-Bass, 1990:177–93.
3. Flanagan, J.C. The critical incident technique. Psychol Bull 1954;51:327–58.
4. Branch, W.T., Arky, R.A., Woo, B., Stoeckle, J.D., Levy, D.B., Taylor, W.C. Teaching medicine as a human experience: a patient-doctor relationship course for faculty and first-year medical students. Ann Intern Med 1991;114:482–9.
5. Tosteson, D.C. New pathways in general medical education. N Engl J Med 1990;322:234–8.
6. Branch, W. Notes of a small-group teacher. J Gen Intern Med 1991;6:573–8.
7. Smith, A.C., Noblit, G.W. The idea of qualitative research in medical education. Teach Learn Med 1989;1:101–8.

Invasions

Perri Klass

∎

Morning rounds in the hospital. We charge along, the resident leading the way, the interns following, the two medical students last, pushing the cart that holds the patients' charts. The resident pulls up in front of a patient's door, the interns stop as well, and we almost run them over with the chart cart. It's time to present the patient, a man who came into the hospital late last night. I did the workup—interviewed him, got his medical history, examined him, wrote a six-page note in his chart, and (at least in theory) spent a little while in the hospital library, reading up on his problems.

"You have sixty seconds, go!" says the resident, looking at his watch. I am of course thinking rebelliously that the interns take as long as they like with their presentations, that the resident himself is long-winded and full of pointless anecdotes—but at the same time I am swinging into my presentation, talking as fast as I can to remind my listeners that no time is being wasted, using the standard hospital turns of phrase. "Mr. Z. is a seventy-eight-year-old white male who presents with dysuria and intermittent hematuria of one week's duration." In other words, for the past week Mr. Z. has experienced pain with urination, and has occasionally passed blood. I rocket on, thinking only about getting through the presentation without being told off for taking too long, without being reprimanded for including nonessential items—or for leaving out crucial bits of data. Of course, fair is fair, my judgment about what is critical and what is not is very faulty. Should I include in this very short presentation (known as a "bullet") that Mr. Z. had gonorrhea five years ago? Well, yes, I decide, and include it in my sentence, beginning, "Pertinent past medical history includes . . ." I don't even have a second to remember how Mr. Z. told me about his gonorrhea, how he made me repeat the question three times last night, my supposedly casual question dropped in between "Have you ever been exposed to tuberculosis?" and "Have you traveled out of the country recently?"

"Five years ago?" The resident interrupts me. "When he was seventy-three? Well, good for him!"

Feeling almost guilty, I think of last night, of how Mr. Z.'s voice dropped to a whisper when he told me about the gonorrhea, how he then went on, as if he felt he had no choice, to explain that he had gone to a convention and "been with a hooker—excuse me, miss, no offense," and how he had then infected his wife, and so on. I am fairly used to this by now, the impulse people sometimes have to confide everything to the person examining them as they enter the hospital. I don't know whether they are frightened by suggestions of disease and mortality, or just accepting me as a medical professional and using me as a comfortable repository for secrets. I have had people tell me about their childhoods and the deaths of their relatives, about their jobs, about things I have needed to ask about and things that have no conceivable bearing on anything that concerns me.

In we charge to examine Mr. Z. The resident introduces himself and the other members of the team, and then he and the interns listen to Mr. Z.'s chest, feel his stomach. As they pull up Mr. Z.'s gown to examine his genitals, the resident says heartily, "Well now, I understand you had a little trouble with VD not so long ago." And immediately I feel like a traitor; I am sure that Mr. Z. is looking at me reproachfully. I have betrayed the secret he was so hesitant to trust me with.

I am aware that my scruples are ridiculous. It is possibly relevant that Mr. Z. had gonorrhea; it is certainly relevant to know how he was treated, whether he might have been reinfected. And in fact, when I make myself meet his eyes, he does not look nearly as distressed at being examined by three people and asked this question in a loud booming voice as he seemed last night with my would-be-tactful inquiries.

In fact, Mr. Z. is getting used to being in the hospital. And in the hospital, as a patient, you have no privacy. The privacy of your body is of necessity violated constantly by doctors and nurses (and the occasional medical student), and details about your physical condition are discussed by the people taking care of you. And your body is made to give up its secrets with a variety of sophisticated techniques, from blood tests to X rays to biopsies—the whole point is to deny your body the privacy that pathological processes need in order to do their damage. Everything must be brought to light, exposed, analyzed, and noted in the chart. And all this is essential for medical care, and even the most modest patients are usually able to come to terms with it, exempting medical personnel from all the most basic rules of privacy and distance.

So much for the details of the patient's physical condition. But the same thing can happen to details of the patient's life. For the remainder of Mr. Z.'s hospital stay, my resident was fond of saying to other doctors, "Got a guy on our service, seventy-eight, got gonorrhea when he was seventy-three, from a showgirl. Pretty good, huh?" He wouldn't ever have said such a thing to Mr. Z.'s relatives, of course, or to any nondoctor. But when it came to his fellow doctors, he saw nothing wrong with it.

I remember another night, 4:00 A.M. in the hospital and I had finally gone to sleep after working-up a young woman with a bad case of stomach cramps and diarrhea. Gratefully, I climbed into the top bunk in the on-call room, leaving the bottom bunk for the intern, who might never get to bed, and who, if she did, would have to be ready to leap up at a moment's notice if there was an emergency. Me, I hoped that, emergency or not, I would be overlooked in the top bunk and allowed to sleep out the next two hours and fifty-five minutes in peace (I reserved five minutes to pull myself together before rounds). I lay down and closed my eyes, and something occurred to me. With typical medical student compulsiveness, I had done what is called a "mega-workup" on this patient, I had asked her every possible question about her history and conscientiously written down all her answers. And suddenly I realized that I had written in her chart careful details of all her drug use, cocaine, amphetamines, hallucinogens, all the things she had said she had once used but didn't anymore. She was about my age and had talked to me easily, cheerfully, once her pain was relatively under control, telling me she used to be really into this and that, but now she didn't even drink. And I had written all the details in her chart. I couldn't go to sleep, thinking about those sentences. There was no reason for them. There was no reason everyone had to know all this. There was no reason it had to be written in her official chart, available for legal subpoena. It was four in the morning and I was weary and by no means clear-headed; I began to fantasize one scenario after another in which my careless remarks in this woman's record cost her a job, got her thrown into jail, discredited her forever. And as I dragged myself out of the top bunk and out to the nurses' station to find her chart and cross out the offending sentences with such heavy black lines that they could never be read, I was conscious of an agreeable sense of self-sacrifice—here I was, smudging my immaculate mega-writeup to protect my patient. On rounds, I would say, "Some past drug use," if it seemed relevant.

Medical records are tricky items legally. Medical students are always being reminded to be discreet about what they write—the patient can demand to see the record, the records can be subpoenaed in a trial. Do not make jokes. If you think a serious mistake has been made, do not write that in the record—that is not for you to judge, and you will be providing ammunition for anyone trying to use the record against the hospital. And gradually, in fact, you learn a set of evasions and euphemisms with which doctors comment in charts on differences of opinion, misdiagnoses, and even errors. "Unfortunate complication of usually benign procedure." That kind of thing. The chart is a potential source of damage; damage to the patient, as I was afraid of doing, or damage to the hospital and the doctor.

Medical students and doctors have a reputation for crude humor; some is merely off-color, which comes naturally to people who deal all day with sick bodies. Other jokes can be more disturbing; I remember a patient whose cancer had destroyed her vocal cords so she could no longer talk. In taking her history from her daughter we happened to find out that she had once been a professional musician, singing and playing the piano in supper clubs. For the rest of her stay in the hospital, the resident always introduced her case, when discussing it with other doctors, by saying, "Do you know Mrs. Q.? She used to sing and play the piano—now she just plays the piano."

As you learn to become a doctor, there is a frequent sense of surprise, a feeling that you are not entitled to the kind of intrusion you are allowed into patients' lives. Without arguing, they permit you to examine them; it is impossible to imagine, when you do your very first physical exam, that someday you will walk in calmly and tell a man your grandfather's age to undress, and then examine him without thinking about it twice. You get used to it all, but every so often you find yourself marveling at the access you are allowed, at the way you are learning from the bodies, the stories, the lives and deaths of perfect strangers. They give up their privacy in exchange for some hope—sometimes strong, sometimes faint—of the alleviation of pain, the curing of disease. And gradually, with medical training, that feeling of amazement, that feeling that you are not entitled, scars over. You begin to identify more thoroughly with the medical profession—of course you are entitled to see everything and know everything; you're a doctor, aren't you? And as you accept this as your right, you move further from your patients, even as you penetrate more meticulously and more confidently into their lives.

Ethical Dilemmas for
House Staff Physicians:
The Care of Critically Ill
and Dying Patients
William Winkenwerder Jr.

∎

The life-sustaining capability of modern medicine, coupled with its difficult ethical choices, has become the physician's most challenging moral dilemma[1-5] (*US News and World Report,* Dec 6, 1982, p 53; *Time,* April 9, 1984, p 68). Caring for critically ill and dying patients is a difficult task that often vacillates between the rational and the absurd, the uplifting and the morbid. Conflicts in values among caretakers are frequently present, and uncertainty is pervasive.

This essay addresses the issue of distinctive ethical dilemmas faced by residents in caring for critically ill and dying patients, a problem that springs from the increasing capabilities of medicine and the peculiar role of residents in our medical hierarchy. Residents are fully licensed to practice medicine, but they are not totally autonomous. They have heavy responsibilities in patients' care, but they are not independent in making many decisions. They are usually the primary caretakers, but usually not the ultimate decision makers. Their job clearly is one of many ambiguities and contradictions as well as great uncertainty. Such a complex role makes it difficult to answer questions regarding residents' rights and responsibilities, particularly in situations of moral dilemma.

Several questions arise when considering choices in care for critically ill and dying patients

from a resident's perspective. Must residents always submit to "the team's" or attending physician's decision when it is in conflict with their personal ethical principles or judgment about the patient's best interests, and is it ever appropriate for house staff physicians to decline, based on ethical reasons, to participate in the life-sustaining care of such patients? What are their legal rights in doing so? What dynamic processes are involved in team decisions concerning critically ill and dying patients, and how do they affect residents' decisions? Finally, how can we deal with conflicts in judgment over ethical questions between house staff and attending physicians and improve ethical decision making?

A Resident's Ethical Dilemma

The patient was a 74-year-old man with a one-year history of recurrent ventricular tachycardia who was admitted for a cavitary right lower lobe mass. A diagnosis of squamous cell carcinoma of the lung was made with a percutaneous needle aspiration. He was evaluated for the possibility of a curative resection. A liver-spleen scan, bone scan, computed tomographic scan of the chest, and bronchoscopy revealed questionably metastatic lesions in the left lung and thoracic vertebrae. However, after a second bronchoscopy and additional spine x-ray films, it was thought that he probably did not have metastatic disease, and a right lower lobectomy was performed. Two days postoperatively, he developed wide complex tachycardia, pulmonary edema, left lung consolidation, and temperature to 39°C.

While artificially ventilated, he was transferred to the medical intensive care unit. He received infusions of dopamine, lidocaine, amiodarone, and antibiotics. The impression was that he had a nosocomial pneumonia, pulmonary edema, and sepsis complicated by recurrent ventricular arrhythmias and congestive heart failure.

One day later, he suffered a cardiac arrest. A

prolonged resuscitation lasting three hours was performed and he survived. During the resuscitation, he suffered multiple rib fractures, resulting in a flail chest. He developed adult respiratory distress syndrome (ARDS) and worsening pneumonia (*Pseudomonas aeruginosa*) to the point that he required maximal ventilation to achieve oxygenation. Several days later, he remained hypotensive despite continuous infusion of dopamine. Neurologically, he became unresponsive. There was concern that he had hypoxic brain damage. Ten days after admission to the intensive care unit (ICU), his renal function declined precipitously and he developed a coagulopathy.

At this time, questions arose concerning further treatment. The patient's wife questioned the staff to determine if anything more could be done for her husband and if there was a treatment for renal failure. A conference ensued, involving the ICU attending physician, the wife, two of the patient's sons, and members of the house staff. All of the medical facts of the situation were carefully explained. It was emphasized that chances of survival were exceedingly slim. The attending physician then presented the wife with the choice of whether to use dialysis, and she decided that it should be used. Her two sons, however, were ambivalent. There was concern, but no proof, that factors of guilt influenced her decision. It was not clear what the patient would have preferred had he been able to voice an opinion.

At this point, as a resident on the ICU team, I became uncomfortable with the decision to employ an additional life-sustaining maneuver. There was only a very small chance that dialysis would make any difference in the patient's immediate, much less short-term, survival. Given this reality, my medical knowledge, my concern for the patient, and my ethical beliefs about patient care, the treatments did not seem to be in his best interests. A further concern was that dialysis could significantly prolong his suffering.

And unfortunately, he had no voice in our decision and was unable to communicate his pain.

Viewing events from a different perspective, it was clear that the decision had been reached in an appropriate manner. Furthermore, I knew that the attending physician had been conscientious in his attempts to serve the patient's interests and meet the family's desires.

Despite these factors, I felt a clear sense of ethical compromise in having to carry out the plans that had been made. But what was I to do as a house staff physician? The options I saw were (1) to continue to participate in the care plan, although doing so would constitute action that opposed my ethics of patient care and judgment about the patient's best interests; (2) to request to not participate further in the patient's care based on my ethical concerns; (3) to discuss the issue with my attending physician; or (4) to seek a higher arbitrator such as the departmental chairman. After discussing the issue with the attending physician, it was clear that, despite our both being committed to the patient's best interests, we had different views concerning my obligations and responsibilities. His perspective was that I had certain moral and professional obligations in this case: to provide treatment as a resident physician in a referral hospital, to abide by the decision to further treat, and to fulfill professional responsibilities to my colleagues. As I wrestled with these thoughts, I was still left with a conscience that was disturbed. It just did not feel right to me to continue aggressive, life-sustaining care in this unfortunate man when it was almost certain that he would soon die. The situation was the most difficult dilemma I had faced as a resident. I was torn and I did not know what to do.

Comment

The dilemma of how much to treat and when to stop medically treating critically ill and dying patients is well recognized[1-7] (*US News and World Report,* Dec 6, 1982, p 53; *Time,* April 9, 1984, p 68; *California,* November 1982, p 79 ff.). However, the house staff physician's role in this relatively recent phenomenon is not, and there are few parallels for it in other areas of medicine. Little attention has been paid to the issue of whether residents are always bound to the decisions of their attending physicians, and whether it may ever be appropriate for residents to decline to participate in the life-sustaining care of patients on the basis of ethical grounds.

How one answers this question may depend on several factors. One's vantage point and level in the hierarchy are likely to influence one's perception, as is one's opinion regarding the rights and duties of residents. Also, an individual's philosophy regarding the moral obligations of physicians is important. In most cases, as in mine, the request to not participate in the life-sustaining care of a patient for ethical reasons comes after a search of one's conscience. However, ethicists and theologians have pointed out that the conscience is not always an infallible guide.[8] When should a physician invoke his conscience? Certainly no one of us can speak for all of us.

The issue is further complicated when the group decision-making process of teaching hospitals is considered. It is not realistic or practical to examine the consciences of a group of attending physicians and residents to make comparisons of their moral validity in circumstances of ethical conflict. Even if this could be done, the issue with respect to residents is not in determining the moral validity of their views on treatment or those of attending physicians, but in allowing residents the freedom to resolve their own conflicts of conscience when obligations of duty that are inherent in a hierarchical structure and those of personal morality are forced into opposition.

How can this be done? One might suggest that residents should be allowed to decline to participate in care if it appeared that their conflicts were truly unresolvable. Granting this right, however, challenges traditional concepts of medical authority and raises questions concerning medical responsibility in the setting of teaching hospitals. The ultimate responsibility for making decisions has always rested with attending physicians. This arrangement is legally sound and it provides for a unified plan of action. The opportunity to oppose an attending physician's or team's decision, even in the form of abstaining from care, has the potential, albeit small, of bringing the walls of authority down. All of us would agree with the illogicality of allowing every physician to unilaterally invoke his preference, but do we have a mechanism for dealing with more serious conflicts of moral opinion, especially since they are so value driven and wrapped in uncertainty?

One effect of the compromises that result from conflicting judgment and values is a personal cost to caretakers. The experience of interns is most illustrative. Many colleagues have remarked that nothing was more painful during this year than to realize that the decision had been made (by a more senior physician or by the team's failure to determine resuscitative status) to "flog" a hopeless patient and that they would be the ones doing the flogging. Because of their proximity to the patient physically and emotionally, they were the caretakers who most felt the patient's suffering and pain. But they were also the physicians who were keeping the patient alive. Other house staff physicians may have experienced similar anxiety when they perceived the actions of the team or attending physician to be undertreatment of salvageable patients.

Also problematic are legal questions surrounding the practices of house staff physicians in caring for critically ill and dying patients. What legal rights do house staff physicians have when declining to participate in the life-sustaining care of such patients on ethical grounds? Similar questions have arisen for nurses, and the answer probably depends on the employee's contract with the hospital. The same reasoning could apply to residents, but the issue is not clear and has not been tested in the courts. Should status as a resident in a teaching hospital influence legal protection in such situations? Does being a house staff physician require that one suspend his or her personal ethical principles in certain situations?

The subject of how group decision making and responsibility influence an individual's acting on his own beliefs and principles has been well studied.[9–11] As Irving Janis has pointed out, there is a "tendency for the collective judgment arising out of group discussions to become polarized, sometimes shifting toward extreme conservatism and sometimes toward riskier courses of action that the individual members would otherwise be prepared to take."[9(p5)] Couple this with the observation of Wanzer et al[4(p956)] that "physicians do not easily accept the concept that it may be best to do less, not more, for a patient," and one may find answers for why "the decision to pull back (especially in intensive care settings) is much more difficult to make than the decision to push ahead with aggressive support."[4(p956)] There are no published data on the subject of how the team decision-making model of residency training programs influences the responses of individual physicians when ethical questions arise. One wonders if a resident's inclination to identify and act on his own beliefs is suppressed in the presence of such a group. The fear of evoking disapproval from colleagues or superiors may play a part in this process.

Part of the problem in making decisions with the critically ill is that medical technology gives us fewer answers than we would like to believe. The most difficult questions are often not those dealing with respirator settings, acid-base balance, or Swan-Ganz catheters, but those having to do with whether or not to continue treating, the assessment of recoverable function and quality of life, the relief of suffering, and the treatment of family members' burdens. Wisdom, good judgment, and experience, too often undervalued, are probably more helpful than expert knowledge in answering these questions.

Suggestions for Dealing With Conflicts and Improving Ethical Decision Making

How can we deal with ethical conflicts within a group of physicians, particularly those involving house staff and attending physicians, and how might medical and ethical decisions in the care of critically ill and dying patients be improved? Others have provided guidelines for responsible behavior with regard to the physician-patient relationship (communication with the patient, promotion of patient autonomy, individualizing treatment in competent and incompetent patients).[4–12] But the following recommendations are directed toward physicians in terms of their interactions with each other and their interactions with other medical caretakers.

1. Recognize value differences when they arise in a group of physicians and recognize the conflicts that might result from these differences. One way to address this important first step in dealing with the problem is to promote discussion of ethical questions and to encourage team members to voice their perspectives. Discussion, question, and dissent have long been part of the medical decision-making process, especially in teaching institutions. The same should hold true for making ethical decisions. Leadership of discussion should be viewed as a major responsibility of all attending physicians. Ethical questions exist for every patient who is critically ill. Not talking about these questions will not make them go away. In fact, the absence of discussion is likely to generate emotional anxiety, add to tension within the team, and lead to poor decisions on patient care. In most cases, all team members should be able to "live with" a careful

and well-reasoned decision. When irreconcilable differences do occur, those in the minority opinion should not be coerced or excluded from the group.

2. Increase formal ethics teaching in medical schools and residency programs. Although there is no firm evidence that formal exposure to issues in medical ethics will produce more compassionate and responsible physicians, it makes educational sense to raise students' sensitivities to moral issues in clinical decision making and to help them clarify their own ethical beliefs. Some advocates believe that formal ethics curriculums should result in physicians having a minimum of certain abilities and knowledge to deal with ethical issues.[13]

3. Utilize consultants or recognized local sages to help resolve differences of ethical opinion. When differences of opinion regarding medical treatment arise, subspecialty consultants are called to provide opinions and delineate choices. Although the ethical consultant's actual function differs somewhat, the same general approach should be followed in resolving ethical differences.

Polarization of opinion among a group of physicians caring for critically ill patients is emotionally exhausting for everyone and detrimental to patient care. An experienced clinician or ethics consultant who is removed from the group but interested in providing guidance may help to bring about a unified management plan. The function of this person should not be to make the actual decision, but to help the primary caretakers, patient, and family reach a mutually agreed-on decision.

4. Attempt to minimize uncertainty and maximize communication. There is considerable uncertainty in caring for patients who are critically ill that must be minimized to facilitate diagnosis and prognosis, but insistence on unreasonable certainty may be detrimental in that it limits treatment options and possibly exposes patients to additional risks.[4]

Uncertainty can be reduced without producing detrimental effects by improving communication among team members. In many cases, poor communication results in suboptimal decisions. Because the patient that one physician perceives is in a nonrecoverable state may be the same one to whom another physician administers life-sustaining or resuscitative care, decisions about the same patient might vary. Care will be improved if every member of the team is familiar with a clear and agreed-on plan for each patient should that patient suddenly decompensate. The plan should exist throughout the entire hospitalization, and it should be reevaluated frequently. Bedell and Delbanco[14] have suggested that this issue is probably far from being clarified in the majority of hospitalized patients.

One possible approach to the problem might be the routine administration of a questionnaire with choices about resuscitation, similar to that described by Wagner,[15] for all patients admitted to acute-care hospitals. If written in simple language and administered with sensitivity, such questionnaires could give patients an opportunity to carefully consider their preferences regarding resuscitation. The use of these questionnaires should not serve as a replacement for patient-physician decision making regarding resuscitation, but rather as an adjunct to improved decision making.

Conclusion

The purpose of this article was to expose and examine certain ethical dilemmas faced by house staff physicians in the care of critically ill and dying patients. Complex ethical issues regarding care for these patients, particularly in the setting of teaching hospitals, are on the rise. Residents, who face unique role demands and obligations of personal conscience, are often presented with hard choices in the care of the critically ill and dying. Medical educators have been slow to recognize these dilemmas, and there has been little effort to develop mechanisms to deal with them. Allowing residents more freedom to resolve their conflicts of conscience is one possible solution, but it challenges traditional concepts of medical authority and responsibility.

Conflicts of moral opinion among physicians at all levels of training are frequently present, but rarely recognized and discussed. Steps are needed to reduce the likelihood of these conflicts and to improve the ethical decision-making process. These include (1) increasing efforts to recognize and resolve value differences when they arise, (2) increasing formal ethics training in medical school and residency programs, (3) utilizing ethics consultants and local sages to resolve differences, and (4) minimizing uncertainty and maximizing communication.

Reluctance on the part of physicians to negotiate and resolve their ethical differences in an open and honest manner concerning the care of critically ill and dying patients may portend an ominous future as other parties seek to impose their solutions. The effects of nonmedical groups' involvement in pediatric intensive care have already been felt. The repercussions of their involvement in the terminal care of elderly and dying patients could be staggering.[16]

Although the outcome of the described case would not have changed, I believed that circumstances would have been better had we recognized our value differences, used a consultant, and sought a clearer understanding of the ethical choices involved. Regarding the fate of our unfortunate patient, he died on the same day as the decision to proceed with dialysis was made. With considerable uneasiness, I remained on the team and directed the final resuscitation attempt.

Notes

The author is indebted to Susan Day, M.D., and Renée Fox, Ph.D., at the University of Pennsylvania and Stuart Bondurant, M.D., and Larry Churchill, Ph.D., at the University of North Carolina for their help and criticism in the preparation of this manuscript. Also, thanks are expressed to Judy Saks for her help in the preparation of the manuscript.

1. Hilfiker, D. Allowing the debilitated to die: Facing our ethical choices. *N Engl J Med* 1983;308:716–719.
2. President's Commission for the Study of Ethical Problems in Medicine and Biomedical and Behavioral Research: *Deciding to Forego Life Sustaining Treatment.* New York, Concern for Dying, 1983, pp. 236–239.
3. Bayer, R., Callahan, D., Fletcher, J. et al. The care of the terminally ill: Mortality and economics. *N Engl J Med* 1983;309:1490–1494.
4. Wanzer, S.H., Adelstein, S.J., Cranford, R.E. et al. The physician's responsibility toward hopelessly ill patients. *N Engl J Med* 1984;310:955–959.
5. Lo, B., Dornbrand, L. Guiding the hand that feeds. *N Engl J Med* 1984;311:402–404.
6. Fried, C. Terminating life support: Out of the closet! *N Engl J Med* 1976;295:390–391.
7. Guidelines for the determination of death: Report of the medical consultants on the diagnosis of death to the President's Commission for the Study of Ethical Problems in Medicine and Biomedical and Behavioral Research. *JAMA* 1981;246:2184–2186.
8. Beauchamp, T., Childress, J.F. Ideals, virtues and conscientious actions, in *Principles of Biomedical Ethics.* New York, Oxford University Press, 1983.
9. Janis, I.L. *Groupthink.* Boston, Houghton Mifflin Co., 1983.
10. Janis, I.L. *Decision Making.* New York, Free Press, 1977, pp 129–133.
11. Cartwright, D. Risk taking by individuals and groups, an assessment of research employing choice dilemmas. *J Pers Soc Psychol* 1971;20:361–378.
12. McCullough, L. Bioethics. *New Physician* 1983;9:31–32.
13. Culver, C.M., Clouser, K.D., Gert, B. et al. Basic curricular goals in medical ethics. *N Engl J Med* 1985;312:253–256.
14. Bedell, S.E., Delbanco, T.L. Choices about cardiopulmonary resuscitation in the hospital: When do physicians talk with patients? *N Engl J Med* 1984;310:1089–1092.
15. Wagner, A. Cardiopulmonary resuscitation in the aged: A prospective survey. *N Engl J Med* 1984;310:1129–1130.
16. Capron, A. The implications of Baby Jane Doe for the internist: The case of Grandpa Doc. Read before the Society for Research and Education in Primary Care Internal Medicine, Washington, DC, May 3, 1984.

A Student's View of a Medical Teaching Exercise

Abenaa Brewster

∎

Physicians are usually careful to explain the purpose and format of a teaching session when asking a patient to take part. Failure to do so when the patient is poorly educated or of a different cultural background may seriously disturb the patient and mislead the other participants. Consider the events at a recent neurology conference at a Boston teaching hospital.

The resident began by describing the case of "a 52-year-old postmenopausal black woman with a history of breast cancer at age 46 treated by mastectomy and radiation." She went on to say:

A year ago the patient had back and leg pain and was found to have diffuse skeletal metastases. She was treated with local radiation and tamoxifen, with moderate relief. The sudden onset of excruciating pain in her right thigh 48 hours ago led to hospitalization. Because of some memory loss and apparent confusion, she was seen by a consulting neurologist, who suggested that she might have cerebral metastases. Her mental status is intact, but she has some difficulty remembering names.

The patient was brought into the room in a wheelchair, accompanied by her daughter and sister. The attending neurologist pulled his chair close to the patient and asked where she was from. She replied in a thick Southern accent that she was from a small town in Arkansas, and she introduced her relatives. She was then asked whether she recognized anyone in the room, to name someone, and to point to those whom she could not name. She seemed bewildered by the request. The conference continued as follows:

Neurologist: How old were you when you had the operation on your breast, and what has happened since?

Patient: Honey, I was maybe 46, but I can't remember all the things from back then that you want me to remember. I want to see the doctor who operated on me, honey. That's who I want to talk to.

Neurologist: What's that about money?

He turned to the room.

Neurologist: What is she saying about money?

Resident: She's calling you "honey."

Everyone in the room laughed, and the neurologist appeared embarrassed.

Patient: I'm not trying to pick you up or nothing, I'm just calling you "honey"; it's just a saying.

Neurologist: Can you try to raise your leg, please.

He leaned forward to hold her leg.

Patient: Don't touch me. Everybody wants me to raise this and raise that. I can't do anything with the leg. Don't ask me to do anything. I'm not doing anything. I'm a smart woman, you know; I'm not stupid. Y'all think that I'm stupid. I don't know anything about those pictures over there [pointing to the x-ray films], but I'm a smart woman, very smart.

The patient started to cry.

Neurologist: It must be very difficult trying to cope with your problems. We will all try to come up with some suitable treatment to help you.

He signaled to the resident that the session was over.

Patient: I know that y'all gonna laugh when I leave, oooh Lord. Y'all gonna laugh, oooh Lord.

The patient was wheeled out of the room as a few people said goodbye.

Neurologist: Well, that was *something.* She is obviously volatile and disinhibited, which probably reflects metastases to her frontal lobes. I thought it best not to persist, for she was obviously being very uncooperative.

A discussion about the patient's medical condition ensued, during which a radiologist indicated that he saw no evidence of brain metastases.

From the beginning of the encounter between the attending neurologist and the patient, a mismatch of agendas was evident. Had time and care been taken at the outset, an agenda could have been set to benefit both parties. The neurologist's goals were to seek additional information about the patient's medical history, to determine her mental status, and to clarify the nature of any neurologic deficits. A further objective might have been to demonstrate to the residents and students a method for establishing a sound patient–doctor relationship.

The patient, for whatever reason, assumed she was to see the doctor who had operated on her years before. Her goal was surely not to be embarrassed for calling a doctor "honey" and not to feel humiliated because she could not recognize faces in the crowd. Similarly, she did not understand why she was asked to answer questions that had been asked several times before, nor why a doctor she had not previously met wished to examine her in front of strangers and to display her lack of motor function.

I could not help but feel that had the patient been a well-educated woman speaking standard English, the demonstration would have been very different. Before the conference, the resident would have explained to the patient what she could expect. During the meeting, the attending neurologist would probably have told her why he was asking her to identify people in the room. And had these simple amenities not been observed, the discussion after her departure might have focused on why she had not been properly informed. The resident would have been asked whether she had forgotten to explain to the patient that questions would be asked and a neurologic examination carried out for the benefit of physicians who had not had the opportunity to read her chart.

Furthermore, I believe that if there had been even one nonwhite doctor in that room, adjectives like "volatile" and "disinhibited" might not have been used so readily. Indeed, an appreciation for the patient's frankness might have replaced "disinhibited," and admiration of her pride and her effort to control her life might have replaced "volatile."

When faced with people who differ from ourselves, or with "difficult" patients, an easy way out is to seek a medical label for behavior that we cannot understand or control. How often do we base differential diagnoses on stereotypes?

Such attitudes and actions on the part of physicians can impede the discovery of nonmedical explanations for what often proves to be, after all, normal behavior. They put us at risk of depriving patients of opportunities to contribute to their own medical care and prevent us from caring properly for people whom we do not understand. They can stifle opportunities to learn more about people of other races, classes, or cultural backgrounds. Finally, they deflect us from giving all our patients unconditional respect.

Note

I am indebted to Dr. Howard Hiatt for his advice and support.

The Libby Zion Case:
One Step Forward or
Two Steps Backward?

David A. Asch

Ruth M. Parker

■

The unexpected death of a young woman at the New York Hospital in 1984 prompted a series of regional investigations that have resulted in recommendations of profound changes in graduate medical education. An initial proposal included the suggestion that work shifts be imposed to limit the long hours traditionally worked by house officers. Although this proposal was sparked by a single event, it did not occur in isolation; a variety of forces from inside and outside the profession gave it support. We examine the political and social pressures that urged the adoption of work shifts in the medical profession and interpret the implications of this trend.

The Libby Zion Case

In March 1984 an 18-year-old woman named Libby Zion died at the New York Hospital a few hours after she had been admitted through the emergency room. Zion's father, an attorney and a writer for *The New York Times,* claimed that his daughter had received inadequate care in the hands of overworked and undersupervised medical house officers. He persuaded New York County District Attorney Robert Morgenthau to begin a grand jury investigation into her death. What follows is a summary of the circumstances in the case, derived from a lengthy report issued in late December 1986 by the grand jury.[1]

In January 1984 Libby Zion began psychiatric treatment for stress. Her therapy included phenelzine, which she took until the day before her arrival at the hospital. In late February she had a tooth extracted, and her dentist prescribed Percodan (aspirin–oxycodone hydrochloride) for pain. A few days later she had a fever and otalgia, and her personal physician prescribed erythromycin and chlorpheniramine. (During the preceding two months she had also been given imipramine, flurazepam, diazepam, tetracycline, and doxycycline, though the circumstances surrounding the prescription of these drugs are not detailed in the grand jury's report.)

Over the next few days, Ms. Zion's fever persisted and she had chills, myalgias, and arthralgias. On March 4 her temperature reached 41°C. That day her father contacted his doctor, an attending physician at the New York Hospital, who suggested that Mr. Zion take his daughter to the emergency room there.

She arrived at the emergency room at 11:30 p.m. The junior medical resident obtained the history noted above, although he was not aware of the previous prescriptions for imipramine, flurazepam, diazepam, tetracycline, and doxycycline. The patient stated that she had not taken erythromycin or phenelzine that day because she had felt too ill. She admitted to frequent use of marijuana but reported no use of cocaine or any other drugs.

The patient was writhing during her physical examination; the resident believed this to be volitional. She had a temperature of 39.7°C and mild orthostatic blood pressure changes. Her right tympanic membrane was hyperemic; she had a soft murmur, a clear chest, and petechiae on her right thigh. The leukocyte count was 18,000 per cubic millimeter, and a chest film was normal. The patient was given intravenous fluids, and one set of blood cultures was obtained.

After a telephone discussion between the resident and the referring physician, the patient was admitted to the medical service at 2:00 a.m. and given acetaminophen. She was examined by both the intern and junior resident, who obtained separate histories. Both their admission notes described her agitation. The junior resident made a tentative diagnosis of "viral syndrome with hysterical symptoms." He recommended that blood, urine, and stool cultures be obtained, antibiotics be withheld, phenelzine be discontinued, therapy be administered for fever, and 25 mg of meperidine be given for agitation and shivering. The intern's tentative diagnosis was "viral syndrome." The admitting orders specified "routine" vital signs.

At 3:30 a.m. the patient was given the meperidine intramuscularly. Shortly thereafter, the house officers left the floor to care for other patients. Between 4:00 and 4:30 a.m., the patient became more restless and confused and began thrashing about in bed. The intern was notified of the patient's status twice during this period and, over the telephone, first ordered the use of physical restraints and later ordered 1 mg of haloperidol. Between 4:30 and 6:00 a.m., the patient was noted to be resting and the restraints were removed. She was calmer and able to take acetaminophen by mouth. Shortly thereafter she again became agitated and was found to have an axillary temperature of 42°C. The intern was called, and cold compresses and a cooling blanket were ordered. At 6:30 a.m. the patient went into respiratory arrest and could not be resuscitated.

The medical examiner's report of March 6, 1984, listed the preliminary cause of death as bilateral bronchopneumonia. The report stated that the patient had "hyperpyrexia and sudden collapse shortly following injection of meperidine and haloperidol while in restraints for toxic agitation." A toxicologist detected acetaminophen and antihistamines in the tissues. Radioimmunoassay revealed trace amounts of cocaine in a specimen from the patient's nostrils. Gas chromatography did not confirm this finding, but serum samples obtained before death were found to be positive for cocaine by radioimmunoassay. The medical examiner considered the evidence of cocaine use to be presumptive but not conclusive.

Although the grand jury returned no criminal indictments against the New York Hospital or its physicians, it found much fault with a system of residency training and physician staffing that could allow such a tragic death to occur. The grand jury's report was, in effect, an indictment of American graduate medical education. In it, the jury emphasized five circumstances it believed contributed to Libby Zion's death and made recommendations for corrective action in five corresponding aspects of hospital care.

First, Libby Zion had initially been evaluated in the emergency room by a junior (second-year) resident, who had discussed her care over the telephone with the referring attending physician; however, she had not been examined in the emergency room by an attending physician. The first recommendation of the grand jury was that

The State Department of Health should promulgate regulations that mandate all level one hospitals to staff their emergency rooms with physicians who have completed at least three years of postgraduate training and who are specifically trained to evaluate and care for patients on an emergency basis.

Second, Ms. Zion had been admitted to the medical service under the immediate care of an intern and a junior medical resident. The grand jury's second recommendation was that

The State Department of Health should promulgate regulations to insure that interns and junior residents in level one hospitals are supervised contemporaneously and in-person by attending physicians or those members of the housestaff who have completed at least a three-year postgraduate residency program. These regulations should narrowly define the circumstances under which interns may practice medicine without direct supervision.

Third, Ms. Zion had been admitted to the medical service at 2:00 a.m., when the intern and junior resident caring for her had each been at work for 18 hours. The third recommendation of the grand jury was that

The State Department of Health should promulgate regulations to limit consecutive working hours for interns and junior residents in teaching hospitals.

Fourth, Ms. Zion had been placed in physical restraints on the orders of the intern, who had examined her an hour earlier but did not reexamine her at the time of the order, which was given by telephone. The fourth recommendation of the grand jury was that

Legislation should be enacted to prescribe when a patient in a medical hospital may be physically restrained and to standardize the care and attention necessary for a patient in restraints.

Fifth, Ms. Zion had been given a dose of meperidine despite the physician's knowledge of her history of treatment with phenelzine. The *Physician's Desk Reference* lists treatment with phenelzine as a contraindication to meperidine. The fifth recommendation of the grand jury was that

The State Department of Health should conduct a study to determine the feasibility of requiring level one hospitals to implement a computerized system to check for contraindicated combinations of drugs.

The grand jury report was issued at a time when media coverage of the Libby Zion case was prompting questions about the quality of care in teaching hospitals. Many questions focused on the long hours that interns and residents work

and on their lack of adequate supervision. At the same time, a sociological study of house officers suggested that long work hours and other intense pressures of clinical training condition physicians to view patients as enemies, in contradiction of the implicit and desired principles of patient care.[2]

Meanwhile, New York City Council President Andrew Stein, who had established himself politically as a consumer advocate for health care in New York City (and who, coincidentally, had employed Libby Zion as a student intern), published a health department study suggesting that mistakes were to blame for many deaths in hospitals in New York City.[3] In that climate David Axelrod, commissioner of the New York State Department of Health, appointed Bertrand Bell to chair the Ad Hoc Advisory Committee on Emergency Services, composed of nine distinguished New York physicians.

The committee reviewed the grand jury's report on the Zion case and released a preliminary statement in early June 1987 that assessed and ultimately endorsed each of the report's five recommendations.[4] The proposed limits on consecutive working hours for interns and residents prompted the committee to suggest that the shifts worked by house staff and attending physicians in emergency services be limited to 12 hours and that physicians caring for patients outside of emergency services work in shifts limited to 16 hours, with at least 8 hours off between shifts.

The committee recognized that its five recommendations would have a profound impact on the health care system. During August, therefore, the committee heard testimony from concerned and informed parties, including the Accreditation Council of Graduate Medical Education, the American College of Physicians, the American College of Surgeons, the American Medical Association, the Association of American Medical Colleges, the Association of Program Directors in Internal Medicine, the Committee of Interns and

Residents, the Greater New York Hospital Association, and the Health and Hospitals Corporation. Much of the testimony concerned potential problems of implementation, including effects on graduate medical education, hospital staffing, malpractice litigation, and health care financing. The Greater New York Hospital Association offered a detailed analysis of the committee's preliminary report and estimated that the proposed recommendations would require an additional 2045 full-time-equivalent attending physicians and 974 full-time-equivalent ancillary personnel in 50 New York City hospitals, at a total annual cost of $203,955,001.[5]

In October the Committee on Emergency Services modified their preliminary statement and issued 19 recommendations to the New York State Department of Health. Its comprehensive report called for on-site supervision of busy emergency rooms by attending physicians and 24-hour supervision of acute care inpatient units by experienced physicians. The committee also called for improved working conditions and greater ancillary support for residents. It suggested guidelines for the use of physical restraints and recommended further study of drug-information systems. The committee upheld its recommendation of a 12-hour limit on coverage of emergency departments by attending physicians and residents. Although it did not suggest that work shifts be abandoned altogether in the inpatient setting, the committee replaced the rigid 16-hour limit with more flexible guidelines. The 13th recommendation of the committee was that

> Individual residents who have direct patient care responsibilities in areas other than the Emergency Department shall have a scheduled work week which will not exceed an average of 80 hours per week over a 4 week period and should not be scheduled to work as a matter of course for more than 24 con-

secutive hours, with one 24 hour period of non-working time per week. . . .[6]

Forces from within the Profession

The political pressures to limit residents' working hours stem from a desire to improve patient care. Parallel to these political pressures is the growing influence of the life-style preferences of graduate medical trainees. As medical industrialization and patient consumerism change traditional concepts of the physician's role, the personal demands of residents and other physicians for more leisure are becoming more compelling. The growing allure of specialties like radiology, anesthesiology, and ophthalmology and the trends toward shared medical practices and employment in health maintenance organizations are easy to explain in economic terms. But these trends may also reflect a desire for predictable working hours and increased leisure time.

The Committee of Interns and Residents, a union of about 5000 residents working in public hospitals in New York, New Jersey, and the District of Columbia, testified to the Ad Hoc Advisory Committee on Emergency Services in favor of the 16-hour limit on work shifts and suggested an additional restriction on cumulative weekly working hours. The Committee of Interns and Residents was instrumental in the 1975 strike by residents in several New York hospitals, when a demand for a 15-hour limit was met only by a reduction in the frequency of overnight on-call duty from every second to every third night.

Why Long Hours?

The long working hours of residency are a tradition in physicians' training. Some believe the tradition is maintained by inertia, in a bow to medicine's historic foundations. Others believe it is a rite of passage that tests residents' worthiness. Still others claim that the long hours are essential to proper training—that an understanding of the evolution of many acute diseases can be gained only through the observation of affected patients over time. Finally, some argue that residents are an elastic source of physician labor and that extended hours are a concession to the economic realities of fiscal temperance.

All these popular arguments hold some truth. But when a house officer attends to an acutely ill patient he admitted 30 hours earlier, the issue is the quality of care—not history, rite, training, or economics. Residents recognize their obligation to provide care and believe that their work with the patient fosters a special understanding that cannot be fully transferred to another, perhaps equally qualified, covering resident. The care another resident provides will at best be a pale form of their own. The concept of shift hours denies this aspect of physicianship.

Shift Hours and the Problem of Continuity

Patients require care 24 hours a day, and although the medical system can operate on a continuous schedule, physicians cannot.[7] Shift work offers one solution to this conflict; however, it subjects patients to a succession of physicians, exposes residents to patients in fragmented blocks of time, and subordinates the Samaritan aspects of physicianship to shift loyalty and the organizational needs of the system.

Doctors form relationships with their patients and have a sense of responsibility to them that does not start and stop at scheduled times. At some point, however, the benefit of having a patient's own physician available is offset by that physician's fatigue. At other times, physicians' personal needs for leisure interfere with their availability to their patients. In these situations, covering residents or attending physicians represent an appropriate compromise for continuity. But if we impose rigid shift hours on graduate medical trainees and make them abandon their

patients' bedsides at preestablished times, we will give future practitioners the wrong message about caring for patients.

These conflicts do not arise in all medical settings. In emergency rooms and walk-in ambulatory care centers, the doctor–patient relationship is defined by acute rather than longitudinal needs, and shift work makes sense. Equally qualified physicians will, in general, provide equivalent and substitutable care in these settings.

In systems in which patient care is performed by physicians working in shifts, the medical profession is reshaped into an industry that follows the traditional models of business organization and management. To this end, Harvard Business School's Theodore Levitt warns that

> If we continue to approach service as something done by individuals rather than by machines or systems, we will continue to suffer from . . . distortions in thinking. . . . Service will be viewed as something residual to the ultimate reality—to a tangible product, to a specific competence (like evaluating loans, writing insurance policies, giving medical aid, preparing on-premises foods).[8]

Administrators have powerful incentives to embrace these systems, because the implementation of shift hours undermines physicians' power: the fragmented, production-line approach to continuous care increases the substitutability of physicians, making each one more replaceable.

The Zion Case in Its Broader Context

The grand jury's recommendations were motivated by a desire to improve hospital care. But the grand jury confused professional incompetence with long working hours. In concentrating on the fact that the residents caring for Libby Zion had been working for 18 hours by the time they evaluated her, the grand jury assumed that the residents were fatigued and that fatigued residents threaten patients' safety. Such assumptions are not well supported: physicians differ in their tolerance for sleeplessness, and it is not easy to prove a correlation between fatigue and medical incompetence.[9,10] Instead, the grand jury might have recommended that working conditions in hospitals not contribute to professional incompetence. Limiting working hours is only one way to improve working conditions for residents. Other ways include ensuring a tolerable balance between residents' medical education and their responsibility for patients; respect from professional staff and allied personnel; adequate ancillary and administrative support services; sufficient educational resources in the form of libraries, conferences, and role models; salaries and benefits commensurate with service; and institutional and departmental recognition of residents' human needs.

Patients should be protected from physicians who are so overworked that their competency is challenged. Residents should work in environments that satisfy their professional and personal needs. Neither goal requires categorical limits on working hours. We must separate the issues of professional incompetence and prolonged hours, and we must distinguish working hours from the larger issue of working conditions. These challenges will best be met through further study.

The Libby Zion case has achieved its profound influence through the political climate surrounding it. In making its recommendations, the grand jury acted as a consumer advocate, expressing to the New York State Department of Health the limits of consumers' tolerance. The rise of consumerism among patients set the stage for the jury's directives.

The heroic image of the physician is fading. As patients are increasingly recognized as consumers of health care and physicians as its producers, physicians are more willing to abandon a tradition of service for an industrial work ethic.

The predictable schedules afforded by time clocks are compelling benefits of this ethic. Although the Ad Hoc Committee on Emergency Services ultimately tempered its suggestion of work shifts for residents, the issue will surface again.

Notes

The opinions expressed are those of the authors and not of the Robert Wood Johnson Foundation.

1. Supreme Court of the State of New York, County of New York: Part 50. Report of the fourth grand jury for the April/May term of 1986 concerning the care and treatment of a patient and the supervision of interns and junior residents at a hospital in New York County, December 1986.
2. Mizrahi, T. Getting rid of patients: contraindications in the socialization of physicians. New Brunswick: Rutgers University Press, 1986.
3. City hospitals cited for patient deaths. Release of the New York City Council President, April 20, 1987.
4. New York State Department of Health Ad Hoc Advisory Committee on Emergency Services, New York, June 2, 1987.
5. Greater New York Hospital Association. Recommendations of the New York State Department of Health's Ad Hoc Advisory Committee on Emergency Services, New York, August 1987.
6. New York State Department of Health Ad Hoc Advisory Committee on Emergency Services. Supervision and residents' working conditions, New York, October 7, 1987.
7. Zerubavel, E. Patterns of time in hospital life: a sociological perspective. Chicago: University of Chicago Press, 1979:37–59.
8. Levitt, T. Production-line approach to service. Harvard Bus Rev 1972;50:41–52.
9. Asken, M.J., Raham, D.C. Resident performance and sleep deprivation: a review. J Med Ed 1983; 58:382–8.
10. Friedman, R.C., Bigger, J.T., Kornfeld, D.S. The intern and sleep loss. N Engl J Med 1971; 285:201–3.

Presidential Address:

The Boundaries of Medicine

Donald W. Seldin

Medical Practice in Social Context

■

Does medicine have social responsibilities and goals, and if so, what are they? Should the physician workforce mirror the social and ethnic makeup of society? What types of relationships are possible between doctors and patients? The series of readings in this section asks these questions and many others about the conduct of medical practice.

We see in these essays doctors who define themselves narrowly as biomedical scientists and doctors who see the social problems of their community as part of the legitimate scope of their medical practice. We also see, in the articles by Arnold Relman and Carola Eisenberg, the increasing representation of women in medicine. This demographic change raises questions about what difference women physicians will make in how medical care is delivered. In the final selection, a short story by Sir Arthur Conan Doyle, Dr. James Ripley is portrayed as he first resists and then adapts to a new woman practitioner setting up a successful practice in his town. Many of the issues raised in this story hold as true now for a contemporary young woman physician starting out in practice as they did when this story was written.

Members of the Association and guests:

At the end of the Second World War, while serving as a medical officer in Munich, Germany, I was called to testify as an expert witness at a trial in the nearby concentration camp of Dachau. A Nazi physician was accused of causing the death, connected somehow with the treatment of infectious hepatitis, of some forty inmates. Previous testimony had established that the patients died following liver biopsies performed by the accused physician. From a legal point of view, a guilty verdict would follow the demonstration that the biopsies were experiments; the physician would be exonerated if the deaths followed, however regrettably, from legitimate medical practice.

The physician was knowledgeable, intelligent, and a former trainee at the Rockefeller Institute. However, some forty consecutive deaths following the performance of an alleged diagnostic procedure, the wholly experimental status of liver biopsy at the time, and the total lack of evidence of informed consent led to a verdict of guilty. The physician was convicted of murder and appropriately sentenced.

The unimaginable horror of the practices of Nazi physicians derives not simply from their viciousness but perhaps more significantly from the appalling degradation of humane values inherent in their behavior. We are, as physicians, concerned not simply with life but with human life—a life endowed with the full capacity for intentionality, free choice, and autonomy, and therefore entitled to respect.

But if medicine is concerned with human life, it is pertinent to inquire in what significantly relevant way such a concern is a medical concern. After all, priests and rabbis, artists, lawyers, sociologists, and economists also have as their focus human beings. A concern for human life is therefore not *ipso facto* a medical concern.

In the remarks that follow I shall argue that medicine is a very narrow discipline. Its goals may be defined as the relief of pain, the prevention of disability, and the postponement of death by the application of the theoretical knowledge incorporated in medical science to individual patients.

Two consequences flow from such a definition. On the one hand, in the restricted domain of biologic malfunction, medicine, although admittedly a comparatively weak scientific discipline, is nevertheless an extremely powerful instrumentality for the mitigation of suffering and in certain instances the prolongation of life. On the other hand, just because of the genuine triumphs of medical science, embedded as they are in a heritage which invests medicine with the priestly function of the counselor and comforter of the sick, there has resulted a tendency to construe all sorts of human problems as medical problems. This medicalization of human experience leads to an enormous hypertrophy of personnel and facilities, massive financial expenditures, and perhaps most tragic of all, frustration and disillusionment when medical intervention fails to eventuate in tranquility, quiescence, and happiness.

Human problems and human agonies are medical problems and medical illnesses only when they can be approached by the theories and techniques of biomedical science. I would like to examine three areas where the boundaries of medicine are blurred.

The Nazi Experience: "Doctors of Infamy"

More than anything else, it was the relevation of medical barbarism conducted by the Nazi government that jolted the world into a scrutiny of the interaction between medical science and human beings.

Medical policy under the Nazis[1-3] is summarized in Table 1. Three programs may be identified. A program of compulsory sterilization was enacted on July 14, 1933. Hereditary health courts were established to enforce sterilization of persons irrespective of racial origin afflicted with hereditary illnesses. This was part of a policy of "race hygiene," and was accompanied by a massive propaganda campaign designed to indoctrinate the medical community in the ideology of racial health. Abortion was in general not countenanced, since the Nazi policy encouraged

Table 1. Medical Policy under the Nazis

I. Sterilization
   A. Hereditary health courts
   B. Abortion
II. Euthanasia
   A. Extermination of the chronically ill: deformed, insane, enfeebled, neurologically impaired
   B. Extermination of the racially "impure": Jews, Gypsies, Poles
   C. Extermination of the socially disruptive
III. Medico-military research
   A. Enhanced blood coagulation
   B. Explosive decompression
   C. Immersion in ice water
   D. Experimental gas gangrene, hepatitis, infected wounds

Derived from: Alexander, L., N. Engl. J. Med. 241:39, 1949, and Dawidowicz, L., Hastings Center Report Supplement, 1976.

Table 2. The Root of Nazi Medical Policy:
Physicians' Attitudes

"Whatever proportions [Nazi] crimes finally assumed, it became evident to all who investigated them that they had started from small beginnings. The beginnings at first were merely a subtle shift in emphasis in the basic attitude of the physicians. It started with the acceptance of the attitude, basic in the euthanasia movement, that there is such a thing as life not worthy to be lived. This attitude in its early stages concerned itself merely with the severely and chronically sick. Gradually the sphere of those to be included in this category was enlarged to encompass the socially unproductive, the ideologically unwanted, the racially unwanted and finally all non-Germans. But it is important to realize that the infinitely small wedged-in lever from which this entire trend of mind received its impetus was the attitude toward the nonrehabilitable sick.

It is, therefore, this subtle shift in emphasis of the physicians' attitude that one must thoroughly investigate."

From Alexander, L., N. Engl. J. Med. 241: 39, 1949.

propagation of the racially pure, and subjected the racially impure to sterilization.

Euthanasia was actually a program of murder of the "racially valueless": deformed children, the mentally ill, and the neurologically impaired were exterminated at killing centers. Killing was done without patient consent, without family notification, and without any consideration of relief of suffering. The program was enormously expanded to involve the extermination of Jews, Gypsies, Poles, and the socially disruptive—groups without biomedical illness of any sort but who were regarded as racially impure. "The Final Solution," the mass murder of European Jews, was the ultimate expression of the policy of racial purity.

Finally, a ruthless program of medico-military research was forcibly imposed on the racially impure with the aim of developing methods of mass extermination and mass sterilization, and experimenting with various bizarre notions of mili-

tary medicine. The experiments, really manipulations, usually had little scientific content and were often clearly conducted so as to inflict torture. Even when an element of rational intellectual content could be discerned, it is obvious that the subjects were not accorded the faintest status as human beings.

What is one to make of Nazi biomedical policy? Granted the unspeakable inhumanity, in what logical domain does the catastrophe reside? In a graphic passage (Table 2), Alexander[1] locates major responsibility in medicine, emphasizing the "wedged-in lever" in the minds of physicians, engendered by a callous attitude toward the sick and infirm. Seen thus, the causal sequence terminating the Nazi terror found its roots in the minds of physicians.

Without in any way exonerating the role of Nazi physicians, the distinguished historian of the Holocaust, Lucy Dawidowicz,[2] offers a dif-

Table 3. The Root of Nazi Medical Policy:
Nazi Racist Ideology

"Sterilization, medical experiments, euthanasia, the Final Solution—all are terms associated with the history of the Nazi regime . . . These terms . . . were integral aspects of Nazi racism. Nazi racism derived from a theory about the ultimate value of the purity of the Volk, a word meaning 'people' or 'nation' which in Nazi usage took on a quasi-mystical sense . . . this Volk, consisting of racially pure Germans, pure 'Aryans,' was destined to rule the world. . . .

"Those persons or groups of persons that were considered harmful to racial health, that is, racial purity, were characterized by the racial ideologists as 'valueless' life, which was slated for destruction. The 'valuelessness' of such life was measured in terms of the health of the Volk, itself an abstract concept, not a physical reality. This health had no bearing on individual health, on family health, even on public health, or the health of society."

From Dawidowicz, L., Hastings Center Report Supplement, 1976.

Table 4. Irrelevance of Nazi Experience for Medicine

Sterilization and euthanasia had nothing to do with "mercy toward the sick . . . or the nonrehabilitable sick, at least in the normal individual sense." (Kohl, M. I., *Beneficent Euthanasia*, Prometheus Books, 1975) "The purpose of Nazi medical experimentation was quite different from the criteria for testing and experimentation that are set elsewhere. Did it serve what we would call a bona fide medical purpose: would the result of the experiment benefit the community at large, would they save lives?" (Dawidowicz, L., Hastings Center Report Supplement, 1976) "The Nazi experience does not enlighten you as to the problems you confront in making decisions today about euthanasia. . . . [The policy] was motivated by the centrality of race and the importance of racial hygiene for the survival of the *Volk*." (Dawidowicz, L., Hastings Center Report Supplement, 1976)

---

ferent framework. The medical policy of the Nazis was principally the catastrophic expression of an appalling social doctrine—the doctrine of the *Herrenvolk,* which reduced anyone considered to contaminate racial purity to subhuman status (Table 3). It was this mystical ideology of racial purity of the *Volk* that justified sterilization and mass extermination of valueless life—whether that life be the chronically ill or mentally infirm or whole populations of different racial or ethnic backgrounds. The Nazi doctrine of euthanasia was racist from the start and had nothing to do with attitudes to the nonrehabilitable sick. She quotes Hitler's statement in *Mein Kampf,* written in 1924, that the *Volkist* state using the most modern medical means "must declare unfit for propagation all who are in any way visibly sick, all who have inherited a disease and can therefore pass it on."

The Nazi medical policy is thus identified as an expression of Nazi racist ideology. The lessons to be learned are political, social, cultural, not primarily medical (Table 4). To ascribe major

causal significance to medicine is to trivialize the enormity of the horror.

Biomedical Ethics

Biomedical ethics has been officially inaugurated into the medical curriculum: the American Board of Internal Medicine now challenges the candidate with a series of questions designed to probe competence in ethical issues. It thus is joined with a burgeoning group of applied ethical disciplines—"business ethics," "legal ethics," "ethics in government"—each constituting a seemingly discrete domain of learning and requiring specialized faculty, courses, and training.

A cardinal feature of ethics is the requirement that principles or codes on the basis of which a person exercises a moral choice must apply to everyone alike, independent of personal or social status (Table 5). If this were not the case, the rich and powerful might successfully escape the moral rules which are applied to those who are weaker or unconventional. Human beings, in Kant's moving formulation, are "members of the Kingdom of Ends" and should never be treated as "means only."

In a recent penetrating analysis,[4] four fundamental principles were identified in terms of which moral problems may be analyzed: auton-

Table 5. The Dignity of the Individual

Categorical imperative:
"Act only according to the maxim by which you can at the same time will that it should become a universal law."
"Act so that you treat humanity, whether in your own person or in that of another, always as an end and never as a means only."

Implication: The moral autonomy of every human being is expressed in self-rule and independence of the will of another.

From Kant, I., *Foundations of the Metaphysics of Morals*, 1764.

omy (right of individuals to believe and act as they choose, independent of the will of others); nonmaleficence (duty not to harm others); beneficence (duty to confer benefits and to promote actions where benefits exceed harms—principle of utility); and justice (requirement that persons should receive what they deserve).

Two features of these moral principles deserve special notice. First, they are all derived from intellectual and social domains having nothing to do with medicine. To be sure, medical issues may be analyzed in terms of these categories. But their study and explication are in general the concern of philosophers of ethics, not physicians. Second, the principles are exceptionally broad and would in the abstract perhaps occasion little dissent. In specific circumstances, however, the same ethical principle may be interpreted in different, even incompatible ways, and different ethical principles may conflict with one another.

The principle of autonomy in Mill's powerful formulation celebrates the widest right of unfettered self-determination, subject only to the constraint that others not be harmed (Tables 6 and 7). Is the requirement to wear airplane seatbelts therefore an intolerable intrusion on personal liberty? Does the legal requirement of motorcyclists to wear helmets constitute unwarranted paternalism? If informed consent is the key to unlock autonomy, when is a patient properly informed and when is consent free of undue pressure? Is informed consent impossible in the relatively closed (perhaps coercive) environment of a prison, so that research on prisoners should be categorically banned? If so, is research in a hospital, or in a research institute, or for that matter in a doctor's office free from subtle, but nevertheless powerful, pressures—the more dangerous, perhaps, for being unsuspected?

It is pertinent to inquire whether the resolution of these issues is greatly facilitated by reference to the four universal ethical principles. To be sure, these principles constitute important frameworks for conceptual analysis. They also serve the vital function of sensitizing individuals to critical ways in which people interact. But the resolution of concrete ethical problems usually follows from a balancing of heterogeneous considerations of a rather specific sort, in accord with which ethical principles are secondarily interpreted.

Consider lying—the deliberate communication of false information in order to deceive. Seriously ill and emotionally fragile patients may be able neither to comprehend nor tolerate the truth about their illnesses. Withholding of information or even a frank lie may mitigate harm. The key question is whether or not lying by the physician was in the overall best interests of the patient. Clearly, there is a conflict of principles between the harm of lying *per se* on the one hand and such benefits as inner quiescence and reassurance that lying may produce. Such an issue is

Table 6. Autonomy (Self-Determination)

" . . . the only purpose for which power can be rightfully exercised over any member of a civilized community, against his will, is to prevent harm to others. His own good, either physical or moral, is not a sufficient warrant. He cannot rightfully be compelled to do or forbear because it will be better for him to do so, because it will make him happier, because, in the opinion of others, to do so would be wise or even right . . . The only part of the conduct of anyone, for which he is amenable to society, is that which concerns others. In the part which concerns himself, his independence is, of right, absolute."

Implications:

1. The only legitimate limitation on an individual's liberty is the prevention of harm to others.
2. Anti-paternalism: interference with a person's liberty by society or by its members for the person's own good is *never* justifiable.

From Mill, J. S., *On Liberty*, 1898.

Table 7. Justification of Autonomy

Utilitarian:

"All errors which the individual is likely to commit against advice and warning are far outweighed by the evil of allowing others to constrain him to what they deem his good."

"Mankind are greater gainers by suffering each other to live as seems good to themselves, than by compelling each other to live as seems good to the rest."

Absolute:

"There is a part of the life of every person who has come to years of discretion, within which the individuality of that person ought to reign uncontrolled by other persons or by the public collectively."

A person's "mode of laying out his existence is the best, not because it is the best in itself, but because it is his mode."

From Mill, J. S., *Utilitarianism*, 1891, and *On Liberty*, 1898.

usually resolved by a sensitive assessment of the emotional stability of patients by physicians entrusted with their care, without recourse to universal ethical principles.

Biomedical ethics seems to embrace two concerns. One is the morality of public policy in medicine. We recognize such issues as abortion, research on the fetus, the just allocation of scarce medical resources, medical care as a right, and the like. A second concern is the moral behavior of individual physicians. Both of these issues are principally centered on conceptual analysis, and might best be placed in a general university department of philosophy, outside the medical school, where formal ethical study can be conducted in an appropriate setting in which biomedical ethics is a component. To be sure, there is need for collaboration and interaction with physicians and medical school faculty to make ethical analysis pertinent to medicine. There is also little doubt that the sophisticated analysis of ethical problems on a philosophical level heightens the sensitivity and sharpens the ana-

lytic tools of individual physicians in their interaction with patients. But it is doubtful that biomedical ethics constitutes a formal domain of learning separate from philosophic ethics and that formal ethical training has great value in the resolution of concrete ethical problems encountered by physicians.

The Care of the Elderly

The phrase, care of the elderly, seems to suggest that old people are in some sense sick and therefore in need of medical care. If this were the case, the problem would be virtually unmanageable. At present, in the United States, some 23,000,000 people are over 65 years of age, and 9,000,000 over 75; by the year 2030, it is projected that the corresponding numbers will be 55,000,000 and 23,000,000, indicating that 18% of the population will be elderly (Table 8). The projected costs for medical care of any substantial fraction of this group would be staggering.

It is by no means clear, however, that the care of the elderly is principally a problem of medical care. Aging seems to entail a certain degree of enfeeblement, causing a diminished capacity for self-care. But old people who are enfeebled are not necessarily patients. To be sure, they may need help of a physical type to ambulate, to feed and dress themselves, to participate in social functions. Appropriate environmental support

Table 8. The Elderly in the United States

Age Group	1977 Millions	1977 % of Total Population	2030 Millions	2030 % of Total Population
>65	23	11	55	18
>75	9	4	23	8

From U.S. Department of Commerce, Bureau of the Census, *1970 Census of the Population*, 1973.

may be required to forestall isolation and depression. The agony and frustration resulting from the physical decay of aging is personified by the poet, William Butler Yeats, as "an enemy [who] has bound and twisted me so that although I can make plans and think better than ever, I can no longer carry out what I plan and think." In beautiful lines he characterizes old age as a seemingly external constraint limiting his capacity for self-realization:

> What shall I do with this absurdity—
> O heart, O troubled heart—this caricature,
> Decrepit age that has been tied to me
> As to a dog's tail?

In the nineteenth century, the care of the elderly was largely a family problem, to be resolved within the bounds of a household. Three forces seem to have been responsible for translocating an increasing fraction of geriatric care into the public domain. Perhaps most important was a change in economic organization in which ownership of homes, previously largely by parents, was now in the hands of children. In consequence, the infirm elderly became dependent on the good will of their children. This transfer of economic power was associated with a social change characterized by a progressive weakening of family bonds. The net result was a collapse of support that family members had previously afforded each other, so we are now confronted with the pathetic spectacle of the enfeebled aged citizenry as constituting a problem of social support in the public domain rather than a family issue to be resolved by warmth and understanding. Finally, entry into and discharge from nursing homes came largely to be supported by Medicaid and similar programs of Federal support which require physician certification of need and thereby increasingly transform the problem of the care of the aged into a medical problem.

In a perceptive analysis, Kane and his associates[5] have set forth several goals for the care of

Table 9. Goals for Health Care of the Elderly

1. Maximizing the independence of the individual
2. Ensuring at least a minimal level of comfort
3. Promoting subjective well-being and morale
4. Avoiding premature deaths
5. Minimizing the cost of care for the elderly

From Kane, R. L., *et al.*, Geriatrics in the United States: Manpower Projections and Training Considerations, 1980.

the elderly (Table 9). They are designed to solve certain personal and social needs of those elderly with a diminished capacity for self-care. Although the term "health care" is used, it is noteworthy that in most instances these measures are not medical measures. They are rather support services that can be rendered as well, or better, by well-trained and motivated personnel who are not physicians. The recommended measures take cognizance of enfeeblement—diminished physical and mental capacity for self-care.

This limitation in the elderly of the full range of normal behavior and expression may well lead to depression, isolation, estrangement. Humane care is clearly necessary. Since expertise in this area requires social and environmental manipulations no less than special physical help for mundane activities, the responsibility for this should logically be placed in the hands of social workers, nurses, and community-based professional personnel rather than physicians.

None of this should be construed to mean that the physician has no role to play in the care of the elderly. Clearly, it is the physician's responsibility to minister to the elderly who are sick. Since these problems can be highly specialized, the care of the elderly sick may well constitute a legitimate domain for a geriatric specialist. Moreover, the geriatric physician can function as a participant in a geriatric team, but need not necessarily be the director or leading figure when the purpose of the group is to design and supervise humane settings for elderly people.

Most of the elderly are not, properly speaking, patients. Medical therapy may not be an essential or critical ingredient for their care. To convert the support of the enfeebled to a medical concern is to incur enormous costs at the same time that their care may be misdirected along narrow biomedical lines. It is not in the best interests of the elderly or of the country to transform every limitation of activity that may beset an elderly person into a medical illness.

Medicine and Health

The central goals of medicine may be defined as the relief of pain, the prevention of disability, and the postponement of death by the application of the theoretical knowledge incorporated in medical science to individual patients. Three features of this definition are of special note.

First, the relief of pain, the prevention of disability, and the postponement of death are specified as distinct objectives. By thus delimiting illness to biomedical derangements expressed in this manner, there is no commitment to include deviant behavior as medical illness. Moreover, the definition makes no statement as to whether such phenomena as pain or disability or death are expressions of a disease or a regulatory disturbance. Diseases, when understood, have causal roots, the elimination of which (in the absence of irreversible damage) is curative. But illnesses are not simply collections of discrete disease entities. Increasingly, illnesses can be analyzed in terms of derangements in regulatory function, the correction of which may restore normal function even when the cause is unknown. This formidable advance in the explanatory power of medical science permits the physician to mitigate or even cure many biomedical disturbances on the basis of understanding the underlying physiologic process.

Second, the definition specifies that the goals of medicine are achieved through the applica-

tion of the knowledge incorporated in biomedical science. Medicine is thus operationally distinguished from other modes of relieving disabilities, such as behavioral therapy, education, and the like. By linking medicine with biomedical science, the basic sciences, such as biochemistry, physiology, cell biology, are seen to furnish the theoretical framework for clinical medicine.

Third, the definition emphasizes that the interaction is a face-to-face encounter between a physician and a patient for the treatment of illness. Aggregate disciplines which influence health through cultural and social forces are thereby excluded from medicine.

These three necessary features of medicine in concert—biomedical science as the underlying basis of medical theory and knowledge, its use for the mitigation of specifically biomedical derangements (pain, disability, premature death), and its application to individual human beings—serve to define the medical model which is summarized in Table 10. There can be no doubt that the application of this model has transformed the physician from a passive, though sympathetic, spectator, to an active agent for the prevention and treatment of illness.

Despite past triumphs and future promise, the medical model is regarded by some as too narrow and restricted. This view is perhaps most dramatically expressed in the definition of health advanced by the World Health Organization

Table 10. The Medical Model: Necessary Features

1. *Interaction*: face-to-face encounter between physician and patient.
2. *Purpose*: relief of pain, prevention of disability, and saving of life by forestalling and treating disease.
3. *Disturbance*: disease viewed as deranged biomedical function.
4. *Intervention*: application of conceptual framework and tools of biomedical science.

(WHO): "Health is a state of complete physical, mental, and social well-being and not merely the absence of disease or infirmity."[6] Such a definition embraces an enormous variety of disparate concerns—ranging from personal maladjustments to social conflicts—within the domain of medicine. Health, so defined, incorporates properties we ordinarily associate with happiness and citizenship.

If health is to include complete mental well-being, then it is quite clear that medicine would be concerned, not "merely" with the elimination of illness, but also with the attainment of happiness. We usually associate happiness with such emotions as pleasure, fulfillment of desires, inner satisfaction. But how can medicine help to achieve such a state? Surely, heredity, lifestyle, social and economic status, and personal expectations have more to do with happiness than anything medicine can offer. The elimination of illness may not be all of the good life, but it is the domain that the physician can address with insight and knowledge. To attempt in some way to impart happiness is not merely beyond the competence of medicine, it is also an unwarranted intrusion on personal privacy.

The concept of social well-being has uncomfortable social overtones. Crime prevention, sexual and racial discrimination, juvenile delinquency are the concern of policemen, legislators, and parents, not physicians. Social well-being also entails the ominous implication that all types of aberrant and antisocial behavior may be construed as disease. Political opposition may thus be interpreted as mental illness requiring hospitalization. Such medicalization may obscure the fact that many patient complaints do not originate in medical causes but rather from deviations from established behavioral and social norms. Alcoholism, sexual deviance, drug habits, antisocial behavior may have appalling medical consequences for the individual, but they usually constitute problems in social, political, and cultural adjustment, not in medicine.

Some issues subsumed under the concept of social well-being are the shared concerns of individuals as citizens. The economic, social, and cultural structure of society influences health profoundly. However, this influence is exerted through forces over which medicine has little control and cannot alter. Incalculable damage will result from a nuclear war with enormous medical consequences. Its prevention, however, is a problem of politics, not of medicine. Mass poverty results in hideous dehumanization and devastating malnutrition, but the problem is primarily economic. The disintegration of family units may eventuate in profoundly disruptive medical consequences, but it is essentially a social problem. Admittedly, disturbances in political, economic, and social organization may express themselves in serious medical disability, yet the causes generating these illnesses lie outside the arena of medicine. The pertinent question for the physician devolves about those health problems that can be influenced by medicine. Health is not synonymous with happiness or tranquility or a noble life or citizenship. Medicine has little power to realize these admirable personal qualities.

When we venture outside the boundaries of our competence, we lose the special status conferred by the command of biomedical science and the promise it holds for the mitigation of a discrete type of human suffering. The tendency to invade areas not encompassed by the explanatory theories of biomedicine leads to a medicalization of all sorts of problems originating in personal, social, and cultural maladjustment—problems which the physician is powerless to alleviate. Sometimes the prestige conferred by medicine leads to pronouncements on broad cultural and social issues wholly outside medical knowledge. The physician then assumes the role of sage. This may be warranted on the basis of the individual's accomplishments as a citizen, but as a physician special competence is conferred only by the command of the explanatory principles of biomedical science.

The Boundaries of Medicine

Medicine is a narrow discipline. It does not promote the realization of happiness, inner tranquility, moral nobility, good citizenship. But it can bring to bear an increasingly powerful conceptual system for the mitigation of human suffering rooted in biomedical disturbances. To some this goal is too restricted. Confronted with mass poverty, the danger of a nuclear war, economic deprivation, and an aging population, the problems addressed by medicine seem insignificant. It is well to remember the view of the British philosopher, Karl Popper, that it is often our misguided moral enthusiasm, our anxiety to create a better world to live in, rather than our moral weakness that is responsible for the main troubles of our time:

> "Our wars are fundamentally religious wars; they are wars between competing theories of how to establish a better world. And our moral enthusiasm is often misguided, because we fail to realize that our moral principles, which are sure to be oversimple, are often difficult to apply to the complex human and political situations to which we feel bound to apply them."[7]

Perhaps, instead of being too narrow, we are too broad. Perhaps we should as physicians acknowledge with some humility our limited arena of expertise and strive to discharge our responsibilities with high competence. To minister to specific patients for the alleviation of that type of human suffering engendered by medical derangements is not a trivial goal. It constitutes the hallowed activity of physicians and defines their unique role in the domain of health.

Notes

1. Alexander, L.: Medical science under dictatorship. N. Engl. J. Med. 241: 39, 1949.
2. Dawidowicz, L.: *In:* Biomedical Ethics and the Shadow of Nazism. Hastings Center Report Supplement, Hastings-on-Hudson, New York, 1976.
3. Kohl, M., Ed.: Beneficent Euthanasia. Prometheus Books, Buffalo, NY, 1975.
4. Beauchamp, T. L., and Childress, J. F.: Principles of Biomedical Ethics. Oxford University Press, New York, 1979.
5. Kane, R. L., Solomon, D. W., Beck, J. C., Keeler, E., and Kane, R. A.: Geriatrics in the United States: Manpower Projections and Training Considerations. Rand Corporation, Santa Monica, CA, 1980.
6. World Health Organization: Basic Documents, 26th ed. World Health Organization, Geneva, 1976.
7. Popper, K. R.: Conjectures and Refutations: The Growth of Scientific Knowledge. Harper & Row, New York, 1965.

The Boundaries of Medicine

Gerald T. Perkoff

■

The nature and limits of medicine have fascinated philosophers and have been the subject of major argument for decades. In recent years, major advances in our understanding of the biomedical nature of many diseases have led some to believe in the biological basis of medicine to the exclusion of other aspects of human illness and disease [1]. Others have emphasized the psychologic, social and cultural context in which disease occurs and include these broader aspects of illness as essential parts of medicine [2]. The existence of a program of research which deals with patient function as a therapeutic goal brings these contrasting views into sharp focus, since many of the interventions used to increase patient function have no known basis in biological science and are viewed by some as being outside the discipline of medicine.

The clearest statement in this running dialogue is an extreme description of medicine as a strictly biomedical discipline. In 1981, at the annual meeting of the Association of American Physicians, the presidential address was given by Dr. Donald Seldin, Chairman of the Department of Medicine at the University of Texas-Southwestern in Dallas [1]. In his talk, which he, too, called the Boundaries of Medicine, he presented a clear and articulate definition of medicine, which excluded from medicine all concepts except those of biomedical science. His address was disturbing to those of us who hold a broader view of medicine, but even more disturbing was the standing ovation he received, indicating general acceptance of his view by the assembled audience of leaders of academic medicine.

Dr. Seldin's clear, sharply defined description of the boundaries of medicine challenges those who have a different view of the nature of our profession. I, for one, am compelled to attempt a contrasting definition of medicine, for in the biomedical view, medicine is narrow, while I believe it is broad. In that view, medicine is based only on biomedical science; I believe it has many bases. That view takes an exclusive view of medicine; my view of medicine is inclusive. To develop a broader definition of medicine more specifically, let me begin by quoting some of the things Dr. Seldin said. In doing so, let me say that my argument is not with Dr. Seldin *per se,* but with the view of medicine for which he has become the leading and most persuasive spokesman.

As a definition of medicine, he stated: ". . . medicine is a very narrow discipline. Its goals may be defined as the relief of pain, the prevention of disability, and the postponement of death by the application of the theoretical knowledge incorporated in medical science to individual patients." Dr. Seldin sought to clarify and sharpen these boundaries of medicine by showing that cultural and social issues, biomedical ethics, even the care of the aged, were not part of medicine.

To demonstrate the separateness of social phenomena from medicine, he talked about the Nazi medical experiments and said: ". . . Nazi medical policy is thus identified as an expression of Nazi racist ideology. The lessons to be learned are political, social, cultural, not primarily medical."

To indicate what he views as an unfortunate blurring of medicine's purpose with subject matter from extraneous disciplines he said: ". . . about biomedical ethics . . . these fundamental moral principles are all derived from intellectual and social domains having nothing to do with medicine." Further, he indicated that ethical principles were not useful for physicians because they often led to conflicting decisions. For this reason, physicians do not need formal training in biomedical ethics. Rather, he says, such issues are "usually resolved by a sensitive assessment of the emotional stability of patients by physicians entrusted with this care, without recourse to universal ethical principles."

And about aged people he said: ". . . (the care of the elderly requires) measures (that) are not medical measures. They are rather support services that can be rendered as well, or better, by well-trained and motivated personnel who are not physicians."

If these statements characterize medicine, what are the consequences? Some of them seem quite good. If medicine really were composed only of the theoretical knowledge of medical science, this would in many ways simplify the job of the physician. Even though biomedical science is complex and difficult to keep up with, such a philosophy permits the physician to exclude from his/her consciousness all ambiguous factors that might come up in patient care, allows him/her to accept only that which can be explained, allows the physician to work in total independence to the exclusion of any other factors but the most basic organization for medical care. Except for biological knowledge, all else is outside medicine. A further, but in this instance, negative, effect of this model is that it lends itself to the unconscious depersonalization of medicine. If it is not part of one's job, one's ethos, to explain or consider the cultural, ethical or social aspects of the human condition, then there is no incentive to learn about them or to include them in medical care. Perhaps this is one of the reasons so many highly sophisticated, biologically

oriented physicians are perceived as being impersonal even while they protest mightily that they have the patients' best interests at heart. They *do* have the patients' best interests at heart to the degree of which they are capable, but without experience and practice using other forms of knowledge than biological knowledge, they are *not* capable.

With regard to a program of research to improve patient function, many of the approaches used in this area of work do not fit in a biomedically defined medicine. Finally, this view represents an enormous boost for the independence of nursing. The strict biomedical definition at one stroke solves the problem of separating medicine and nursing, and ends the boundary conflict that has bedeviled all those who work at the interface between the two professions in patient care and in research. The biomedical view gives nurses free rein in nursing homes, in health assessment, in prevention, and in various forms of nursing counselling, which many now view as overlapping medicine.

As is so often true of complex subjects, there is some truth in each of Dr. Seldin's points. But the view of medicine that he describes is not only very narrow, it is also unappealing from an intellectual point of view. It accepts current truth as whole truth, leaving little room for new concepts or ideas that may come to the fore to explain human illness phenomena, which biological science cannot now, and may never, explain. If anything, it is an anti-intellectual approach to medicine.

I propose to describe a different kind of medicine. To do so, I will refute some of the major examples given above, hoping in the process to provide a convincing argument for the importance of non-biological phenomena in the many aspects of human illness for which physicians are responsible. I will attempt to show that many of the most vexing of today's ethical issues are, in fact, iatrogenic, caused to appear by spectacular advances in medical science, and therefore the responsibility of medicine. I will make the point that the principles which help us to understand the doctor/patient relationship also help us to identify broader, if more ambiguous, boundaries for medicine than those Dr. Seldin circumscribes.

The first task I have set for myself is to understand the first major example Dr. Seldin chose. To illustrate the separateness of social from medical phenomena, he chose the most dramatic and perhaps the most horrifying known example of conflicting views about medicine. Everyone should be familiar with the fact that in Central Europe in the 1930's and 40's, Germany carried out the killing of so-called undesirable people under the euphemism of "euthanasia," with the underlying purpose of the purification of an abstract concept of race called *Volk*. First the mentally retarded and old senile, then the incurably ill, then the racially and politically undesirable, were killed in what ultimately became the Final Solution: the murder of over six million Jews, and, along the way, an equal number of non-Jews of various political and national origins. In the course of these horrors, so-called medical experiments were undertaken. Initially, these activities were carried out under the guise of aiding the German war effort. But such things as decompression chamber experiments, immersion of people in ice water and the production of battlefield-like wounds and gangrene without anesthesia, were really immoral tortures, which finally led to large scale experiments with various kinds of poisons, conducted to learn how to kill large numbers of people most efficiently.

Two major schools of thought exist to explain physicians' participation in these activities. One, espoused by Leo Alexander in the New England Journal of Medicine in 1949 [3], was that the underlying cause of physicians' participation in these so-called experiments was the initial small "subtle shift in emphasis in the basic attitude of physicians. It started with the acceptance of the attitude . . . that there is such a thing a life not worthy to be lived." Later he says "it is important to realize that the infinitely small wedged-in lever from which this entire trend of mind received its impetus was the attitude toward the nonrehabilitable sick." Alexander believed that if physicians had not taken that initial step in ethical reasoning they would not have been able to countenance such work. His view would place the social and ethical implications of this kind of activity squarely within medicine.

Seldin, however, sides with Lucy Davidowicz, a distinguished historian of the holocaust, who believes that physicians' attitudes had nothing to do with this. Instead, she believes that the basic racism of the Nazi regime was at fault [4]. According to this view, the Nazi medical experiments were the result of social and cultural forces beyond the control of the physicians or anyone else, and that therefore the blame for these same events cannot be laid at the foot of medicine, or on these physicians. It was a social, not a medical series of events. I don't know who is right, but whichever view holds, Dr. Alexander's or Dr. Davidowicz's, could a more potent example of the intertwining of society, social morals, culture, politics and medicine be chosen than the Nazi experience?

If I had been trying to make a strong case for the importance of these non-biological influences on medicine and on human health and illness, I probably would have described a different series of events, perhaps the astute observations of John Snow, who observed the frequency of cholera around the Broad Street pump, a milestone in the history of modern epidemiology [5]. Or I might have chosen the work of Berkman and Syme [6] or of John Cassel [7], demonstrating that people undergoing life changes in an environment deficient in social support have higher incidence of such diverse and serious disorders as cancer, tuberculosis and heart disease, and use more medical services than other people. Such examples illustrate well the intertwining of social phenomena and medicine and argue for the importance of non-biological subjects in the education for, and the practice of medicine.

Instead, to help make this point even further, let me tell you of a different, quite interesting, and fortunately for us, a yet undeveloped parallel between very recent events in our country and physician participation in the Nazi medical experiments. In the resurgence of interest in capital punishment over the past several years, several states have passed laws requiring that executions be carried out by intravenous injection of lethal doses of drugs. In at least one instance, the initial wording of the bill authorizing such executions contained the requirement that the lethal dose be injected by a physician. The outcry by members and friends of the medical profession in that particular state led to change in the wording so that the physician-administration requirement was deleted. What would we think of the physician who accepted this kind of direction arising, in strict terms, from social causes? How could we reconcile physicians' commitment to healing with purposeful execution? How can we understand Nazi medical behavior and its conflict with medical ideas or, indeed with medicine itself, without knowing something about the social, cultural and, especially ethical influences upon those physicians? No one seems uncomfortable when we apply classic criteria of consent, research design, sample size and analytic plan to the Nazi experiments to declare them unscientific. Is this what makes them immoral? How can we understand them without recourse to other fields of knowledge that become part of medicine as they are needed for that understanding?

Such considerations lead me directly into the next example, the identification of biomedical ethics as an area of knowledge outside the domain of medicine. Certainly ethical considerations in medicine are not in and of themselves medical in nature. But it is equally certain that, if it were not for major biological advances which have made possible new and powerful technologic, pharmacologic and physiological tools, few of the major bioethical issues we face today would be with us. These issues can be considered side effects of medical advances in a quite reasonable analogy to the side effects of drug therapy, such as urticarial eruptions and anaphylactic shock, or the deleterious effects of hormonal overdose, like Cushing's Syndrome resulting from excess steroid administration, or malabsorption following the Whipple procedure for carcinoma of the pancreas, or countless others. Were it not for the successes of our science, we would not be faced with the whole issue of death and dying, or the problem of allocation of scarce resources. We would have nothing with which to treat the Baby Jane Does. Genetic engineering, cloning and test tube pregnancies would not exist; and we would not need to be concerned with the propriety of experimentation on products of abortions. The list is almost endless.

According to the biomedical view, ethical principles are not helpful in such matters, because they often lead to controversy over what should be done. Are we to be less interested in these things because they are difficult and controversial, or more interested in them because they represent challenging problems in patient care? More to the point, why is it unhelpful, and outside medicine, that adherence to ethical principles we now believe to be important leads to controversy, and does not always point directly to a decision with which all can agree?

There are many examples in medicine of situations in which reasoning according to agreed upon sets of biological information leads to markedly different opinions, but these are considered part and parcel of the everyday practice of medicine. We may be faced with a patient with a form of leukemia for which there is only partially effective therapy. Further, we may know that for those patients who do not respond to the initial course of therapy, life span may be shortened by treatment compared to the life span of patients not treated. But if the patient who is treated makes an initial response to therapy, then life span may be prolonged for an average, perhaps, of six to eight months. Does the fact that different consultants make different recommendations about therapy detract from the usefulness of the information at hand? Does it matter if the etiology of leukemia turned out to be more complex than an as yet unknown biological cause, perhaps a viral particle, plus some as yet unrecognized social influence or support system? Would these complexities or differences of opinion make the care of leukemia any less a part of medicine than it is now? What about other examples? We know a great deal about the pathogenesis of post-menopausal osteoporosis. There is general agreement that decreased bone density is associated with minimal but longstanding negative calcium balance and that this can be corrected, at least partially, by small doses of vitamin D and calcium. Though still disputed, both the post-menopausal occurrence and the responses to therapy suggest strongly that estrogen deficiency plays a role. Yet there is marked disagreement about the course to follow in post-menopausal women.

These disagreements seem no different to me than do those which arise from disagreement about ethical principles. Moreover, if physicians are encouraged to have sound biological information to reason effectively about the side effects of their major therapeutic advances, why should they not have the same level of sound information about ethical issues? The same reasoning process is just as useful for ethical issues as it is for biomedical problems. Doctors can include in their thinking, and in communication with patients, the religious beliefs of both patient and doctor, as well as their views about autonomy, consent, and justice. At the same time, they can keep in mind the physician's responsibility to do

good and to do no harm. These factors clarify—but do not decide for the physician, any more than biological information decides for the physician—what courses of action exist for the physician and patient to choose among. There seems little logic in a position which maintains that the physician should be trained in biology because he deals with biology, but not be trained for other areas of doctor/patient interaction and that such matters should be considered outside medicine.

This point of view has been expressed in more formal terms by Pellegrino and Thomasma, in their book titled "A Philosophical Basis of Medical Practice," published in 1981 [8]. Their language is not the language of medicine, and their terms require explanation, but their views accord with a much broader view of medicine. They say that medicine is a "relation of mutual consent to effect individualized well being by working, in, with, and through the body." They go on to indicate that in the "relation" they speak of, the job of the physician and patient is to discover necessary analogies between scientific pathogenesis and the individual patient, i.e. the transactions take place within the confines of the doctor/patient relationship. Nowhere in this definition does it say that only biological science can provide the tools for medicine, nor does it overlook the powerful influence of the physician on this process. In other words, it provides a place for the doctor/patient relationship, one of the strongest therapeutic tools the physician has. To our knowledge, neither the function nor the effectiveness of the doctor/patient relationship is dependent upon biological science.

The next example was the care of the aged. Everyone can agree with Dr. Seldin that most elderly people are not patients. They are people who live in a community and who function in effective or ineffective ways more often than not the results of factors other than disease. One also can agree that the political medicalization of the national approach to the elderly has led to enormous expense, which comes from involving physicians in most decisions related to their interactions with governmental agencies. However, Seldin then goes on to say that the only role a physician has to play in the care of the elderly is in the care of disease within the cited definition of medicine, i.e. within the model of the application of the theoretical knowledge of medical science to the relief of pain, the postponement of death, and the prevention of disability. The care of the chronically ill aged is left entirely to non-physician health professionals, predominantly nurses and social workers. It is almost certain that we could benefit if competent nurses were permitted a more independent, judgemental role in nursing homes, day care centers, or in the homes of older people under this model [9]. But it is only fair to point out that nurses need physicians, even physicians whose only interest is diseases of the aged, as much as physicians need nurses interested in the broad issues of the care of the elderly person. Who will the nurse turn to for coordination of illness care with disease treatment, if not the physician? And which physician is more likely to function well in this role of consultant to the primary care nurse—someone whose only interest and expertise is in biomedical science, or a physician who knows and understands biomedical science in the context of social and cultural issues, and who can use more expertise than mere personal sensitivity to reason about the vexing ethical issues of aging? Here we are dealing with the interaction of the physician with other health professionals and with the community.

Again a physician with a different, broader point of view has described such relationships by means of a broader definition of medicine. In 1972 Robert Haggarty published a paper entitled the "Boundaries of Health Care" [10]. He chose the term "Health Care" instead of "Medical Care" on purpose, in line with his view that traditional medical care leads to a very restricted and all-

too-often, an ineffective approach to the care of people. Haggarty reviews the major advances in biological science and describes some of their strengths as well as their inadequacies for the solution of the problems of human illness. He asks in a very practical way "where does medicine end and where does public health and the other health professions begin?"

Haggarty uses lead poisoning as a major example—a condition in which the etiologic agent and the biological sequellae are known, and for which an effective biomedical treatment is available. However, exclusive application of biological treatment only leads to return of the victim, usually a small child, back into the environment in which the lead poisoning is almost certain to recur. It is not incongruous that as biomedical physicians we would be satisfied only to take care of the end state of a disorder that we could affect in a more positive way if we understood something of infant behavior, parental problems, poverty and politics? I don't suggest that physicians run to the ghetto and take lead paint off the walls, but why should a physician not understand these factors so he/she can participate in effective programs for detection and correction of the problems which cause lead poisoning? Indeed, it was physician use of biomedical science which made possible the development of modern lead screening programs. Their ineffectiveness is the result of our inability to effect social change. If we know nothing of the social and economic causes of lead poisoning, we might be more complacent physicians, but would we be better physicians? I think not. Instead, it seems that the more effectively we understand other professions and the concepts upon which they are based, and the more effectively we learn to incorporate those concepts in patient care, the better job we do as physicians. Once again, the broader view seems to fit.

Fortunately, a very articulate physician has given his attention to the divergence between the strictly biomedical view of medicine so clearly stated by Dr. Seldin, and the open-ended view of Dr. Haggarty. The case of psychiatry has many lessons for us and provided the basis for Dr. George Engel's biopsychosocial model of medicine. He has incorporated both biological and non-biological disciplines and methods into a description of the boundaries of medicine.

Psychiatry is a very interesting specialty. It had its modern origin in the pioneer work of Freud, Jung, and others who conceptualized psychiatric illness as resulting from certain important life experiences external to the individual. Until recent times, treatment methods in psychiatry consisted mainly of talking and listening. Beginning with electro-shock and insulin treatment, but especially after we learned about neurotransmittors and psychopharmacologic agents, drug therapy for psychiatric disease entered medical practice. This divergence between traditional treatment methods and modern physiologic information is paralleled by divergence in view about the nature of psychiatry. In an article titled "The Need for a New Medical Model: A Challenge for Biomedicine," published in Science in 1977 [11], Dr. Engel reviews the consequences of such divergent views about the nature of psychiatric illness and its relationship to medicine.

At one extreme are the views of Thomas Szasz, who views mental illnesses as behavioral problems, not as diseases, and therefore not part of medicine [12]. The opposite view, propounded most effectively by workers at Harvard and Washington Universities, is that psychiatric illnesses are diseases of biological origin [13, 14]. Thus, there is strong evidence for the biological basis of some psychiatric diseases, notably manic depressive disease. If this condition is hereditary, it therefore is primarily the result of single or multiple gene abnormality in the same way as is sickle cell anemia, muscular dystrophy or any one of the many other disorders everyone accepts as having a biomedical nature. But

manic-depressive disease was manic-depressive disease 200 years ago, before we knew that relatives of manic patients had a high frequency of the same disorder. What was it then? Was it a disease, and part of medicine, or was it a behavioral disorder outside medicine?

The same can be said for the severe disorders of anxiety. Patients with panic reactions and with generalized anxiety have been recognized for centuries. Their symptoms often are incapacitating, their need for assistance repeatedly acute and severe. Is anxiety not a medical condition just because it is not yet proved, and may be incorrect, that abnormalities of lactic acid metabolism cause these conditions [15]? When and if such metabolic abnormalities are proved to be causal, does that make the anxiety disorders something that physicians will welcome as diseases they should take care of? What determines that switchover? At a more interesting social and ethical level, what do we think about placebo effect? Is it unethical to use placebos, or is such use a justifiable, relatively safe and innocuous form of treatment? Does it make a difference that we now know that some placebos cause the secretion of endorphins [16]? Does understanding that placebo effect may have a biological origin make placebos legitimate therapy, part of biological medicine, or does use of therapies without informed consent still have the same importance as before we knew they might be "effective"?

Engel points out that the biomedical model was devised by medical scientists, not for the treatment of disease, but for its study. Broadly speaking, models are nothing more than belief systems utilized to explain natural phenomena, to make sense out of what is puzzling. Though the biomedical model is a scientific one, he makes clear that not all models are scientific. There also are folk models that bear no certain relationship to science. The more disturbing a phenomenon is, the more we feel compelled to have a model to explain it; disease fills the bill as a particularly disturbing "phenomenon" which requires explanation. Engel further points out that in our culture the scientific or medical model to explain disease has become the dominant folk model as well. Physicians are conditioned by the general acceptance of the folk model to accept it themselves long before they become physicians. They give little thought to its greater applicability to the *study* of disease than to its *treatment.*

Engel makes a very important point which helps to explain the marked differences of opinion characterized by Seldin's view, Haggarty's and mine. Because the biomedical model has acquired the characteristics of what Engel calls a cultural imperative, it has acquired the status of dogma, causing most people to overlook its limitations. He says that, in science, a model is revised or abandoned when it fails to account adequately for all the data. A dogma, on the other hand, requires that discrepant data be forced to fit the model or be excluded. Biomedical dogma, therefore, requires that all disease, including psychiatric disease, be conceptualized in terms of derangement of underlying physical mechanisms. This leads to only two responses physicians can make to incongruities between behavior, disease, illness and therapy. Either one takes a reductionist approach, which says that all illness phenomena must be conceptualized in terms of physiochemical principles, or the exclusionist approach, which says that whatever is not capable of being so explained must be excluded from the definition of disease.

This view of the nature of the argument explains why Dr. Seldin says that so many of the ambiguous things medicine deals with are the business of other professionals, and why he excludes social, ethical and cultural phenomena from physicians' activities. In placing his challenge to biomedicine, Engel proposes a much more inclusive model, which he calls the *biopsychosocial model.* The relationship implied by this complex word takes into account the traditional biomedical aspects of patients' illnesses, the social context in which the patient lives, and the not-yet-known-to-be-and-perhaps-permanently-non-biological aspects of the patient's psyche that affect illness behavior and outcomes. This model uses information from these seemingly disparate areas of human knowledge to understand the cause of human illness and what to do about it. The model allows for the powerful influence of the doctor/patient relationship in the diagnostic and treatment aspects of patient care. Most exciting, it says explicitly that various aspects of knowledge form the basis for understanding and affecting human illness and therefore are the business of medicine and of competent physicians.

Perhaps the most succinct statement of the way that clinical medicine combines the biomedical and non-biomedical was made by Dr. Walsh McDermott [17]: "The physician seeks to do two main things: to manage biomedical knowledge of practical use—its technology—in an effective and discriminating fashion for the prevention and management of illness and disease and to help establish peace of mind." With regard to the latter point, McDermott continued as follows: "Medicine itself is deeply rooted in a *number* of sciences, but it is also deeply rooted in the samaritan tradition. The science and the samaritanism are both directed toward the same goal of tempering the harshness of illness and disease. Medicine is thus *not a science* but a learned profession that attempts to blend affairs of the spirit and the cold objectivity of science.... These two functions, the technologic and the samaritan, are *separable in the world of analysis but not in the world of real life.* . . . A doctor cannot get a passing grade by being proficient at one or the other; he must be good at both, for they are to be regarded as opposite sides of the coin." Walsh McDermott was as committed as anyone I ever knew to the primacy of biomedical science as a basis for medicine, but this view expresses his clear understanding of the fact that more than biomedical science is involved in medicine.

To sum up, my definition of medicine is as follows: Medicine is a broad discipline, a helping profession, which has a constantly growing body of knowledge to call upon. Of the component parts of medicine's knowledge, biomedical science is the most powerful and best developed portion yet known, but biomedical science is but the centerpiece of an amalgam of concepts useful in the care of patients. The method through which this amalgam is applied is the doctor/patient relationship, a human inter-activity which has ameboid rather than sharp borders, drawing into its corpus those things that most logically fulfill the patients' needs.

Medicine deals with mind/body, disease/illness and person/society as a continuum. It is strong because its boundaries are blurred, fluid and opportunistic, not because they are sharply defined. It deals with biomedical, social and cultural function. It is in the strength of its inclusive character that medicine can prevent disability, relieve pain, cure disease, care for illness and promote life, even for those in the process of dying. In all these ways it is human service of the highest order.

Notes

1. Seldin, D.W. Presidential address: the boundaries of medicine. Trans Assoc Am Phys 94: 75–84, 1981
2. Eisenberg, L. The subjective in medicine. Perspect Biol Med 27: 48–61, 1983
3. Alexander, L. Medical science under dictatorship. N Engl J Med 241: 39–47, 1949
4. Davidowicz, L. In Biomedical Ethics and The Shadow of Nazism: Hastings Center Report Supplement, Hastings-on-Hudson, New York, 1976
5. Snow, J. On the mode of communication of cholera. In Snow on Cholera. New York: The Commonwealth Fund, 1936. pp. 1–175
6. Berkman, L., Syme, S.L. Social networks, host resistance, and mortality. A nine-year follow up study of alameda county residents. Am J Epid 109: 186–203, 1979.
7. Cassel, J. The contribution of the social environment to host resistance. Am J Epid 104: 107–123, 1975
8. Pellegrino, E., Thomasma, D. A Philosophical Basis of Medical Practice. New York: Oxford University Press, 1981
9. Mechanic, D., Aicken, L. A cooperative agenda for medicine and nursing. N Engl J Med 307: 747–750, 1982
10. Haggarty, R.J. The boundaries of health care. Pharos 35: 106–111, 1972
11. Engel, G.L. The need for a new medical model: a challenge for biomedicine. Science 196: 129–136, 1977
12. Szasz, T.S. The Myth of Mental Illness. New York: Harper & Row, 1961
13. Kety, S. Am J Psychiat 131: 957–963, 1974
14. Reich, T., Clayton, P., Winokur, G. Family history studies, V. The genetics of mania. Am J Psychiat 125: 1358–1369, 1969
15. Pitts, F.N. Jr., McClure, J.N. Jr. Lactate Metabolism in anxiety neurosis. N Engl J Med 30: 895–904, 1967
16. Berg, A. The placebo effect reconsidered. J Family Pract 17: 647–650, 1983
17. McDermott, W. Medicine: the public good and one's own. Perspect Biol Med 21: 167–187, 1978

The Changing Demography of the Medical Profession

Arnold S. Relman

■

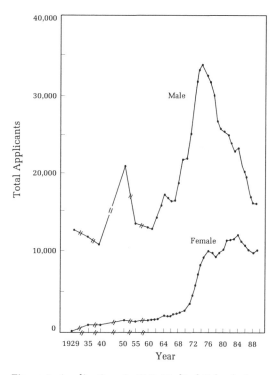

Figure 1. Applications to U.S. Medical Schools from 1929 to 1989. Source: Association of American Medical Colleges.

Nearly 10 years ago I called attention to the rapid increase in the number of women entering U.S. medical schools and speculated on the changes in the medical profession that might ensue if this trend were to continue.[1] Since then, the increase in the number of women medical students has continued,[2] but it is now clear that this change is occurring against a background of declining numbers of white male applicants. We seem to be witnessing the beginnings of a demographic revolution of major proportions, which is bound to have great importance for the future of our health care system.

The percentage of female applicants and matriculants began to rise abruptly in 1970–1971, and this trend has continued to the present. In 1969–1970 approximately 9 percent of new first-year students were women, in 1979–1980 28 percent, and in 1989–1990 38 percent. The number of applications from women appears to have leveled off during the past decade, but the number of applications from men, which had been rising steeply before and after the influx of women began, reached a peak in 1974–1975 and has been falling precipitously ever since. These contrasting changes in numbers of male and female applicants are shown in Figure 1. Since 1974–1975, the total number of applications from men has fallen by over 17,000, nearly 50 percent.

Most of this is due to a reduction in the number of white men applying to medical school. (Since 1974, applications from black men dropped by about 700 [41 percent], but applications from Asian-American men rose by nearly 1200 [133 percent].) A generation or more ago, over 90 percent of medical students and physicians were white men. Ten years ago, nearly two thirds of entering medical students were white men; the most recent figure, for the freshman class of 1988–1989, is 48 percent. In short, if recent trends continue, the medical profession in the United States, which not too long ago was composed almost entirely of white men, will soon have a majority consisting of men from racial minorities and women.

Two articles in the *Journal* (vol. 321, no. 22) deal with the recent influx of women into medi-

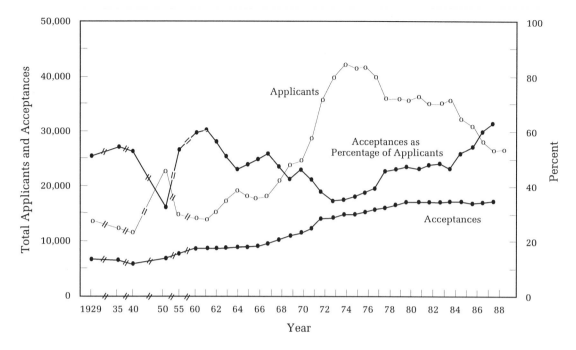

Figure 2. Applications and Acceptances to U.S. Medical Schools and Acceptances as a Percentage of Applications. Source: Association of American Medical Colleges.

cine, with particular reference to the problems they face as members of medical school faculties. Levinson et al.[3] conducted a national survey of women holding full-time appointments in departments of medicine, the majority of whom were married and had children. The survey provides interesting data on how women cope with the competing demands of family and profession. Most were satisfied with their decision to have children, despite feeling that their professional progress had been slowed. Eisenberg[4] urges that women in academic medicine be given equal opportunity for professional success, by which she means not only parental leaves and day care but a tenure policy that allows for childbearing and child rearing. She also advocates an "affirmative action" policy in academic appointments and promotions: "If there is only one tenure slot and there are both men and women fully qualified to fill it, a woman should be appointed."

Eisenberg also observes that without the influx of women, medical education would now be facing a severe crisis because there would not be enough male applicants even to fill existing first-year positions.[4] The increase in female applicants, shown in Figure 1, has cushioned the impact of the decline in male applicants on the availability of acceptable candidates to fill medical school places. Nevertheless, the ratio of acceptances to applicants is now higher than it has ever been—over 65 percent. Figure 2 shows the changes since 1929 in the total number of applicants, total acceptances, and acceptances as a percentage of applicants. The number of acceptances to the first year of medical school (a close approximation of the number of available places) has been essentially constant for the past decade, but applications have declined substantially (entirely because fewer men have been applying), so that the fraction of applicants admitted has been increasing. So far, as judged by college grade-point averages and scores on the medical college aptitude tests, the shrinking pool of applicants has been associated with only a slight reduction in the academic qualifications of those entering medical school. However, the implications are worrying medical educators,[5,6] as well they should.

It seems clear that medicine is now viewed by white male college graduates in the United States as a much less attractive career than heretofore. Many explanations have been offered, all of them probably valid to a degree, but I believe the most important of these are the rising cost of medical education and a growing concern about future professional autonomy and economic opportunity. Women have shown a greater preference for salaried practice and the less remunerative specialties, so the latter consideration is likely to weigh less heavily with them than with men. On the other hand, the sudden flattening of the curve in Figure 1 describing applications by women suggests the possibility that women may also be getting discouraged about the prospects of a medical career. It is interesting that in Canada the demand for medical education has not fallen during the past decade and the present ratio of available places to applicants (24 percent) is much lower than in the United States. Canada has also seen a recent increase in the numbers of women applicants, but applications from men have fallen only slightly, so the total number of applicants is higher now than a decade ago.[7] Medical education in Canada is heavily subsidized by government and is therefore less costly to students than in the United States, but its continued appeal may also be explained by differing social values in the two countries.

To understand the changes in our medical care system that are likely to ensue when women and members of racial minorities constitute more than half the medical profession, one needs to look at the different practice choices of men and women physicians.[1,8] Women have traditionally chosen primary care specialties, obstetrics and gynecology, and psychiatry more frequently, and all of the surgical specialties less frequently, than men. Judging from the results of the most recent National Resident Matching Program, these preferences persist. Women also more frequently choose to practice in salaried group arrangements than men, and their income, adjusted for age, hours worked, and specialty, is lower.[8]

In 1980 I said that the influx of women might well lead to a "softening of the profession's traditional resistance to experimentation with different economic arrangements for medical practice." I also suggested that "major transformations in professional attitudes and styles of medical practice are in the offing, and . . . young women physicians will have an important role in bringing them about."[1] Today, nearly a decade later, the signs of change are growing clearer, and the demographic transformation of the medical profession is quickening its pace. As government and private insurers seek to control costs while ensuring general access to good-quality care, it seems more likely now that there is going to be greater emphasis on primary care and on salaried group-practice arrangements. Doctors will have to be more concerned with the social and economic problems of health care; they will either participate in developing constructive solutions they can support or be forced to accept arrangements imposed by third-party payers.

A changing younger profession, more broadly representative of American society, with more moderate economic expectations and a greater commitment to the primary care specialties, will be in a better position to meet the needs for health care in the next century. Still, the successful practice of medicine will always require brains, compassion, and hard work. We must therefore bend every effort to attract qualified students of both sexes and all racial and ethnic

origins who can respond to the unique challenges and rewards of our profession.

Notes

I am grateful to Richard R. Randlett, assistant vice president for Student Services, Association of American
Medical Colleges, and deputy director, National Resident Matching Program, for his help in providing data
from the files of these organizations.

1. Relman, A.S. Here come the women. N Engl J Med 1980;
   302:1252–3.
2. Bickel, J. Women in medical education: a status report.
   N Engl J Med 1988; 319:1579–84.
3. Levinson, W., Tolle, S.W., Lewis, C. Women in academic
   medicine: combining career and family. N Engl J Med
   1989; 321:1511–7.
4. Eisenberg, C. Medicine is no longer a man's profession:
   or, when the men's club goes coed it's time to change the
   regs. N Engl J Med 1989; 321:1542–4.
5. The declining applicant pool: proceedings: implications
   for the selection of medical students. AAMC Invitational
   Conference, Washington, D.C., June 13–14, 1988. Washington, D.C.: Association of American Medical Colleges,
   1989.
6. Geokas, M.C., Branson, B.J. Recruiting students for medicine. Ann Intern Med 1989; 111:433–6.
7. Ryten, E. Trends in the demand for medical education in
   Canada. Association of Canadian Medical Colleges
   Forum 1989; 22:1–8.
8. Wilson, M.P. Making a difference: women, medicine,
   and the twenty-first century. Yale J Biol Med 1987;
   60:273–88.

Medicine Is No Longer a Man's Profession, Or, When the Men's Club Goes Coed It's Time to Change the Regs

Carola Eisenberg

∎

The influx of women into medicine during the
past two decades has rescued the profession
from a serious threat to its quality. Given what
women have done for medicine, the time is over-
due for the changes medicine must make to accommodate its new demography.

Let's look at the facts.[1] In 1967–1968, when
women made up only 10 percent of the applicant
pool and the size of the entering class was 9702,
the ratio of applicants to first-year places was 1.9.
This ratio should be at least 1.5, many think, to
ensure the selection of well-qualified medical
students. Had there been no women, the ratio
would have been 1.7—still quite acceptable. Ten
years later, the number of applicants had risen to
40,569 and the size of the entering class to 15,977;
again, had no women applied, the ratio would
have fallen from 2.5 to 1.9, but it would have been
more than high enough to permit the selection of
a satisfactory class. By 1984–1985, however,
when first-year places numbered 17,194, there
were only 32,893 applicants, of whom a third
were women. The ratio of male applicants to first-
year positions had dropped to 1.2, which is far
below the proportion needed to fill all classes
with competent students. By 1988–1989, the
pool of male applicants had declined so far
(16,457) that it numbered 324 fewer than the prospective first-year class (16,781).[2]

Thus, had the number of women applicants (and acceptances) not risen sharply, medical education would have been in a severe crisis by the middle of the decade. The United States would have faced an unpalatable choice between a precipitous drop in the number of medical students and the acceptance of students of uncertain quality.

The consequences of increasing female participation in medicine have not yet been appropriately addressed. Women now make up more than a third of the enrollees in medical schools. Although they constitute only one sixth of all physicians (a legacy of past discrimination), the ratio of female to male practitioners will continue to rise each year. Medicine is no longer an overwhelmingly male profession.

It will not have escaped the notice of *Journal* readers that women are the ones who bear children. That is a biologic fact that will not change. A more important aspect of contemporary life is that women continue to make a considerably larger investment in child rearing than men do, for reasons that probably have little to do with biology; the ways boys and girls are socialized for adulthood allow men to be more willing than women to have a smaller parental role. This disparity may change, but there is little likelihood that it will change very much in the near term. And it is the near term with which we must be concerned.

Given the demographics of the medical profession, parental leave and day care must become part of the standard package of fringe benefits available to women (and to men who wish to make use of it) from the time they enter medical school, through their residency training, and during their employment in any large medical group or institution. Although family decisions about the timing and number of offspring are made individually, the aggregate need for day care slots and flexible coverage by residents at academic medical centers is predictable.[3] Support for parenting is a fundamental desideratum, like pensions or health insurance, for all working women and men in two-worker families.[4] What is at stake in every industrial society is the right of children to have suitable conditions for their development.

Full justice for women requires that they have an equal opportunity for professional success after acceptance to medical school. That means offering not only parental leave and day care, but in academic medicine stopping or slowing the tenure clock during the period the doctor-parents choose to take off for bearing and rearing children. Time devoted to parenting should be subtracted in appropriate proportion from the years counted under the up-or-out rule for full-time faculty. The playing field is hardly level if only superwomen, rather than most women, can satisfy the needs of their families and meet their professional goals.

Although the proportion of women serving on medical faculties has risen from 13 to 19 percent over the past 20 years, women continue to be clustered at the lower ranks; 71 percent of faculty women are at the level of assistant professor or lower, in contrast to only 43 percent of the men.[5] In part, this can be ascribed to the recent appearance of women on the academic ladder in more than token numbers. A more accurate measure of the speed with which women climb the ladder can be obtained by following the women and men who joined the faculty in a given year. For the cohort appointed in 1976, Bickel[5] finds that 12 percent of the men but only 3 percent of the women had been promoted to full professor by 1987. Is this entirely attributable to bias? Certainly not. Available data from departments of radiology[6,7] and internal medicine[7] indicate that on average female faculty members have had somewhat less research training and involvement in research and somewhat fewer publications than their male counterparts, although they are equally likely to be engaged in patient care (in both specialties) and administrative responsibilities (in internal medicine). However, it strains credulity to believe that a fourfold difference in rates of achieving full professorship is explicable solely by a difference in academic productivity that, insofar as it is measurable, is much less than fourfold.

An effective remedy requires affirmative action. Medical schools should increase the number of women in senior academic ranks and should do so explicitly. If there is only one tenure slot and there are both men and women fully qualified to fill it, a woman should be appointed. That is the only way to offset the prevailing pattern of discrimination. The credentials of women are subtly discounted because of prejudice so thoroughly inculcated in men (and in all too many women) that it operates automatically, often altogether without awareness.

The problem with this recommendation is that two candidates are never exactly the same—that is, equally "qualified." It is always possible to find ostensibly legitimate reasons for preferring John X to Helen Y when both are excellent. John will have conducted research at the molecular level, whereas Helen, perhaps, is a cell biologist. Although Helen is a very effective teacher of small groups, John is a charismatic lecturer. Moreover, Helen has not supervised as large a project as John has; yet, it is true that her department chairman never asked her to, but the fact is that John has the track record and she does not. Besides, Helen has not published as many papers as John has. Granted, she had done more teaching and has served on more medical school committees, but still, the published record is the published record. Add it all up, and the promotions committee chooses John. The members are sad about Helen, whom they all like, but, they report to the dean, the record "compelled" their decision.

Members of search committees should recognize that the Helens on our faculties are being denied promotion partly because bias in the committee members' very bones makes it hard for them to take women as seriously as men. That acknowledgment is a prerequisite for meaningful change in sex distribution among faculty members that is badly skewed. Neither I nor any other advocate of women's rights wants to see mediocre women promoted; there are all too many mediocre men around already. Agreed, there are not enough fully qualified women today for a one-to-one ratio at senior levels. But there will be in the next century if we act now to make full academic careers for women generally achievable. Let me offer a modest proposal: the nationwide percentage of women among faculty members with tenure should be increased from the current 6.7 to 10 within the next three years. Does anyone really believe that 500 qualified women cannot be found among the 8000 now at the level of assistant or associate professor[5] to make this goal realistic?

The day is not far off when half of all medical students will be women. This is not because all women harbor a secret longing to be doctors, any more than all men do. It is simply this: given that talent is distributed equally between the two sexes, an environment in which there is equal opportunity is likely to elicit equal interest. The sixfold increase in the number of female applicants during the past 20 years is due not to a sudden change in women's natures but to the encouragement given women who undertake professional careers and the removal of barriers to their attainment. At present, an equal number of men and women enter premedical programs in colleges, but fewer women stay the course.[6] When not only the front doors but also the corridors of power are open to them, women will persist in pursuing medical careers to the same extent as men.

Women will bring into academic medicine a greater emphasis on the importance of the physician's family life. The beneficiaries of this concern will be men as well as women. During my years as a child psychiatrist on three successive medical faculties, I became all too well aware of the extent to which many male physicians fail to meet their responsibilities as fathers and husbands. Restructuring medical careers to recognize the legitimate needs of physicians' families will be to the advantage of all.[9] I am not arguing for a "daddy track" to parallel the existing "mommy track," which reaches a dead end before the professorial level. Rather, I urge that men and women alike be offered a single academic track, compatible with both a rewarding family life and professional success.

The record is clear that female physicians in academic medicine or clinical practice have been remarkably productive professionally, home and child care responsibilities notwithstanding. Studies carried out over the past several decades of the work patterns of male and female physicians demonstrate that sex-related differences in work output are diminishing rapidly. Using data on physicians who graduated between 1931 and 1956, when women in the profession were few, Powers et al.[10] reported that men worked an average of 30 percent more hours, a finding similar to that obtained a decade earlier by Dykman and Stalnaker.[11] By contrast, in data collected by the American Medical Association in a 1986 survey of physicians, Silberger et al.[12] found a sex-related difference in work time of no more than 10 percent, much as was reported by Bobula[13] from data collected nationally by the American Medical Association in 1978 and by Heins et al.[14] in a sample from the Detroit metropolitan area. A substantial part of the remaining difference stems from the higher ratio of men to women in private practice (which has longer hours than salaried practice), a career option chosen by fewer graduates of both sexes each year. Curry's study[15] of physicians in the Canadian Maritime Provinces may be an augury of the future; over the professional lifetime of

physicians, she found no sex-related difference in numbers of hours worked per week or weeks worked per year. The equalization, Curry suggests, reflects a reduction in the number of hours worked by men more than it does an increase in those worked by women.

Whether women as women bring something special to medical practice is an open question. The so-called feminine qualities—nurturance, concern for other persons, sensitivity, and the like—are found in both sexes. If male doctors are on average more detached and impersonal, as is popularly believed, it is equally true that a number of women doctors outdistance just about any man on those dimensions; if female physicians are on average more nurturant, quite a few male physicians are more caring than the majority of women. Given the fine mesh of the admissions sieve and the rigorous training to which medical students are exposed, female and male physicians are more likely to resemble each other on a number of important dimensions than they are other members of their own sexes.[16] If medicine is to become more humane, admitting more women into the profession will not be enough. The task will be to cultivate the humane qualities in all health professionals by making career paths, and the reward structure that reinforces them, consonant with that goal.

Notes

1. Jonas, H.S., Etzel, S.I. Undergraduate medical education. JAMA 1988; 260:1063–71.
2. Jonas, H.S., Etzel, S.I., Barzansky, B. Undergraduate medical education. JAMA 1989; 262:1011–9.
3. Sayres, M., Wyshak, G., Denterlein, G., Apfel, R., Shore, E., Federman, D. Pregnancy during residency. N Engl J Med 1986; 314:418–23.
4. Kamerman, S.S., Kahn, A.J. Income transfers, work and the economic well-being of families with children. Int Soc Sec Rev 1982; 3:345–82.
5. Bickel, J. Women in medical education: a status report. N Engl J Med 1988; 319:1579–84.
6. Whitley, N.O., Evens, R.G., Moody, M.A., Putnam, C.E.,

Sackett, J.F., Vydareny, K.H. Advancement of women in academic radiology. Invest Radiol 1987; 22:431–5.

7. Dial, T.H., Bickel, J., Lewicki, A.M. Sex difference in rank attainment among radiology and internal medicine faculty. Acad Med 1989; 64:198–202.

8. Florentine, R. Men, women and the premed persistence gap: a normative alternatives approach. Am J Sociol 1987; 92:1118–39.

9. Angell, M. Women in medicine: beyond prejudice. N Engl J Med 1981; 304:1161–3.

10. Powers, L., Parmelle, R.D., Weisenfelder, H. Practice patterns of women and men physicians. J Med Educ 1969; 44:481–91.

11. Dykman, R.A., Stalnaker, J.M. Survey of women physicians graduating from medical school 1925–1940. J Med Educ 1957; 32(3):3–38.

12. Silberger, A.B., Marder, W.D., Willke, R.J. Practice characteristics of male and female physicians. Health Aff (Millwood) 1987; 6(4):104–9.

13. Bobula, J.D. Work patterns, practice characteristics, and incomes of male and female physicians. J Med Educ 1980; 55:826–33.

14. Heins, M., Smock, S., Martindale, L., Jacobs, J., Stein, M. Comparison of the productivity of women and men physicians. JAMA 1977; 237:2514–7.

15. Curry, L. The effect of sex on physician work patterns. In: Proceedings of the 22nd Annual Conference on Research in Medical Education. Washington, D.C.: Association of American Medical Colleges, 1983:144–8.

16. Eisenberg, C. Women as physicians. J Med Educ 1983; 58:534–41.

The Doctors of Hoyland

Sir Arthur Conan Doyle

■

Dr. James Ripley was always looked upon as an exceedingly lucky dog by all of the profession who knew him. His father had preceded him in a practice in the village of Hoyland, in the north of Hampshire, and all was ready for him on the very first day that the law allowed him to put his name at the foot of a prescription. In a few years the old gentleman retired, and settled on the South Coast, leaving his son in undisputed possession of the whole country-side. Save for Dr. Horton, near Basingstoke, the young surgeon had a clear run of six miles in every direction, and took his fifteen hundred pounds a year, though, as is usual in country practices, the stable swallowed up most of what the consulting-room earned.

Dr. James Ripley was two-and-thirty years of age, reserved, learned, unmarried, with set, rather stern features, and a thinning of the dark hair upon the top of his head, which was worth quite a hundred a year to him. He was particularly happy in his management of ladies. He had caught the tone of bland sternness and decisive suavity which dominates without offending. Ladies, however, were not equally happy in their management of him. Professionally, he was always at their service. Socially, he was a drop of quicksilver. In vain the country mammas spread out their simple lures in front of him. Dances and picnics were not to his taste, and he preferred during his scanty leisure to shut himself up in his study, and to bury himself in Virchow's Archives and the professional journals.

Study was a passion with him, and he would have none of the rust which often gathers round a country practitioner. It was his ambition to keep his knowledge as fresh and bright as at the moment when he had stepped out of the examination hall. He prided himself on being able at a moment's notice to rattle off the seven ramifications of some obscure artery, or to give the exact percentage of any physiological compound. After a long day's work he would sit up half the night performing iridectomies and extractions upon the sheep's eyes sent in by the village butcher, to the horror of his housekeeper, who had to remove the *débris* next morning. His love for his work was the one fanaticism which found a place in his dry, precise nature.

It was the more to his credit that he should keep up to date in his knowledge, since he had no competition to force him to exertion. In the seven years during which he had practised in Hoyland three rivals had pitted themselves against him, two in the village itself and one in the neighbouring hamlet of Lower Hoyland. Of these one had sickened and wasted, being, as it was said, himself the only patient whom he had treated during his eighteen months of ruralising. A second had bought a fourth share of a Basingstoke practice, and had departed honourably, while a third had vanished one September night, leaving a gutted house and an unpaid drug bill behind him. Since then the district had become a monopoly, and no one had dared to measure himself against the established fame of the Hoyland doctor.

It was, then, with a feeling of some surprise and considerable curiosity that on driving through Lower Hoyland one morning he perceived that the new house at the end of the village was occupied, and that a virgin brass plate glistened upon the swinging gate which faced the high road. He pulled up his fifty guinea chestnut mare and took a good look at it. "Verrinder Smith, M.D.," was printed across it in very neat, small lettering. The last man had had letters half a foot long, with a lamp like a fire-station. Dr. James Ripley noted the difference, and deduced from it that the newcomer might possibly prove a more formidable opponent. He was convinced of it that evening when he came to consult the current medical directory. By it he learned that Dr. Verrinder Smith was the holder of superb degrees, that he had studied with distinction at Edinburgh, Paris, Berlin and Vienna, and finally that he had been awarded a gold medal and the Lee Hopkins scholarship for original research, in recognition of an exhaustive inquiry into the functions of the anterior spinal nerve roots. Dr. Ripley passed his fingers through his thin hair in bewilderment as he read his rival's record. What on earth could so brilliant a man mean by putting up his plate in a little Hampshire hamlet?

But Dr. Ripley furnished himself with an explanation to the riddle. No doubt Dr. Verrinder Smith had simply come down there in order to pursue some scientific research in peace and quiet. The plate was up as an address rather than as an invitation to patients. Of course, that must be the true explanation. In that case the presence of this brilliant neighbour would be a splendid thing for his own studies. He had often longed for some kindred mind, some steel on which he might strike his flint. Chance had brought it to him, and he rejoiced exceedingly.

And this joy it was which led him to take a step which was quite at variance with his usual habits. It is the custom for a new-comer among medical men to call first upon the older, and the etiquette upon the subject is strict. Dr. Ripley was pedantically exact on such points, and yet he deliberately drove over next day and called upon Dr. Verrinder Smith. Such a waiving of ceremony was, he felt, a gracious act upon his part, and a fit prelude to the intimate relations which he hoped to establish with his neighbour.

The house was neat and well appointed, and Dr. Ripley was shown by a smart maid into a dapper little consulting-room. As he passed in he noticed two or three parasols and a lady's sunbonnet hanging in the hall. It was a pity that his colleague should be a married man. It would put them upon a different footing, and interfere with those long evenings of high scientific talk which he had pictured to himself. On the other hand, there was much in the consulting-room to please him. Elaborate instruments, seen more often in hospitals than in the houses of private practitioners, were scattered about. A sphygmograph stood upon the table and a gasometer-like engine, which was new to Dr. Ripley, in the corner. A book-case full of ponderous volumes in French and German, paper-covered for the most part, and varying in tint from the shell to the yolk of a duck's egg, caught his wandering eyes, and he was deeply absorbed in their titles when the door opened suddenly behind him. Turning round, he found himself facing a little woman, whose plain, palish face was remarkable only for a pair of shrewd, humorous eyes of a blue which had two shades too much green in it. She held a *pince-nez* in her left hand, and the doctor's card in her right.

"How do you do, Dr. Ripley?" said she.

"How do you do, madam?" returned the visitor. "Your husband is perhaps out?"

"I am not married," said she simply.

"Oh, I beg your pardon! I meant the doctor—Dr. Verrinder Smith."

"I am Dr. Verrinder Smith."

Dr. Ripley was so surprised that he dropped his hat and forgot to pick it up again.

"What!" he gasped, "the Lee Hopkins prizeman! You!"

He had never seen a woman doctor before, and his whole conservative soul rose up in revolt at the idea. He could not recall any Biblical injunction that the man should remain ever the doctor and the woman the nurse, and yet he felt as if a blasphemy had been committed. His face betrayed his feelings only too clearly.

"I am sorry to disappoint you," said the lady drily.

"You certainly have surprised me," he answered, picking up his hat.

"You are not among our champions, then?"

"I cannot say that the movement has my approval."

"And why?"

"I should much prefer not to discuss it."

"But I am sure you will answer a lady's question."

"Ladies are in danger of losing their privileges when they usurp the place of the other sex. They cannot claim both."

"Why should a woman not earn her bread by her brains?"

Dr. Ripley felt irritated by the quiet manner in which the lady cross-questioned him.

"I should much prefer not to be led into a discussion, Miss Smith."

"Dr. Smith," she interrupted.

"Well, Dr. Smith! But if you insist upon an answer, I must say that I do not think medicine a suitable profession for women and that I have a personal objection to masculine ladies."

It was an exceedingly rude speech, and he was ashamed of it the instant after he had made it. The lady, however, simply raised her eye-brows and smiled.

"It seems to me that you are begging the question," said she. "Of course, if it makes women masculine that *would* be a considerable deterioration."

It was a neat little counter, and Dr. Ripley, like a pinked fencer, bowed his acknowledgment.

"I must go," said he.

"I am sorry that we cannot come to some more friendly conclusion since we are to be neighbours," she remarked.

He bowed again, and took a step toward the door.

"It was a singular coincidence," she continued, "that at the instant that you called I was reading your paper on 'Locomotor Ataxia,' in the *Lancet*."

"Indeed," said he drily.

"I thought it was a very able monograph."

"You are very good."

"But the views which you attribute to Professor Pitres, of Bordeaux, have been repudiated by him."

"I have his pamphlet of 1890," said Dr. Ripley angrily.

"Here is his pamphlet of 1891." She picked it from among a litter of periodicals. "If you have time to glance your eye down this passage—"

Dr. Ripley took it from her and shot rapidly through the paragraph which she indicated. There was no denying that it completely knocked the bottom out of his own article. He threw it down, and with another frigid bow he made for the door. As he took the reins from the groom he glanced round and saw that the lady was standing at her window, and it seemed to him that she was laughing heartily.

All day the memory of this interview haunted him. He felt that he had come very badly out of it. She had shown herself to be his superior on his own pet subject. She had been courteous while he had been rude, self-possessed when he had been angry. And then, above all, there was her presence, her monstrous intrusion to rankle in his mind. A woman doctor had been an abstract thing before, repugnant but distant. Now she was there in actual practice, with a brass plate up just like his own, competing for the same patients. Not that he feared competition, but he objected to this lowering of his ideal of womanhood. She could not be more than thirty, and had a bright, mobile face, too. He thought of her humorous eyes, and of her strong, well-turned chin. It revolted him the more to recall the details of her education. A man, of course, could come through such an ordeal with all his purity, but it was nothing short of shameless in a woman.

But it was not long before he learned that even her competition was a thing to be feared. The novelty of her presence had brought a few curious invalids into her consulting-rooms, and, once there, they had been so impressed by the firmness of her manner and by the singular, new-fashioned instruments with which she tapped, and peered, and sounded, that it formed the core of their conversation for weeks afterward. And soon there were tangible proofs of her powers upon the countryside. Farmer Eyton, whose callous ulcer had been quietly spreading over his shin for years back under a gentle *régime* of zinc ointment, was painted round with blistering fluid, and found, after three blasphemous nights, that his sore was stimulated into healing. Mrs. Crowder, who had always regarded the birthmark upon her second daughter Eliza as a sign of the indignation of the Creator at a third helping of raspberry tart which she had partaken of during a critical period, learned that, with the help of two galvanic needles, the mischief was not irreparable. In a month Dr. Verrinder Smith was known, and in two she was famous.

Occasionally, Dr. Ripley met her as he drove upon his rounds. She had started a high dog-cart, taking the reins herself, with a little tiger behind. When they met he invariably raised his hat with punctilious politeness, but the grim severity of his face showed how formal was the courtesy. In fact, his dislike was rapidly deepening into absolute detestation. "The unsexed woman," was the description of her which he permitted himself to give to those of his patients who still remained stanch. But, indeed, they were a rapidly-decreasing body, and every day his pride was galled by the news of some fresh defection. The lady had somehow impressed the country folk with almost superstitious belief in her power, and from far and near they flocked to her consulting-room.

But what galled him most of all was, when she did something which he had pronounced to be impracticable. For all his knowledge he lacked nerve as an operator, and usually sent his worst cases up to London. The lady, however, had no weakness of the sort, and took everything that came in her way. It was agony to him to hear that she was about to straighten little Alec Turner's club foot, and right at the fringe of the rumour came a note from his mother, the rector's wife, asking him if he would be so good as to act as chloroformist. It would be inhumanity to refuse, as there was no other who could take the place, but it was gall and wormwood to his sensitive nature. Yet, in spite of his vexation, he could not but admire the dexterity with which the thing was done. She handled the little wax-like foot so gently, and held the tiny tenotomy knife as an artist holds his pencil. One straight insertion, one snick of a tendon, and it was all over without a stain upon the white towel which lay beneath. He had never seen anything more masterly, and he had the honesty to say so, though her skill increased his dislike of her. The operation spread her fame still further at his expense, and self-preservation was added to his other grounds for detesting her. And this very detestation it was which brought matters to a curious climax.

One winter's night, just as he was rising from his lonely dinner, a groom came riding down from Squire Faircastle's, the richest man in the district, to say that his daughter had scalded her hand, and that medical help was needed on the instant. The coachman had ridden for the lady doctor, for it mattered nothing to the Squire who came as long as it were speedily. Dr. Ripley rushed from his surgery with the determination that she should not effect an entrance into this stronghold of his if hard driving on his part could prevent it. He did not even wait to light his lamps, but sprang into his gig and flew off as fast as hoof could rattle. He lived rather nearer to the Squire's than she did, and was convinced that he could get there well before her.

And so he would but for that whimsical element of chance, which will forever muddle up the affairs of this world and dumfound the prophets. Whether it came from the want of his

lights, or from his mind being full of the thoughts of his rival, he allowed too little by half a foot in taking the sharp turn upon the Basingstoke road. The empty trap and the frightened horse clattered away into the darkness, while the Squire's groom crawled out of the ditch into which he had been shot. He struck a match, looked down at his groaning companion, and then, after the fashion of rough, strong men when they see what they have not seen before, he was very sick.

The doctor raised himself a little on his elbow in the glint of the match. He caught a glimpse of something white and sharp bristling through his trouser leg half way down the shin.

"Compound!" he groaned. "A three months' job," and fainted.

When he came to himself the groom was gone, for he had scudded off to the Squire's house for help, but a small page was holding a gig-lamp in front of his injured leg, and a woman, with an open case of polished instruments gleaming in the yellow light, was deftly slitting up his trouser with a crooked pair of scissors.

"It's all right, doctor," said she soothingly. "I am so sorry about it. You can have Dr. Horton to-morrow, but I am sure you will allow me to help you to-night. I could hardly believe my eyes when I saw you by the roadside."

"The groom has gone for help," groaned the sufferer.

"When it comes we can move you into the gig. A little more light, John! So! Ah, dear, dear, we shall have laceration unless we reduce this before we move you. Allow me to give you a whiff of chloroform, and I have no doubt that I can secure it sufficiently to—"

Dr. Ripley never heard the end of that sentence. He tried to raise a hand and to murmur something in protest, but a sweet smell was in his nostrils, and a sense of rich peace and lethargy stole over his jangled nerves. Down he sank, through clear, cool water, ever down and down into the green shadows beneath, gently, without

effort, while the pleasant chiming of a great bel-
fry rose and fell in his ears. Then he rose again,
up and up, and ever up, with a terrible tightness
about his temples, until at last he shot out of
those green shadows and was in the light once
more. Two bright, shining, golden spots gleamed
before his dazed eyes. He blinked and blinked
before he could give a name to them. They were
only the two brass balls at the end posts of his
bed, and he was lying in his own little room, with
a head like a cannon ball, and a leg like an iron
bar. Turning his eyes, he saw the calm face of Dr.
Verrinder Smith looking down at him.

"Ah, at last!" said she. "I kept you under all the
way home, for I knew how painful the jolting
would be. It is in good position now with a strong
side splint. I have ordered a morphia draught for
you. Shall I tell your groom to ride for Dr. Horton
in the morning?"

"I should prefer that you should continue the
case," said Dr. Ripley feebly, and then, with a half
hysterical laugh,—"You have all the rest of the
parish as patients, you know, so you may as well
make the thing complete by having me also."

It was not a very gracious speech, but it was a
look of pity and not of anger which shone in her
eyes as she turned away from his bedside.

Dr. Ripley had a brother, William, who was assistant surgeon at a London hospital, and who
was down in Hampshire within a few hours of
his hearing of the accident. He raised his brows
when he heard the details.

"What! You are pestered with one of those!" he
cried.

"I don't know what I should have done without her."

"I've no doubt she's an excellent nurse."

"She knows her work as well as you or I."

"Speak for yourself, James," said the London
man with a sniff. "But apart from that, you know
that the principle of the thing is all wrong."

"You think there is nothing to be said on the
other side?"

"Good heavens! do you?"

"Well, I don't know. It struck me during the
night that we may have been a little narrow in
our views."

"Nonsense, James. It's all very fine for women
to win prizes in the lecture room, but you know
as well as I do that they are no use in an emergency. Now I warrant that this woman was all
nerves when she was setting your leg. That reminds me that I had better just take a look at it
and see that it is all right."

"I would rather that you did not undo it," said
the patient. "I have her assurance that it is all
right."

Brother William was deeply shocked.

"Of course, if a woman's assurance is of more
value than the opinion of the assistant surgeon of
a London hospital, there is nothing more to be
said," he remarked.

"I should prefer that you did not touch it," said
the patient firmly, and Dr. William went back to
London that evening in a huff.

The lady, who had heard of his coming, was
much surprised on learning of his departure.

"We had a difference upon a point of professional etiquette," said Dr. James, and it was all
the explanation he would vouchsafe.

For two long months Dr. Ripley was brought in
contact with his rival every day, and he learned
many things which he had not known before.
She was a charming companion, as well as a
most assiduous doctor. Her short presence during the long, weary day was like a flower in a
sand waste. What interested him was precisely
what interested her, and she could meet him at
every point upon equal terms. And yet under all
her learning and her firmness ran a sweet, wom-
anly nature, peeping out in her talk, shining in
her greenish eyes, showing itself in a thousand
subtle ways which the dullest of men could read.
And he, though a bit of a prig and a pedant, was
by no means dull, and had honesty enough to
confess when he was in the wrong.

"I don't know how to apologise to you," he said in his shame-faced fashion one day, when he had progressed so far as to be able to sit in an armchair with his leg upon another one; "I feel that I have been quite in the wrong."

"Why, then?"

"Over this woman question. I used to think that a woman must inevitably lose something of her charm if she took up such studies."

"Oh, you don't think they are necessarily unsexed, then?" she cried, with a mischievous smile.

"Please don't recall my idiotic expression."

"I feel so pleased that I should have helped in changing your views. I think that it is the most sincere compliment that I have ever had paid me."

"At any rate, it is the truth," said he, and was happy all night at the remembrance of the flush of pleasure which made her pale face look quite comely for the instant.

For, indeed, he was already far past the stage when he would acknowledge her as the equal of any other woman. Already he could not disguise from himself that she had become the one woman. Her dainty skill, her gentle touch, her sweet presence, the community of their tastes, had all united to hopelessly upset his previous opinions. It was a dark day for him now when his convalescence allowed her to miss a visit, and darker still that other one which he saw approaching when all occasion for her visits would be at an end. It came round at last, however, and he felt that his whole life's fortune would hang upon the issue of that final interview. He was a direct man by nature, so he laid his hand upon hers as it felt for his pulse, and he asked her if she would be his wife.

"What, and unite the practices?" said she.

He started in pain and anger.

"Surely you do not attribute any such base motive to me!" he cried. "I love you as unselfishly as ever a woman was loved."

"No, I was wrong. It was a foolish speech," said she, moving her chair a little back, and tapping her stethoscope upon her knee. "Forget that I ever said it. I am so sorry to cause you any disappointment, and I appreciate most highly the honour which you do me, but what you ask is quite impossible."

With another woman he might have urged the point, but his instincts told him that it was quite useless with this one. Her tone of voice was conclusive. He said nothing, but leaned back in his chair a stricken man.

"I am so sorry," she said again. "If I had known what was passing in your mind I should have told you earlier that I intend to devote my life entirely to science. There are many women with a capacity for marriage, but few with a taste for biology. I will remain true to my own line, then. I came down here while waiting for an opening in the Paris Physiological Laboratory. I have just heard that there is a vacancy for me there, and so you will be troubled no more by my intrusion upon your practice. I have done you an injustice just as you did me one. I thought you narrow and pedantic, with no good quality. I have learned during your illness to appreciate you better, and the recollection of our friendship will always be a very pleasant one to me."

And so it came about that in a very few weeks there was only one doctor in Hoyland. But folks noticed that the one had aged many years in a few months, that a weary sadness lurked always in the depths of his blue eyes, and that he was less concerned than ever with the eligible young ladies whom chance, or their careful country mammas, placed in his way.

3

Relationships between Doctors

and Patients

The readings in this section examine the relationships between physicians and patients. Thomas Szasz and Marc Hollender's classic piece on the three models of the doctor-patient relationship asks whether one model or another is most effective at producing "good medicine" and offers a mechanism to analyze what patients want in relationships with physicians. The reading portrays physicians who are consciously considering the nature of their relationship to their community and their patients. In David Hilfiker's essay the meaning of uncertainty and risk become apparent in a wrenching revelation of mistakes he had made in caring for a pregnant young woman. He discusses the chances that even a good physician will, on occasion, err in judgment and end up causing more harm than good, and asks how doctors can in those circumstances best manage to heal themselves spiritually and continue to practice.

Maureen Flannery's essay explores how a rural practice context and its scarce resources affect the doctor-patient relationship and the range of care. She uses her rural Appalachian practice experience to discuss the impacts of poverty; isolation, age structure, and resources on medical ethics and physician values. Flannery vividly describes working and living in a community where anonymity is impossible and in which her lifestyle, earnings, and roles are visible and determined by her community membership. The William Carlos Williams short story that closes part III depicts the physician as a patient advocate seeking to exert influence on powerful community institutions. The physician's limited success in helping a worker burned on the job to deal with his employer demonstrates the limited capacity that doctors have to improve the lives of patients with medical interventions.

The Basic Models of the Doctor-Patient Relationship

Thomas S. Szasz and Marc H. Hollender

∎

When a person leaves the culture in which he was born and raised and migrates to another, he usually experiences his new social setting as something strange—and in some ways threatening—and he is stimulated to master it by conscious efforts at understanding. To some extent every immigrant to the United States reacts in this manner to the American scene. Similarly, the American tourist in Europe or South America "scrutinizes" the social setting which is taken for granted by the natives. To scrutinize—and criticize—the pattern of other peoples' lives is obviously both common and easy. It also happens, however, that people exposed to cross cultural experiences turn their attention to the very customs which formed the social matrix of their lives in the past. Lastly, to study the "customs" which shape and govern one's day-to-day life is most difficult of all.[1]

In many ways the psychoanalyst is like a person who has migrated from one culture to another. To him the relationship between physician and patient—which is like a custom that is taken for granted in medical practice and which he himself so treated in his early history—has become an object of study. While the precise nature and extent of the influence which psychoanalysis and so-called dynamic psychiatry have had

on modern medicine are debatable, it seems to us that the most decisive effect has been that of making physicians explicitly aware of the possible significance of their relationship to patients.

The question naturally arises as to "What is a doctor-patient relationship?" It is our aim to discuss this question and to show that certain philosophical preconceptions associated with the notions of "disease," "treatment," and "cure" have a profound bearing on both the theory and the practice of medicine.

What Is a Human Relationship?

The concept of a relationship is a novel one in medicine. Traditionally, physicians have been concerned with "things," for example, anatomical structures, lesions, bacteria, and the like. In modern times the scope has been broadened to include the concept of "function." The phenomenon of a human relationship is often viewed as though it were a "thing" or a "function." It is, in fact, neither. Rather it is an abstraction, appropriate for the description and handling of certain observational facts. Moreover, it is an abstraction which presupposes concepts of both structure and function.

The foregoing comments may be clarified by concrete illustrations. Psychiatrists often suggest to their medical colleagues that the physician's relationship with his patient per se helps the latter. This creates the impression (whether so intended or not) that the relationship is a thing, which works not unlike the way that vitamins do in a case of vitamin deficiency. Another idea is that the doctor-patient relationship depends mainly on what the physician does (or thinks or feels). Then it is viewed not unlike a function.

When we consider a relationship in which there is joint participation of the two persons involved, "relationship" refers to neither a structure nor a function (such as the "personality" of

Table 1. Three Basic Models of the Physician–Patient Relationship

Model	Physician's Role	Patient's Role	Clinical Application of Model	Prototype of Model
1. Activity–passivity	Does something to patient	Recipient (unable to respond or inert)	Anesthesia, acute trauma, coma, delirium, etc.	Parent–infant
2. Guidance–cooperation	Tells patient what to do	Cooperator (obeys)	Acute infecticus processes, etc.	Parent–child (adolescent)
3. Mutual participation	Helps patient to help himself	Participant in "partnership" (uses expert help)	Most chronic illnesses, psychoanalysis, etc.	Adult–adult

the physician or patient). It is, rather, an abstraction embodying the activities of two interacting systems (persons).[5]

Three Basic Models of the Doctor-Patient Relationship

The three basic models of the doctor-patient relationship (see Table 1), which we will describe, embrace modes of interaction ubiquitous in human relationships and in no way specific for the contact between physician and patient. The specificity of the medical situation probably derives from a combination of these modes of interaction with certain technical procedures and social settings.

1. The Model of Activity-Passivity

Historically, this is the oldest conceptual model. Psychologically, it is not an interaction, because it is based on the effect of one person on another in such a way and under such circumstances that the person acted upon is unable to contribute actively, or is considered to be inanimate. This frame of reference (in which the physician does something to the patient) underlies the application of some of the outstanding advances of modern medicine (e.g., anesthesia and surgery, anti-

biotics, etc.). The physician is active; the patient, passive. This orientation has originated in—and is entirely appropriate for the treatment of emergencies (e.g., for the patient who is severely injured, bleeding, delirious, or in coma). "Treatment" takes place irrespective of the patient's contribution and regardless of the outcome. There is a similarity here between the patient and a helpless infant, on the one hand, and between the physician and a parent, on the other. It may be recalled that psychoanalysis, too, evolved from a procedure (hypnosis) which was based on this model. Various physical measures to which psychotics are subjected today are another example of the activity-passivity frame of reference.

2. The Model of Guidance-Cooperation

This model underlies much of medical practice. It is employed in situations which are less desperate than those previously mentioned (e.g., acute infections). Although the patient is ill, he is conscious and has feelings and aspirations of his own. Since he suffers from pain, anxiety, and other distressing symptoms, he seeks help and is ready and willing to "cooperate." When he turns to a physician, he places the latter (even if only in some limited ways) in a position of power. This is due not only to a "transference reaction" (i.e., his regarding the physician as he did his father when he was a child) but also to the fact that the physician possesses knowledge of his bodily processes which he does not have. In some ways it may seem that this, like the first model, is an active-passive phenomenon. Actually, this is more apparent than real. Both persons are "active" in that they contribute to the relationship and what ensues from it. The main difference between the two participants pertains to power, and to its actual or potential use. The more powerful of the two (parent, physician, employer, etc.) will speak of guidance or leadership and will expect cooperation of the other member of the pair (child, patient, employee, etc.). The patient is expected to "look up to" and to "obey" his doctor. Moreover, he is neither to question nor to argue or disagree with the orders he receives. This model has its prototype in the relationship of the parent and his (adolescent) child. Often, threats and other undisguised weapons of force are employed, even though presumably these are for the patient's "own good." It should be added that the possibility of the exploitations of the situation—as in any relationship between persons of unequal power—for the sole benefit of the physician, albeit under the guise of altruism, is ever present.

3. The Model of Mutual Participation

Philosophically, this model is predicated on the postulate that equality among human beings is desirable. It is fundamental to the social structure of democracy and has played a crucial role in occidental civilization for more than two hundred years. Psychologically, mutuality rests on complex processes of identification—which facilitate conceiving of others in terms of oneself—together with maintaining and tolerating the discrete individuality of the observer and the observed. It is crucial to this type of interaction that

the participants (1) have approximately equal power, (2) be mutually interdependent (i.e., need each other), and (3) engage in activity that will be in some ways satisfying to both.

This model is favored by patients who, for various reasons, want to take care of themselves (at least in part). This may be an overcompensatory attempt at mastering anxieties associated with helplessness and passivity. It may also be "realistic" and necessary, as, for example, in the management of most chronic illnesses (e.g., diabetes mellitus, chronic heart disease, etc.). Here the patient's own experiences provide reliable and important clues for therapy. Moreover, the treatment program itself is principally carried out by the patient to help himself.

In an evolutionary sense, the pattern of mutual participation is more highly developed than the other two models of the doctor-patient relationship. It requires a more complex psychological and social organization on the part of both participants. Accordingly, it is rarely appropriate for children or for those persons who are mentally deficient, very poorly educated, or profoundly immature. On the other hand, the greater the intellectual, educational, and general experiential similarity between physician and patient, the more appropriate and necessary this model of therapy becomes.

The Basic Models and the Psychology of the Physician

Consideration of why physicians seek one or another type of relationship with patients (or seek patients who fit into a particular relationship) would carry us beyond the scope of this essay. Yet, it must be emphasized that as long as this subject is approached with the sentimental viewpoint that a physician is simply motivated by a wish to help others (not that we deny this wish), no scientific study of the subject can be undertaken. Scientific investigation is possible only if value judgment is subrogated, at least temporarily, to a candid scrutiny of the physician's actual behavior with his patients.

The activity-passivity model places the physician in absolute control of the situation. In this way it gratifies needs for mastery and contributes to feelings of superiority.[6,7] At the same time it requires that the physician disidentify with the patient as a person.

Somewhat similar is the guidance-cooperation model. The disidentification with the patient, however, is less complete. The physician, like the parent of a growing child, could be said to see in the patient a human being potentially (but not yet) like himself (or like he wishes to be). In addition to the gratifications already mentioned, this relationship provides an opportunity to recreate and to gratify the "Pygmalion Complex." Thus, the physician can mold others into his own image, as God is said to have created man (or he may mold them into his own image of what they should be like, as in Shaw's "Pygmalion"). This type of relationship is of importance in education, as the transmission of more or less stable cultural values (and of language itself) shows. It requires that the physician be convinced he is "right" in his notion of what is "best" for the patient. He will then try to induce the patient to accept his aims as the patient's own.

The model of mutual participation, as suggested earlier, is essentially foreign to medicine. This relationship, characterized by a high degree of empathy, has elements often associated with the notions of friendship and partnership and the imparting of expert advice. The physician may be said to help the patient to help himself. The physician's gratification cannot stem from power or from the control over someone else. His satisfactions are derived from more abstract kinds of mastery, which are as yet poorly understood.

It is evident that in each of the categories mentioned the satisfactions of physician and patient complement each other. This makes for stability

in a paired system. Such stability, however, must be temporary, since the physician strives to alter the patient's state. The comatose patient, for example, either will recover to a more healthy, conscious condition or he will die. If he improves, the doctor-patient relationship must change. It is at this point that the physician's inner (usually unacknowledged) needs are most likely to interfere with what is "best" for the patient. At this juncture, the physician either changes his "attitude" (not a consciously or deliberately assumed role) to complement the patient's emergent needs or he foists upon the patient the same role of helpless passivity from which he (allegedly) tried to rescue him in the first place. Here we touch on a subject rich in psychological and sociological complexities. The process of change the physician must undergo to have a mutually constructive experience with the patient is similar to a very familiar process: namely, the need for the parent to behave ever differently toward his growing child.

What Is "Good Medicine"?

Let us now consider the problem of "good medicine" from the viewpoint of human relationships. The function of sciences is not to tell us what is good or bad but rather to help us understand how things work. "Good" and "bad" are personal judgments, usually decided on the basis of whether or not the object under consideration satisfies us. In viewing the doctor-patient relationship we cannot conclude, however, that anything which satisfies—irrespective of other considerations—is "good." Further complications arise when the method is questioned by which we ascertain whether or not a particular need has been satisfied. Do we take the patient's word for it? Or do we place ourselves into the traditional parental role of "knowing what is best" for our patients (children)?

The shortcomings and dangers inherent in

Table 2. Analysis of the Concepts of "Disease," "Treatment," and "Therapeutic Result"

Doctor–Patient Relationship	The Meaning of "Treatment"	The "Therapeutic Result"
1. Activity–passivity	Whatever the physician does; the actual operations (procedures) which he employs	Alteration in the structure and/or function of the patient's body (or behavior, as determined by the physician's judgment); the patient's judgment does not enter into the evaluation of results; e.g., T & A is "successful" irrespective of how patient feels afterward
2. Guidance–cooperation	Whatever the physician does; similar to the above	Similar to the above, albeit patient's judgment is no longer completely irrelevant; success of therapy is still the physician's private decision; if patient agrees, he is a good patient, but if he disagrees he is bad or "uncooperative"
3. Mutual participation	An abstraction of one aspect of the relationship, embodying the activities of both participants; "treatment" cannot be said to take place unless both participants orient themselves to the task ahead	Much more poorly defined than in the previous models; evaluation of the result will depend on both the physician's and the patient's judgments and is further complicated by the fact that these may change in the very process of treatment

these and in other attempts to clarify some of the most basic aspects of our daily life are too well known to require documentation. It is this very complexity of the situation which has led, as is the rule in scientific work, to an essentially arbitrary simplification of the structure of our field of observation. (We omit any discussion of the physician's technical skill, training, equipment, etc. These factors, of course, are of importance, and we do not minimize them. The problem of what is "good medicine" can be considered from a number of viewpoints [e.g., technical skill, economic considerations, social roles, human relationships, etc.]. Our scope in this essay is limited to but one—sometimes quite unimportant—aspect of the contact between physician and patient.)

Let us present an example. A patient consults a physician because of pain and other symptoms resulting from a duodenal ulcer. Both physician and patient assume that the latter would be better off without these discomforts. The situation now may be structured as follows: healing of the ulcer is "good," whereas its persistence is "bad." What we wish to emphasize is the fact that physician and patient agree (explicitly or otherwise) as to what is good and bad. Without such agreement it is meaningless to speak of a therapeutic relationship.

In other words, the notions of "normal," "abnormal," "symptom," "disease," and the like are social conventions. These definitions often are set by the medical world and are usually tacitly

The Notions of Disease and Health	In Medicine (Illustrative Examples)	In Psychiatry (Illustrative Examples)
The presence or absence of some unwanted structure or function The actual state of affairs The same state without the disability	1. Treatment of the unconcious patient; for example, the patient in diabetic coma; cerebral hemorrhage; shock due to acute injury; etc. 2. Major surgical operation under general anesthesia	1. Hypnosis 2. Convulsive treatments (electroshock, insulin, etc.) 3. Surgical treatments (lobotomy, etc.)
The presence or absence of "signs" and "symptoms"; the physician's particular concept of "Disease" (e.g., infection), "Health" (usually no disease; e.g., no infection)	Most of general medicine and the postoperative care of surgical patients (e.g., prescription of drugs, "advice" to smoke less, etc.)	1. "Suggestion," counseling, therapy based on "advice," etc. 2. Some modifications of psychoanalytic therapy 3. So-called psychotherapy "combined" with physical therapies (e.g., electric shock)
The notions of disease and health lose most of their relevance in this context; the notions of more-or-less successful (for certain purposes) modes of behavior, adaptation, or integration take the place of the earlier, more categorical concepts	The treatment of patients with certain chronic diseases or structural defects; for example, the management of diabetes mellitus or of myasthenia gravis; "rehabilitation" of patients with orthopedic defects, such as learning the use of prostheses, etc.	1. Psychoanalysis 2. Some modifications of psychoanalytic therapy

accepted by others. The fact that there is agreement renders it difficult to perceive their changing (and relativistic) character. A brief example will clarify this statement. Some years ago—and among the uneducated even today—fever was regarded as something "bad" ("abnormal," a "symptom"), to be combated. The current scientific opinion is that it is the organism's response to certain types of influences (e.g., infection) and that within limits the manifestation itself should not be "treated."

The issue of agreement is of interest because it has direct bearing on the three models of the doctor-patient relationship. In the first two models "agreement" between physician and patient is taken for granted. The comatose patient obviously can not disagree. According to the second model, the patient does not possess the knowledge to dispute the physician's word. The third category differs in that the physician does not profess to know exactly what is best for the patient. The search for this becomes the essence of the therapeutic interaction. The patient's own experiences furnish indispensable information for eventual agreement, under otherwise favorable circumstances, as to what "health" might be for him.

The characteristics of the different types of doctor-patient relationships are summarized in Table 2. In this connection, some comments will be made on a subject which essentially is philosophical but which continues to plague many medical discussions; namely, the problem of comparing the efficacy of different therapeutic measures. Such comparisons are implicitly based on the following conceptual scheme: We postulate disease "A," from which many patients suffer. Therapies "B," "C," and "D" are given to groups of patients suffering with disease "A," and the results are compared. It is usually overlooked that, for the results to be meaningful, significant conceptual similarities must exist between the operations which are compared. The three categories of the doctor-patient relationship are concretely useful in delineating areas within which meaningful comparisons can be made. Comparisons between therapies belonging to different categories are philosophically (and logically) meaningless and lead to fruitless controversy.

To illustrate this thesis let us consider some examples. A typical comparison, with which we can begin, is that of the various agents used in the treatment of lobar pneumonia: type-specific antisera, sulfonamides, and penicillin. Each superseded the other, as the increased efficacy of the newer preparations was demonstrated. This sort of comparison is meaningful because there is agreement as to what is being treated and as to what constitutes a "successful" result. There should be no need to belabor this point. What is important is that this conceptual model of therapeutic comparisons is constantly used in situations in which it does not apply; that is, in situations in which there is clear-cut disagreement as to what constitutes "cure." In this connection, the problem of peptic ulcer will exemplify a group of illnesses in which several therapeutic approaches are possible.

This question is often posed: Is surgical, medical, or psychiatric treatment the "best" for peptic ulcer? Such a question is roughly comparable to asking, "Is an automobile or an airplane better?" —without specifying for what.[8] Unless we specify conditions, goals, and the "price" we are willing to pay (in the largest sense of the word), the question is meaningless. In the case of peptic ulcer, it is immediately apparent that each therapeutic approach implies a different conception of "disease" and correspondingly divergent notions of "cure." At the risk of slight overstatement, it can be said that according to the surgical viewpoint the disease is the "lesion," treatment aims at its eradication (by surgical means), and cure consists of its persistent absence (nonrecurrence). If a patient undergoes a vagotomy and all evidence of the lesion disappears, he is considered cured even if he develops another (apparently unrelated) illness six months later. It should be emphasized that no criticism of this frame of reference is intended. The foregoing (surgical) approach is entirely appropriate, and accusations of "narrowness" are no more (nor less) justified than they would be against any other specialized branch of knowledge.

To continue our analysis of therapeutic comparisons, let us consider the same patient (with peptic ulcer) in the hands of an internist. This specialist might have a somewhat different idea of what is wrong with him than did the surgeon. He might regard peptic ulcer as an essentially chronic disease (perhaps due to heredity and other "predispositions"), with which the patient probably will have to live as comfortably as possible for years. This point is emphasized to demonstrate that the surgeon and the internist do not treat the "same disease." How then can the two methods of treatment and their results be compared? The most that can be hoped for is to be able to determine to what extent each method is appropriate and successful within its own frame of reference.

If we take our hypothetical patient to a psychoanalyst, the situation is even more radically different. This specialist will state that he is not treating the "ulcer" and might even go so far as to say that he is not treating the patient for his ulcer. The psychoanalyst (or psychiatrist) has his own ideas about what constitutes "disease," "treatment," and "cure."[9,10]

Conclusions

Comments have been made on some factors which provide satisfactions to both patient and physician in various therapeutic relationships. In conclusion, we call attention to two important considerations regarding the complementary situations described.

First, it might be thought that one of the three basic models of the doctor-patient relationship is in some fundamental (perhaps ethical) way "better" than another. In particular, it might be considered that it is better to identify with the patient than to treat him like a helplessly sick person. We have tried to avoid such an inference. In our opinion, each of the three types of therapeutic relationship is entirely appropriate under certain circumstances and each is inappropriate under others.

Secondly, we will comment on the therapeutic relationship as a situation (more or less fixed in time) and as a process (leading to change in one or both participants). Most of our previous comments have dealt with the relationship as a situation. It is, however, also a process in that the patient may change not only in terms of his symptoms but also in the way he wishes to relate to his doctor. A typical example is the patient with diabetes mellitus who, when first seen, is in a coma. At this time, the relationship must be based on the activity-passivity model. Later, he has to be educated (guided) at the level of cooperation. Finally, ideally, he is treated as a full-fledged partner in the management of his own health (mutual participation). Confronted by a problem of this type, the physician is called upon to change through a corresponding spectrum of attitudes. If he cannot make these changes, he may interfere with the patient's progress and may promote an arrest at some intermediate stage in the evolution toward relative self-management. The other possibility in this situation is that both physician and patient will become dissatisfied with each other. This outcome, however unfortunate, is probably the commonest one. Most of us can probably verify it firsthand in the roles of both physician and patient.[11]

At such juncture, the physician usually feels that the patient is "uncooperative" and "difficult," whereas the patient regards the physician as "unsympathetic" and lacking in understanding of his personally unique needs. Both are correct. Both are confronted by the wish to induce changes in the other. As we well know, this is no easy task. The dilemma is usually resolved when the patient seeks another physician, one who is more attuned to his (new) needs. Conversely, the physician will "seek" a new patient, usually one who will benefit from the physician's (old) needs and corresponding attitudes. And so life goes on.

The pattern described accounts for the familiar fact that patients often choose physicians not solely, or even primarily, on the basis of technical skill. Considerable weight is given to the type of human relationship which they foster. Some patients prefer to be "unconscious" (figuratively speaking), irrespective of what ails them. Others go to the other extreme. The majority probably falls somewhere between these two polar opposites. Physicians, motivated by similar personal "conflict" form a complementary series. Thus, there is an interlocking integration of the sick and his healer.

Summary

The introduction of the construct of "human relationship" represents an addition to the repertoire of fundamental medical concepts.

Three basic models of the doctor-patient relationship are described with examples. The models are (a) Activity-passivity. The comatose patient is completely helpless. The physician must take over and do something to him. (b) Guidance-cooperation. The patient with an acute infectious process seeks help and is ready and willing to cooperate. He turns to the physician for guidance. (c) Mutual participation. The patient with a chronic disease is aided to help himself.

The physician's own inner needs (and satisfactions) form a complementary series with those of the patient.

The general problem usually referred to with the question "what is good medicine?" is briefly considered. Different types of doctor-patient relationships imply different concepts of "disease," "treatment," and "cure." This is of importance in comparing diverse therapeutic methods. Meaningful comparisons can be made only if interventions are based on the same frame of reference.

It has been emphasized that different types of doctor-patient relationships are necessary and appropriate for various circumstances. Problems in human contact between physician and patient often arise if in the course of treatment changes require an alteration in the pattern of the doctor-patient relationship. This may lead to a dissolution of the relationship.

Notes

In our approach to this subject we have been influenced by psychologic (psychoanalytic), sociologic, and philosophic considerations. See in this connection References 2–4 below and Szasz, T.S.: On the Theory of Psychoanalytic Treatment, Internat. J. Psychoanal., 38:166, 1957.

1. Ruesch, J., and Bateson, G.: Communication: The Social Matrix of Psychiatry, New York, W. W. Norton & Company, Inc., 1951.

2. Dewey, J., and Bentley, A.F.: Knowing and the Known, Boston, Beacon Press, 1949.

3. Russell, B.: Power: A New Social Analysis, New York, W. W. Norton & Company, Inc., 1938.

4. Szasz, T. S.: Entropy, Organization, and the Problem of the Economy of Human Relationships, Internat. J. Psychoanal. 36:289, 1955.

5. Dubos, R. J.: Second Thoughts on the Germ Theory, Scient. Am. 192:31, 1955.

6. Jones, E.: The God Complex, in Jones E.: Essays in Applied Psychoanalysis, London, Hogarth Press, 1951, Vol. 2, p. 244.

7. Marmor, J.: The Feeling of Superiority: An Occupational Hazard in the Practice of Psychotherapy, Am. J. Psychiat. 110:370, 1953.

8. Rapoport, A.: Operational Philosophy, New York, Harper & Brothers, 1954.

9. Zilboorg, G.: A History of Medical Psychology, New York, W. W. Norton & Company, Inc., 1941.

10. Bowman, K. M., and Rose, M.: Do Our Medical Colleagues Know What to Expect from Psychotherapy? Am. J. Psychiat. 111:401, 1954.

11. Pinner, M., and Miller, B. F., Editors: When Doctors Are Patients, New York, W. W. Norton & Company, Inc., 1952.

Facing Our Mistakes

David Hilfiker

■

Looking at the appointment book for July 12, 1978, I notice that Barb Daily will be in today for her first prenatal examination. "Wonderful," I think, remembering my joy as I helped her deliver her first child two years ago. Barb and her husband Russ are friends, and our relationship became much closer with the shared experience of that birth. With so much exposure to disease every day in my rural family practice, I look forward to today's appointment with Barb and to the continuing relationship over the next months.

Barb seems to be in good health with all the symptoms and signs of pregnancy, but her urine pregnancy test is negative. I reassure Barb and myself that she is fine and that the test just hasn't turned positive yet. Rescheduling another test for the following week, I congratulate her on her condition and promise to get all her test results to her promptly.

But the next urine test is negative, too, which leaves me troubled. Isn't Barb pregnant? Has she had a missed abortion? I could make sure right now, of course, by ordering an ultrasound, but the new examination is available only in Duluth, 110 miles away from our northern Minnesota village, and it is expensive. I am aware of the Dailys' modest income. Besides, by waiting a few weeks, I'll find out for sure without the ultrasound. I call Barb on the phone and tell her about the negative

test, about the possible abortion, and about the necessity of a repeat appointment in a few weeks if her next menstrual period does not occur on schedule.

It is, as usual, a hectic summer, and I almost forget about Barb's situation until a month later when she returns. Still no menstrual period, no abortion. She is confused and upset, since, she says, "I feel so pregnant." I am bothered, too, especially because her uterus continues to be enlarged. Her urine test remains definitely negative.

I break the bad news to her. "I think you have a missed abortion. You were probably pregnant, but the baby appears to have died some weeks ago, before your first examination. Unfortunately, you didn't have the miscarriage to get rid of the dead tissue from the baby and the placenta. If a miscarriage does not occur within a few weeks, I'd recommend a reexamination, another pregnancy test, and if nothing shows up, a dilation and curettage to clean out the uterus."

Barb is disappointed and saddened; there are tears. Both she and Russ have sufficient background in science to understand the technical aspects of the situation, but that doesn't alleviate the sorrow. We talk in the office at some length and make an appointment for two weeks later.

When Barb returns, Russ is with her. Still no menstrual period, no miscarriage, and a negative pregnancy test. It is difficult, but it also feels right to be able to share in friends' sadness. Thoroughly reviewing the situation with both of them, I schedule the D and C for later in the week.

Friday morning, when Barb is wheeled into the operating room, we chat before she is put to sleep. The surgical nurses in our small hospital are all friends, too, so the atmosphere is warm and relaxed. After induction of anesthesia, I examine Barb's pelvis. To my hands, the uterus now seems bigger than it had two days previously, but since all the pregnancy tests were negative, the uterus couldn't have grown. I continue the operation.

But this morning there is considerably more blood than usual, and it is only with great difficulty that I am able to extract any tissue. The body parts I remove are much larger than I had expected, considering when the fetus died, and they are not the decomposing tissue I'd anticipated. These are body parts that were recently alive! I suppress the rising panic in my body and try to complete the procedure. I am unable to evacuate the uterus completely, however, and after much sweat and worry, I stop, hoping that the uterus will expel the rest within a few days.

Russ is waiting outside the operating room, so I sit with him for a few minutes, telling him that Barb is fine but that there were some problems with the procedure. Since I haven't completely thought through what has happened, I can't be very helpful in answering his questions. I leave hurriedly for the office, promising to return that afternoon to talk with them once Barb has recovered from the anesthesia.

In between seeing other patients in the office that morning, I make several rushed phone calls, trying to figure out what has happened. Despite reassurances from the pathologist that it is statistically "impossible" for four consecutive pregnancy tests to be negative during a viable pregnancy, the horrifying awareness is growing that I have probably aborted Barb's living child. I won't know for sure until several days later, when the pathology report is available. In a daze I walk over to the hospital and try to tell Russ and Barb as much as I know, without telling them all that I suspect. I tell them that there may be more tissue expelled and that I won't know for sure about the pregnancy until the next week.

I can't really face my own suspicions yet.

That weekend I receive a tearful call from Barb. She has just passed some recognizable body parts of the baby; what is she to do? The bleeding has stopped, and she feels physically well, so it is apparent that the abortion I began on Friday is now over. I schedule a time in midweek to meet with them and review the entire situation.

The pathology report confirms my worst fears: I have aborted a living fetus at about 13 weeks of age. No explanation can be found for the negative pregnancy tests. My consultation with Barb and Russ later in the week is one of the hardest things I have ever done. Fortunately, their scientific sophistication allows me to describe in some detail what I have done and what my rationale was. But nothing can obscure the hard reality: I have killed their baby.

Politely, almost meekly, Russ asks whether the ultrasound examination could not have helped us. It almost seems that he is trying to protect my feelings, trying to absolve me of some of the responsibility. "Yes," I answer, "if I had ordered the ultrasound, we would have known that the baby was alive." I cannot explain to him why I didn't recommend it.

Over the next days and weeks and months, my guilt and anger grow. I discuss the events with my partners, with our pathologist, and with obstetric specialists. Some of my mistakes are obvious: I relied too heavily on one particular test; I was not skillful in determining the size of the uterus by pelvic examination; I should have ordered the ultrasound before proceeding with the D and C. Other mistakes become apparent as we review my handling of the case. There is simply no way I can justify what I have done. To make matters worse, complications after the D and C have caused much discomfort, worry, and expense. Barb is unable to become pregnant again for two years.

As physicians our automatic response to reading about such a tragedy is to try to discover what went wrong, to analyze why the mistakes occurred, and to institute corrective measures so that such things do not happen again. This response is important, indeed necessary, and I spent hours in such a review. But it is inadequate if it does not address our own emotional and spiritual experience of the events.

Although I was as honest with the Dailys as I could be in those next months, although I told them everything they wanted to know and described to them as completely as I could what had happened, I never shared with them the agony that I underwent trying to deal with the reality of the events. I never did ask for their forgiveness. I felt somehow that they had enough sorrow without having to bear my burden as well. Somehow, I felt, it was my responsibility to deal with my guilt alone.

Everyone, of course, makes mistakes, and no one enjoys the consequences. But the potential consequences of our medical mistakes are so overwhelming that it is almost impossible for practicing physicians to deal with their errors in a psychologically healthy fashion. Most people—doctors and patients alike—harbor deep within themselves the expectation that the physician will be perfect. No one seems prepared to accept the simple fact of life that physicians, like anyone else, will make mistakes.

By the very nature of our work, we physicians daily make decisions of extreme gravity. Our work in the intensive-care unit, in the emergency room, in the surgery suite, or in the delivery room offers us hundreds of opportunities daily to miscalculate, often with drastic consequences.

And it is not only in these settings but also in the humdrum of routine daily care that a physician can blunder into tragedy. One evening, for instance, a local boy was brought to the emergency room after an apparently minor automobile accident. One leg and foot were injured, but he was otherwise fine. After examining him, I consulted by telephone with an orthopedic surgeon in Duluth, and we decided that I would try to correct what appeared on the x-ray film to be a dislocated foot. As usual, I offered the patient and his mother (who happened to be a nurse with whom I worked regularly) a choice: I could reduce the dislocation in our small hospital or they could travel to Duluth to see the specialist. I was somewhat offended when they decided they would go to Duluth. My feelings changed considerably when the surgeon called me the next

morning to thank me for the referral. He reported that the patient had not had a dislocation at all but a severe posterior compartment syndrome, which had hyperflexed the foot, causing it to appear dislocated. The posterior compartment had required immediate surgery the previous night in order to save the muscles of the lower leg. I felt physically weak as I realized that this young man would have been permanently injured had his mother not decided on her own to take him to Duluth.

Although much less drastic than the threat of death or severe disability, perhaps the most frequent result of physician misjudgment is the wasting of money, often in large amounts. Every practicing physician spends thousands of dollars of patients' money every day in the costs for visits, laboratory examinations, medications, and hospitalizations. An unneeded examination, the needless admission of a patient to the hospital, even the unnecessary advice to stay home from work can waste large amounts of money—frequently, the money of people who have little to spare. One comes to feel that any decision may have important consequences.

The cumulative impact of such mistakes (and the ever-present potential for many others) has had a devastating effect on my own emotional health, as it does, I believe, for most physicians. For it is not only the obvious mistakes with obvious results that trouble us. Such mistakes as I made with Barb are fortunately rare occurrences for any physician, and an emotionally mature person may learn to cope with them. But there are also those frequent times when an obvious mistake may lead to less obvious consequences, when the physician errs in judgment, never to know how important the error was.

Some years ago, as I was rushing to an imminent delivery, a young woman stopped me in the hospital hall to tell me that her mother had been having chest pains all night. Should she be brought to the emergency room? I knew her mother well, had examined her the previous week, and knew of her recurring angina. "No," I responded, thinking primarily of my busy schedule and the fact that I was already an hour late because of the unexpected delivery. "Take her over to the office, and I'll see her there as soon as I'm done here." It would be a lot more convenient to see her in the office, I thought. About 20 minutes later, as I was finishing the delivery, our clinic nurse rushed into the delivery room, her face pale and frantic. "Come quick! Mrs. Martin just collapsed." I sprinted the 100 yards to the office to find Mrs. Martin in cardiac arrest. Like many physician offices at that time, ours was not equipped with the advanced life-support equipment necessary to handle the situation. Despite everything we could do, Mrs. Martin died.

Would she have survived if I had initially agreed to see her in the emergency room where the requisite staff and equipment were available? No one will ever know for sure, but I have to live with the possibility that she might have lived if I had made a routine decision differently, a decision similar to many others I would make that day, yet one with such an overwhelming outcome.

There is also the common situation of the seriously ill, hospitalized patient who requires almost continuous decision making on the part of the physician. Although no "mistake" may be evident, there are always things that could have been done better: a little more of this medication, starting that treatment a little earlier, recognizing this complication a bit sooner, limiting the number of visitors, and so forth. If the patient dies, the physician is left wondering whether the care provided was adequate. There is no way to be certain, for no one can know what would have happened if things had been done differently. Usually, in fact, it is difficult to get an honest opinion from consultants and other physicians about what one could have done differently. (Judge not, that you not be judged?) In the end, the physician has to swallow the concern, suppress the guilt, and move on to the next patient. He or she may simply be unable to discover whether the mistakes were responsible for the patient's death.

Worst of all, the possibility of a serious mistake is present with each patient the physician sees. The inherent uncertainty of medical practice creates a situation in which errors are always possible. Was that baby I just sent home with a diagnosis of a mild viral fever actually in the early stages of a serious meningitis? Could that nine-year-old with stomach cramps whose mother I just lectured about psychosomatic illness come into the hospital tomorrow with a ruptured appendix? Indeed, the closest I have ever come to involvement in a courtroom malpractice case was the result of my treatment of an apparently minor wrist injury one week after it happened: I misread a straightforward x-ray film and sent the young boy home with a diagnosis of sprain. I next heard about it five years later, when after being summoned to a hearing, I discovered that the fracture I had missed had not healed, and the patient had required extensive treatment and difficult surgery years later.

As practicing primary-care physicians, then, we work in an impossible situation. Each of the myriad decisions to be made every day has the potential for drastic consequences if it is not determined properly. And it is highly likely that sooner or later we will make the mistake that kills or seriously injures another person. How can we live with that knowledge? And after a serious mistake has been made, how can we continue in daily practice and expose ourselves again? How can we who see ourselves as healers deal with such guilt?

Painfully, almost unbelievably, we physicians are even less prepared to deal with our mistakes than the average lay person is. The climate of medical school and residency training, for instance, makes it nearly impossible to confront the emotional consequences of mistakes; it is an environment in which precision seems to pre-dominate. In the large centers where doctors are trained, teams of physicians discuss the smallest details of cases; teaching is usually conducted to make it seem "obvious" what decisions should have been made. And when a physician does make an important mistake, it is first whispered about in the halls, as if it were a sin. Much later, a case conference is called in which experts who have had weeks to think about the situation discuss the way it should have been handled. The environment in which physicians are trained does not encourage them to talk about their mistakes or about their emotional responses to them.

Indeed, errors are rarely admitted or discussed once a physician is in private practice. I have some indication from consultants and colleagues that I am of at least average competence as a physician. The mistakes I have discussed here represent only a fraction of those of which I am aware. I assume that my colleagues at my own clinic and elsewhere are responsible for similar numbers of major and minor errors. Yet we rarely discuss them; I cannot remember a single instance in which another physician initiated a discussion of a mistake for the purpose of clarifying his or her own emotional response or deciding how to follow up. (I do not wish to imply that we don't discuss difficult cases or unfortunate results; yet these discussions are always handled so delicately in the presence of the "offending" physician that there is simply no space for confession or absolution.)

The medical profession simply seems to have no place for its mistakes. There is no permission given to talk about errors, no way of venting emotional responses. Indeed, one would almost think that mistakes are in the same category as sins: it is permissible to talk about them only when they happen to other people.

If the profession has no room for its mistakes, society seems to have even more rigid expectations of its physicians. The malpractice situation

in our country is symptomatic of this attitude. In what other profession are practitioners regularly sued for hundreds of thousands of dollars because of a misjudgment? A lawyer informed me I could be sued for $50,000 for misreading the x-ray film that led to the young man's unhealed fracture. I am sure the Dailys could have successfully sued me for large amounts of money, had they chosen to do so. Experienced physicians who are honest with themselves can count many potential malpractice suits against them. Even the word "malpractice" carries the implication that one has done something more than make a natural mistake; it connotes guilt and sinfulness.

It is easy, of course, to understand why this situation has arisen. These mistakes are terrible; their consequences are drastic; and the victim or family should be compensated for medical bills, time lost from work, and suffering or death. But in our society, rather than establish a "patient compensation fund" (similar to worker's compensation) from which a deserving patient can be compensated for an injury that results from a legitimate mistake, we insist that the doctor be sued for "malpractice," judged guilty, and forced to compensate the patient personally. An atmosphere of denial is created: the "good physician" doesn't make mistakes.

The drastic consequences of our mistakes, the repeated opportunities to make them, the uncertainty about our own culpability when results are poor, and the medical and societal denial that mistakes must happen all result in an intolerable paradox for the physician. We see the horror of our own mistakes, yet we are given no permission to deal with their enormous emotional impact; instead, we are forced to continue the routine of repeatedly making decisions, any one of which could lead us back into the same pit.

Perhaps the only adequate avenue for dealing with this paradox is spiritual. Although mistakes are not usually sins, they engender similar feelings of guilt. How can I not feel guilty about the death of Barb's baby, the lack of adequate emergency care for Mrs. Martin, the fracture that didn't heal? Whether I "ought" to feel guilty is a moot point; most of us do feel guilty under such circumstances.

The only real answer for guilt is spiritual confession, restitution, and absolution. Yet within the structure of modern medicine there is simply no place for this spiritual healing. Although the emotionally mature physician may find it possible to give the patient or family a clinical description of what happened, the technical details are often so difficult for the lay person to understand that the nature of the mistake is hidden. Or if an error is clearly described, it is presented as "natural," "understandable," or "unavoidable" (which, indeed, it often is). But there is no place for real confession: "This is the mistake I made; I'm sorry." How can one say that to a grieving mother, to a family that has lost a member? It simply doesn't fit into the physician-patient relationship.

Even if one were bold enough to consider such a confession, strong voices would raise objections. When I finally heard about the unhealed fracture in my young patient, I was anxious that the incident not create antagonism between me and the family, since we live in a small town and see each other frequently. I was tempted to call the family and express my apologies and the hope that a satisfactory settlement could be worked out. I mentioned that possibility to a malpractice lawyer, but he was strongly opposed, urging me not to have any contact with the family until a settlement was reached. Even if a malpractice suit is not likely, the nature of the physician-patient relationship makes such a reversal of roles "unseemly." Can I further burden an already grieving family with the complexities of my feelings, my burden?

And if confession is difficult, what are we to say about restitution? The very nature of our work means that we are dealing with elements that cannot be restored in any meaningful way. What can I offer the Dailys in restitution?

I have not been successful in dealing with the paradox. Any patient encounter can dump me back into the situation of having caused more harm than good, yet my role is to be a healer. Since there has been no permission to address the paradox openly, I lapse into neurotic behavior to deal with my anxiety and guilt. Little wonder that physicians are accused of having a God complex; little wonder that we are defensive about our judgments; little wonder that we blame the patient or the previous physician when things go wrong, that we yell at the nurses for their mistakes, that we have such high rates of alcoholism, drug addiction, and suicide.

At some point we must bring our mistakes out of the closet. We need to give ourselves permission to recognize our errors and their consequences. We need to find healthy ways to deal with our emotional responses to those errors. Our profession is difficult enough without our having to wear the yoke of perfection.

Simple Living and

Hard Choices

Maureen A. Flannery

■

As a family physician in rural Appalachia, I do not confront many of the issues that pervade the literature of contemporary medical ethics. In my county, we do not debate which facilities should have CAT scanners; we are just trying to replace an outmoded x-ray machine so that we can obtain clearer chest films while exposing our patients to less scatter radiation.

Amniocentesis is not much of an issue in my practice. My patients are astonished at the suggestion that they drive three hours to the university medical center to have a risky procedure simply because they are pregnant past the age of thirty-five or forty, because childbearing into these years remains common in Appalachia. Within large families, it is not unexpected that one or two of the children will be "slow" or "strange"; most women reject an invasive test to predict whether a subsequent child might turn out similarly.

For most Appalachian women, abortion is not an option, even in the case of an unplanned and desperately unwanted pregnancy. This is partly because of strong family ties and the value placed on children within the extended mountain family; and perhaps because Appalachian women are resigned to the fact that motherhood is one of the few potentially fulfilling roles available to them in their home communities. The un-availability of abortions, physically and economically, within the region is less of a factor; the unusual woman who elects abortion as a solution to an unwanted pregnancy prefers that the procedure be done far from the gossip of her home community and without the knowledge of the local "welfare office."

I do not see the daughters or sons of women who took DES during pregnancy and are therefore at risk for a rare cancer. The mothers of most of my patients received little, if any, prenatal care, thereby avoiding that particular pharmacologic tragedy. Decisions around "exotic medical lifesaving therapy" and "scarce lifesaving medical resources," to use the jargon of bioethics, are issues only in their general unavailability, sparing me from difficult decisions about the individual allocation of these technologies. Even medical ethics in the sense of professional etiquette is largely irrelevant in an area where physicians are scarce and isolated. When a city friend asked me whether the medical community had criticized my midwife-attended home birth, I responded, "What medical community?"

The ethical issues I face daily are less dramatic than those involved in decisions around critically ill neonates, organ transplants, and brain death; but they are no less difficult to resolve. Some of them are peculiar to practice in a rural and impoverished area; some are shared by practitioners in other poor areas, such as urban slums; many are faced by all primary-care providers. And with the current health budget cuts, ethical issues around allocation of resources are concerns for all health workers.

My definition of medical ethics is simple: it is ordinary ethics applied to the practice of medicine. Medical ethics is what I do when I stop short in the middle of a busy day in the clinic or have difficulty returning to sleep after an early-morning telephone call from the emergency room because I am asking myself, "What ought I to do in this case?" or "What is the right solution to this problem?"—where the answer to my question cannot be found by checking *Medical Letter* or dialing the neonatologist on the medical center hotline.

Sometimes the situation is a new one, like having a member of one of my families with *osteogenesis imperfecta* (a genetic disease in which the bones are abnormally brittle) become pregnant, despite contraceptive and genetic counseling. More often the problem the patient presents is familiar, but something about the patient or the family situation confounds me, calls my assumptions into question, makes me stop and think.

The nature of the situations that present ethical dilemmas are quite different for the family physician than for the specialist. They tend to be personal and unpredictable. As one family doctor described her practice in North Carolina, "I never did specialize in anything except just people and what came along next."[1] I. R. McWhinney's description of the family medicine perspective is useful:

Family physicians have in common the fact that they obtain fulfillment from personal relations more than from the technical aspects of medicine. Their commitment is to a group of people more than to a body of knowledge. . . . It is difficult for a doctor to commit himself [or herself, throughout] to a person and at the same time to limit his commitment to certain diseases or certain types of problem . . . the kind of commitment I am speaking of implies that the physician will "stay with" a person whatever his problem may be, and he will do so because his commitment is to people more than to a body of knowledge or a branch of technology. To such a physician, problems become interesting and important not only for their own sake but because they are Mr. Smith's or Mrs. Jones's problem. Very often in such relations

there is not even a very clear distinction between a medical problem and a nonmedical one. The patient defines the problem.[2]

For a family physician in a rural area, often the only limit to practice is geographic; everyone within a one- or two-hour driving distance may be the doctor's responsibility. Depending upon the other resources of the area, the physician's commitment may even extend beyond human patients. When I worked with a young physician in Jackman, Maine, the summer after my first year of medical school, I was amazed to find myself confronted in the emergency room of the tiny local hospital with a puppy that had been attacked by a porcupine. Fortunately, the county where I now practice has a veterinarian; she does, however, sometimes send her patients over to our clinic to have their broken limbs x-rayed because she has no x-ray machine.

Given the general commitment a rural family physician has to the surrounding community, the realities of life for the people nearby largely determine the issues that arise in practice. Survival in rural America involves a unique set of struggles, many of which influence health.[3]

One major factor is *low income.* A disproportionate number of the nation's poor live in rural America. About 25 percent of the U.S. population lives in non-metropolitan areas, yet the rural population accounts for 40 percent of those people living below the poverty level. Furthermore, of this 40 percent, ethnic minority groups and the elderly make up a significant proportion. Fifty percent of rural Native Americans, 27 percent of rural Hispanics, and 41 percent of rural blacks have incomes below the poverty level, as compared to 11 percent of rural whites.[4] Poverty increases health problems because of its association with poor nutrition, inadequate housing, unsafe living conditions, and inability to purchase health services.

Low income becomes a greater liability when wages are earned in a *hazardous occupation.* According to 1976 Department of Labor statistics, rural Americans represented the majority of workers in those industries that rank first and second in job-related fatalities: mining and agriculture.[5] Despite the well-known health and safety risks of these occupations, they often represent the only available or the only well-paying jobs for rural Americans.

Not only are rural occupations more likely to be low paying and hazardous, these industries generally provide *fewer health benefits* for their employees. Many rural workers cannot get workers' compensation and they are rarely provided with health insurance. In Texas, for instance, workers' compensation is mandatory for all workers except the farmworkers, who constitute the majority of the rural population of the state. Farm workers are rarely provided with health insurance.[6] Employed rural residents in low-benefit industries are often unable to make payments for their health care, generating insufficient revenue for the facilities that provide them services.

A related disadvantage for rural dwellers is a *lower-than-average educational level,* a characteristic that correlates closely with poor usage of health services.[7] Less-educated persons tend not to have had the opportunity to learn about health, hygiene, and preventive measures. Often they are not informed about governmental programs for which they are eligible, programs that might help with some of the costs or remove some of the obstacles to needed health care services.

Rural dwellers tend to have *closer family ties* than city dwellers because of the preservation of traditional values and also because other societal structures upon which a family can depend are limited in rural areas. Divorce is less common than in urban areas; traditional nuclear and/or extended families are the rule. Since 70 percent of rural families have two parents in the home, compared to 39 percent in the inner cities, the rural poor often fail to meet eligibility criteria for governmental insurance programs that were designed to deal with urban poverty, such as Medicaid and Aid to Dependent Children.[8]

The *particular age structure* of rural America affects the health care of its inhabitants. The number of elderly persons and of children under ten is proportionately higher in rural areas. Since women not only constitute the largest number of health care consumers in general, but also live longer than men and bear children, they are disproportionately represented among rural persons in need of health care. Institutions that care for dependent members of society, such as nursing homes and day care centers, are not prevalent in rural areas; nor are they well accepted, since traditional rural families "care for their own."

In addition to these epidemiological characteristics that militate against good health care, many rural areas have a history of *substandard health care providers.* In Appalachia, the most dramatic example is the coal company doctor. In many communities, the first "professional" health provider was a physician brought in by the local coal company to treat all its employees and their families. There was no alternative to the company doc; he was part of the paternalistic monopoly, just like the company store. Rather than health insurance benefits workers received free care or else scrip for the company doc's services. Since miners were poorly paid and other health providers were scarce, there was essentially no consumer choice for health care. For a variety of reasons, the coal companies did not attract particularly qualified physicians. And patients saw quite clearly that their doctor's allegiance was to the company management, not to their health. (It was not until the United Mine Workers developed its visionary system of hospitals and clinics in the late 1950s that qualified physicians came in any number to the mountains.)

"Bad Nerves" and "Smothering"

I became particularly aware of the influence of all these characteristics on the health of rural dwellers this fall when my partner and I taught a self-care course for the patients in our clinic, modifying a curriculum taught in several Kentucky cities. In dealing with our class of twenty layfolk, we came up against the many conditions that hinder outpatients in taking care of themselves—poverty, environmental hazards, dangerous occupations, lack of education, unemployment, socialization into dependence upon "experts," and lack of support for healthy behavior within a society that condones and often encourages self-destructive habits. Trying to modify a curriculum developed for urban middle-class folk to our rural participants made me realize that much of the self-care and holistic health movements does not apply to people who lack control over many of the basic conditions of their lives.

For instance, self-responsibility is a basic concept of the holistic health movement. The notion that individuals are responsible for their health is sometimes extended to assume that people are also responsible for their diseases. Although this idea can be useful for individuals seeking to understand the meaning of their illnesses—particularly illnesses with significant psychological components—much of the popular self-care literature fails to acknowledge that there are some factors over which we have control in our lives and other factors (known and unknown) over which we have little or no control. For the people in our class, the latter often clearly dominated. Black lung victims, for instance, do not create their health problems (unless they also smoke heavily); unhealthy working conditions do. It is wrong to suggest that the victims must change themselves in order to survive; it is the work-

place that must be changed. The problem and its treatment are not individual but societal.[9]

Many specifics of the curriculum were as inappropriate to our class as the underlying philosophy. For example, how do you start a jogging regimen when you live up a creekbed, when the nearby public roads have no shoulders and are dominated by overfull and uncovered coal trucks? When "just getting by" occupies most of your time, leaving little for leisure activities, however healthful? And when jogging itself is a foreign concept: in the mountains, anyone who would run for any reason other than to get somewhere—or else to get away from something—is a fool.

For a family physician with a commitment to a group of people who have relatively little control over the overwhelming realities of their lives, fostering "self-care" is difficult. Nothing illustrates that better than an examination of two chief complaints that I see often in my practice, "bad nerves" and "smothering."

Many of the female patients I see tell me that they have come to my office because of "bad nerves"; or else they may use it as a tag-on at the visit's end ("By the way, doc, I've got these bad nerves. . . ."). A doctor who practiced nearby several years ago recorded a number of interviews with "bad nerves" patients in which she explored the origin of the diagnosis and the patient's concept of the nature of the malady.[10] Her discovery was that "bad nerves" was largely an iatrogenic complaint. Asked when they became aware of their bad nerves, patients generally said that they had visited a physician with a somatic complaint, say a headache or a stomach ache, and had been told, "No, you don't have a brain tumor," or "There's no ulcer causing your stomach to hurt," but rather, "What you have is *bad nerves*." And the treatment in most cases was a prescription for "nerve pills." Patients took this medical diagnosis and its pharmacological treatment very seriously, seeing "bad nerves" as an illness as physical and concrete as a tumor or an ulcer. One woman vividly described her concept of the nerves coursing through her body as "frayed and tarnished" rather than "silvery smooth" as in a fifth-grade health book picture. Another understood the doctor who performed her hysterectomy to say that he saw her nerves "all aquiver" on the operating table, clearly the worst case of "bad nerves" he had witnessed.

The response of the participants in our self-care course to the treatment game we played during the first session confirms this view of "bad nerves." In the game, each participant has pinned to his or her back the name of a common symptom. The class members then mill around describing "treatments" for the symptom on the other participants' backs, while each participant tries to guess the other's "disease." The purpose of the game is to emphasize the variety of remedies that are available for common symptoms. Interestingly, although "vomiting" and "cold" elicited a variety of treatments, including non-drug and folk cures, the woman who had "bad nerves" pinned to her back encountered only one remedy: "nerve pills."

A common dilemma I face in my practice is what to do when a woman comes in requesting (and requests unmet soon escalate to demands) drug treatment for her "bad nerves." A thorough history usually confirms the iatrogenic labeling of the "bad nerves" and in addition uncovers a difficult and complex social situation that perpetuates the symptoms. Given a busy practice, a bare-bones staff, and poor human service resources in the area; given that patients who discontinue benzodiazepine tranquilizers after more than four months of regular use have a physiological as well as psychological addiction to overcome; and given that there are no transcendental meditation sessions, yoga or exercise classes, or even competent individual or group therapists within a reasonable driving distance, is it right for me to refuse to refill the patient's

Valium, cutting off her way of dulling her responses to the problems of her life? Is it right for me to support her habit? Must a good family physician in a rural area play the roles of counselor, social worker, recreation therapist, and scout leader as well as doctor? Is it possible for one person, however committed, to handle such multiple and demanding roles?

Another frequent complaint, one so common that it is difficult to get patients to clarify it, is "smothering." In the mountains, "smothering" describes everything from the sudden shortness-of-breath of an acute asthmatic attack to the labored breathing of poor physical condition to the short-windedness of chronic obstructive lung disease. I imagine that the frequency of this description is related to the prevalence of black lung, an occupational disease of enormous significance in our single-industry region. Almost everyone knows a neighbor or relative, retired from years in the coal mines, spending his days bound to his home "breathing machine," coughing into a cutoff milk carton in front of the television set. The image is so familiar that even children pick it up: the other day an asthmatic five-year-old described his problem to me as "smothering." I can't help but think that the image is metaphorical for a group of people as oppressed and accustomed to outside control of their lives, their money, and their land as Appalachians. Is it right for a physician simply to treat "smothering" with epinephrine or aminophylline without attempting to deal with the root causes of the oppression? Must a good rural family physician also be a political activist?

And what do patients' rights mean when dealing with people so oppressed and unassertive that they are reluctant to take any responsibility for the care that they receive? It takes hard work and time to bring such folk to demand any of the rights that they have traditionally signed away, just as their foreparents signed away the mineral rights to the land on which they live.[11] In the midst of a busy practice, it is far easier to lapse into the paternalistic pattern to which patients are accustomed. Must a conscientious rural doc also be a part-time community organizer?

A patient came to me the other day to see whether I could "do something" about the dust accumulation in her parents' home. They live up an isolated holler near the clinic, and the dirt road that once ended at their cabin now provides access to a newly developed strip mine. Huge coal trucks now rumble past day and night—their daughter counted five in the space of an hour. Since her parents are the only inhabitants along the road, the coal company ignores the requirement that it "water" the road several times a day to reduce dust accumulation. My patient was concerned that the particles in the air were exacerbating her father's severe chronic obstructive pulmonary disease, a result of thirty-five years of coal dust exposure in underground mines. And it was certainly affecting the couple's quality of life: her elderly mother, a fastidious housekeeper with an early organic brain syndrome, was wearing herself out in a hopeless situation.

Certainly this is an appropriate problem for a family physician. But how far do I go? Write a letter to the owner of the coal company? Report the violation to the Office of Surface Mining when the owner does not respond? Pursue the matter to the state or federal level when lower officials do not act because they are in league with one of the biggest coal operators in the region? How much time and energy can I consume hassling a nonresponsive bureaucracy to benefit one family? Would it be right for me to do nothing?

Limitation of commitment is a very real issue for rural primary health care providers. Responsible to a group of people limited only by geography, in an area with overwhelming needs and relatively few resources to help meet them, the rural physician must constantly ask, how much can one individual do? Can one be a good and ethical physician just by treating symptoms, or

must a doctor become deeply involved in addressing the sources of disease in the people she or he cares for? And if a doctor neglects continuing medical education because of political involvements, or "burns out" from the stress of trying to do too much, do the patients and community ultimately benefit or not?

The Wise Old Woman of the Village

In struggling with the issue of setting limits to commitment, a rural health care provider must deal with a related question: personal survival in a rural community. For a physician in a rural area, there is no boundary between professional and private life. Living among the people whom I serve in a close-knit community, I do not have the luxury of retreating to a suburban lifestyle surrounded by other "young professionals" when I end my day at an inner-city clinic. I am one of a few professionals in my county, and everyone knows where I live, how I spend my days off, and whether I dug up my potatoes before the first frost. Values I hold or reject in my personal life are clear to my patient-neighbors. Questions like those Robert Coles asks,

> How much money is too much money? Who commands one's time, and who does not? What balance is there to one's commitment of energy?[12]

become not just matters of individual lifestyle but vital issues in medical ethics.

Physicians have traditionally considered their private lives immune to this sort of public scrutiny. Although they have almost unlimited access to patients' minds and bodies, an unwritten ethic of the relationship generally prevents patients from intruding into their doctors' private lives.[13] But is it unreasonable for patients to demand that I connect my public and private lives? To challenge me to be consistent in the values I profess in the clinic and at home? How I spend my time and money, what political convictions I hold—do these not affect my doctoring?

Many urban physicians make a sharp distinction between the people with whom they spend social or after-hours time and those they see as patients. The director of my residency program felt very strongly that a doctor should not accept friends as patients. He believed that confusing friend-friend and doctor-patient relationships created problems for both physician and patient: the blurring made medical judgments more difficult for the physician and detracted from the role of "authority figure" that the physician plays. He also believed in the value of friends who relate to the physician as a person, and who can help him or her escape from medicine after hours. Whatever the merits of that position, a rural physician has little choice in the matter I would have to drive a long way for friends or my friends would have to travel a long way for their medical care if I followed his advice. Instead, I trust my patient/friends to understand that I need "time off" in order to be there for them as physician/friend.

Given the high visibility of a physician in a small community, anonymity is impossible. From an income disproportionately higher than that of hard-working neighbors to preferential treatment in scheduling a haircut, the "myriad and often subtle privileges of physician status" are striking in a rural community.[14] Should I accept these favors as compensation for the pressing and demanding work I do? Or should I refuse them as elitist and unnecessary? The absence of boundaries between personal and public lives makes it difficult for the rural physician to lead a "well-rounded" life in the sense of an urban or suburban colleague. Yet those of us who are content with our lives as country docs discover ways of dealing with our situations. Mary Howell describes a model that works for me:

My vision of how I like to work and relate to the people I serve does not correspond to the usual understanding of the professional role. I have found a different "role model" altogether—that of the wise old woman of the village, the witch healer, who has been privileged to learn from her predecessors and to share with many generations of village folk their experiences as family members, and who can convey what she has distilled (what she "knows") to others so that they too can use that wisdom.[15]

For rural primary health care providers, finding the wisdom to cope with work that specializes only in "people and what comes along next" is often an overwhelming task. How well we seek that wisdom and resolve the everyday ethical issues that arise in our work ultimately determines our effectiveness in helping the people with whom we live and whom we serve.

Notes

1. Mary Frances Shuford, M.D., b. 1900, Asheville, N.C. cited in Sara Jean Wilhelm, *On Her Own Terms,* unpublished manuscript.

2. I.R. McWhinney, "Family Medicine in Perspective," *New England Journal of Medicine* 293 (July 24, 1975), 176.

3. This section is based upon Chapter 1 of Rural Health Issues Committee, *Patterns for Change* (Washington D.C.: National Women's Health Network, 1981), pp. 9–22.

4. Sandra Lichty and Ann Zuvekas, "Rural Health: Policies, Progress, and Challenges," *Urban Health* (September 1980), p. 45.

5. U.S. Department of Labor, 1978.

6. United Farm Workers, *Facts about the Farm Workers of Texas* (San Juan, Texas, 1980).

7. M.C. Ahearn, *Health Care in Rural America* (Washington D.C.: U.S. Department of Agriculture, Bulletin 428, July 1979), p. 7.

8. *Ibid.,* pp. 9–10.

9. Sally Guttmacher, "Whole in Body, Mind, and Spirit: Holistic Health and the Limits of Medicine," *Hastings Center Report,* April 1979, p. 16.

10. Laurie Dornbran, unpublished data.

11. The recently documented corporate and absentee

ownership of much of Appalachia contributes to the
lack of control that many Appalachians feel over their
lives. See Appalachian Land Ownership Task Force,
*Land Ownership Patterns and Their Impacts on Appa-
lachian Communities* (Washington, D.C.: Appalachian
Regional Commission, February 1981).

12. Robert Coles, "Medical Ethics and Living a Life," *New
England Journal of Medicine* 301 (August 23, 1979),
446.

13. Chase Patterson Kimball, "The Ethics of Personal Medicine," *Medical Clinics of North America* 61 (July
1977), 876.

14. Mary C. Howell, "Can We Be Feminist Physicians? Mi-
rages, Dilemmas, and Traps," *Journal of Health Politics, Policy and Law* 2 (Summer 1977), 169.

15. Mary C. Howell, *Helping Ourselves: Families and the
Human Network* (Boston: Beacon Press, 1975), p. xvi.

The Paid Nurse

William Carlos Williams

■

When I came in, approaching eleven o'clock
Sunday evening, there had been a phone call for
me. I don't know what it is, Mrs. Corcoran called
up, said Floss, about an accident of some sort
that happened to George. You know, Andy's
friend. What kind of an accident? An explosion, I
don't know, something like that, I couldn't make
it out. He wants to come up and see you. She'll
call back in a minute or two.

As I sat down to finish the morning paper the
phone rang again as usual. His girl friend had
heard about it and was taking him up to her doctor in Norwood. Swell.

But next day he came to see me anyhow. What
in hell's happened to you, George? I said when I
saw him. His right arm was bandaged to the
shoulder, the crook of his left elbow looked like
overdone bacon, his lips were blistered, his nose
was shiny with grease and swollen out of shape
and his right ear was red and thickened.

They want me to go back to work, he said. They
told me if I didn't go back I wouldn't get paid. I
want to see you.

What happened?

I work for the General Bearings Company, in
Jersey City. You know what that means. They're a
hard-boiled outfit. I'm not kidding myself about
that, but they can't make me work the way I feel.
Do you think I have to work with my arms like

this? I want your opinion. That fellow in Norwood said it wasn't anything but I couldn't sleep last night. I was in agony. He gave me two capsules and told me to take one. I took one around three o'clock and that just made me feel worse. I tried to go back this morning but I couldn't do it.

Wait a minute, wait a minute. You haven't told me what happened yet.

Well, they had me cleaning some metal discs. It wasn't my regular job. So I asked the boss, What is this stuff? Benzol, he said. It is inflammable? I said. Not very, he said. We use it here all the time. I didn't believe him right then because I could smell it, it had a kind of smell like gasoline or cleaning fluid of some kind.

What I had to do was to pick those pieces out of a pail of the stuff on this side of me, my left side, and turn and place them in the oven to dry them. Two hundred degrees temperature in there. Then I'd turn and pick up another lot and so on into the dryer and back again. I had on long rubber gauntlets up almost to my elbow.

Well, I hadn't hardly started when, blup! it happened. I didn't know what it was at first. You know you don't realize those things right away—until I smelt burnt hair and cloth and saw my gloves blazing. The front of my shirt was burning too—lucky it wasn't soaked with the stuff. I jumped back into the aisle and put my hands back of me and shook the gloves off on the floor. The pail was blazing too.

Everybody came on the run and rushed me into the emergency room. Everybody was excited, but as soon as they saw that I could see and wasn't going to pass out on them they went back to their jobs and left me there with the nurse to fix me up.

Then I began to feel it. The flames from the shirt must have come up into my face because inside my nostrils was burnt and you can see what it did to my eyebrows and eyelashes. She called the doctor but he didn't come any nearer than six feet from me. That's not very bad, he

said. So the nurse put a little dressing, of tannic acid, I think she said it was, on my right arm which got the worst of it. I was just turning away from the oven when it happened, lucky for me, so I got it mostly on my right side.

What do I do now? I asked her. Go home? I was feeling rotten.

No, of course not, she told me. That's not bad. Go on back to work.

What! I said.

Yes, she said. And come back tomorrow morning. If you don't you won't get paid. And, by the way, she said, don't go to any other doctor. You come back here tomorrow morning and go to work as usual. Do you think that was right?

The bastards. Go ahead. Wasn't there someone you could appeal to there? Don't you belong to a union?

No, said George. There's nothing like that there. Only the teamsters and the pressmen have unions, they've had them long enough so that the company can't interfere.

All right. Go ahead.

So I went back to the job. They gave me something else to do but the pain got so bad I couldn't stand it so I told the boss I had to quit. All right, he said, go on home but be back here tomorrow morning. That would be today.

You went back this morning?

I couldn't sleep all night. Look at my arm.

All right. Let's look at it. The worst was the right elbow and forearm, almost to the shoulder in fact. It was cooked to about the color of ham rind with several areas where the Norwood doctor had opened several large blisters the night before. The arm was, besides that, swollen to a size at least a third greater than its normal volume and had begun to turn a deep, purplish red just above the wrist. The ear and nose were not too bad but in all the boy looked sick.

So you went back this morning?

Yes.

Did they dress it?

No, just looked at it and ordered me on the floor. They gave me a job dragging forty-pound cases from the stack to the elevator. I couldn't use my right arm so I tried to do it with my left but I couldn't keep it up. I told 'em I was going home.

Well?

The nurse gave me hell. She called me a baby and told me it wasn't anything. The men work with worse things than that the matter with them every day, she said.

That don't make any difference to me, I told her, I'm going home.

All right, she said, but if you don't show up here tomorrow for work you don't get any pay. That's why I'm here, he continued. I can't work. What do you say?

Well, I said, I'll call up the Senator, which I did at once. And was told, of course, that the man didn't have to go to work if I said he wasn't able to do so. They can be reported to the Commission, if necessary. Or better perhaps, I can write them a letter first. You tell him not to go to work.

You're not to go to work, I told the boy. O.K., that settles it. Want to see me tomorrow? Yeah. And quit those damned capsules he gave you, I told him. No damned good. Here, here's something much simpler that won't at least leave you walking on your ear till noon the next day. Thanks. See you tomorrow.

Then it began to happen. Late in the afternoon the nurse called him up to remind him to report for duty next morning. I told her I'd been to you, he said, and that you wanted the compensation papers. She won't listen to it. She says they're sending the company car for me tomorrow morning to take me in to see their doctor. Do I go?

Not on your life.

But the next day I was making rounds in the hospital at about ten A.M. when the office reached me on one of the floors. Hold the wire. It was George. The car is here and they want me to go back with them. What do I do?

Wait a minute, I said. What's their phone number? And what's that nurse's name? I'll talk to them. You wait till I call you back. So I got the nurse and talked to her. I hear you had an explosion down at your plant, I told her. What do you mean? she said. What are you trying to do, cover it up, I asked her, so the insurance company won't find out about it? We don't do that sort of thing in this company. What are you doing now? I asked her again. She blurted and bubbled till I lost my temper and let her have it. What is that, what is that? she kept saying. You know what I'm talking about, I told her. Our doctors take care of our own cases, she told me. You mean they stand off six feet from a man and tell him he's all right when the skin is half-burned off of him and the insides of his nostrils are all scorched? That isn't true, she said. He had no right to go to an outside doctor. What! I said, when he's in agony in the middle of the night from the pains of his burns, he has no right to get advice and relief? Is that what you mean? He has the privilege of calling our own doctor if he needs one, she says. In the middle of the night? I asked her. I tell you what you do, I said, you send me the compensation papers to sign. You heard me, I said, and make it snappy if you know what's good for you. We want our own doctor to see him, she insisted. All right, I said, your own doctor can see him but he's not to go to work. Get that through your head, I said. And that's what I told him.

He went back to their doctor in the company car.

It was funny. We were at supper that evening when he came to the house door. I didn't have any office hours that night. Floss asked him to come in and join us but he had eaten. He had a strange look on his face, half-amused and half-bewildered.

I don't know, he said. I couldn't believe it. You ought to see the way I was treated. I was all ready to be bawled out but, oh no! The nurse was all smiles. Come right in, George. Do you feel all right, George? You don't look very well. Don't you want to lie down here on the couch? I thought she was kidding me. But she meant it. What a difference! That isn't the way they treated me the first time. Then she says, It's so hot in here I'll turn on the fan so as to cool you a little. And here, here's a nice glass of orange juice. No kiddin'. What a difference!

Floss and I burst out laughing in spite of ourselves. Oh, everything's lovely now, he said. But you're not working? No, I don't have to work. They sent me back home in the company car and they're calling for me tomorrow morning. The only thing is they brought in the man who got me the job. That made me feel like two cents. You shouldn't have acted like that, George, he told me. We'll take care of you. We always take care of our men.

I can take it, sir, I told him. But I simply couldn't go back to work after the burning I got. You didn't have to go back to work, he said. Yes, I did, I said. They had me dragging forty-pound cases around the floor. . . .

Really? he said.

He didn't know that, did he? I interposed. I'm glad you spoke up. And they want you to go back tomorrow?

All right, but don't work till I tell you. But he did. After all, jobs aren't so easy to get nowadays even with a hard-boiled firm like that. I won't get any compensation either, they told me, not even for a scar.

Is that so?

And they said they're not going to pay you, either.

We'll see what the Senator says about that.

He came back two days later to tell me the rest of it. I get it now, he said. It seems after you've been there a year they insure you, but before that you don't get any protection. After a year one of the fellows was telling me—why, they had a man there that just sprained his ankle a little. It wasn't much. But they kept him out on full pay for five months, what do you know about that? They wouldn't let him work when he wanted to.

Good night!

Geez, it was funny today, he went on. They were dressing my arm and a big piece of skin had all worked loose and they were peeling it off. It hurt me a little, oh, you know, not much but I showed I could feel it, I guess. My God! the nurse had me lie down on the couch before I knew what she was doing. And do you know, that was around one-thirty. I didn't know what happened to me. When I woke up it was four o'clock. I'd been sleeping all that time! They had a blanket over me and everything.

Good!

How much do I owe you? Because I want to pay you. No use trying to get it from them. If I make any trouble they'll blackball me all over the country they tell me.

PART IV

Health Care Ethics and

the Provider's Role

Many textbooks and readers exclusively devoted to health care ethics already exist. Why, then, devote a part to ethics in a reader like this? The answer is simple: ethics has meaning only in context.

Aristotle (1941) observed that a person living outside of human society is either a beast or a god. This is to say, first, that morality is a distinctively human capacity, and, second, that belief and behavior cannot be truly moral except in the context of a community of persons. Similarly, what we consider moral and how we think and feel about what morality is are deeply affected by both the membership and the history of the community with which we are concerned.

This reader offers insights into the various communities that play roles in determining the morality of health care decisions. Without the context provided by the other disciplines and perspectives represented here, moral deliberation lacks the depth and richness, the appreciation of difference, and the keen sense of roles and relationships that characterize modern health care ethics. And without a discussion of ethics that grounds moral reasoning not only in cases but also in an understanding of theory, principles, character, virtue, narrative, and the relationship between law, ethics, and policy, this reader would risk perpetuating the misconception that ethics is merely relative, a matter of taste.

Part IV addresses some key relationships, issues, and conflicts in health care ethics. It makes no claim to exhaustiveness; instead, it seeks to promote reflection, which may then be turned toward other questions. The selection of readings reflects our collective teaching experience with medical students, students in other health professions, and health care practitioners in a variety of fields. Basic questions about the provider-patient relationship are examined, as well as some of the most divisive issues that have arisen as a result of medical progress. The readings in this part have been chosen to work as well on their own as they will in tandem with any of the many good health care ethics texts and anthologies currently available.

Ethical issues in health care have been a focus of public fascination since at least the 1970s, when our attention was drawn to them by developments like the public discussion of treatment withdrawal after the Karen Quinlan case, or the patients' rights movement. What helps to make "bioethics" (as it is usually called) so compelling is that its issues, conflicts, and stories belong both to health care professionals and to everyone else. We relate to health care ethics as patients, members of patients' families, potential patients, and representatives of a society that has some say in the activities of health care professionals and some interest in fostering public discussion of health care issues. We each read about the latest "hot topic" in health care and ask ourselves, not only, "What do I think?" but also, "What would I do if it were me?" "What would I want my doctor to do?" and "What should society do?" Thus, health care ethics has the capacity to engage our individual moral sensibilities, our vision of professional ethics, and our public policy concerns all at once. This complexity is compounded by the "scientific" component of health care, which makes us acutely aware of

how new problems, and new twists on old problems, are created as part of medical progress, and which also gives rise to a sometimes strongly felt, but nonetheless largely illusory, dichotomy between "hard" data and "soft" ethics. Health care professionals and students can become particularly frustrated in their search for answers to questions of ethics, because they sometimes tend to view the examination of moral questions as utterly different from the fact-based training that forms the bedrock of their professional knowledge. Viewing health care ethics in a social medicine context, however, as this volume does, confronts students with uncertainty, not only in ethics, but in medicine and science as well.

Health care ethics is generally understood as applied ethics: that is, as moral theory applied to a specific domain of issues, relationships, and practices. Traditionally, then, health care ethics has begun from the study of moral theory and moved to its application in the health care setting. In Western moral tradition, theories of ethics have fallen into two domains: principle and virtue. Principle-based theories of ethics apply principles to the resolution of moral quandaries. Reasoning through principles is very familiar in Western thought; it is mathematical in style, it forms the basis of much of American law and public policy, and it has strongly influenced modern medical ethics. Many professional codes of ethics are made up of principles, and some of the legal principles underlying the Bill of Rights—freedom of speech, freedom of religion, liberty and privacy, due process, and equal protection of the laws—have become thoroughly identified with health care ethics as a result of their importance in defining the rights of patients. The triumvirate of particular principles that shape most discussions of medical ethics—autonomy, beneficence, and justice—has been the centerpiece of medical ethics theory for several decades (Beauchamp and Childress 1994).

The principle of autonomy, which is also

often labeled respect for persons, or self-determination, is the principle most often associated with "patients' rights." Respecting the autonomy of patients means viewing their decisions and choices as valid; it means not interfering with them (the "negative" right to be left alone) unless their actions injure others; and it means assisting them in the exercise of their autonomy (for example, by providing information about health care decisions).

In contrast, the principle of beneficence focuses on the duty of health care providers to act in the best interests of the patient. Beneficence, which entails both "doing no harm" and trying to do good, is generally seen by health care providers as the most important moral principle in health care. Many moral quandaries in health care present themselves as conflicts between the principles of autonomy and beneficence, which are often dichotomized as representing, respectively, the patient's values and the doctor's values. It is important to recognize, however, that a number of key concepts and issues in health care ethics—in particular, informed consent, truth telling, and confidentiality—combine and weigh considerations of autonomy and beneficence, and careful analysis will uncover the relationships between them. Autonomy and beneficence are better understood not as inevitably competing but as frequently complementary principles.

Justice, on the other hand, is not so easy to grasp. Usually understood to mean fairness, justice introduces a wider social dimension to individual caregiver-patient relationships than those aspects emphasized by autonomy and beneficence. Justice sometimes means addressing questions about the distribution of health care resources, and what it means to do so equally or fairly. It sometimes means considering whether health care should have a role in remedying injustices, past or present. Justice also focuses on questions like whether health care is (or should be) a right, and what that might mean. Growing

recognition of the limits of America's financial and material resources is helping to bring the larger political and social dimensions of health care ethics into the forefront of discussion and concern; the meaning of justice in health care is a central concern of that inquiry.

Most of the traditional moral theories that have been applied to medical ethics are principle-based. The "deontological" or rule-based moral theory of Immanuel Kant (1985), which emphasizes treating persons as "ends in themselves," rather than as objects to be used for the ends of others, has been influential in medical ethics' understanding of the principle of autonomy. Jeremy Bentham and John Stuart Mill's "consequential" theory of utilitarianism (Mill 1957), which focuses on the consequences of choices and actions, holds that moral actions are those that result in the greatest good for the greatest number; it considers beneficence to be central (but also prescribes that actions which do not harm others should not be interfered with by society, thus establishing autonomy as a good). These two theories—Kantian deontology and utilitarianism—are the ones most often cited in health care ethics. They are generally viewed as being in opposition, but are often seen to be combined as the basis of much law and public policy (Arras and Steinbock 1995).

Virtue (or character) is very different from principle as a way of thinking about ethics. It is not quandary-focused; it does not present a set of tools to apply to a problem. Virtue theory looks at persons. Its moral language is different; instead of saying, "But it's the right thing to do," moral actors who think in terms of virtue and character are more likely to say "I'm the kind of person who couldn't do that," or "I wouldn't feel right if I did that." Health professionals' codes and statements of ethics are often cast in virtue language rather than, or in addition to, the language of principles (for example, "The nurse should be honest" instead of "The nurse should tell the truth"). Western virtue theory has Greek roots, with Aristotle's ethics being the best-known exemplar. Patients often focus on virtue and character more than on principles; it is the language of many religious traditions, and forms the basis of much of the moral instruction that families pass on to children. After all, that familiar childhood moral instruction "be good" is virtue language. In part because of its familiarity and in part because it is more challenging to apply to problems—where modern medical ethics focuses its attention—virtue theory has tended to be devalued. Its revival by philosophers like Alasdair MacIntyre (1984) has raised many interesting questions about the role of the virtues in modern multicultural societies, where different social and historical influences may result in different conceptions of good character and right action.

Importantly, the question of whether there is a "medical ethic"—that is, whether there is a specific professional ethic for doctors and other health care providers that sets moral standards unique to health care professionals—attempts to sidestep this problem of diversity by drawing on virtue theory. What it means to be a good doctor, and how good doctoring is taught, are in this view inquiries about virtue in medicine. A peculiarly medical ethic might be conceived as universal, transcending particular social and cultural influences. Physician-philosopher Leon Kass's examination of the Hippocratic Oath (1985) offers a thoughtful example of this kind of approach, proposing that the oath provides a definition of good medicine that takes precedence over individual physicians' preferences in professional life and practice. The challenge to such an account of medical virtue lies in whether and how the "universal physician" understands the effects of society and culture on the patient's illness and on medicine's role.

Quite naturally, most people in their personal and professional lives mix the language of principles with the language of virtues. Most of us also mix moral theories together when we are addressing issues, using them to shape a container that fits the discussion, rather than stuffing the quandary into a box labeled "autonomy" or "utilitarianism" and cutting off the parts that won't go in. The almost instinctive eclecticism of practical moral agency represents a problem for traditional, all-encompassing theories of ethics—despite our (also practical) longing for a single, simple formula that will provide moral answers. As a result, some new moral theories have emerged, claiming to offer a better "fit" for medical ethics. One of these is casuistry, an analytical method revived by Albert Jonsen and Stephen Toulmin from Catholic moral theology (1988). Casuistry means, simply, reasoning by cases. It employs cases, not principles, precepts, or virtues, as the unit of moral analysis, and reaches judgments on a case-by-case basis, rather than attempting to apply or extract general rules. Casuistry is particularly attractive for health care ethics because health care is case-focused.

Cases are also stories, and narrative ethics has recently come to give a name to a way of doing ethics that focuses not just on the case but on the story (Hunter 1991). Stories have storytellers, principal and minor characters, relationships, dramatic structure, and history. Stories can also often be told from multiple viewpoints, employing frames of reference of varying sizes: family, institution, community, and society. Using a narrative theory of ethics emphasizes not the facts but their context as integrally important to understanding. For example, the patient's history, as presented by the doctor according to the conventions of medicine, may be different in highly significant ways from the patient's story, told by the patient, even when the factual details of the patient's "chief complaint" are identical in both accounts. Casuistry and narrative ethics thus both provide new insights and approaches to moral analysis, without necessarily providing new analytical tools or suggesting new answers.

Another new cluster of moral theories, even more difficult to characterize, might be loosely called "difference ethics." Theories of difference ethics do two things. They challenge the definitive position of Western moral theories, asserting the superiority of moral traditions other than those derived from the Greeks, Western religious traditions, or the Enlightenment—they may, for example, champion a "feminine" ethics of care, compassion, and relationship over a traditional ethics based on reason and justice; or they may argue that individual autonomy has no meaning in non-Western cultures where family and community are central or where religious traditions are not focused on the individual self. Some theories of difference ethics go on to make a deeper critique of moral philosophy in general, by highlighting power and inequality as a central but undiscussed issue in moral relationships both individual and societal, and by bringing questions about the uses of power to the forefront of moral agency. Though most often associated with feminist ethics, power analysis is common also to the search for an African American perspective on bioethics, and to inquiries about the relationship between ethics and ethnicity and culture (Flack and Pellegrino 1992, Tong 1993). It also has visible roots in modern medical ethics. For example, the recognition of inequality of power and knowledge between patients and physicians formed the basis for the doctrine of informed consent as it developed in the 1950s and 1960s (Faden, Beauchamp, and King 1986).

The new perspectives offered by narrative ethics and difference ethics in particular parallel very usefully the social medicine context for health care ethics offered by this book. What is most exciting and daunting about adding new moral theories to the traditional palette is that we don't know yet what kind of difference they will make to the developing portrait of moral agency in health care. The process of bringing different perspectives to bear on cases, issues, and stories thus enriches not only the individual reader but the field as a whole. Therefore, all of the selections in part IV invite discussion and analysis from a multiplicity of perspectives, with the goal of promoting the development of individual moral sensibility and a broad and deep capacity for recognizing and addressing moral issues, in study, in practice, and in life.

Nancy M. P. King

The Provider-Patient Relationship

Section 1 has two concerns. First, it examines what moral reasoning is and what it means to have a moral life as a health care professional in relationships with patients. Second, it examines three bedrock precepts of that relationship—truth telling, informed consent, and confidentiality—and explores their differences and similarities. The readings chosen for this section should deepen capacities for moral analysis of both everyday and exotic ethical problems, and help to develop new skills incorporating more information and different perspectives into the moral context of common problems.

The first two readings address the first concern of this section, focusing on the nature of ethical problems, different ways of thinking about ethics, and the moral framework of the physician-patient relationship. Larry Churchill's "Bioethics in Social Context" lays a groundwork of moral vocabulary and analysis. He invites us to consider the complexity of moral experience, and the limitations of traditional moral theory as means of addressing moral quandaries. He challenges us to broaden and deepen our sense of how to approach moral quandaries in health care, both personally and professionally.

Next, physician and writer William Carlos Williams provides an account of a complex and highly emotional encounter between a physician

and a child patient. This famous story, "The Use of Force," clearly and passionately conveys the emotional tension between *being* right and *doing* right that characterizes the choices between the principles of autonomy and beneficence and highlights the issue of power. The story permits us to enlarge upon Churchill's admonition to consider the patient's voice, by inviting analysis from a variety of perspectives and by providing a richly detailed factual, psychological, and emotional context for the doctor's actions. Together these readings suggest that there is always a moral dimension to consider in the structure of the encounter and the goals of the relationship between caregivers and patients.

The first of three classic issues in medical ethics, truth telling, is a principle that must be balanced against both beneficence and autonomy in different circumstances. This set of readings provides a variety of applications: a case that asks how long the arm of informed consent should be; a pair of articles considering whether truth telling interferes with patients' well-being; and an article that tries to balance truth telling with the choice not to know. Taken together, these readings promote discussion about the following concerns: what "the truth" is; why truthfulness matters; how caregivers do, or should, make judgments about what to tell, when, and how; and whether truthfulness is a value in all cultures.

Informed consent (or, to use a more descriptive but less popular term, informed choice) follows closely from concerns about truth, and the moral and legal doctrine of informed consent attempts to balance autonomy and beneficence. The readings cover a range of perspectives. First, Raymond Carver's poem (which is also concerned with truth telling) allows us to consider the emotional impact of receiving information and making decisions and to examine how physicians manage disclosure and how patients respond. Like the Williams story and the Churchill essay,

"What the Doctor Said" helps to prevent the all-too-common maneuver of separating the "psychosocial" from the "factual" or "rational," thus pushing us toward a more realistic picture of health care decision making. The poem can be interpreted in a variety of ways. Is it an endorsement of beneficence-based nondisclosure, or is it an exploration of the emotional content of "rational" discourse for both physicians and patients? The poem offers an opportunity to consider what might be done differently to support the informed consent process. George Annas's short essay continues by illustrating the relationship between the law of informed consent and informed consent as a moral doctrine, using the example of disclosure of statistical prognosis information and focusing on why patients need information. These readings might be supplemented by examination of state laws governing informed consent.

The last issue, confidentiality, is addressed by two very short readings. One considers the moral meaning of sharing stories without the subject's permission, even if no "harm" is done; the other offers several analyses of a case example of the classic confidentiality problem in which the patient's right to confidentiality must be balanced against the risk of harm to another. The nature of the physician's duty is explored, and in addition a feminist perspective is offered. This focus on the nature of the harm caused by breaches of confidentiality, on the nature of the virtue of keeping confidences, and on different ways of analyzing a case that pits the harms of breaching confidentiality against the possible harm of not informing an affected person reflect themes raised in part III of this reader, especially in Perri Klass's memoir, "Invasions."

Bioethics in Social Context

Larry R. Churchill

■

I. Mapping the Moral Terrain

What is it like to be in a moral quandary? How do people describe this kind of experience? They often say they feel anxious, as well as intellectually perplexed. They describe themselves as emotionally vulnerable and conflicted. Typically, there is a sense that a great deal is at stake in terms of how others will view them or how they view themselves, as well as what their future life prospects may hold. The affective dimensions center on being ambivalent, anxious, perhaps guilty, and sometimes overwhelmed. The cognitive aspects are uncertainty, ambiguity, or lack of clarity about values—a sense of facing problems that resist simple resolution or exceed one's capacities. Overall, the experience is not high on the hedonic scale. Anyone who has wrestled with a serious moral dilemma, or who works with persons who do, will recognize this list and could extend it at some length.

I begin with this abbreviated description of the human experience of ethical conflict in order to emphasize that ethics is about a concrete human phenomenon, or set of phenomena. Ethics is about what happens to people in the process of living a life, not a matter of what happens in the heads of academics in their studies. Ethics is first and foremost a matter of bumps and bruises encountered as people seek moral direction, as they strive to live lives they can respect, or at least tolerate upon reflection. And it is indelibly part of human nature to so reflect, to make judgments about ourselves and others which can only be called *value* judgments—judgments not reducible to facts, and of much greater importance than matters of taste or decorum. I begin in this way as a reminder that we are the species who says "ought," and to refresh our memories about what the experience of saying "ought" is like. For if the academic study of bioethics is to be helpful in illuminating the choices and guiding the actions of patients and doctors, it will have to be responsive to these experiences, which are the basic ingredients of moral life.

A related question is equally important to keep before us. How do people resolve moral quandaries? What sorts of strategies, maneuvers, processes, and steps do they take to get themselves out of the experience of value conflict? These strategies and maneuvers, like the experience of a moral quandary, are constantly in evidence, and are of an endless variety. There are, no doubt, common features among persons stemming from cultural or social similarities. Yet on careful examination, the movements in each ethical problem-solving process display unique configurations, just as each person has a unique signature, and no person ever quite duplicates exactly his or her own signature.

How do people resolve moral quandaries? Often they tell stories about themselves, about the sort of persons they are or hope to become. They tell such stories for many reasons—as a means of reassurance, as imaginative rehearsals, as trial balloons, or with aspirations for finding a course of action that will fit what they take to be the on-going narrative thread of their lives. They ask what others would think of them were they to pursue one course of action or another. They consult the living and the dead, and, in certain biomedical situations, even the unborn, trying to configure their relationships appropriately. They

seek advice from authorities—kinship networks, friends, people they respect, people in whom they mirror themselves, from communities to which they belong, or hope to belong. These communities may be specifically identifiable as one's neurosurgical colleagues, or as utilitarians, or orthodox Jews, or one's family, and so on. However designated, a reference community is composed of the important others who might approve or disapprove a choice, and accept or reject the person involved. These sorts of strategies are typical of the moves encouraged by those ethical philosophies which focus on character and virtues. But people consult not only reference communities. They also consult rules and principles, and occasionally oaths sworn in professional initiations. Ethical problem-solving usually involves critical, applied analysis of such rules and principles, as well as reflective talking, remembering and imagining.

The style, and not just the content, of individual problem-solving varies also. Some persons seek, primarily, to think themselves out of moral difficulty, looking for consistency between situations. They may employ formal tests, such as asking what choices they would approve in others as a measure of what they should choose for themselves. Those who identify strongly with formal codes of ethics may do strenuous intellectual work in interpreting and applying these codes. For example, doctors often work to parse the meaning of "Do no harm," and Christians often seek actions which embody "the love of God." For others, the essence of moral problem-solving is getting "in touch" with one's true feelings, with the idea that deep emotions are morally instructive, but not readily accessible.

This list of strategies and styles of moral problem-solving is, of course, far from complete. I intend it only as a reminder of the "stuff" of ethics—the real world thoughts and actions which bioethical theories and analyses are intended to address and refine.

My point here is that human moral activity is complex and multi-faceted. It includes decision and action, reflection and contemplation, sustaining habits over time, nurturing character, and many other kinds of activity. It is part logic, part acts of will, part turning and tuning emotional sensibilities, part feats of imagination. Because moral activity is complex and multi-faceted, ethical theory must be multi-faceted as well. Since there is no single, uniform, subject matter in view when we say "morality," since it is always necessary to probe to discover just what aspect of morality is being considered, the need for diverse kinds of ethical theory should be evident. Yet often this need for theoretical diversity is not recognized, and a mismatch results. For example, moral theories designed to clarify the thinking of the muddle-headed are sometimes brought to bear on the emotional facets of a situation, or on what are better described as failures of character or will. Or a rule or principle that is clarifying and insightfully used in one context is misapplied in another. Such mismatches and misapplications are an inevitable part of every person's struggle for morally mature judgments, for ethical wisdom. Yet often bioethics exhibits just the opposite of careful attention to the complexity of moral experience, and fails to engage persons as they seek resolution to their moral quandaries. This failure to engage is not just unfortunate. It is damaging. Bioethicists too often do not simply fail to read complex moral situations, they also oversimplify them. They tend to substitute their own idealized version of experience for the moral phenomena described above.

Using the metaphor of cartography, let me put this in another way. Because moral experience is complex, it requires careful mapping. Yet often in the study of bioethics, academics bring their own maps and ignore the sketches provided by the natives. Instead of constructing a map after walking across the terrain and talking with those who live there, academics often arrive in the territory with their own requirements for what the lay of the land must be. Such preconceived moral topography is of interest to other academics, but of little use to persons who are trying to find their way. When academics or professionals have power to impose their maps on moral travelers the problems become acute, as I will illustrate in the two scenarios that follow.

II. Nobody Said Hello

In a regular feature of the *Cambridge Quarterly of Healthcare Ethics* called "Bedside Story," an ethics committee meeting is recounted from the perspective of the patient (1992a, pp. 185–186).

The patient was a young HIV-positive woman. After she underwent exploratory surgery for pelvic pain, it was discovered that her fallopian tubes were blocked. She requested surgery to remove the obstruction, explaining to her gynecologist that she and her husband wanted the opportunity to have a child in the future, in case a cure for AIDS is found. Because this patient was HIV positive, any baby would have a 30% risk of being born with HIV, and the patient herself might not live to raise the child. (This case preceded 1993 studies indicating that zidovudine can reduce HIV transmission to newborns by two-thirds.) The patient's request for surgery became an ethics "case" when her physician referred her request to an ethics committee.

The patient's perceptions of her interaction with the ethics committee are given in some detail, and make distressing reading. According to the patient "Nobody said hello . . ." and the demeanor of the committee embodied many of the standard complaints directed toward physicians in tertiary-care settings—impersonal, businesslike exchanges, directed by anonymous professionals, and questions which presumed the priority of the professionals' agenda. But the agenda, at least as the patient perceived it, was overtly moralistic rather than professional, as the committee probed the cause of the patient's HIV infection and her reasons for wanting to bear a child. Some committee members "seemed angry at me and asked how I could be making plans so far into the future . . ." Finally, the committee made, not a recommendation to the physician, but a decision, delivered to the patient by the ethics committee chair.

In sum, in this patient's view the committee treated her like "a child," put her "on trial," found her "guilty" and denied her medical services. She summarized her feelings: "I didn't need them practicing morality on me."

The patient's story was followed in the next issue of the *Cambridge Quarterly* by a response from the ethics committee chair (1992b, pp. 285– 286). While acknowledging that the patient may have felt as if the committee "ganged up" on her, the chair portrayed the patient as ambivalent in her desire for surgery. She maintained that "the consultation process did facilitate this couple's ability to resolve their dilemma." The chair also listed ways the committee could improve the consultation process, which she portrayed as too dominated by the "didactic manner" of experts.

What is distressing about the ethics committee chair's response is the subtle discrediting of the patient's perspective and the ease with which this chair dismissed legitimate moral concerns as matters of process and protocol. The chair repeatedly said of the patient's views that they were "interesting." But most telling is the summary statement of the chair following her list of proposed improvements: "We feel that instituting some or all of these measures will improve the consultation process and help to make it a positive and rewarding experience for all concerned." The chair seemed oblivious to the connection between the consultation process and the conclusion the committee reached, as if an encounter which left the patient feeling infantilized and morally judged can be separated from whether the committee rendered good advice. It

is unclear whether this ethics committee did more harm than good.

Can an ethics consultation be good when nobody says hello, that is, when the discussion about what is good or right lacks human qualities of respect and sympathy? A decision on the part of the patient to do what most persons might agree is "best" is morally bankrupt if the price of getting the patient to this decision is questioning the patient's character. Not just the decision, but the decisional process, must be patient-centered. The only person likely to have been well-served by this consultation was the physician, who was given the ethics committee's approval for not doing what he apparently did not want to do.

These brief accounts from a patient and an ethics committee chair raise profound questions about whether ethics committees can serve both patients and caregivers, to say nothing of institutions. But my concern here is with whose notion of "ethics" is at work in this committee. We are not told exactly what the ethics committee's understanding of "ethics" is, except that, in the chair's words, it involved "principles" and a "process." Yet whatever principles or process were in use, it is clear that the committee's concept of ethics was dominant over the patient's. The committee effectively substituted their own version of "the case" for the patient's moral experiences. It should not be surprising that the patient felt disenfranchised and angry. If this is how ethics committees work, patients will correctly view them as representing only the interests of doctors and hospitals, and as indifferent or at worst hostile to their perspectives.[1]

III. Sacrificial Atonement

Fifteen years ago a patient-physician interaction was pivotal in demonstrating to me the inadequacy of much that goes under the name "bioethics."[2] This interaction involved a sixty-year-old woman being seen in the clinic for pain in the groin area and a palpable lump. Some years earlier, she had undergone amputation of her left leg but remained ambulant through the aid of a prosthesis and crutches. The physician strongly suspected that the mass represented a recurrence of the malignancy which had required taking her leg, but the patient, after hearing a careful explanation of the need for surgery, refused. A deeply religious person, she believed that God afflicted her with cancer in order to save souls. She saw the amputation of her leg as a "giving up to the Lord," an offering, or sacrifice, in order that through her example others could be reconciled to God. The loss of her leg was an atonement for the transgressions of a member of her local congregation—an interpretation which she announced and which was affirmed within her community. As an example of her witness, she told of a dream in which she was again whole, walking to visit a neighbor whom she knew to have end-stage carcinoma of the head and neck. Interpreting this dream as a sign to her, she and her husband went the following day to visit this neighbor. She later reported that this visit had a conversional and healing quality.

The physician interpreted this patient's refusal of treatment as a problem of noncompliance. He saw a clear need for a biopsy, and very probably surgery and/or radiation. The principle-oriented bioethicist in attendance saw the situation as a classic conflict of respect for autonomy with paternalism. The "issue" was how aggressively to test the authenticity of the patient's refusal, and whether beneficent paternalism (pressing for treatment) might be justified in this situation.

What is impressive here is just how wide of the mark both the physician *and* the bioethicist were. Neither "noncompliance" nor "autonomy" were meaningful terms for this patient. To suggest that either of them captured the true significance of her choice would be like treating a myth as a propositional statement, for example, treating the creation stories in Genesis as literal accounts, or Aesop's fable of the hare and the tortoise as an historical occurrence. As Maurice Merleau-Ponty put it, it would be "like applying our own grammar and vocabulary to a foreign language" (1964, p. 121).

The first and most basic task in ethics is paying attention to the moral phenomena. Paying attention requires not only suspending immediate judgments of right and wrong, but also suspending our usual categories of interpretation. If ethics is not one thing but many—not one kind of human activity, but a complex variety of activities held together for each person in unique ways—then it is essential to let people speak for themselves, and in their own terms, about the moral dimensions of their lives. Interpretation, of course, always follows, but it should not precede and preempt the voices of the morally perplexed, nor should it presume finality of interpretive power over these voices.

The patient requesting surgery for tubal blockage may have been heard by the ethics committee, but there is no evidence for it, in either her comments or those of the committee chair. The chair analyzed the difficulties as administrative in nature, a problem of how to handle a demanding and distraught patient. Judging from the written record, the ethical problem was defined and then managed by the committee, not *with* the patient, but *for* the patient. The patient never appeared; "Nobody said hello."

The patient who refused surgery in order to continue her evangelical mission simply went unheard. The key interpretive concepts of her life (sin, and salvation through sacrificial atonement) had priority for neither physician nor philosopher. Neither shared her universe of discourse. To the physician she appeared as noncompliant, and irrational. To the philosopher her decision took the form of an ill-advised exercise of autonomy. Neither physician nor philosopher was prepared to see (much less affirm) her refusal of treatment as part of a larger healing ritual for her and her community.

IV. Bioethics in Social Context

The two scenes described above display presumptions of professional privilege, both medical and bioethical. These presumptions have practical implications; they not only distort, they disable as well. They distort patient (and professional) experiences, and they disable persons from using their own moral resources at critical life junctures when they need these resources most.

Bioethics conceived as a part of a larger social inquiry can help to disabuse us of this sort of parochialism. Social research places physicians and patients in a cultural and historical, and not just a medical and moral, interaction. It attends to power differentials and to the nuanced exchanges that characterize physician-patient interaction. Socially informed perspectives see illnesses not just as standard pathological entities but as dynamic concepts, dependent for their meaning on personal and institutional settings. Social research recognizes the powerful ways that relationships can either enhance or defeat a therapeutic course. Bioethics conceived as a part of this larger social location of disease and illness, patients and doctors, brings into focus the local and distinctive meanings of moral quandaries, meanings forged in social exchanges rather than in theoretical systems. The typical mode of doing bioethics neglects these dimensions in favor of the search for general meanings (rather than particular ones) and sees these as the products of intellectual acumen and logical rigor (rather than social meanings and institutional forces).[3]

Historically, ethics in medicine has been a construct of physicians. As such it has emphasized the development of character, typically in terms of the given period's orthodox requirements for custom and decorum. The influx of philosophically trained ethicists over the past two decades has substantially changed this focus, away from character, custom and decorum, and toward the application of rules and principles. At the same time, a reaction against principled approaches is evident in the emphasis on narrative ethics. Yet narrative approaches still frequently carry an assumption typical of principled approaches about application, viz., that biomedical ethics is fundamentally "applied ethics"—if not the application of antecedently known principles, then the application of narrative methods and concepts to moral problems. The idea that the experiences of patients and doctors might themselves be key formative items for ethics, altering expectations for methods and requiring multiple approaches, has been only a minor note in the bioethics movement to date.

The philosophical, principle-oriented, version of "applied ethics" is the most familiar. Here bioethics means the uses of Kant, Mill, or Rawls (or pick your favorite theorist!) in the context of medicine and the health sciences. Tom Beauchamp and James Childress have done the most to popularize this view. Their book, *Principles of Biomedical Ethics,* is now in its fourth edition. The title bespeaks the methodology. Principles, they say in the first edition preface, bring "order and coherence" to the frequently "disjointed approach" that relies on discussion of cases (1979, p. vii). Principles provide a way to justify choices, to say why one action is morally preferable to another. Principles save us from ad hoc decisional processes and moral inconsistency. Biomedical ethics is, then, largely defined as the skillful use of the principles of autonomy, nonmaleficence, beneficence and justice in situations of moral complexity in health care. The fourth edition of *Principles of Biomedical Ethics* (1995) is less revisionist in its tone, and more eclectic in its approach, with greater attention to non-principled methods. Moreover, Beauchamp and Childress never claim that their approach describes the whole of the moral life, but only the justification of choices when faced with dilemmas. Those who employ their methods, however, are seldom as careful, or as cognizant of the limits of this approach.

Narrative ethics, with its emphasis on stories, substitutes what Stephen Crites calls the "narrative quality of experience" for principled reason (1971, pp. 291–311). Narrative ethics broadens what will count as morally significant, but it often retains a key prejudice characteristic of the heavy-handed use of principles. It retains the universalizing assumption of principled reasoning—the conviction that the job of ethics is to describe, if not the universal values, the universally correct metaethical position. It is this assumption that often gives the theoretical debates between Kantian deontologists, Benthamite utilitarians and narrative theologians such passion. Each is contending for dominance of the entire field, not just the validity of their perspective *among* others, but *over* all others. Crites, for example, working from the Augustinian notion that human experience is always time-laden or "tensed," extends this observation into a requirement for ethics, claiming that "ethical authority . . . is always a function of a common narrative coherence of life" (1971, p. 310). Stanley Hauerwas, with a more direct critical focus on bioethics, says that principled reason always functions in a story context, explicitly or implicitly, and that "character and moral notions only take on meaning in a narrative" (1977, p. 15). Alasdair MacIntyre asserts in *After Virtue,* "I can only answer the question 'What am I to do?' if I can answer the prior question 'Of what story or stories do I find myself a part?' " (1981, p. 201).

So while narrative bioethicists give us new concepts with which to work, they tend to overextend the range of these concepts, making them the new methodological requirements for ethics generally, and bioethics in particular. It may be true, as J. Hillis Miller claims, that "without storytelling there is no theory of ethics" (1987, p. 3), but ethical theorizing is not reducible to storytelling. Again, it is the overextension of a valid moral insight that is the source of the problem. As much as the principle-oriented bioethics which it eschews, narrative bioethics is too often in the service of an urge to provide not only A model *of* moral experience, but THE definitive model *for* moral experience.[4]

I criticize principled and narrative approaches because of their prominence, but the same criticism could be directed at the superordinate claims that occasionally come from those who espouse casuistry, hermeneutical approaches, feminist theories, and a variety of others.[5] Each of these approaches can add a valuable dimension to bioethics, but none alone has adequate range or depth to encompass the field or fold the others under its interpretive grid.

The universalizing urge of bioethical theorists blocks recognition of a central, empirical datum, viz., that the moral experiences of human life are more varied and complex than the theories we employ to grasp them conceptually. This is true generally, but especially apparent in the moral experiences that are part of health care. Practice continues to outrun and elude theoretical encapsulation. Ethical theories are best seen, then, not as competitors for the whole of moral life, but as potentially complementary modes of approach, each with a useful, but limited, range of application. In bioethics this means that no one theory can do full justice to the experiences of patients who are ill and those who care for them. We should be suspicious of theories that claim universal purchase, and cautious about the drive for all-encompassing formulations. The theories will prove to be procrustean beds, and the drive will distract us from attending carefully to the variety of human moral dynamics.

The appropriate methodological stance for dealing with this experiential complexity is not an anti-theoretical posture, but one open to the multiplication of theories. What our experiences require is not *the* theory (or no theories), but several theories. Differing theories are best seen as complements rather than competitors, with each describing a facet of moral life, each supplying something other theories lack. Bioethicists do us a disservice if they make us choose between Kant and Mill, or Rawls and MacIntyre, or suggest that the resolution of competing theories (deontological vs. utilitarian, etc.) should be sought in a supertheory that transcends the others. If human moral experiences were simple and shallow, a single theoretical framework might capture them all. Since they are not, we are free to welcome many theories, and perhaps periodically revive old ones and concoct new ones to keep the variety and depth of moral experience displayed before us. We must resist the philosopher's platonic hankerings for moral ideals or decisional processes that will both transcend human experiences and somehow become the measure of them all.

The urge for theoretical hegemony can take several forms. Some bioethicists have suggested that the inadequacy of any single type of theory to cover the wide diversity of moral experiences should lead us to devise a supertheory that will teach us how to use the right theory in the right way at the right time. For example, in the introduction to the second edition of their widely used anthology, *Ethical Issues in Modern Medicine,* John Arras and Robert Hunt say "It is our contention that, if answers to ethical issues are to be found, they are to be found through the development of a cogent and comprehensive ethical theory—a theory that will both explain the principles of morality and give us a guide to their application" (1983, p. vii). While recognizing the need for theoretical pluralism, these authors seem to be holding out the hope that the problems of skillful use of the tools and methods of

ethics can still be resolved at the theoretical level, in some sort of "comprehensive" theory. While this is an improvement over the view that some single principle or theory will have universal validity, it still seeks resolution in the conceptual realm, rather than through a closer and more perceptive grasp of the social and cultural factors of the situations in which theories are used. Interestingly, the most recent edition of *Ethical Issues in Modern Medicine,* drops the aspiration for comprehensiveness. Here Arras and his new collaborator, Bonnie Steinbock, make more modest claims and affirm the dynamic flux of experience and judgments, saying the best we can hope for is greater, but not complete, systematic coherence (1995, p. 39). This recognition is the beginning step to the more full contextualization of ethics I am arguing for in this essay.

How does ethics in the context of a larger social inquiry help to avoid this tendency toward universalist assumptions and superordinate theoretical processes in ethics? By insisting that ethics be done in a cross-disciplinary fashion, using the tools and perspectives of disciplines like literary criticism, medical sociology, and cultural anthropology. Let me explain what I mean through an example, an example of moral exchange central to health care, but one which is elusive to the usual ways of doing ethics.

John Berger and Jean Mohr's account of a British GP, entitled *A Fortunate Man*, contains the following scene:

> Once he was putting a syringe deep into a man's chest: there was little question of pain but it made the man feel bad: the man tried to explain his revulsion: "That's where I live, where you're putting the needle in." "I know," Sassell said, "I know what it feels like. I can't bear anything done near my eyes, I can't bear to be touched there. I think that's where I live, just under and behind my eyes" (1976, pp. 47, 50).

What is interesting about this slice of conversation is how it conveys experiences of suffering and empathy—items central to the moral life of medicine. But notice, there are no decisions portrayed here, no problems delineated, no priorities sorted. Rather what is displayed is what sociologist Arthur Frank calls "recognition" (1991, pp. 49–55).[6]

Describing his own experiences first with a heart attack, then with cancer, Frank says that a critical illness is like a journey that takes its travelers to the margins of life. He believes that the central task in giving care to patients is recognizing the journey they are on. He reserves the name "caregivers" to people who listen to the ill, witness to the particulars of patients' illnesses and "recognize" them—a feat Frank believes most hospital staff have little time for (1991, pp. 48–49). Frank concludes that the power to recognize others on their journey of suffering is "fundamental to our humanity" (1991, p. 104).

My point in this example is that bioethical inquiry which is methodologically conceived and practiced in the context of the other social sciences and humanities stands a better chance of noticing and accrediting these non-decisional aspects, like "empathy," "journey," and "recognition"—aspects which are not peripheral, but central to medicine and the health professions, and which figure heavily in the shape and meaning of moral quandaries. Ethics has as much to do with how well we attend as with how well we decide, and this is a skill characteristic of good field work in sociology and anthropology. Conceptions of ethics which pay no attention to attending, which have no category called "recognition," are weakened by this absence.

Principle-oriented, applied-ethics bioethicists do, of course, use terms like "empathy" and "recognition" in their analyses. Yet they are usually pressing to get beyond these items to a formulation of "the problem" or "the issue" that will allow them to apply their principles. They tend to see empathy and recognition as preliminaries to the real work of ethics. In the gadarene rush to proper formulation, they sometimes miss the items of major importance.[7]

Ludwig Wittgenstein put it well in *Zettel:*

Here we come up against a remarkable and characteristic phenomenon in philosophical investigation: the difficulty—I might say—is not that of finding the solution but rather that of recognizing as the solution something that looks as if it were only a preliminary to it. "We have already said everything.—Not anything that follows from this, no, *this* itself is the solution!"

This is connected, I believe, with our wrongly expecting an explanation, whereas the solution of the difficulty is a description, if we give it the right place in our considerations. If we dwell upon it, and do not try to get beyond it.

The difficulty here is: to stop (1967, parag. 314).

The difficulty Wittgenstein attributed to philosophical investigation is also characteristic of bioethical inquiry. The difficulty in "recognizing" persons, in stopping and accrediting the great variety of moral experiences and valid problem-solving strategies, is part of American bioethics. I am not, to be sure, arguing that bioethics need *only* describe and not explain or guide. I am arguing that privileging theory in the way described above gives description too little place in ethics. And giving description a more robust place will enhance our skills in recognizing and accrediting what we are prone to rush past.

In summary, I have argued that this difficulty in attending and recognizing is tied to restrictive methodological assumptions about the fields of bioethics. These restrictive assumptions are not just unfortunate blindspots, but potentially disabling forces to those who are most vulnerable and powerless in medical interactions. I have also argued that placing bioethical inquiry in the larger context of other humanities and social science disciplines will help to counter this methodological parochialism. The distinct advantage of placing bioethics in social context is that an interdisciplinary setting makes it less likely that we will be seduced by the intellectual glamor, or the intuitive emotional appeal, of any single approach to moral problems. Resisting a hypertheoretical approach to the methods of bioethics will make for greater agility in problem-solving, and more resilience in facing those problems that cannot be solved. It will, in the end, make for better health professionals, and for better patient care.

Notes

1. An interesting move in the right direction is Susan M. Wolf's "Toward A Theory of Process," *Law, Medicine and Health Care* 20 (Winter, 1992): 278–289. Wolf argues that the lack of attention to process poses a serious threat to patients.
2. I have discussed this experience previously in "Bioethical Reductionism and Our Sense of the Human," *Man and Medicine* 5 (November 4, 1980): 229–242.
3. Thomas H. Murray, writing in a spirit congenial to this essay, analyzes the Dax Cowart films with attention to the social, psychological, and political detail (and not just the conflicting principles) in "Moral Reasoning in Social Context." *Journal of Social Issues* 49 (1993): 185–200.
4. In contrast to the sweeping claims of some narrative bioethicists, Rita Charon articulates a more balanced view, signaled in the title of her essay "Narrative Contributions to Medical Ethics." Here she argues for a necessary place for narrative among other methods of ethics, and that bioethicists need as much facility in listening and interpreting as they have in applying principles; "narrative competence is among the required capacities of any biomedical ethicist" (1994, p. 275). Charon's point of view is entirely congenial with the perspective I argue for in this essay.
5. See, for example, the excellent work by Albert Jonsen and Stephen Toulmin, *The Abuse of Casuistry* (Berkeley, Cal.: University of California Press, 1988). Toulmin, however, occasionally carries his zeal for practical rea-

soning to an antitheoretical extreme. For example, he has recently claimed that the casuistical analysis of actual cases in clinical medicine is "pretheoretical," by which he means that the moral significance of these cases can be stated in a way that is neutral as between theoretical constructs. See here his essay "Casuistry and Clinical Ethics," in *A Matter of Principles,* ed. Edwin R. DuBose, Ron Hamel, and Laurence J. O'Connell (Valley Forge, Penn.: Trinity Press International, 1994), 310ff. Yet I think it can be shown that casuistry is not pretheoretical, or neutral, but theory-laden, insofar as it is committed to a tradition of naturalistic, Aristotelian interpretations about how ethical problems arise and how they are properly solved. Casuistry is, after all, one ethical method of problem-formulation and problem-solving among others, not the theory-free description Toulmin claims. Rather than try to get behind, or beyond, ethical theory, the more productive effort lies in spotting the *misuses* of theory. Theories, of course, can obscure and frustrate, as well as illuminate and facilitate problem-solving. The trick lies in using theories judiciously. In brief, Toulmin is on target with his criticisms, but wrong in his view that somehow casuistry is exempt from these criticisms.

An alternative, and perhaps more accurate, interpretation of Toulmin is that the target of his criticism is only the kind of theorizing that assumes hegemony over the terms of moral debate and insight, and that he would allow for the kind of low-altitude theorizing I want to endorse here, and which I find evident in his own embrace of casuistry. If this is the correct interpretation of Toulmin's polemic against theory, then I share his critical agenda, but remain skeptical about the preeminence of casuistical analysis.

6. For an excellent development of the concept "recognition" that also draws from Arthur Frank's work see Ronald A. Carson's "Beyond Respect to Recognition and Due Regard," in *Chronic Illness: From Experience to Policy,* edited by S. Kay Toombs, David Barnard, and Ronald Carson (Bloomington, Ind.: Indiana University Press, 1995).
7. The original "gadarene rush" is recorded in Matthew 8:27ff., and refers to the manner in which a demon-possessed herd of swine found their way down a steep bank and into the Sea of Galilee.

References

Anonymous: 1992a, "Bedside Story," *Cambridge Quarterly of Healthcare Ethics* 2, 185–186.

Anonymous: 1992b, "Bedside Story," *Cambridge Quarterly of Healthcare Ethics* 3, 285–286.

Arras, J. and Hunt, R. (eds.): 1983 (2nd ed.), *Ethical Issues in Modern Medicine,* Mayfield Publishing Company, Palo Alto.

Arras, J. and Steinbock, B. (eds.): 1995 (4th ed.), *Ethical Issues in Modern Medicine,* Mayfield Publishing Company, Palo Alto.

Beauchamp, T. and Childress, J.: 1979 (1st ed.), 1995 (4th ed.), *Principles of Biomedical Ethics,* Oxford, New York.

Berger, J. and Mohr, J.: 1976, *A Fortunate Man,* Writers and Readers Publishing Cooperative, London.

Crites, S.: 1971, "The Narrative Quality of Experience," *Journal of the American Academy of Religion* XXXIX, 291–311.

Frank, A.: 1991, *At the Will of the Body,* Houghton Mifflin Company, Boston.

Hauerwas, S.: 1977, *Truthfulness and Tragedy,* University of Notre Dame, Notre Dame, Ind.

MacIntyre, A.: 1981, *After Virtue,* University of Notre Dame, Notre Dame, Ind.

Merleau-Ponty, M.: 1964, *Signs,* R. McLeary (trans.) Northwestern, Evanston, Ill.

Wittgenstein, L.: 1967, *Zettel,* G. Anscombe (trans.), Basil Blackwell, Oxford.

The Use of Force

William Carlos Williams

■

They were new patients to me, all I had was the name, Olson. Please come down as soon as you can, my daughter is very sick.

When I arrived I was met by the mother, a big startled looking woman, very clean and apologetic who merely said, Is this the doctor? and let me in. In the back, she added. You must excuse us, doctor, we have her in the kitchen where it is warm. It is very damp here sometimes.

The child was fully dressed and sitting on her father's lap near the kitchen table. He tried to get up, but I motioned for him not to bother, took off my overcoat and started to look things over. I could see that they were all very nervous, eyeing me up and down distrustfully. As often, in such cases, they weren't telling me more than they had to, it was up to me to tell them; that's why they were spending three dollars on me.

The child was fairly eating me up with her cold, steady eyes, and no expression to her face whatever. She did not move and seemed, inwardly, quiet; an unusually attractive little thing, and as strong as a heifer in appearance. But her face was flushed, she was breathing rapidly, and I realized that she had a high fever. She had magnificent blonde hair, in profusion. One of those picture children often reproduced in advertising leaflets and the photogravure sections of the Sunday papers.

She's had a fever for three days, began the father and we don't know what it comes from. My wife has given her things, you know, like people do, but it don't do no good. And there's been a lot of sickness around. So we tho't you'd better look her over and tell us what is the matter.

As doctors often do I took a trial shot at it as a point of departure. Has she had a sore throat?

Both parents answered me together, No . . . No, she says her throat don't hurt her.

Does your throat hurt you? added the mother to the child. But the little girl's expression didn't change nor did she move her eyes from my face.

Have you looked?

I tried to, said the mother, but I couldn't see.

As it happens we had been having a number of cases of diphtheria in the school to which this child went during that month and we were all, quite apparently, thinking of that, though no one had as yet spoken of the thing.

Well, I said, suppose we take a look at the throat first. I smiled in my best professional manner and asking for the child's first name I said, come on, Mathilda, open your mouth and let's take a look at your throat.

Nothing doing.

Aw, come on, I coaxed, just open your mouth wide and let me take a look. Look, I said opening both hands wide, I haven't anything in my hands. Just open up and let me see.

Such a nice man, put in the mother. Look how kind he is to you. Come on, do what he tells you to. He won't hurt you.

At that I ground my teeth in disgust. If only they wouldn't use the word "hurt" I might be able to get somewhere. But I did not allow myself to be hurried or disturbed but speaking quietly and slowly I approached the child again.

As I moved my chair a little nearer suddenly with one catlike movement both her hands clawed instinctively for my eyes and she almost reached them too. In fact she knocked my glasses flying and they fell, though unbroken, several feet away from me on the kitchen floor.

Both the mother and father almost turned themselves inside out in embarrassment and apology. You bad girl, said the mother, taking her and shaking her by one arm. Look what you've done. The nice man . . .

For heaven's sake, I broke in. Don't call me a nice man to her. I'm here to look at her throat on the chance that she might have diphtheria and possibly die of it. But that's nothing to her. Look here, I said to the child, we're going to look at your throat. You're old enough to understand what I'm saying. Will you open it now by yourself or shall we have to open it for you?

Not a move. Even her expression hadn't changed. Her breaths however were coming faster and faster. Then the battle began. I had to do it. I had to have a throat culture for her own protection. But first I told the parents that it was entirely up to them. I explained the danger but said that I would not insist on a throat examination so long as they would take the responsibility.

If you don't do what the doctor says you'll have to go to the hospital, the mother admonished her severely.

Oh yeah? I had to smile to myself. After all, I had already fallen in love with the savage brat, the parents were contemptible to me. In the ensuing struggle they grew more and more abject, crushed, exhausted while she surely rose to magnificent heights of insane fury of effort bred of her terror of me.

The father tried his best, and he was a big man but the fact that she was his daughter, his shame at her behavior and his dread of hurting her made him release her just at the critical moment several times when I had almost achieved success, till I wanted to kill him. But his dread also that she might have diphtheria made him tell me to go on, go on though he himself was almost fainting, while the mother moved back and forth behind us raising and lowering her hands in an agony of apprehension.

Put her in front of you on your lap, I ordered, and hold both her wrists.

But as soon as he did the child let out a scream.

Don't, you're hurting me. Let go of my hands. Let them go I tell you. Then she shrieked terrifyingly, hysterically. Stop it! Stop it! You're killing me!

Do you think she can stand it, doctor! said the mother.

You get out, said the husband to his wife. Do you want her to die of diphtheria?

Come on now, hold her, I said.

Then I grasped the child's head with my left hand and tried to get the wooden tongue depressor between her teeth. She fought, with clenched teeth, desperately! But now I also had grown furious—at a child. I tried to hold myself down but I couldn't. I know how to expose a throat for inspection. And I did my best. When finally I got the wooden spatula behind the last teeth and just the point of it into the mouth cavity, she opened up for an instant but before I could see anything she came down again and gripping the wooden blade between her molars she reduced it to splinters before I could get it out again.

Aren't you ashamed, the mother yelled at her. Aren't you ashamed to act like that in front of the doctor?

Get me a smooth-handled spoon of some sort, I told the mother. We're going through with this. The child's mouth was already bleeding. Her tongue was cut and she was screaming in wild hysterical shrieks. Perhaps I should have desisted and come back in an hour or more. No doubt it would have been better. But I have seen at least two children lying dead in bed of neglect in such cases, and feeling that I must get a diagnosis now or never I went at it again. But the worst of it was that I too had got beyond reason. I could have torn the child apart in my own fury and enjoyed it. It was a pleasure to attack her. My face was burning with it.

The damned little brat must be protected against her own idiocy, one says to one's self at such times. Others must be protected against her. It is social necessity. And all these things are true. But a blind fury, a feeling of adult shame, bred of a longing for muscular release are the operatives. One goes on to the end.

In a final unreasoning assault I overpowered the child's neck and jaws. I forced the heavy silver spoon back of her teeth and down her throat till she gagged. And there it was—both tonsils covered with membrane. She had fought valiantly to keep me from knowing her secret. She had been hiding that sore throat for three days at least and lying to her parents in order to escape just such an outcome as this.

Now truly she *was* furious. She had been on the defensive before but now she attacked. Tried to get off her father's lap and fly at me while tears of defeat blinded her eyes.

Case Study:

The "Student Doctor" and

a Wary Patient

Marc D. Basson, Gerald Dworkin,

and Eric J. Cassell

■

Like many medical schools, State Medical College permits its third-year students to rotate through Anesthesiology for a month. During the first week, students follow Anesthesiology residents as they visit patients. Then students are assigned their own patients. After obtaining informed consent, they administer anesthesia under supervision.

James Denton is one such third-year student, rotating through the Smithville VA, an affiliated hospital. His first solo patient is Robert Criswell, a sixty-four-year-old man with metastatic prostate cancer who is scheduled to undergo bilateral orchiectomy (castration) in the morning. Criswell has a history of heavy smoking and poor pulmonary function, so James reasons that a spinal anesthetic would be safer than general anesthesia.

The attending anesthesiologist tentatively agrees to this plan. "You've done lumbar punctures before, haven't you?" the anesthesiologist asks. James says that he has done one spinal tap previously, but had great difficulty with it. He adds that he has seen three others performed. "Well, you've got to learn some time," responds the anesthesiologist. "Don't worry, I'll be with you."

James returns to the ward and finds Mr. Criswell. The residents have advised him to introduce himself as "Doctor" Denton so as not to frighten the patient unnecessarily. Some of James's fellow students use deliberately ambiguous phrases such as "one of the anesthesiology team that will be taking care of you." James selects a popular alternative, introducing himself as "a student doctor from Anesthesiology."

James tells Mr. Criswell that he would like to use spinal anesthesia and explains the procedure for lumbar puncture. "You should know," he says as he fills in the consent sheet, "that like any other medical procedure a lumbar puncture has risks, including bleeding, infection, paralysis, pain, and perhaps even death. Also, a few people develop severe headaches after such a procedure and we will ask you to lie flat for twenty-four hours afterwards to lessen the chances of this happening."

"Tell me, doctor," Criswell asks, "have you ever had any of these problems with your patients?" James feels uneasy at being called a doctor and at Criswell's assumption that he has done many lumbar punctures before, but he decides that this is not the time to bring up his inexperience. "No, never, although I have seen one moderately severe spinal headache lasting for three days in a friend's patient," he responds.

"That's OK, I can take a headache," Criswell says as he signs the consent form. "I didn't want to insult you or anything. It's just that I've heard all kinds of stories about those medical students from the university coming over here to practice on the vets and leaving them paralyzed for life."

How should James Denton introduce himself? Is he morally or legally obligated to discuss his inexperience in obtaining an informed consent? Would it make a difference if the patient had never raised the issue of experience?
Marc D. Basson

Commentary
Gerald Dworkin

Considering the frequency with which situations similar to the one described in this case arise in everyday medical practice, it is surprising that the legitimacy of what occurs has not occasioned greater ethical scrutiny. Perhaps this is a specific instance of the generalization that the amount of attention paid to ethical issues is inversely proportional to their frequency in practice. Abortions performed because the life of the mother is threatened by pregnancy account for a minuscule proportion of the total, but occupy a fairly high proportion of the philosophical literature. This case, involving the training of students by allowing them to practice technical procedures on patients under supervision, occurs routinely. Yet the only public discussion I have seen concerned the bizarre case of a salesman from a medical instrumentation company who was allowed to operate on patients—without their knowledge—in order to demonstrate the nature and value of his company's products.

We are not faced here with a moral dilemma. This is not a situation in which there are good reasons of a fairly weighty nature for and against a certain course of action. A patient is being misled as to the qualifications, experience, and competence of his "healer." He thinks that James is a doctor (when he is not). He thinks that James has performed this procedure many times before (when he has not). He thinks that James has fairly wide experience with the possible side effects of the procedures (when he has not). While the violation of informed consent is not as gross as that which occurs very commonly when a surgeon does not tell his patient that the operation will actually be performed by a resident or intern (under the surgeon's supervision), the interference with the patient's ability to make an informed choice is clear. In the absence of exceptions to the principle of informed consent, we must condemn this practice.

By exceptions to the principle of informed consent, I mean factors such as impossibility (the patient is unconscious or an infant), waiver (the patient has waived the right to be informed), ex-

ternal justification (getting the consent of the patient would violate more important rights of others), internal justification (the ends served by the rule would be better served by making an exception).

In this case I do not see that such factors are present, and I conclude therefore that James ought to inform his patient of his status, experience, and qualifications. The patient then could either decide to go ahead or ask for a more experienced physician. The fact that the patient has explicitly raised the issue of experience is only relevant insofar as it offers empirical evidence that this patient is particularly worried about this matter. But it is reasonable to assume that all patients have a concern about their doctor's experience and competence, and would want to know that this is the first time he or she is performing a fairly risky procedure.

This answer to the particular issue does not, however, address the more general concern underlying the practice; namely, that we would all be worse off if surgeons and anesthesiologists could not be trained and training requires "hands on" experience. The solution is not deception, but finding ways to make it attractive for patients to agree to being the subjects of such training. It is reasonable for teaching hospitals to claim that the quality of care they provide is better than that of nonteaching hospitals, and that the "price" for this is that patients agree to being part of the training process. As long as this is done forthrightly, and patients have some degree of choice as to the hospitals they enter, I see no objection. Or perhaps there could be a price differential, depending on whether a doctor performed the operation or merely supervised it. This is common practice for analysts-in-training, who charge their patients a greatly reduced fee.

It is worth noting that the problem of "hands on" training is not confined to the medical profession. Airline pilots, automobile mechanics, sushi chefs, student drivers, hairdressers, psychotherapists—all have to impose risks on others in order to learn their skills. But those who bear the risks ought to be aware that they are doing so and be compensated in some fashion for their cooperation.

Commentary
Eric J. Cassell

This case raises two distinct questions. The first is how the medical student, James Denton, should respond to the patient who questions his qualifications. The second is the more general question of whether medical educators are justified in allowing trainees to have primary responsibility for the care of the sick when more qualified physicians are available.

James Denton is obligated to tell the patient, Robert Criswell, the truth. But that is not the end of the matter, it is merely the beginning. Ethical issues such as truth-telling are too often dealt with as though they stood alone and timeless, like public monuments. These problems achieve their importance because of their place in human relations—of persons to themselves and to others. In medical practice, telling the truth serves something larger than itself. It is, for example, an important aspect of trust, and trust is fundamental in the doctor-patient relationship. But trust is a complex, poorly understood matter and so it is easier to discuss truth-telling in the same over-simplified way that we often discuss other ethical issues like autonomy.

Consider this case again. Robert Criswell has metastatic cancer of the prostate and he is about to have his testicles removed. From this history we do not know much about him, but if he is like most of us, he may be frightened by his situation. He is in a VA hospital where the care is sometimes impersonal and where his need for reassurance and for the information that might reduce his uncertainties may not be met.

Into that setting walks James Denton, third-year student cum anesthesiologist, also frightened and unsure. The way this case history is recounted suggests that they are adversaries. On the contrary, they are natural allies (like many, perhaps most, doctors and sick patients) because they need each other. Should Denton be honest? Of course he must tell the truth. But then he must actively set out to win Criswell's trust because both he and the patient need it. He must make it clear that he is a novice, but just because of that he will be more attentive and more concerned about Criswell's well-being than another, more experienced anesthesiologist might be. For this and other reasons (including the fact that information can itself be therapeutic when properly employed) he will carefully explain what is to be done, why it is being done, and what it means to Criswell, answering each of the patient's questions (and getting the correct information when he does not know). He will point out that the attending physician will be watching over them to make sure nothing goes wrong, and that he, James Denton, will visit Criswell while he is in the hospital.

For the rest of his life, if he takes care of patients, James Denton will be talking people into doing things that, while for their benefit, may be fraught with risk and fear. And on many of those occasions he will be pursued by doubts and well aware that others might do things better. That is the nature of medical care. Of course, when trust has been created and nurtured, it must not be betrayed because that is worse than lying.

This case does not describe an isolated instance, although "see one, do one, teach one" is an exaggeration of the problem. It is the strength of American medical education that physicians learn while taking care of patients under the guidance of more experienced teachers. However, the teachers, especially attending physicians, could often give better, more efficient, and less costly care to a particular patient than their trainees. Indeed, the student or house officer may be learning on someone who has been the patient of the teacher for many years. In that case the attending physician further helps the doctor in training by including him or her within the bonds of trust that have developed over those years. How, then, can we justify this method of education? Without this system of supervised learning by doing, teachers themselves would not be well trained and the qualifications of the whole profession would suffer.

What I have touched on so briefly describes a complex system of relationships and bonds that are part of the moral nature of the institution of medicine. Many would be quick to point out the ethical error if James Denton lied to Robert Criswell about his professional status. Those same critics, both inside and outside of the profession, might consider it old-fashioned, "hierarchical," or too conservative to worry about such important moral flaws as the failure to give deference to attending physicians and patients, the failure to protect the bonds of trust between patient and doctor, and the failure to protect both the past and the future of the profession of medicine. But a lie by James Denton threatens only Denton and Criswell, while those other "old-fashioned" flaws endanger the integrity of the profession without which no one would take this case seriously.

Truth Telling to the Patient
Antonella Surbone

■

And you shall know the truth, and the truth shall make you free.—John 8:32

When I started writing this letter last year, I was practicing medical oncology in the United States. My work, based on providing thorough information to every patient, was that of an expert in a particular field as well as an educator. By explaining diagnosis, prognosis, and treatment options to the patient, I was creating the basis for freedom: freedom not only from symptoms and disease, but also freedom to make informed choices. At the same time, I grew to believe that truth telling goes far beyond providing mere information. Truth is not just the opposite of a lie, not just the sum of correct statements, but a reciprocal state in the patient-physician relationship. This relationship is established on the basis of mutual responsibilities. In such a context, information should never become a way of delegating the entire burden of medical decisions to the patient, thus limiting medical responsibilities. Truth should expand rather than limit professional responsibilities.

The Italian Deontology Code and Withholding Truth

While reflecting on my responsibility to provide patients with information, which is an ethical duty of American physicians,[1] I often thought of the different approaches used in my country of origin, Italy, where patients are not always informed of their diagnosis and prognosis. In medical school at the University of Turin in the late 1970s, I learned the Italian Deontology Code, written by the Italian Medical Association, which included the following statement: "A serious or lethal prognosis can be hidden from the patient, but not from the family."[2]

During my first year of oncology fellowship in Italy in 1983, a middle-aged businessman was told he had gastritis, when dying of cachexia from end-stage carcinoma; a young, divorced housewife was told she had arthritis while receiving palliative radiation therapy for chemotherapy-resistant metastatic breast cancer; and a college student was told he had drug-induced hepatitis, but he was indeed progressing toward liver failure from widespread hepatic involvement with lymphoma. In each case the patient's family or only one family member was informed of the true diagnosis and prognosis. A ritual started, composed of sotto voce conversations between the physician and family members outside the patient's room: "Doctor, don't speak too loud" or "Doctor, tell me how much time is left for my husband, because I have to prepare." In each case, the patients knew or at least strongly suspected the truth, but they were part of a generally accepted farce of deception that prevented open discussion about the truth and how to act on it. Consequences of such deception varied from the unresolved financial problems left at the businessman's death, to the stressful, secret, and unsuccessful attempt of the dying single mother to find a way to provide for the future of her four children.

In 1986, an Italian public television survey of a sample population representative of the entire nation showed that Italians were more or less equally divided in their preferences for truth telling in medicine. A 1991 study of 1171 breast cancer patients and their physicians and surgeons in general hospitals in Italy evaluated the frequency of disclosure of the diagnosis of operable breast cancer.[3] Only 47% of these patients reported having been told that they had cancer, and 25% of their physicians stated they had not given accurate information. After reading the results of this study, I asked myself, from an assimilated American perspective, how could such women not participate in the decision to undergo mastectomy or breast-conserving surgery, especially in those cases where we predict the outcomes to be equivalent?[4]

Later in 1991, I accepted my present position as vice-chairman in the oncology department of Santa Chiara Hospital in Pisa, Italy. The situation in the Italian medical world is rapidly evolving, with malpractice lawsuits increasing and the public skepticism of physicians on the rise.[5,6] It is in this reality that bioethical issues, including patients' rights to information, are the subject of frequent discussions among physicians.

The Deontology Code was revised in 1989 and it now reads as follows:

The physician has the duty to provide the patient—according to his cultural level and abilities to understand—the most serene information about the diagnosis, the prognosis and the therapeutic perspectives and their consequences; in the awareness of the limits of medical knowledge, in the respect of the person's rights, to foster the best compliance to the therapeutic proposals. Each question asked by the patient has to be accepted and answered clearly. The physician might evaluate, specifically in relationship with the patient's reactions, the opportunity not to reveal to the patient or to mitigate a serious or lethal prognosis. In this case it will have to be communicated to the family. In any event, the patient's will, freely expressed, should represent for the physician [an] element to which he will inspire his behavior.[7]

With regard to informed consent and participation in clinical studies, the Code states "experimentation is subordinated to the consent of the subject which has to be—if possible—freely expressed in writing."[8] In each of these statements the possibility of truth withholding still exists, and I think this can only be understood by considering the Italian cultural background.

I must first stress that I believe that ethics is inevitably connected to cultural values and, therefore, varies in different societies. This requires an implicit understanding of the dichotomy between believing in absolute values and respecting the pluralism of different cultures. This is to say, as difficult as it may sound for someone only used to one culture, that both the Italian and the American ways are ethical in their context.

Autonomia e Isolamento

First, the Italian culture is strongly bound to the Greek and Latin approaches to medicine. "To benefit, at least not to harm," wrote Hippocrates. Benefit is the priority in the patient-physician relationship. In a recent public debate in Rome among physicians and journalists on truth telling, even those stating that information is the basis for the contract between patient and physician stressed that the first aim of such a contract is not information, but what is good for the patient.[9] In bioethics, practical directions derive from a balance between the two principles of beneficence and autonomy. While the concept of beneficence is quite similarly perceived in Italy and in the United States, autonomy is certainly viewed in different ways.

In the Italian culture, autonomy (*autonomia*) is often synonymous for isolation (*isolamento*). The Italian patient is frequently viewed as being unable to learn enough to make appropriate autonomous health care decisions. Autonomy thus would easily become isolation for a person overwhelmed by complicated and frightening information that does not develop into knowledge. If information does not create knowledge, it does not create a positive autonomy. Protecting the ill family member from painful information is seen as essential for keeping the family together and not allowing the ill member to suffer alone. In addition, many Italians find it difficult to openly confront sickness and death.

Today, many Americans usually demand and are given information that enables them to make decisions either autonomously or with a physician's advice about their health care. Ancient Greek philosophers disputed the possibility of effectively communicating knowledge. Contemporary Italian attitudes perpetuate the belief that patients will never acquire enough knowledge to enable them to fully and appropriately participate in their care. As a result, the Italian physician remains a powerful, distant figure exercising unilateral decisions on the basis of knowledge that is assumed incommunicable.[10] "It is difficult to remain Imperator in the presence of a physician," said the Roman Emperor Hadrian in the second century,[11] and this seems to hold true even today.

Truth and the Therapeutic Relationship

We should never forget that the ill person, because of the nature of disease itself, is in a "uniquely dependent state."[12] The Italian Deontology Code thus allows physicians to use their experience and expertise to understand each patient and to establish how much information the patient can accept and process and in what manner the information is best conveyed. Any connection between patient and physician should be therapeutic. I firmly believe that truth is essential for a therapeutic relationship,[13] but I have to acknowledge that the Italian society is not prepared for the American way.

On the other hand, the Italian medical scene is

rapidly changing, and physicians are now confronted with medicolegal issues that did not exist a few years ago. Although strongly believing in the truth, I am concerned that Italian physicians may communicate vast amounts of complicated information to unprepared patients only out of fear of litigation. Should this happen, it probably will not give rise to real truth telling and may result in exhaustive lists of information that will not improve the patient-physician relationship.

The Italian bioethical situation regarding truth telling to patients is often compared with the US situation a few decades ago.[14] I believe Italians should not borrow the American way, but they should learn from Americans and try to find a better Italian way. I already see signs of this happening. There are now courses in bioethics at the universities of Florence and Rome, updates on bioethics in some regions of Italy,[15] medical meetings on truth telling[16] and communicating with patients,[17] and a project to establish a database for national and international bioethical issues.[18] From the patients' side, a spontaneous organization called "Tribunale per i Diritti del Malato" (Court for the Patient's Rights) now exists.[19]

For now, when dealing with my patients, I try to tell them the complete truth. But there are times when this is not so easy. For example, when faced with a family repeatedly asking me not to use the word "cancer," I rely on nonverbal communication to establish a truthful and therapeutic relationship with the patient. In all instances, I make an effort to listen to the patients and to respect their need for information. Since I believe the suffering person knows the truth, I think the only way to respect both Italian ethical principles and the patient's autonomy and dignity is to let the patient know that there are no barriers to communication and to the truth.

I hope all my Italian patients will soon ask me for the truth, and I hope I will never give information just for medicolegal reasons. Moreover,

I hope I will contribute—together with my colleagues—to a positive change in our society.

Notes

1. Ad Hoc Committee on Medical Ethics. American College of Physicians Ethics Manual, I. History of medical ethics, the physician and the patient, the physician's relationship to other physicians, the physician and society. *Ann Intern Med.* 1984;101:129–137.

2. Federazione Nazionale degli Ordini dei Medici Chirurghi e degli Odontoiatri. *Guida all'Esercizio Professionale per i Medici-Chirurghi e degli Odontoiatri.* Turin, Italy: Edizioni Medico Scientifiche; 1987:66–67.

3. Mosconi, P., Meyerowitz, B.E., Liberati, M.C. et al. Disclosure of breast cancer diagnosis: patient and physician reports. *Ann Oncol.* 1991;2:273–280.

4. Treatment of early-stage breast cancer. *JAMA.* 1991; 265:391–395. NIH Consensus Conference.

5. Sabbioni, M.E.E. Speech is silver, silence is gold? *Ann Oncol.* 1991;2:234.

6. Boeri, S. Medici e no. *Panorama.* 1992;1349:38–42.

7. Codice Deontologico 1989. Informazione e consenso del paziente, art 39. In: Ordine dei Medici, ed. *Annuario dell'Ordine dei Medici della Provincia di Torino.* Turin, Italy: Ordine dei Medici; 1990:27.

8. Codice Deontologico 1989. Sperimentazione, art 49. In: Ordine dei Medici, ed. *Annuario dell'Ordine dei Medici della Provincia di Torino.* Turin, Italy: Ordine dei Medici; 1990:28.

9. Il Medico d'Italia. Informazione al malato: come, quando e perché. *Organo Ufficiale della Federazione Nazionale degli Ordini dei Medici Chirurghi e degli Odontoiatri.* 1991;41:1–2.

10. Zittoun, R. Patient information and participation. In: Holland, J.C., Zittoun, R. eds. *Psychosocial Aspects of Oncology.* Berlin, Germany: Springer-Verlag; 1990:27–44.

11. Yourcenar, M. *Memoires d'Hadrien suici de Carnets de notes de memoires d'Hadrien.* Paris, France: Gallimard; 1974.

12. Pellegrino, E.D. Altruism, self-interest, and medical ethics. *JAMA.* 1987;258:1939–1940.

13. Suchman, A.L., Matthews, D.A. What makes the patient-doctor relationship therapeutic? exploring the connexional dimension of medical care. *Ann Intern Med.* 1988;108:125–130.

14. Novack, D.H., Plumer, R., Smith, R.L. et al. Changes in physicians' attitudes toward telling the cancer patient. *JAMA.* 1979;241:897–900.

15. Corso di formazione sulle tematiche bioetiche connesse al trattamento sanitario. Unitá Sanitaria Locale 12, Pisa, Italy. January–February 1992.

16. Il Medico d'Italia. Come informare il paziente grave. *Organo Ufficiale della Federazione Nazionale degli Ordini dei Medici Chirurghi e degli Odontoiatri.* 1992; 30:17.

17. Il Medico d'Italia. Come costruire e migliorare il rapporto medico-paziente. *Organo Ufficiale della Federazione Nazionale degli Ordini dei Medici Chirurghi e degli Odontoiatri.* 1992;26:16.

18. Il Medico d'Italia. Al via una banca dati sulla bioetica. *Organo Ufficiale della Federazione Nazionale degli Ordini dei Medici Chirurghi e degli Odontoiatri.* 1992;40:4.

19. Tribunale per i Diritti del Malato. Sezione di Pisa, Ospedale Santa Chiara. Carta dei diritti del cittadino malato. Pisa, Italy, 1984.

Is Truth Telling to the Patient a Cultural Artifact?

Edmund D. Pellegrino

◼

In the previous selection, Antonella Surbone, MD, describes her dilemma in trying to transfer the ideals of medical ethics she learned in the United States to her native Italy.[1] From her experience in the United States, she found that truth telling and respect for autonomy have become virtual moral absolutes. On the other hand, in Italy, families and physicians often shield patients from painful truths and difficult decisions. As Dr. Surbone points out, what is beneficent in one country may seem maleficent in another country.

This contrast in moral perspectives, of course, is not unique to the differences between Italy and North America. It has become a worldwide problem as newer models of medical ethics nurtured in the individualistic soil of North America are introduced to other countries with different moral traditions.[2] But similar contrasts may exist within a country, for example, between northern and southern Italy, or between the multiple ethnic groups in the United States.[3] Everywhere, as cultural groups attain freedom of expression, physicians and patients must relate with each other across ethical barriers especially with respect to the importance of autonomy.

These contrasts raise some provocative questions. Is medical ethics a cultural artifact such that a universal medical ethic is not viable? How should physicians who are dedicated to the best interests of their patients conduct therapeutic relationships with patients whose cultural values differ materially from their own?

These questions invite a critical reexamination of the foundation and meaning of autonomy and its relationship with truth telling. Such reflection suggests that autonomy is not and cannot be unequivocally interpreted. Some of the dilemma is more superficial than real and derives from a narrow interpretation of the concept of autonomy.

Autonomy entered medical ethics as part of a system of prima facie principles devised to deal with moral pluralism. Prima facie principles, such as autonomy, nonmaleficence, beneficence, and justice, are those that ought to be respected unless powerful reasons for overriding them can be adduced.[4,5] In this system, each principle is given equal weight. Priorities among principles can be established only when the detailed circumstances of a particular decision are known. No principle, including autonomy, is granted a priori moral hegemony over the others.

The principle of autonomy is grounded in respect for persons and the acknowledgment that as rational beings we have the unique capability to make reasoned choices. Through these choices we plan and live lives for which we are morally accountable. Inhibiting an individual's capability to make these personal choices is a violation of his or her integrity as a person and thus a maleficent act.

Autonomy, therefore, is not in fundamental opposition with beneficence as is too often supposed, but in congruence with it. Problems arise when the content of what is beneficent is defined by others such as family members or physicians. This may be warranted when we are mentally incompetent, when our choices harm others, or when we make choices that contravene good medical practice or harm us seriously. In the absence of these limitations, competent humans are owed the freedom to define beneficence in terms of their own values. This does not mean

that all values are morally equivalent or defensible, but only that as humans we are owed respect for the choices we voluntarily make.

In North America, in the United States in particular, autonomy has tended to become a moral absolute. The reasons for this are multiple. They include improved education of the public, a strong tradition of privacy rights and personal liberty, a distrust of authority and the possibilities of medical technology, and the loosening of family and community identification. In this context, truth telling is a necessary corollary, since human capability for autonomous choices cannot function if truth is withheld, falsified, or otherwise manipulated. Truth telling is essential to informed consent, the instrument whereby personal autonomy is expressed in concrete decisions.

Respect for autonomy and truth telling are intrinsic to beneficent medical care for many people in the North American context. It does not follow, however, that this concept of autonomy is always beneficent or that it must be accepted by, or imposed on, everyone living in the United States or elsewhere.

For one thing, autonomous patients are free to use their autonomy as they see fit—even to delegate it when this fits their own concept of beneficence. Some patients need a more authoritative approach than others. This approach is legitimate when, for example, despite efforts to inform and empower patients to make their own decisions, patients find themselves unable or unwilling to cope with choices. Such patients may feel sincerely that a close friend or family member would be able to make decisions that better protect their values than they could make themselves. Such a delegation of decision-making authority may be explicit or implicit depending on the dominant ethos.

In some parts of Italy, among many ethnic groups in the United States, and in large parts of the world, this delegation of authority is culturally implicit. In such contexts, the uniformity of the practice suggests that delegation of decision making is an expectation of the sick person that need not be explicit. To thrust the truth or the decision on a patient who expects to be buffered against news of impending death is a gratuitous and harmful misinterpretation of the moral foundations for respect for autonomy. In many cultures clinicians encounter patients who are fully aware of the gravity of their condition but choose to play out the drama in their own way. This may include not discussing the full or obvious truth. This is a form of autonomy, if it is implicitly and mutually agreed on, between physician and patient. However, autonomy should not be violated by a misconceived attempt to be morally rigorous. Withholding the truth from a patient demands, of course, the utmost care in responding to any occasion when the patient wishes to exert more control.

Among most North American physicians, the withholding of truth, in whole or in part, is a therapeutic privilege accepted as morally licit when we have substantial evidence that offering the patient the truth has a significant probability of causing harm, for example, emotional damage or suicide. This "privilege" must be used rarely and with utmost care since it is so easily abused.

Treating patients within the conception of beneficence defined by their own cultural ideas is a form of therapeutic privilege. However, a palpable risk of harm in knowing the truth must exist that must not be outweighed by the risk of withholding the truth. The amount, manner, and timing of truth telling or truth withholding are crucial factors for which there is no ready formula.

Thus, autonomy cannot be an absolute principle with a priori precedence over other prima facie principles. Rather, the judicious exercise of respect for autonomy means that health professionals must act in a manner that enables and empowers patients to make decisions and act in a way that is most in accord with their values.

That the patient may draw these values from the circumambient culture does not make autonomy or medical ethics a cultural artifact. Autonomy is still a valid and universal principle because it is based on what it is to be human. The patient must decide how much autonomy he or she wishes to exercise, and this amount can vary from culture to culture.

It seems probable that the democratic ideals that lie behind the contemporary North American concept of autonomy will spread and that something close to it will be the choice of many individuals in other countries. What then does the physician do when a society is in transition as Dr. Surbone suggests is the case in Italy today, or when many different cultures make up one society as is the case in the United States? To preserve both autonomy and beneficence, physicians must get to know their patients well enough to discern when, and if, those patients wish to contravene the mores of prevailing medical culture. This requires a degree of familiarity and sensitivity increasingly difficult to come by, but morally inescapable for every physician who practices in today's morally and culturally diverse world society.

Notes

1. Surbone, A. Truth telling to the patient. *JAMA*. 1992; 268:1661–1662.
2. Pellegrino, E.D., Mazzarella, P., Corsi, P., eds. *Transcultural Dimensions in Medical Ethics*. Frederick, Md: University Publishing Group. 1993.
3. Flack, H.E., Pellegrino, E.D., eds. *African American Perspectives on Biomedical Ethics*. Washington, DC: Georgetown University Press; 1992.
4. Beauchamp, T.L., Childress, J.F. *Principles of Bioethics*. 3rd ed. New York, NY: Oxford University Press; 1989.
5. Ross, W.D. *The Right and the Good*. Indianapolis, Ind: Hackett Publishing Company; 1988:33–34.

Offering Truth: One Ethical
Approach to the Uninformed
Cancer Patient

Benjamin Freedman

■

Medical and social attitudes toward cancer have evolved rapidly during the last 20 years, particularly in North America.[1,2] Most physicians, most of the time, in most hospitals, accept the ethical proposition that patients are entitled to know their diagnosis. However, there remains in my experience a significant minority of cases in which patients are never informed that they have cancer or, although informed of the diagnosis, are not informed when disease progresses toward a terminal phase. Although concealment of diagnosis can certainly occur in cases of other terminal or even nonterminal serious illnesses, it seems to occur more frequently and in more exacerbated form with cancer because of the traditional and cultural resonances of dread associated with cancer.

These cases challenge our understanding of and commitment to an ethical physician-patient relationship. In addition, they are observably a significant source of tension between health-care providers. When the responsible physician persists in efforts to conceal the truth from patients, consultant physicians, nurses, social workers, or others may believe that they cannot discharge their functions responsibly until the patient has been told. Alternatively, when a treating physician decides to inform the patient of his or her diagnosis, strong resistance from family mem-

bers who have instigated a conspiracy of silence may be anticipated.

This article outlines one approach, employed in my own ethical consultations and at some palliative care services or specialized oncology units. This approach, offering truth to patients with cancer, affords a means of satisfying legal and ethical norms of patient autonomy, ameliorating conflicts between families and physicians, and acknowledging the cultural norms that underlie family desires.

Common Features of Cases

Mrs. A is a woman in her 60s with colon cancer, with metastatic liver involvement and a mass in the abdomen. She is not expected to survive longer than weeks. Other than a course of antibiotics, which she was just about to complete, no active treatment is indicated or intended. She is alert. She knows that she has an infection; her family refuses to inform her that she has cancer. The precipitating cause of the ethical consultation, requested by the newly assigned treating physician (Dr. H), is his ethical discomfort with treating Mrs. A in this manner.

When one is confronted with a case of concealment, it is worth wondering how it came about that everyone but the patient has been told of the diagnosis, so that similar situations may be avoided in the future. Often, a diagnosis is defined in the course of surgery and disclosed to waiting relatives; this may most appropriately be handled by a prior understanding with the patient, communicated to the family, as to whether and how much they will be told before the patient awakens. But there are at least two other major ways in which a situation of concealment might develop.

A patient might be admitted in medical crisis, at a time when he or she is obtunded and incapable of being informed of his or her condition and treatment options. Law and ethics alike require that the medical team inform and otherwise deal with the person who is most qualified to speak on the patient's behalf (usually, the next of kin), until the patient has recovered enough to speak for himself or herself. Unfortunately for this plan, though, a patient will often fail to cross, at one moment, the bright line from incompetent to competent. Consequently, patterns of communicating with the relative instead of with the patient may persist beyond the intended period. Such situations have their own momentum. Later disclosure to the patient will need to deal both with the burden of providing bad news and with the fact that this information has been concealed from the patient up to that point.

A second typical way in which concealment develops is the following. A patient with close family ties is always attended by a relative (commonly, spouse or child) at medical appointments. Before a firm diagnosis is established, that relative manages to elicit a promise from the physician not to tell the patient should the tests show that the patient has cancer. Faced with a distraught and deeply caring relative, the physician goes along, at least as a temporizing tactic, only to discover, as described above, how the situation develops its own inertia. The cycle may be broken in a number of ways. Sometimes the physician simply decides to call a halt to concealment; often the patient's care is transferred to another physician who has not been a party to the conspiracy, as had happened with Mrs. A.

> As clinical ethicist, I met with Dr. H and the relevant family members (husband, daughter, and son). Most of the discussion was held with the son; the husband, a first-generation Greek-Canadian immigrant, knows little English and was at any rate somewhat withdrawn. As expected, they are a close family, deeply solicitous of the patient, and con-

vinced that she will suffer horribly were she to be told she has cancer. They confirmed my sense that the Greek cultural significance of cancer equals death—something that in this case is in all likelihood true.

> At this time the family was willing to sign any document we wanted them to, assuming all responsibility for the decision to conceal the truth from Mrs. A. "Do us this one favor" was a plea that punctuated the discussion.

Although other factors, such as the context of treatment and the patient's own idiosyncratic personality, may cause the same kind of problem in communication, my experience suggests the situation is often, as here, mediated by cultural factors. As one text on ethnic factors in family counseling puts it, "Greek Americans do not believe that the truth shall make you free, and the therapist should not attempt to impose the love of truth upon them."[3] (And compare Dalla-Vorgia et al.[4]) I often find other immigrant families of Mediterranean or Near Eastern origin reacting similarly, for example, Italian families and those of Sephardic Jews who have immigrated from Morocco. In all cases, in my experience, there is a special plea on the part of families to respect their cultural pattern and tradition. Health-care providers often feel the force of this claim and its corollary: informing the patient would be an act of ethical and cultural imperialism. Moreover, the family not uncommonly feels strongly enough that legal action is threatened unless their wishes are respected. Mrs. A's family, in fact, threatened to sue at one point when they were told that Mrs. A's diagnosis would be revealed.

Telling Families Why the Patient Should Be Informed

By the time a clinical ethical consultation is requested, the situation has often become highly charged emotionally. In addition to the unpleasantness of threats of legal action, there may have been some physical confrontation.

Mrs. S was a Sephardic woman in her 70s with widespread metastatic seedings in the pleura and pericardium from an unknown primary tumor. Her family insisted that she not be informed of her diagnosis and prognosis. Suffering from a subjective experience of apnea, she was to have a morphine drip begun to alleviate her symptoms. The family physically expelled the nurse from the room. If their mother were to learn she was getting morphine, they said, she would deduce that her situation was grave.

Such aberrant behavior cannot fairly be understood without realizing that these families may be acting out of uncommonly deep concern for the well-being of the patient, as they (perhaps misguidedly) understand it. The healthcare team shares the same ultimate goal, to care for the patient in a humane, decent, caring manner. This commonality can serve as the basis for continuing discussion, as in the above case of Mrs. A, the Greek patient.

Discussion with the family was long and meandering. The usual position of the healthcare team was explained in some detail: patients in our institution are generally told their diagnosis; we are accustomed to telling patients that they have cancer, and we know how to handle the varied normal patient reactions to this bad news; patients do not (generally) kill themselves immediately on being told, or die a voodoo death, in spite of the family's fears and cultural beliefs about patient reaction to this diagnosis. Patients have a right to this information and may have the need to attend to any number of tasks pending death: to say goodbye, to make arrangements, to complete unfinished business. As her illness progresses, decisions will likely need to be made about further treatment, for example, of infections or blockages that develop. Already, one of Mrs. A's kidneys is blocked and her urine is backing up. If the mass should obstruct her other kidney, for example, should a catheter be placed directly into the kidney or not? These decisions of treatment management for dying patients are dreadful and should if possible be made by the patient, with awareness of her choices and prospects. In addition, Mrs. A is very likely already suspicious that she is gravely ill, and we have no means of dealing with her fears without the ability to speak to her openly. Finally, the fears that the family expresses about the manner of informing her—"How can we tell our mother, 'You have cancer, it will kill you in weeks' "—are groundless: she must be told that she is very ill, but we would never advise telling her she has a period of x weeks to live—a statement that is never wise or medically sound—nor will we try to remove her hope.

The physician or other health-care provider may be primarily motivated by the ethical principle of respect for patient autonomy, grounding a patient's right to know of his or her situation, choices, and likely fate. Connected with this may be the correct belief that any consent to treatment that the patient provides without having an opportunity to learn the reason for that treatment is legally invalid. To be properly informed, consent must be predicated on information about the nature and consequences of treatment, which must in turn be understood in the context of the patient's illness. A patient cannot validly consent to the passing of a tube into the kidney without being informed that her urinary tract is blocked, or of the reason for that blockage.

These reasons, so determinative for the physician, often carry no weight with the family. In

Mrs. A's case, for example, the family pledged to sign anything we would like to free us of liability. Our response, that their willingness cannot affect either our moral or legal obligation, which vests in the patient directly, was similarly unpersuasive; nonetheless, it was a fact and had to be said.

The direct negative impact on the patient's care and comfort that results from her being left in the dark represents more in the way of common ground between family and health-care provider. It is often quite clear that failure to reveal the truth causes a variety of unfortunate psychosocial results. As in all such cases, we highlighted for Mrs. A's family the strong possibility that she already suspects she is ill and dying of cancer but is unable to speak about this with them because all of us, in our concealment and evasions, had not given her "permission" to broach the topic. Mrs. A is dying, but there are things worse than dying, for example, dying in silence when one needs to speak.

It is also important to emphasize to families that the patient may have "unfinished business" that he or she would like to complete. For example, after one of my earliest consultations of this nature, the patient in question chose to leave the hospital for several weeks to revisit his birthplace in Greece.

Finally, it is sometimes the case that the failure to discuss with the patient his or her diagnosis can directly result in inadequate or inappropriate medical care. Mrs. S, above, was denied adequate comfort measures because the institution of morphine might tip her off to her condition. In another case, the son and daughter-in-law of a patient insisted that she not receive chemotherapy for an advanced but treatable blood cancer so that she would be spared the knowledge of her disease and the side effects of treatment. In such cases, great injury is added to the insult of withholding the truth from a patient. Often, it is this prospect that serves as the trigger to mobilize the health-care team to seek an ethical consultation.

Offering Truth to the Uninformed Patient with Cancer

A patient's knowledge of diagnosis and prognosis is not all-or-nothing. It exists along a continuum, anchored at one end by the purely theoretical "absolute ignorance" and at the other by the unattainable "total enlightenment." Actual patients are to be found along this continuum at locations that vary in response to external factors (verbal information, nonverbal clues, etc.) as well as internal dynamics, such as denial.

The approach called here "offering truth" represents a brief dance between patient and health-care provider, a pas de deux, that takes place within that continuum. When offering truth to the patient with cancer, rather than simply ascertaining that the patient is for the moment lucid, and then proceeding to explain all aspects of his or her condition and treatment, both the physician(s) and I attempt repeatedly to ascertain from the patient how much he or she wants to know. In dealing with families who insist that the patient remain uninformed, I explain this approach, a kind of compromise between the polar stances. I also explain that sometimes the results are surprising, as indeed happened with Mrs. A.

In spite of all the explanations we provided to Mrs. A's family of the many reasons why it might be best to speak with her of her illness, they continued to resist. Mrs. A, the son insisted, would want all the decisions that arise to be made by the physicians, whom they all trusted, and the family itself.

If their assessment of Mrs. A is correct, I pointed out, we have no problem. Dr. H agrees with me that while Mrs. A has a *right* to know, she does not have a *duty* to know. We would not force this information on her—indeed, we cannot. Patients who do not want to know will sometimes deny ever having been told, however forthrightly they have been spoken to. So Mrs. A will be offered this information, not have it thrust on her—and if they are right about what she wants, and her personality, she will not wish to know.

Mrs. A was awake and reasonably alert, although not altogether free of discomfort (nausea). She was told that she had had an infection that was now under control, but that she remains very ill, as she herself can tell from her weakness. Does she have any questions she wants to ask; does she want to talk? She did not. We repeated that she remains very ill and asked if she understands that—she did. Some patients, it was explained to her, want to know all about their disease—its name, prognosis, treatment choices, famous people who have had the disease, etc.—while others do not want to know so much, and some want to leave all of the decisions in the hands of their family and physicians. What would she like? What kind of patient is she? She whispered to her daughter that she wants to leave it alone for now.

That seemed to be her final word. We repeated to her that treatment choices would need to be made shortly. She was told that we would respect her desire, but that if she changed her mind we could talk at any time; and that, in any event, she must understand that we would stay by her and see to her comfort in all possible ways. She signified that she understood and said that we should deal with her children. Both Dr. H and I understood this as explicitly authorizing her children to speak for her with respect to treatment decisions.

The above approach relies on one simple tactic: a patient will be offered the opportunity to learn the truth, at whatever level of detail that patient desires. The most important step in these attempts is to ask questions of the patient and then listen closely to the patient's responses. Since the discussion at hand concerns how much information the patient would like to receive, here, unlike most physician-patient interchanges, the important decisions will need to be made by the patient.

Initiating discussion is relatively easy if the patient is only recently conscious and responsive; it is more difficult if a conspiracy of silence has already taken effect. The conversation with the patient might be initiated by telling him or her that at this time the medical team has arrived at a fairly clear understanding of the situation and treatment options. New test results may be alluded to; this is a fairly safe statement, since new tests are always being done on all patients. These conversational gambits signal that a fresh start in communication can now be attempted. (At the same time it avoids the awkwardness of a patient's asking, "Why haven't you spoken to me before?")

The patient might then be told that, before we talk about our current understanding of the medical situation, it is important to hear from the patient himself or herself, so that we can confirm what he or she knows or clear up any misunderstanding that may have arisen. The patient sometimes, with more than a little logic, responds, "Why are you asking me what is wrong? You're the doctor, you tell me what's wrong." A variety of answers are possible. A patient might be told that we have found that things work better if we start with the patient's understanding of the illness; or that time might be saved if we know what the patient understands, and go from there; or that whenever you try to teach someone, you have to start with what they know. Different approaches may suggest themselves as more fitting to the particular patient in question. The important thing is to begin to generate a dynamic within which the patient is speaking and the physician responding, rather than vice versa. Only then can the pace of conversation and level of information be controlled by the patient. The structure of the discussion, as well as the content of what the physician says, must reinforce the message: We are now establishing a new opportunity to talk and question, but you as the patient will have to tell us how much you want to know about your illness.

The chief ethical principle underlying the idea that patients should be offered the truth is, of course, respect for the patient's personal autonomy. By holding the conversation, the patient is given the opportunity to express autonomy in its most robust, direct fashion: the clear expression of preference. Legal systems that value autonomy will similarly protect a physician who chooses to offer truth and to respect the patient's response to that offer; "a medical doctor need not make disclosure of risks when the patient requests that he not be so informed."[5] A patient's right to information vests in that patient, to exercise as he or she desires; so that a patient's right to information is respected no less when the patient chooses to be relatively uninformed as when full information is demanded.[6] This stance is entirely consistent with the recent adoption of the widely noted (and even more widely misconstrued) Patient Self-Determination Act.[7] The major innovation this entails has been to involve institutions in the process of informing patients of their rights. However, the Patient Self-Determination Act has not changed state laws about informed consent to treatment in any way,[8] and as such the basic question here addressed—a physician's responsibility to inform patients of their diagnoses—remains entirely unaffected.

When offering truth, we are forced to recognize that patients' choices should be respected not because we or others agree with those choices (still less, respected *only* when we agree with those choices), but simply because those are the patient's choices. Indeed, the test of autonomy comes precisely when we personally disagree with the path the patient had chosen. If, for example, patient choice is respected only when the patient chooses the most effective treatment, when respecting those choices we would be respecting only effective therapeutics, not the person who has chosen them.

Many physicians hold to the ideal of an informed, alert, cooperative, and intelligent patient. But the point of offering truth—rather than inflicting it—is to allow the patient to choose his or her own path. As a practical matter, of course, it could scarcely be otherwise. A physician with fanatic devotion to informing patients can lecture, explain, even harangue, but cannot force the patient to attend to what the physician is saying, or think about it, or remember it.

Families need to confront the same point. Ambivalence and conflict are often observed among family members concerning whether the patient who has not been informed "really" knows (or suspects, etc.), and by offering the patient the opportunity to speak, this issue may be settled. More fundamentally, though, the concealing family—which is after all characterized by deep concern for the patient's well-being—will rarely (has never, in my experience to date) maintain that even if the patient demands to know the truth, the secret should still be kept. The family rather relies on the patient's failure to make this explicit demand as his or her tacit agreement to remain ignorant. Families can be helped to see that there may be many reasons for the patient's failure to demand the truth (including the fact that the patient may believe the lies that have been offered). If the patient wishes to remain in a state of relative ignorance, he or she will tell us that when asked; and if the patient states an explicit desire to be informed, families will find it hard to deny his or her right to have that desire respected.

Some families, naturally enough, suspect chicanery, that this approach is rigged to get the patient to ask for the truth. To them I respond that my experience proves otherwise: to my surprise and that of the physicians, some patients ask to leave this in the family's hands; to the surprise of families, some patients who seemed quietistic in fact strongly wish to be told the truth (which many of them had already suspected). We cannot know what the patient wants until we ask, I tell them, and we all want to do what the patient wants.

Having held the discussion, it is important to move on to its resolution as soon as possible.

> I met with Mrs. S's children, together with a nurse, medical resident, and medical student, for about an hour and a half; the treating oncologist also made a brief appearance. The discussion featured a lengthy and eloquent exposition by the resident of why Mrs. S. needs to be spoken to, and a passionate and equally eloquent appeal by one son to respect the different culture from which they come. Finally, I introduced the idea that we offer her the truth, and then follow her lead. This was agreed to by the family, and I left.

The medical student thanked me some days later and told me the rest of the story. The tension that had existed between health-care team and family had largely dissipated; as the student put it, "People were able to look each other in the eye again." Mrs. S was lucid but fatigued that evening; for that reason, and probably because they had already spent so much time talking at our meeting, the family delayed the agreed-on discussion. Unexpectedly, Mrs. S did not survive the night.

Conclusion

The problem of the uninformed patient with cancer can be described in many different ways, for example, as faulty physician-patient communication; as an obstacle to good medical care; as a cause of stress among hospital staff; and as

a failure to respect patient autonomy. A dimension at least as important as these, but rarely acknowledged, is the clash it may represent between diverse cultures and their basic moral commitments.

The approach presented above reflects an effort to maintain accepted standards of the physician-patient relationship while respecting the cultural background and requirements of families. This form of respect involves reasonable accommodation to these cultural expectations but should not be confused with uncritical acquiescence. The critical question is, perhaps, this: How should we react to a family that refuses to allow the patient an offering of truth, that maintains that discussion itself to be contrary to cultural norms? Under those circumstances, I believe the offering must be made notwithstanding family demands. My reasons have as much to do with my beliefs about the nature of ethnic and religious moral norms themselves as with the view that in cases of conflict, our public morality (as concretized in law) should prevail.

First, I believe that members of a cultural community are as prone to mistaking what their own norms require of them as we within the broader culture are to mistaking our own moral obligations. The norm of protecting the patient clearly requires rather than prohibits disclosure in some cases, including some described above, to prevent physical or psychological damage or to enable some final task to be consummated. All of the factors that we recognize sometimes to derange our own moral judgments—inertia, ill-grounded prejudices and generalizations, lack of the courage to confront unpleasant situations, and many more—may operate as powerfully in deranging the views of those from another culture. Their initial sense of what ethics require may, that is, be mistaken, from the point of view of their own norms as well as those of modern, Western, secular culture.

Second, even if a family's judgment of what

their culture requires is accurate, we must not presume that a patient like Mrs. A will choose, in extremis, to abide by her own cultural norms. Like any immigrant, she may have adopted the norms of broad society, or, acculturated to some lesser degree, she may act according to some hybrid set of values. Concretely, the offering of truth is about her diagnosis; symbolically, it is a process that allows her to declare her own preference regarding which norms shall be respected and how.

A last word is in order about the view implicit in this approach regarding the nature of a bioethical consultation. As these cases illustrate, patients, families, and health-care professionals come to a meeting from different moral worlds, as well as different backgrounds and biographies; and these worlds involve not simply rights and privileges, but duties as well. A successful consultation attempts to clarify on behalf of the different parties their own moral principles and associated moral commitments. It needs to proceed from the premise that all present ultimately share a common goal: the well-being of the patient.

Notes

I am grateful to Eugene V. Bareza, MD, CM, and to Charles Weijer, MD, for valuable advice in the preparation of the manuscript. All errors are my own.

1. Oken, D. What to tell cancer patients: a study of medical attitudes. *JAMA*. 1961;175:1120–1128.

2. Novack, D.H., Plumer, R., Smith, R.L., Ochitil, H., Morrow, G.R., Bennett, J.M. Changes in physicians' attitudes toward telling the cancer patient. *JAMA*. 1979;241:897–900.

3. Welts, E.P. The Greek family. In: McGoldrick, M.M., Pearce, J.K., Giordano, J. *Ethnicity and Family Therapy*. New York, NY: Guilford Press: 1982:269–288.

4. Dalla-Vorgia, P., Katsouyanni, K., Garanis, T.N. et al. Attitudes of a Mediterranean population to the truth-telling issue. *J Med Ethics*. 1992;18:67–74.

5. *Cobbs v Grant*. 502 P2d 1 (Cal 1972) (a similar provision for a patient's right to waive being informed was established by the Supreme Court of Canada in *Reibl v Hughes* 2SCR 880 [1980]).

6. Freedman, B. The validity of ignorant consent to medical research. *IRB Rev Hum Subjects Res*. 1982;4(2):1–5.

7. The Patient Self Determination Act, sections 4206 and 4751 of the Omnibus Reconciliation Act of 1990, Pub L 101–508.

8. McCloskey, E. Between isolation and intrusion: the Patient Self Determination Act. *Law Med Health Care*. 1991;19:80–82.

What the Doctor Said

Raymond Carver

■

He said it doesn't look good
he said it looks bad in fact real bad
he said I counted thirty-two of them on one lung
    before
I quit counting them
I said I'm glad I wouldn't want to know
about any more being there than that
he said are you a religious man do you kneel
    down
in forest groves and let yourself ask for help
when you come to a waterfall
mist blowing against your face and arms
do you stop and ask for understanding at those
    moments
I said not yet but I intend to start today
he said I'm real sorry he said
I wish I had some other kind of news to give you
I said Amen and he said something else
I didn't catch and not knowing what else to do
and not wanting him to have to repeat it
and me to have to fully digest it
I just looked at him
for a minute and he looked back it was then
I jumped up and shook hands with this man
    who'd just given me
something no one else on earth had ever given
    me
I may even have thanked him habit being so
    strong

Informed Consent, Cancer, and Truth in Prognosis

George J. Annas

■

Barbara Tuchman records that during the Black
Death epidemic in the early 14th century, "doctors were admired, lawyers universally hated
and mistrusted."[1] The great plagues and wars of
the Middle Ages produced a "cult of death," including a vast popular literature that had death
as its theme. As the 20th century closes, our emphasis is on the denial of death, and the honest
discussion of death remains rare both in popular
literature and in conversations between physicians and patients. This is one reason why Shana
Alexander shocked a national conference of bioethicists last year by saying, "I trust my lawyer
more than I trust my doctor." What she meant,
she explained, was that she trusted her lawyer to
tell her the truth about her alternatives and to
execute faithfully the one she chose; she did not
have this confidence in her physician, at least
not if she were critically ill.

To the extent that Alexander's attitude is
shared by Americans, it is an indictment, because nowhere in medicine is trust so necessary
as in physician–patient conversations near
death. The national survey conducted by Louis
Harris for a presidential commission on bioethics in 1982 supports her view. It found that 96
percent of Americans wanted to be told if they
had cancer, and 85 percent wanted a "realistic
estimate" of how long they had to live if their

type of cancer "usually leads to death in less than a year."[2] On the other hand, fewer than half the physicians surveyed said they would either give a "straight statistical prognosis" (13 percent) or "say that you can't tell how long [the patient] might live, but stress that in most cases people live no longer than a year" (28 percent) if the patient had a "fully confirmed diagnosis of lung cancer in an advanced stage."[2]

The country's most recent important case involving informed consent, *Arato* v. *Avedon,*[3] centers on whether the law should require physicians to report statistical life-expectancy data to their patients in cases of illness that is likely to be terminal.

The Case of Miklos Arato

On July 21, 1980, Miklos Arato, a 43-year-old electrical contractor, was operated on to remove a nonfunctioning kidney. During surgery a tumor was found in the tail of his pancreas, and the tumor, along with the surrounding tissue and lymph nodes, was removed. Several days later, the surgeon met with Mr. Arato and his wife. He told them that he thought he had removed all of the tumor and referred them to an oncologist. The surgeon did not tell them that only about 5 percent of patients with pancreatic cancer survive for five years or give Mr. Arato either a prognosis or a reasonable estimate of his life expectancy. The oncologist told the Aratos that there was a substantial chance of a recurrence, and that a recurrence would mean that the disease was incurable. He recommended experimental chemotherapy and radiation treatment, acknowledging that this might produce no benefit. The oncologist was not asked for and did not volunteer a prognosis.

While the chemotherapy and radiation treatment were continuing, on April 22, 1981, a recurrence was detected. Even though the physicians believed Mr. Arato's life expectancy could then be measured in months, they did not tell him so. Mr. Arato died on July 25, 1981, approximately one year after his cancer had been diagnosed. After his death, his wife and two adult children brought suit against the surgeons and oncologists, alleging that they had had an obligation, under California's informed-consent doctrine, to tell Mr. Arato, before asking him to consent to chemotherapy, that approximately 95 percent of people with pancreatic cancer die within five years.

The Proceedings in the Lower Court

At trial it was shown that at the first meeting with his oncologist, Mr. Arato had filled out an 18-page questionnaire in which he answered "yes" to the question, "If you are seriously ill now or in the future, do you want to be told the truth about it?"[3] The physicians who treated Mr. Arato justified their nondisclosure of the statistical prognosis on a variety of grounds, most based on traditional medical paternalism. His surgeon, for example, thought Mr. Arato had shown such great anxiety about his cancer that it was "medically inappropriate" to disclose specific mortality rates. The chief oncologist said he understood that patients like Mr. Arato "wanted to be told, but did not want a cold shower." He thought that reporting extremely high mortality rates might "deprive a patient of any hope of a cure," and that this was medically inadvisable. His physicians also said that during his 70 visits with them over a one-year period, Mr. Arato had avoided ever specifically asking about his own life expectancy and that this indicated that he did not want to know the information. In addition, all the physicians testified that the statistical life expectancy of a group of patients had little predictive value when applied to a particular patient.[3,4]

Mrs. Arato argued that the statistical prognosis should have been disclosed because it indicated that even with successful treatment (the physicians measured success in terms of added months of survival), Mr. Arato would probably live only a short time. If Mr. Arato had known the facts, she believed, he would not have undergone the rigors of the experimental treatment, but would instead have chosen to live out his final days at peace with his wife and family and would have made final arrangements for his business affairs. Mr. Arato had failed to order his financial affairs properly before his death, which had resulted in the eventual failure of his contracting business and substantial tax losses after his death.

On the basis of standard California jury instructions on informed-consent requirements, the jury returned a verdict in favor of the physicians. The Aratos appealed. A California court of appeals reversed the decision in a two-to-one opinion, stating that physicians were under an obligation to disclose statistics concerning life expectancy to patients so that they might take timely action to plan for their deaths, including the financial aspects of their deaths.[4] The physicians then appealed.

The California Supreme Court

The California Supreme Court unanimously reversed the appeals court's decision. The justices began their analysis by reviewing their own most important previous cases related to informed consent: *Cobbs* v. *Grant,*[5] *Truman* v. *Thomas,*[6] and *Moore* v. *Regents of the University of California.*[7] The court noted, as it had in *Cobbs,* that the doctrine of informed consent is "anchored" in four postulates:

—patients are generally ignorant of medicine;
—patients have a right to control their own body and thus to decide about medical treatment;

—to be effective, consent to treatment must be informed;
—patients are dependent upon their physicians for truthful information and must trust them (making the doctor-patient relationship a "fiduciary" or trust relationship rather than an arms-length business relationship).[5]

In *Truman,* a case about the refusal of a patient to have a Pap smear, the court decided that information had to be disclosed even if the patient refused treatment "so that patients might meaningfully exercise their right to make decisions about their own bodies."[6] And in *Moore,* a case about creating an immortal cell line from a diseased spleen, the court held that the physician must disclose "personal interests unrelated to the patient's health, whether research or economic, that may affect the physician's personal judgment."[7] Instead of taking the opportunity to resolve what the California Supreme Court described as a "critical standoff" in the development of the doctrine of informed consent between the extremes of absolute patient sovereignty and medical paternalism, the court focused on one very narrow question: whether California's standard instructions to juries should be revised to require the specific disclosure of a patient's life expectancy as predicted by mortality statistics.[3]

Framing the question so narrowly made answering it relatively easy. The court described the physician–patient relationship as "an intimate and irreducibly judgment-laden one" that had to be judged within "the overall medical context."[3] As for statistics on life expectancy, the court found them of little use to individual patients. The court thought, for example, that "statistical morbidity values derived from the experience of population groups are inherently unreliable and offer little assurance regarding the fate of the individual patient."[3]

Perhaps most important, the court described this case as one that was "fairly litigated" and properly put in the hands of "the venerable American jury," which had rendered a reasonable verdict that it was not prepared to second-guess.[3] The court concluded:

> Rather than mandate the disclosure of specific information as a matter of law, the better rule is to instruct the jury that a physician is under a legal duty to disclose to the patient all material information—that is, information which would be regarded as significant by a reasonable person in the patient's position when deciding to accept or reject a recommended medical procedure—needed to make an informed decision regarding a proposed treatment.[3]

The patient's desire to be told the truth, as evidenced by his answer on the questionnaire, was found to be irrelevant, since the physician has an independent legal duty to tell the "truth" (although a patient can waive the right to information). The court also dealt with the issue of expert testimony, noting that in addition to the information required to be disclosed by *Cobbs*[5] (the nature and benefits of the proposed treatment, its risks of death or serious harm, reasonable alternatives and their risks, and problems of recuperation), physicians must also disclose any other information that another skilled practitioner would disclose. The court ruled that specific data on life expectancy fell within this standard. Thus, the defendant physicians were properly permitted to call expert medical witnesses to testify that it was not standard practice in the medical community in 1980 to disclose specific life-expectancy data.

Prognosis and Success

If the only issue is whether the law should require physicians always to disclose statistical life-expectancy data to critically ill patients as part of the informed-consent process, the conclusion of the court is defensible. But this is much too narrow a basis for the decision. Although by itself the statistical probability of survival for an individual patient may not be material, it is material if it indicates whether the patient is likely to survive and the probable quality of life with and without treatment. In other words, the issue of informed consent in this instance centers on the disclosure of the success rate of the proposed treatment in terms of both the prospects for long-term survival and the patient's quality of life. This is what patients need to know, and this is the type of material information patients have a right to—not only because it is the patient's body, but, more important, because it is the patient's life.[8]

It is unfortunate that the plaintiff did not argue the case on the grounds of the necessity to explain success rates, because the results could have (and should have) been different. In *Cobbs,* which *Arato* affirms, the California Supreme Court had said:

> A medical doctor, being the expert, appreciates the risks inherent in the procedure he is prescribing, the risks of a decision not to undergo the treatment, and the probability of a successful outcome of the treatment. . . . The weighing of these risks against the individual subjective fears and hopes of the patient is not an expert skill. Such evaluation and decision is a nonmedical judgment reserved to the patient alone.[5]

This language explicitly requires physicians to explain the probability that a proposed treatment will be successful and implicitly requires the physician to tell the patient what the physician means by "success."[9] In this case, for example, the court seems correct in concluding that a statistical life-expectancy profile of all patients with pancreatic cancer, by itself, might not have been required to inform Mr. Arato of his prognosis properly. But such information is very valuable when coupled with an explanation of why the physician thinks the patient's case is or is not typical. Group data are the basis for predictions in individual cases—including both treatment recommendations and statements about probable risks and benefits. The physicians relied on group data, for example, to tell Mr. Arato that if his cancer recurred it would be "incurable." The court should have made it clearer that it is always material to a reasonable person to know both the probability of success of a proposed treatment and the meaning of success. Without this information, it is the physician, not the patient, who is making the treatment decision, and that is precisely what the doctrine of informed consent is designed to prevent.

Culture and Death

A culture's general attitude toward death strongly influences what information about their prognosis will be provided to terminally ill patients. In the Middle Ages, for example, "when death was to be met any day around the corner, it might have been expected to become banal; instead it exerted a ghoulish fascination."[1] There was an emphasis on "worms and putrefaction and gruesome physical details"; instead of emphasizing a spiritual journey, the culture concentrated on the rotting of the body.[1] In our culture, with its unprecedented life expectancy, we tend to deny death altogether and celebrate new forms of medical technology designed to forestall death. In this context, it is not surprising that physicians often conceal prognostic information from their patients, just as most physicians once refused to use the word "cancer."[9] But concealment of prognosis from patients near death makes them feel abandoned and makes physicians feel estranged.[10,11] Candor toward the dying is an old problem, which Tolstoy described so well in "The Death of Ivan Ilych":

> What tormented Ivan Ilych most was the deception, the lie . . . that he was not dying but was simply ill, and that he only need keep quiet and undergo treatment and then something very good would result.[12]

Ilych, a former prosecutor, also recognized that his physician's manner, which implied "if only you put yourself in our hands we will arrange everything—we know indubitably how it has to be done, always the same way for everybody alike," was "just the same air towards him as he himself put on towards an accused person."[12] Of course, the doctrine of informed consent is based on the recognition that people are not all the same and that physicians must let patients decide about treatment options so that they do not treat them "always the same way for everybody alike." In the treatment of cancer, the problem is especially acute because it is complicated by the financial conflicts of interest of oncologists. The chief beneficiaries of unproved cancer treatments are often the "appointment book of the oncologist" and "the pharmaceutical companies and their stockholders."[13] It is also likely that there would be far less aggressive treatment at the end of life if patients were honestly informed of the "sheer futility" of such experimental interventions.[13]

After more than two decades of legal and ethical debate, neither the idea nor the ideal of informed consent governs the doctor–patient relationship.[9,10,11,13] Jay Katz has properly noted that for conditions in which

> prognosis is dire and fatal outcome a likely prospect . . . physicians should be guided by the strongest presumption in favor of disclosure and consent which can be modified only by clear and carefully documented evidence that patients do not wish to be fully informed.[14]

In affirming *Cobbs,* the court's decision in *Arato,* although very narrow, is consistent with Katz's vision and should be understood as an affirmation of information sharing and patient-centered decision making in the context of a physician–patient relationship based on trust.

Notes

1. Tuchman, B.W. A distant mirror: the calamitous 14th century. New York: Ballantine Books, 1978:58.
2. President's Commission for the Study of Ethical Problems in Medicine and Biomedical and Behavioral Research. Making health care decisions: the ethical and legal implications of informed consent in the patient-practitioner relationship. Vol. 2. Appendices. Washington, D.C.: Government Printing Office, 1982:245–6.
3. Arato v. Avedon, 5 Cal. 4th 1172, 23 Cal. Rptr.2d 131, 858 P.2d 598 (1993).
4. Arato v. Avedon, 13 Cal. App. 4th 1325, 11 Cal. Rptr.2d 169 (1992).
5. Cobbs v. Grant, 8 Cal.3d 229, 104 Cal. Rptr. 505, 502 P.2d 1 (1972).
6. Truman v. Thomas, 27 Cal.3d 285, 165 Cal. Rptr. 308, 611 P.2d 902 (1980).
7. Moore v. Regents of the University of California, 51 Cal.3d 120, 271 Cal. Rptr. 146, 793 P.2d 479 (1990).
8. Capron, A.M. Duty, truth, and whole human beings. Hastings Cent Rep 1993;23(4):13–4.
9. Annas, G.J. The rights of patients: the basic ACLU guide to patient rights. 2nd ed. Carbondale: Southern Illinois University Press, 1989.
10. Cassel, C.K., Meier, D.E. Morals and moralism in the debate over euthanasia and assisted suicide. N Engl J Med 1990;323:750–2.
11. Katz, J. The silent world of doctor and patient. New York: Free Press, 1984.
12. Tolstoy, L. The death of Ivan Ilych. New York: New American Library, 1960.
13. Moertel, C.G. Off-label drug use for cancer therapy and national health care priorities. JAMA 1991;266:3031–2.
14. Katz, J. Physician-patient encounters "On a darkling plain." W N Engl Law Rev 1987;9:207–26.

Swapping Stories:
A Matter of Ethics
Judith Andre

■

"Just promise you'll never write about me," pleaded a friend of mine. There was nothing ethically unusual about his life, and he knew that identities are disguised in case studies—nevertheless, he felt strongly, and I have honored his request. (I feel slightly uneasy even quoting him here.)

Stories are one of the joys of life. In some sense stories are life, for through them we make sense out of what happens. Professionals, like all people, tell stories. We talk about friends, family, colleagues, and clients. Waitresses talk about customers, architects about clients, teachers about students. By telling stories we let off steam, we ask for moral support, we check our judgments against those of others. We entertain: with a good story, the saying goes, one can dine out for weeks.

In some fields stories are also the raw materials with which we work. In ethics and in health care, case studies are crucial. They illustrate, challenge, suggest and anchor all our theory. So we have professional reasons as well as the ubiquitous personal reasons to share what we've been part of.

There are limits, personal and professional, to what can be shared. Most professions hold their members to strict standards of confidentiality, because clients need to talk freely in order to get much help from us, and they talk more freely when they believe their secrets will be kept. Something similar could be said of friendship: the good it provides depends on mutual trust.

And here's the tension: as professionals, as co-workers, and as friends, we need to protect confidences. Revealing what we have been told often violates implicit promises, abuses trust and destroys relationships. Yet as professionals and simply as human beings, we want and need to share our experiences.

Most writing about confidentiality looks at dramatic situations, and looks at conflicts between professional commitments to confidentiality and general obligations to prevent harm. Gunshot wounds, child abuse, and sexually transmitted diseases must by law be reported. Credible threats to harm people must usually be made known. HIV and AIDS create particularly intense conflicts between privacy and the right to know.

I'm interested in more mundane questions: the dangers posed by our human need to talk about one another. I want to evaluate different ways of swapping stories, about clients but also about one another.

The Moral Variables

The following factors make a moral difference.

(1) Whether the people who figure in the story want it told.

(2) Whether we have committed ourselves to confidentiality.

(3) The good and the harm that may result.

(4) Our intentions.

(5) How easily the people in it can be identified.

(6) Whether the audience needs to know.

The worst case would be something like this: a professional passes on to the world at large a story about his client, a story that names her and injures her. He does so against her wishes, and

wanting to cause her pain. Could such a thing ever be justified? It might be the only way to prevent still more serious harm. The Tarasoff case comes to mind: a therapist's patient threatened to kill someone, and eventually did so. The therapist was held liable for not telling the victim of the threats he had heard. Yet even in this case the therapist would not have been justified in telling the world at large. Factor (6) is at work: only a few people needed to know of the threats. At the other extreme, there is no ethical problem with a story in which identities are disguised, the client has agreed, and only good is intended and expected.

Harder Cases

As usual, it is the middle ground where hard and interesting questions arise. Some might argue, for instances, that someone's wishes alone do not count; that factors (2) through (6) above matter, but (1) does not. Such a position would let me write about the friend I mentioned earlier, particularly if I disguised his identity. Yet I do not, and not only because I made the promise he asked me of me. My reluctance stems partly from the fact that any story can get back to anyone; if he should someday read a story which he knew was his, he would feel betrayed. What if I disguised his identity so thoroughly that he could not recognize himself? Even here I would hesitate; I suppose what grounds that hesitation is a sense that one's story is private property. I do not have permission to use his.

Others might argue that factor (3), harm to the figures in the story, does not count, especially where the only harm is knowledge of unflattering facts. Recently, for instance, I heard of a health care professional who refused to care for an AIDS patient. If I added a few more details, knowledgeable readers could track down the provider involved. Does s/he have a right for the story not to be known? Partly that depends on how the story first "got out." If I learned of it through serving on an ethics committee, then I have probably made an implicit promise not to reveal what I learned. If I learned of it from the patient, however, my telling would violate no commitment, no professional obligation. Refusal of treatment is, in some sense, a public act.

Yet I do not feel free to pass on what I know, without significantly disguising the details. Why? For one thing, "what I know" overstates the case: I heard the story from someone who had heard the story from someone else. Every fable, every child's game, about gossip reminds us that stories mutate in being told; in every ethics consultation I've taken part in, it has taken 30 to 45 minutes to arrive at a reasonable grasp of the basic facts, and I've always thought that another 30 or 45 minutes would alter my understanding still further. What is morally relevant here is not any promise I've made, but the chance of harm to someone who does not deserve it. In fact I would make a still stronger claim: even if the provider were without question in the wrong—say, a cardiologist who refused to put her stethoscope to an AIDS patient's chest—I do not think the story should be told without disguise. People do not usually "deserve" to be thought poorly of, even when those thoughts are accurate. More precisely, the advantages of having people understand one another's faults rarely outweigh the harm to the maligned and the danger of exaggeration. We *do* love to talk.

Finally, there are our intentions (factor (4) above). These are notoriously hard to get hold of. Here I will use "intentions" loosely, to include all that one hopes to accomplish. In cases like Tarasoff one's intentions seem morally irrelevant: the threat has to be made known, even if one secretly takes delight in harming the threatener. Yet even here intentions may matter, not to the rightness of the disclosure, but to the character of the discloser. Morally speaking, it's not great to delight in someone else's suffering.

Intentions also play a deeper and more practical role. We need to be suspicious of our motives. We may think we're telling a story because it's funny—but just under the surface we may be telling it from anger, and a desire to ridicule.

Here we come full circle. Story telling allows us to discharge our anger, check our perceptions, sort out feelings, share our lives. It would be puritanical to deny those needs. Yet stories can easily hurt, and hurt badly; we are likely to underestimate how much they can, and how much we may want them to.

Can we keep our stories and tell them, too? With several cautions, I think we can. Ideally stories are told only with the subjects' permission. Of course groups of friends develop norms, as do cultures, and it becomes understood what is private and what is public. (Watch out, though, for the norms professionals develop about sharing among themselves. Clients may have no idea of the kind of story-swapping their professionals take for granted.)

Without the subjects' permission, implicit or explicit, stories should be so heavily disguised that its characters would not recognize themselves. (In clinical sciences variables should not be changed: age, sex, history all can have clinical significance. What serves as a disguise here is abstraction: a "67-year old female with chronic obstructive pulmonary disease" is too spare a description to pick out anyone. When the combination of physical facts *is* unique, the client's permission should be gotten.)

Stories that (apparently) can hurt no one need less care.

But sometimes we speak from anger and pain; sometimes we need to. And catharsis demands that names be used. Here the best protection is choosing and limiting one's audience. A single trusted friend, bound to confidence, is the best choice.

Final Thoughts

The position for which I argue may seem rigorous, even rigid. But I have seen communities of friends and workers which flourish within its protection, and I have seen others damaged for lack of it. I would be glad to hear what others have to say—your thoughts and your stories (!).

Case Study:

Please Don't Tell!

Leonard Fleck and

Marcia Angell

■

The patient, Carlos R., was a twenty-one-year-old Hispanic male who had suffered gunshot wounds to the abdomen in gang violence. He was uninsured. His stay in the hospital was somewhat shorter than might have been expected, but otherwise unremarkable. It was felt that he could safely complete his recovery at home. Carlos admitted to his attending physician that he was HIV-positive, which was confirmed.

At discharge the attending physician recommended a daily home nursing visit for wound care. However, Medicaid would not fund this nursing visit because a caregiver lived in the home who could adequately provide this care, namely, the patient's twenty-two-year-old sister Consuela, who in fact was willing to accept this burden. Their mother had died almost ten years ago, and Consuela had been a mother to Carlos and their younger sister since then. Carlos had no objection to Consuela's providing this care, but he insisted absolutely that she was not to know his HIV status. He had always been on good terms with Consuela, but she did not know he was actively homosexual. His greatest fear, though, was that his father would learn of his homosexual orientation, which is generally looked upon with great disdain by Hispanics.

Would Carlos's physician be morally justified in breaching patient confidentiality on the grounds that he had a "duty to warn"?

Commentary
Leonard Fleck

If there were a home health nurse to care for this patient, presumably there would be no reason to breach confidentiality since the expectation would be that she would follow universal precautions. Of course, universal precautions could be explained to the patient's sister. In an ideal world this would seem to be a satisfactory response that protects both Carlos's rights and Consuela's welfare. But the world is not ideal.

We know that health professionals, who surely ought to have the knowledge that would motivate them to take universal precautions seriously, often fail to take just such precautions. It is easy to imagine that Consuela could be equally casual or careless, especially when she had not been specifically warned that her brother was HIV-infected. Given this possibility, does the physician have a duty to warn that would justify breaching confidentiality? I shall argue that he may not breach confidentiality but he must be reasonably attentive to Consuela's safety. Ordinarily the conditions that must be met to invoke a duty to warn are: (1) an imminent threat of serious and irreversible harm, (2) no alternative to averting that threat other than this breach of confidentiality, and (3) proportionality between the harm averted by this breach of confidentiality and the harm associated with such a breach. In my judgment, none of these conditions are satisfactorily met.

No one doubts that becoming HIV-infected represents a serious and irreversible harm. But, in reality, is that threat imminent enough to justify breaching confidentiality? If we were talking about two individuals who were going to have sexual intercourse on repeated occasions, then the imminence condition would likely be met. But the patient's sister will be caring for his wound for only a week or two, and wound care does not by itself involve any exchange of body fluids. If we had two-hundred and forty surgeons operating on two-hundred and forty HIV-infected patients, and if each of those surgeons nicked himself while doing surgery, then the likelihood is that only one of them would become HIV-infected. Using this as a reference point, the likelihood of this young woman seroconverting if her intact skin comes into contact with the blood of this patient is very remote at best.

Moreover in this instance there are alternatives. A frank and serious discussion with Consuela about the need for universal precautions, plus monitored, thorough training in correct wound care, fulfills what I would regard as a reasonable duty to warn in these circumstances. Similar instructions ought to be given to Carlos so that he can monitor her performance. He can be reminded that this is a small price for protecting his confidentiality as well as his sister's health. It might also be necessary to provide gloves and other such equipment required to observe universal precautions.

We can imagine easily enough that there might be a lapse in conscientiousness on Consuela's part, that she might come into contact with his blood. But even if this were to happen, the likelihood of her seroconverting is remote at best. This is where proportionality between the harm averted by the breach and the harm associated with it comes in. For if confidentiality were breached and she were informed of his HIV status, this would likely have very serious consequences for Carlos. As a layperson with no professional duty to preserve confidentiality herself, Consuela might inform other family members, which could lead to his being ostracized from the family. And even if she kept the information confidential, she might be too afraid to provide the care for Carlos, who might then end up with no one to care for him.

The right to confidentiality is a right that can be freely waived. The physician could engage Carlos in a frank moral discussion aimed at persuading him that the reasonable and decent thing to do is to inform his sister of his HIV status. Perhaps the physician offers assurances that she would be able to keep that information in strict confidence. The patient agrees. Then what happens? It is easy to imagine that Consuela balks at caring for her brother, for fear of infection.

Medicaid would still refuse to pay for home nursing care because a caregiver would still be in the home, albeit a terrified caregiver. Consuela's response may not be rational, but it is certainly possible. If she were to react in this way it would be an easy "out" to say that it was Carlos who freely agreed to the release of the confidential information so now he'll just have to live with those consequences. But the matter is really more complex than that. At the very least the physician would have to apprise Carlos of the fact that his sister might divulge his HIV status to some number of other individuals. But if the physician impresses this possibility on Carlos vividly enough, Carlos might be even more reluctant to self-disclose his HIV status to Consuela. In that case the physician is morally obligated to respect that confidentiality.

Commentary
Marcia Angell

It would be wrong, I believe, to ask this young woman to undertake the nursing care of her brother and not inform her that he is HIV-infected.

The claim of a patient that a doctor hold his secrets in confidence is strong but not absolute. It can be overridden by stronger, competing claims.

For example, a doctor would not agree to hold in confidence a diagnosis of rubella, if the patient were planning to be in the presence of a pregnant woman without warning her. Similarly, a doctor would be justified in acting on knowledge that a patient planned to commit a crime. Confidentiality should, of course, be honored when the secret is entirely personal, that is, when it could have no substantial impact on anyone else. On the other hand, when it would pose a major threat to others, the claim of confidentiality must be overridden. Difficulties arise when the competing claims are nearly equal in moral weight.

In this scenario, does Consuela have any claims on the doctor? I believe she does, and that her claims are very compelling. They stem, first, from her right to have information she might consider relevant to her decision to act as her brother's nurse, and, second, from the health care system's obligation to warn of a possible risk to her health. I would like to focus first on whether Consuela has a right to information apart from the question of whether there is in fact an appreciable risk. I believe that she has such a right, for three reasons.

First, there is an element of deception in *not* informing Consuela that her brother is HIV-infected. Most people in her situation would want to know if their "patient" were HIV-infected and would presume that they would be told if that were the case. (I suspect that a private nurse hired in a similar situation would expect to be told—and that she would be.) At some level, perhaps unconsciously, Consuela would assume that Carlos did not have HIV infection because no one said that he did. Thus, in keeping Carlos's secret, the doctor implicitly deceives Consuela—not a net moral gain, I think.

Second, Consuela has been impressed to provide nursing care in part because the health system is using her to avoid providing a service it would otherwise be responsible for. This fact, I believe, gives the health care system an additional obligation to her, which includes giving her all the information that might bear on her decision to accept this responsibility. It might be argued that the information about her brother's HIV infection is not relevant, but it is patronizing to make this assumption. She may for any number of reasons, quite apart from the risk of transmission, find it important to know that he is HIV-infected.

Finally, I can't help feeling that this young woman has already been exploited by her family and that the health care system should not collude in doing so again. We are told that since she was twelve, she has acted as "mother" to a brother only one year younger, presumably simply because she is female, since she is no more a mother than he is. Now she is being asked to be a nurse, as well as a mother, again presumably because she is female. In this context, concerns about the sensibilities of the father or about Carlos's fear of them are not very compelling, particularly when they are buttressed by stereotypes about Hispanic families. Furthermore, both his father and his sister will almost certainly learn the truth eventually.

What about the risk of transmission from Carlos to Consuela? Many would—wrongly, I believe—base their arguments solely on this question. Insofar as they did, they would have very little to go on. The truth is that no one knows what the risk would be to Consuela. To my knowledge, there have been no studies that would yield data on the point. Most likely the risk would be extremely small, particularly if there were no blood or pus in the wound, but it would be speculative to say how small. We do know that Consuela has no experience with universal precautions and could not be expected to use them diligently with her brother unless she had some sense of why she might be doing so. In any case, the doctor has no right to decide for this young woman that she should assume a risk,

even if he believes it would be remote. That is for her to decide. The only judgment he has a right to make is whether *she* might consider the information that her brother is HIV-infected to be relevant to her decision to nurse him, and I think it is reasonable to assume she might.

There is, I believe, only one ethical way out of this dilemma. The doctor should strongly encourage Carlos to tell his sister that he is HIV-infected or offer to do it for him. She could be asked not to tell their father, and I would see no problem with this. I would have no hesitation in appealing to the fact that Carlos already owes Consuela a great deal. If Carlos insisted that his sister not be told, the doctor should see to it that his nursing needs are met in some other way. In sum, then, I believe the doctor should pass the dilemma to the patient: Carlos can decide to accept Consuela's generosity—in return for which he must tell her he is HIV-infected (or ask the doctor to tell her)—or he can decide not to tell her and do without her nursing care.

Interests in Conflict

Section 2 presents two common instances of conflicting interests in health care ethics, for comparison and contrast.

There are occasions when the interests of the pregnant woman conflict with those of her fetus. Powerful arguments have been made on all sides of this issue. Out of the volumes of readings available on the subject, we have chosen only two. Nancy Rhoden argues that intervening on behalf of the fetus over the pregnant woman's objection is both immoral and impractical; Frank Chervenak and Laurence McCullough defend the position that favors medicine's authority to intervene. Is this conflict, as it is presented by cesarean section cases, similar to or different from the case of the pregnant woman's use of illegal (or legal) drugs, exposure to environmental toxins, diet, lifestyle, or genetic contribution to the fetus? How is this conflict affected by the issue of gender? Is pregnancy unique, or should the lives and choices of the fathers of fetuses raise similar concerns?

The second instance of conflicting interests lies in the area of research and treatment. The two readings in this section ask how medicine and science fit together, by examining where the line between research and treatment becomes blurred. In fact, in some cases there may be no line at all, but rather a no-man's-land that

may be surprisingly large. In the first reading, George Annas discusses the distinction between research and treatment and some of the history of the federal Food and Drug Administration's regulation of new drug testing, and sharply criticizes moves to make new AIDS drugs available more quickly. He addresses the role of scientific evidence in medicine and argues that the rules of research should not change for persons with fatal diseases.

The last reading is a case study that juxtaposes the viewpoint of the patient with a fatal disease and the viewpoint of the physician who seeks to do the best for that patient, when in the physician's view the best treatment is available only through enrollment in a clinical trial. The central matters of how we balance risks against potential benefits and of how autonomy stacks up against beneficence in this context are illuminated by comparing the physician's goal of benefiting individual patients and the scientist's goal of determining whether a treatment is sufficiently beneficial. Are the judgments involved individual, medical, or social? What is the physician's role in making, facilitating, or curtailing them? Though these readings are perhaps more detailed and dependent on the understanding of technical matters than any others in this part of the reader, they permit a thorough exploration of the relationship between research and treatment, of the complex conflict between science and hope, and of how researchers, physicians, and patients use information and balance roles when making difficult choices.

There is a large body of literature on this topic as well. The readings in this section could be supplemented by excerpts from the *Belmont Report* (National Commission for the Protection of Human Subjects of Biomedical and Behavioral Research 1978) and from the Federal Regulations for the Protection of Human Subjects of Medical Research, as well as by many other writings. In addition, these readings could form the basis for a discussion of some larger issues, including the nature of medical progress, the question of informed consent to unprecedented treatments, and the policy problem of how and by whom medical innovation should be regulated.

Cesareans and Samaritans

Nancy K. Rhoden

∎

Until recently, if one asked the proverbial person on the street to list maternal-fetal conflicts, he or she would have mentioned abortion and, when pressed to continue, looked at the questioner blankly. Now, however, the populace is becoming aware of a host of maternal-fetal conflicts. Indeed, mother-and-child, long a somewhat romanticized unity, are increasingly being treated by physicians, courts, and the media as potential adversaries, locked in battle on the rather inconvenient battleground of the woman's belly.

Some of these newly publicized conflicts— pregnant women abusing drugs or alcohol, or continuing to work in occupations hazardous to fetal health—are not all that new: the hazards of various substances have been known for years. Other of the conflicts are new, inasmuch as doctors could not recommend Cesareans or other procedures for the fetus' benefit until they could detect fetal problems during or before labor. But probably what is most unprecedented is that now, suddenly, physicians are seeking court intervention to protect these imperiled fetuses— intervention that, inevitably, constitutes a significant intrusion into the woman's conduct during pregnancy or birth.

This essay will discuss just one of the proliferating array of maternal-fetal conflicts—the question whether courts should have the power to authorize doctors to perform Cesarean deliveries against the woman's will. Doctors typically seek these orders when they believe, based on diagnostic techniques, that vaginal delivery risks death or neurological damage to the fetus. (In some cases, vaginal delivery is a risk for the woman as well.) Women who refuse most commonly do so based on religious beliefs opposed to surgery, though they may refuse because they fear surgery, do not believe the doctor's prognoses, or whatever.

I have restricted my focus to this issue for several reasons. First, these cases are more common than the absence of reported judicial decisions would make one believe, because many of them are completely unreported.[1] Some make the local newspapers,[2] but many don't. For example, during my year as a visiting professor at Albert Einstein College of Medicine, such a case arose at North Central Bronx, one of the college's affiliated hospitals. It was litigated, and a nonconsensual Cesarean was authorized.[3] But there was no reported decision, no coverage in local newspapers and, indeed, no way anyone not involved in the case or present at the hospital would know of it. Second, these cases are extraordinarily difficult. They pit a woman's rights to privacy and bodily integrity, normally more than sufficient to allow a competent adult to refuse major surgery, against the possibility of a lifetime of devastating disability to a being who is within days or even hours of independent existence. Finally, as more and more techniques for diagnosing and treating problems in utero are developed, it is likely that doctors will seek authorization for other nonconsensual treatments.[4] The Cesarean cases, inasmuch as they rest on technology that is standard and routine right now, will constitute important precedents for such future controversies.

The position I will defend is that courts should not order competent women to have Cesareans, despite the potentially tragic consequences to the fetus. This is neither an easy position nor a fully satisfactory one. Indeed, it is the sort of hard-line civil libertarian position that I ordinarily find oversimplified in bioethics issues. Yet I believe that it is the morally and legally correct position—albeit merely the "least worst" one—because these orders (1) impose an unparalleled intrusion upon pregnant women; (2) undermine the teachings of the informed consent doctrine that only the individual being subjected to a procedure can assess its risks and benefits; and (3) contain within them the seeds of widespread and pernicious usurpation of women's choices during obstetrical care.

Justifications for Nonconsensual Cesareans

Abortion Law

In the cases of which I am aware, every judge but one who has ruled on an application for nonconsensual Cesarean delivery has granted the request.[5] Interestingly, *Roe v. Wade,*[6] which has stood firmly for a woman's right to privacy and right to make her own decisions about pregnancy, is the case most commonly invoked by courts to justify these orders.[7] Under *Roe,* women must be allowed to choose abortion prior to fetal viability (subject to state regulation to protect the mother's health in the second trimester). But once a fetus is capable of independent life outside the womb, albeit with artificial aid, the state's interest in potential life becomes compelling.[8] Then the state can prohibit abortion, unless it is necessary to protect the woman's life or health. Courts invoking *Roe* to support nonconsensual Cesarean delivery reason that since states can prohibit the intentional termination of fetal life after viability, they can likewise protect viable fetuses by preventing vaginal delivery when it will have the same effect as abortion.[9]

At first glance this analysis appears attractive. Attempting a vaginal delivery when responsible medical opinion says that surgical delivery is necessary for the fetus may cause a stillbirth or, perhaps worse, profound neurological damage to the child. These consequences are clearly ones that states have an interest in preventing. But the fact that states have an interest in preventing certain consequences does not mean that any and all action to prevent such consequences is constitutional. For example, states have an interest in preventing use of illicit drugs, and they can make such conduct criminal. But this doesn't mean that they can take any and all other steps to prevent drug use, such as ordering random strip searches at airports (though the way things are going, we may soon see random urine samples). Similarly, the Court in *Roe* said that in the third trimester, the state can even "go so far as to proscribe abortion,"[10] unless the woman's health is at stake. That the state can go this far, prohibiting intentional fetal destruction, doesn't necessarily mean that it can go even farther, and mandate major surgery to protect and preserve the fetus' life. There is a quantum leap in logic between prohibiting destruction and requiring surgical preservation that courts and commentators relying on abortion law have ignored.

In fact, if one reads *Roe* and its progeny more closely, it becomes apparent that court-ordered Cesareans violate *Roe*'s constitutional schema. *Roe* emphasizes that even after the fetus is viable, the woman's life and health come first. If her health is threatened by her pregnancy even after the fetus is viable, she must be allowed to abort.[11] In *Colautti v. Franklin,*[12] the Supreme Court discussed the primacy of maternal health even more specifically. It invalidated a statute that required doctors performing postviability abortions to use the technique least harmful to the fetus, unless another technique was necessary for the woman's health. Among other infirmities, this statute impermissibly implied that the more hazardous technique had to be *indispensable* to the woman's health, and suggested that doctors could be required to make trade-offs between her health and additional percentage points of the fetus' survival.[13] Abortion law makes clear that such trade-offs cannot be required.

Thus a state could not, under *Colautti,* require that all abortions after viability be done by hysterotomy, a surgical technique that is basically a mini-Cesarean, on the grounds that this is safest for the fetus. A state could not require this because such a technique is less safe for the woman. It may not be immediately apparent that this proscription of compulsory maternal-fetal trade-offs in late abortion applies to the Cesarean dilemma. Yet this becomes quite clear when one realizes that after a fetus is viable, the methods of abortion and of premature delivery simply merge.[14] Although the Supreme Court in *Roe* and subsequent cases has spoken of post-viability abortion, doctors have historically thought of late terminations necessitated by a health problem on the woman's part as premature deliveries—deliveries that may put the fetus at great risk but that are not specifically intended to destroy it. In other words, post-viability terminations of pregnancy are simply inductions of labor, just as might be done at full term.

Once we recognize this, we see that what the Court says about third-trimester abortion should apply to delivery methods as well. When that yardstick is applied, it yields the conclusion that a state clearly could not enact a statute requiring Cesarean over vaginal delivery to protect the fetus. Inasmuch as surgical delivery involves approximately four times the maternal mortality rate of vaginal delivery,[15] such a statute would impermissibly mandate trade-offs between maternal and fetal health. The state could not statutorily mandate surgical delivery even in those cases where the fetus' health was seriously threatened by vaginal delivery, because the mother's health will still almost always be somewhat threatened by surgical delivery. Likewise, it violates the Constitution for courts to authorize nonconsensual Cesarean delivery in individual cases, since it seems clear that courts should not issue orders in individual cases that, if generalized in the form of a statute, would be unconstitutional.

The Child Neglect/Fetal Neglect Analogy

Despite the strong argument that nonconsensual Cesareans are at odds with the teachings of *Roe* and other Supreme Court abortion cases, it may be objected that in rejecting maternal-fetal trade-offs, the Supreme Court was thinking only about abortions, not about full-term deliveries. Given the state's strong interest in preservation of life, why, one might ask, must doctors stand by while a baby who could be fine if delivered surgically dies or suffers irreversible brain damage? What-ever abortion law says, should women really have a right to make this potentially lethal choice, when the risk to them is quite minimal?

Courts and commentators have frequently re-lied on the law of child neglect to argue that harmful choices such as these are not the wom-an's to make.[16] Parents, of course, cannot refuse needed medical care for their children, even if the provision of such care violates their most cherished religious beliefs.[17] Likewise, it is often argued, pregnant women cannot refuse care nec-essary for their fetus' well-being. To do so is the prenatal equivalent of child neglect (and, accord-ing to this theory, taking substances such as her-oin while one is pregnant is the prenatal equiv-alent of child abuse).

There's a simple charm to this notion that if parents cannot deny care to a child, neither can a pregnant woman deny it to a fetus, at least to a fetus that is fully formed and clearly viable. When analyzed, however, this notion is far from charming. It has far-reaching and very alarming implications, and it is far less simple than it ap-pears. Child neglect is, of course, the failure to perform one's legal duties to one's children. The term "fetal neglect" implies that there are legally enforceable duties to fetuses. But while parents have historically owed a whole panoply of duties to their children, women have not heretofore been held to have legally enforceable duties to fetuses. Of course, we have until recently lacked the technology for visualizing the fetus, diag-nosing its problems, and hence recommending procedures for its benefit. Some writers have suggested that the development of such technol-ogies is sufficient to create new maternal duties to the fetus.[18] But before we let technology create entirely new sets of duties, we should at least stop and ask what technology hath wrought.

The technology for treating the fetus as a pa-tient within a patient has transformed the unity of pregnancy into an uneasy duality. Two gestalts are now at work. One sees the pregnant woman as primary and the fetus as secondary; the other reverses the roles. "Fetal neglect" proponents unquestionably see the fetus as primary. They would discern the fetus' needs and then hold the woman responsible for either meeting those needs or justifying her failure to do so. Although they might argue that this is as good a way of reconciling the mother–fetus duality as subor-dinating the fetus' needs to the mother's, there are good reasons why, under the law, it is not. For one thing, while many women may place the best interests of their fetuses first and foremost, for the law to mandate this approach denies the full import of the fact that the fetus is located inside the woman.

Obviously, "fetal neglect" proponents recog-nize the *fact* of the fetus' internal location. They then draw the analogy with child neglect by stat-ing that this difference in location is the only difference between a fetus and a child. True, it is (at least for very late-term fetuses). But in terms of what a state must do to end "fetal neglect" as opposed to ending child neglect, this "slight dis-analogy" is like the difference between night and day. Children can simply be treated, in opposi-tion to parental demands. But "fetal neglect" cannot be remedied without, as it were, "breaching the maternal barrier"—restraining and physically invading the woman. If one approaches this issue looking to what the fetus needs, there is a tendency to forget the woman is there—or to forget that she is more than, as George Annas puts it, a "fetal container."[19] Instead, one must approach the issue by asking if the woman's privacy can be violated—with the reason for violation being the state's important interest in protecting the life within her.

Giving due weight to the respective locations of mother and fetus debars us from using the simple (and simplistic) child neglect/fetal neglect analogy. It does not, however, answer the question of whether nonconsensual surgery can be imposed. For this, we must consider other cases in which the state's interests may oppose a patient's right to refuse treatment.

The State's Interest in the Well-Being of Third Parties

Competent persons can refuse medical treatment, even when it means their death. Their rights to privacy and bodily integrity are increasingly respected, even though the state has interests, such as in preserving life, that are arrayed against virtually all treatment refusals.[20] In other words, while the state's interests are neither negligible nor forgotten, the patients' privacy rights trump them. But most refusals do not have a direct and devastating effect upon third parties. How do we weigh the individual's right to refuse in these cases against the state's interest in preserving a third party's life—an interest that puts these cases in a class by themselves?

Courts have not taken the interests of third parties lightly, even when the goal was to preserve their emotional welfare rather than to protect them from physical harm. Some courts have overridden treatment refusals by parents of dependent children (usually Jehovah's Witnesses

refusing blood transfusions), on the grounds that the parent should not be allowed to orphan his or her child.[21] It can readily be argued that if a parent's privacy right can be overridden to spare his child emotional or financial loss, surely it can be overridden to prevent a stillbirth or a birth injury that may cause profound impairment. The only problem with this argument is that these cases are, in my opinion, clearly wrong.[22] Although the practice is frowned upon, parents can abandon their children by putting them in foster care or even up for adoption; some parents de facto abandon their children by, for example, divorcing and leaving the jurisdiction; and parents take health risks, such as hang gliding, sky diving, or joining the U.S. army, that could potentially result in their children being orphaned. Why, in the one sphere of medical treatment, should they be required to violate their faith and adhere to medical orthodoxy? I see no good reason why here, but not elsewhere, parenthood should obliterate personal autonomy.

Of course, even if one accepted this line of cases, they could still readily be distinguished from the Cesarean dilemma. First, a blood transfusion is a less serious intrusion, involving far less pain, risk, bodily invasion, and recovery time. Second, the imposition of blood transfusions to prevent child abandonment does benefit the parent, in objective or secular terms: it saves his life, even though it does so, according to his faith, at the cost of his future salvation. Except in cases involving conditions such as placenta previa, where vaginal delivery threatens the lives of both woman and fetus, a Cesarean will benefit the fetus but not the woman. Indeed, rather than benefiting, the woman will typically be placed at somewhat greater risk by the proposed surgery. This makes the Cesarean cases truly unusual: one must ask when, if ever, the state can override a treatment refusal and impose a risk upon one person so as to preserve the life or health of another person.

Having recognized that the true analogue to imposed Cesareans is nonconsensual surgery sought to benefit a third party, we now confront a significant dearth of caselaw. One reason is that there are few fact patterns in which a medical procedure performed on A will save B. Another reason is that compelling A to undergo risks so as to save B has always been considered beyond the reaches of state authority. In setting forth the limits of state authority, philosophers and legal scholars frequently note that the state could not require one citizen to give up a kidney to save another citizen, or to give up an eye so another could see.[23] The idea is outrageous enough to have been burlesqued in a *Monty Python* skit, where a woman minding her own business at home is interrupted by a loud knock on the door. The official-looking man at the door announces, "We've come for your kidney." When she protests, he says, "But you signed a donor card, didn't you?" She stammers that she meant to donate only after she was dead. Looking solemn, he says, unsheathing his surgical tools, "But someone needs it now."

In this country there is no general duty to rescue. There are exceptions, which include a special relationship between the parties such as that of innkeeper and guest, common carrier and passenger, and, most importantly, parent and child.[24] But even when a special relationship gives rise to a duty to rescue, there is still no duty to undertake *risky* rescues.[25] Nor is there such a duty in countries where there is a general duty to rescue.[26] It is easy to see that a demand for someone's kidney falls under the law of rescue (Samaritan law) and goes far beyond what is ever required of potential rescuers. In the one case on point, *McFall v. Shimp,*[27] a man dying of aplastic anemia asked the court to mandate that his cousin donate bone marrow to save him. The court called the relative's refusal to donate morally reprehensible, but held that for the law to "sink its teeth into the jugular vein or neck of

one of its members and suck from it sustenance for *another* member, is revolting to our hard-wrought concepts of jurisprudence. Such would raise the spectre of the swastika and the Inquisition, reminiscent of the horrors this portends."[28] Although there are no *McFall*-type cases involving parent-child donation, I think we can say with a fair degree of certainty that the outcome would and should be the same. Parents have a duty to rescue their children—i.e., to be basic Good Samaritans—but they have no duty to be "Splendid Samaritans,"[29] embarking upon rescues that risk their life or health.

The Illegitimacy of Interpersonal Risk-Benefit Comparisons

If what a court does in mandating a Cesarean is no different from mandating a bone marrow transfusion to save a dying relative, it clearly exceeds the state's legitimate authority. While the two seem equivalent to me, they certainly haven't seemed so to most of the courts that have considered requests for nonconsensual Cesareans. For various reasons, court-ordered Cesareans strike many people as legitimate, while court-ordered bone marrow transfusions or kidney donations (a more equivalent intrusion), even from parent to child, seem outrageous. These reasons are important and cannot be ignored—they are what makes this situation so agonizing. However, I will try to show that while these reasons go to the woman's conduct, the appropriate question concerns the nature of the *state's* conduct. When we look to it, all nonconsensual risks imposed on one person to save another are equally illegitimate.

The Cesarean cases unquestionably *feel* different from cases or hypotheticals involving forced intrusions on parents to save children. For one thing, the woman is going to give birth anyway, and if she just does it surgically instead of vaginally the baby will probably be fine. Cesareans are common and relatively safe, and the potential harm from delivering the baby vaginally is very serious. Moreover, it seems to some that women who choose not to abort thereby assume certain obligations to their fetuses, a by no means unreasonable suggestion. Finally, pregnancy simply is a unique situation. A dying relative, even a child, is a separate, independent person. However dire his need, he is not a tiny, helpless, totally dependent creature.

Emotional responses should certainly not be disregarded in bioethics. But neither should they necessarily rule. Physicians understandably become very uncomfortable when a woman appears ready to risk her fetus' life and health for the sake of her religious faith, and they feel even stronger when her reasons appear less weighty. Indeed, trivial reasons for running this risk may justify our casting moral aspersions on the woman's conduct. Despite the uniqueness of pregnancy, however, and despite the strength or weakness of the woman's reason for refusal (assuming she is competent), what the *state* does when it orders a compulsory Cesarean is no different from what it does when it orders compulsory bone marrow or kidney "donation," and what the state does is wrong.

The most significant feature of decisions ordering Cesareans is that the court, explicitly or implicitly, finds that the potential harm to the fetus overrides the woman's rights to privacy, autonomy, and bodily integrity, and justifies imposing a physical harm upon her (because surgery is a harm even if it has no untoward consequences). The court, in other words, takes two people, looks at the potential consequences of a bad situation, and says that the probably severe harm to X warrants imposing a lesser physical harm on Y. The legitimacy of this argument depends upon the assumption that a third party can step in and weigh the risks of surgery for someone who has competently chosen to forego them, and can then order that these risks be run. This is an assumption that has always been rejected in

American jurisprudence, and that, if accepted, has far-reaching and extraordinarily frightening implications.

There is something special about the body. In theory, we can all recognize that everyone's body is equally special. But in practice, somehow our own seems far more special than anyone else's. It is very easy for us to say, as objective third parties, that a patient really should have needed surgery, because its risks are minute—perhaps only 1 in 10,000. But when we are thinking about that same surgery for ourselves, the minuteness of that chance may somehow seem less pertinent than the ghastly thought that we might be that one. This different attitude toward low statistical risks when run by a group of strangers and when run by oneself explains the old saying, "Minor surgery is surgery performed on somebody else." Perhaps this difference also explains why even countries with general duties to rescue never require risky rescues. While cowardice may not be admired, it is too human a quality to be formally punished by law.

Needless to say, a court can contemplate surgery for a pregnant woman only as a third-party bystander, albeit a careful and concerned bystander. It can assess the objective risks of surgery to the woman and the corresponding benefits to the fetus. But its ability truly to understand the situation is radically limited. Some limitations are simply due to the impossibility of extrapolating from statistical statements of risks, which apply to groups, to the risks faced by a particular individual. The court cannot know the exact risks it is planning to impose on the individual woman, because statistics don't tell us this. Other limitations relate to the particular, and undoubtedly unusual, circumstance: the risks may be increased if the surgery is done on an emergency basis,[30] and likewise may be magnified by its nonconsensual nature. But perhaps the most significant limitation is that a judge cannot possibly know or take into account the woman's subjective response to these risks, or to the proposed violation of her deeply held religious beliefs. In short, these decisions simply cannot be rendered objective. That is, after all, the whole point of the informed consent doctrine: people should be able to make their own decisions about surgery, even if their choices are idiosyncratic or even harmful.

In ordering surgery, the court is thus rendering objective a determination that cannot rightfully be anything but subjective. Although it is doing so for the best of reasons, its action nonetheless denies to a disturbing extent the woman's uniqueness and individuality. It denies her special fears or her special spiritual reasons for rejecting surgery and "leaving things in the hands of God." When it subjugates her views about having her body invaded (or about interfering with Providence) to its assessment of the "right" action based on potential consequences, it is making an interpersonal risk-benefit comparison and holding that she must run the risk to prevent the greater risk to the baby. Objectively, this may well be the proper assessment. But decisions about major surgery on unconsenting adults simply are not delegated to third parties, and delegating this one is no different from delegating a decision about bone marrow extraction or kidney transplant. I can think of no other instance where a state feels it has the authority to compare the risks faced by one individual to those faced by the other. The court compromises its integrity in making these orders, because whether it realizes it or not, it is treating the woman as a means—a vehicle for rescuing an imperiled fetus—and not as an end in herself.

Two disturbing potential scenarios will help illustrate why a nonconsensual Cesarean is inevitably a wrong against the woman. First, imagine surgery has been authorized, and the woman struggles to try to avoid it. In the case at North Central Bronx, doctors repeatedly asked what they should do if this occurred. Should they hold her down and anesthetize her? Some proponents of intervention would characterize this as merely

a practical problem in enforcement—some injunctions being easier to enforce than others. Yet this is much more than a mere enforcement issue. It illustrates the violence lurking here, whether or not it is ever actually committed. The court is at one remove from the violence, because its role is limited to issuing the order. Nonetheless, the court has authorized an act of violence against the woman, even if the violence is obscured by her cowed compliance in the face of judicial power.

Second, imagine that the highly unexpected happens, and the woman is killed or injured by the surgery. Although this is exceedingly unlikely, its possibility raises an interesting moral issue. The court cannot, of course, be held legally responsible for this harm, nor can the doctors, assuming they were not negligent. Yet the court would be, it seems, morally responsible, because it chose to subject the woman to this risk. There is no comparison between the state's responsibility under this scenario and its responsibility if the woman's refusal is upheld and the baby is harmed. If the baby suffers, the woman is causally responsible (assuming surgery would have prevented the harm) and in some cases, at least, will be morally to blame. But the state won't be implicated, because the state does not normally intervene in a person's medical decisions. In other words, a private wrong will have occurred. But if the state has the hubris to intervene in what is ordinarily a private (albeit potentially tragic) choice, it takes on the moral responsibility for the outcome as well. Although the chances of maternal injury are low, the moral risk is great, and this possibility should make courts think twice before mandating surgery.

Some Additional Social Concerns

For purposes of analyzing nonconsensual Cesareans, I have been assuming that the physicians' predictions of harm to the infant are correct. In any individual case, of course, the doctor's alarm is most likely warranted—although it is interesting to note that in *Jefferson, Headley,* and *Jeffries,* the women delivered vaginally and the infants were fine. But when we think of mandatory Cesareans not simply as individual cases but as a social policy, we must recognize that some of the operations will be unnecessary. This is because the tools upon which doctors rely to diagnose problems during pregnancy or labor detect abnormally high risks, but do not necessarily distinguish cases in which the risks will materialize from those in which they will not.

Some tools and diagnoses are better than others. For example, ultrasonography is highly reliable in detecting placenta previa, and diagnosis of complete placenta previa reliably dictates Cesarean delivery. But even here prediction is not 100-percent accurate: both Ms. Jefferson and Ms. Jeffries, who were diagnosed as having complete placenta previa, delivered vaginally. Other tools are as likely to be wrong as right. Electronic fetal monitoring detects abnormal fetal heart patterns during labor that suggest an inadequate flow of oxygen to the fetus. According to the Office of Technology Assessment, the false positive rate of this technology is between 18.5 and almost 80 percent.[31] The rate is around 44 percent even when combined with fetal scalp blood sampling, another test that is believed to be more reliable.[32] A number of controlled studies have shown no difference in perinatal outcome when low-risk women were monitored electronically and when nurses performed intermittent ascultation (listening for heart rate changes).[33]

Physicians should be risk-averse and reluctant to gamble with the lives of babies, and fears of legal liability naturally enhance these traits. However, technological limitations combined with a cautious, risk-averse approach virtually ensure that some of the Cesareans doctors recommend will turn out not to have been required. While the vast majority of women would far rather risk an unnecessary operation than an im-

paried infant, it is not so clear that, given the technological limitations, it is irrational or immoral to take a different approach to risk. At any rate, mandatory Cesareans will mean that the judicial system requires this risk-averse approach, and forces pregnant women as a group to run some unnecessary risks to ensure healthy babies.

Although it might be suggested that courts can distinguish truly risky situations from only somewhat risky ones, this suggestion unfortunately puts more faith in the judicial system than it deserves, at least in these types of cases. The doctors bringing them will undoubtedly believe that surgery is necessary. The courts will have little choice but to accept the doctor's assessment—especially since in the typical Cesarean case the woman is either not present at all (and of course not represented by counsel) or represented by an attorney appointed only hours or days before and patently incapable of presenting contrary medical evidence even if it could be obtained.[34] These cases have thus far been very one-sided, and given the time constraints will almost surely continue to be so. This may account in part for the fact that most courts have issued the orders. It is interesting to note that in the Pamela Rae Stewart case, where Ms. Stewart was criminally prosecuted for prenatal conduct that allegedly caused her child to be born with brain damage and then to die, there was for once a two-sided debate. Here the American Civil Liberties Union came to Ms. Stewart's defense, and all charges against her were dismissed.[35]

Another social consequence of mandatory Cesareans might well be harm to the babies themselves. When the court authorized nonconsensual surgery for Ms. Jeffries, she went into hiding and could not be found even by a police search. When the court authorized the surgery for Ms. Headley, she avoided the hospital by having a home birth with a lay midwife. If women with unorthodox religious beliefs know that their beliefs will not be honored, they may avoid physicians during delivery or even during their entire pregnancy, thus placing their babies at greatly increased risk. Presumably the informed consent doctrine would dictate that physicians tell women, early on in prenatal care, that they will not honor their religious beliefs if their fetus is endangered. This disclosure, however, will only serve to make such women avoid prenatal care (much as the reporting of drug abuse will make pregnant drug users avoid doctors and hospitals). Hence as a general social policy, mandatory fetal protection will have questionable success in protecting fetuses.

Conclusion

Emotionally compelling cases often make bad law. It is very hard for physicians and judges to resist the urge to save fetuses threatened by what appears to be the irrational conduct of the mother. The benevolence they feel is deeply rooted and deserves our respect. Unfortunately, mandatory rescue of the fetus requires an imposition upon the mother that goes far beyond what our society has imposed, or should impose, on others. Our historical restraint regarding such impositions has strong constitutional and ethical bases. Technology threatens this restraint, by making mandatory intervention possible. But technology cannot change the ethical principles that make mandatory intervention wrong.

Notes

This article is a shortened version of "The Judge in the Delivery Room: The Emergence of Court-Ordered Cesareans," which appeared in the California Law Review 1987, 74: 1951.

1. Only one of these cases—Jefferson v. Griffin Spalding County Hospital Authority, 274 S.E.2d 457 (Ga. 1981)—has been officially reported. Another case—In re Unborn Baby Kenner, No. 79 JN 83 (Colo. Juv. Ct. Mar. 6, 1979)—has been reported in medical literature; see Bowes, W.A., Selgestad, B., Fetal versus maternal

rights: Medical and legal perspectives, Obstetrics & Gynecology 1981, 58(2): 209, 211. A report of a large-scale survey indicates that courts in eleven states have ordered Cesarean deliveries. Kolder, V.E.B., Gallagher, J., Parsons, M.T., Court-ordered obstetrical interventions, New England Journal of Medicine 1987, 316(19): 1192–96, 1194.

2. See, e.g., In re Baby Jeffries, No. 14004 (Mich. P. Ct. May 24, 1982). Developments in the *Jeffries* case are described in a series of newspaper articles. See Detroit Free Press, May 29, 1982; June 13, 1982; and June 16, 1982.

3. North Central Bronx Hospital Authority v. Headley, No. 1992–85 (N.Y. Sup. Ct. Jan. 6, 1986).

4. For discussions of in utero therapy, see, e.g., Robertson, J.A., The right to procreate and in utero fetal therapy, Journal of Legal Medicine 1982, 3(3): 333–66; Ruddick, W., Wilcox, W., Operating on the fetus, Hastings Center Report 1982, 12(5): 10–14; Barclay, W.R. et al., The ethics of in utero surgery, Journal of the American Medical Association 1981, 246(14): 1550–55.

5. Jefferson v. Griffin Spalding County Hospital Authority, 274 S.E.2d 457 (Ga. 1981); In re Unborn Baby Kenner, No. 79-JN-83 (Colo. Juv. Ct. Mar. 6, 1979); In re Baby Jeffries, No. 14004 (Mich. P. Ct. May 24, 1982) (order authorizing surgery); North Central Bronx Hospital Authority v. Headley, No. 1992-85 (N.Y. Sup. Ct. Jan. 6, 1986) (order authorizing surgery). There is no written decision in the case where the judge refused to authorize surgery. Interview with Judge Margaret Taylor, Family Court, in New York City (Nov. 6, 1985) (describing 1982 case where attorneys for St. Vincent's Hospital sought an order, but she refused to issue one).

6. 410 U.S. 113 (1973).

7. Jefferson v. Griffin Spalding County Hospital Authority, 274 S.E.2d 457 (Ga. 1981); North Central Bronx Hospital Authority v. Headley, No. 1992-85 (N.Y. Sup. Ct. Jan. 6, 1986), slip op. at 5; In re Unborn Baby Kenner, No. 79-JN-83 (Colo. Juv. Ct. Mar. 6, 1979), slip op. at 6–9.

8. 410 U.S. at 163–64.

9. North Central Bronx Hospital Authority v. Headley, No. 1992-85 (N.Y. Sup. Ct. Jan. 6, 1986); In re Unborn Baby Kenner, No. 79-JN-83 (Colo. Juv. Ct. Mar. 6, 1979).

10. 410 U.S. at 163–64.

11. Id.

12. 439 U.S. 379 (1979).

13. Id. at 400.

14. Late abortion methods include induction of labor with substances such as prostaglandin or oxytocin—proce-

dures likewise used to induce labor when a live birth is desired (especially oxytocin)—and hysterotomy, a procedure similar to a Cesarean. Pritchard, J., Macdonald, P., Gant, N., Williams' obstetrics, 17th ed., 1985: 428.

15. National Institute of Health, U.S. Dept. of Health and Human Services, Pub. No.82-2067, Cesarean childbirth: Report of a consensus development conference, Oct. 1981: 268.

16. See, e.g., Jefferson v. Griffin Spalding County Hospital Authority, 274 S.E.2d 457 (Ga. 1981); Myers, D.B.E., Abuse and neglect of the unborn: Can the state intervene?, Duquesne Law Review 1984, 23(1): 1, 26–31; Robertson, supra note 4, at 352, 357–58.

17. For example, in Matter of Jensen, 633 P.2d 1302 (Or. App. 1981), despite the parents' religious objections, the court ordered surgery for a fifteen-month-old child with hydrocephalus (accumulation of fluid in the brain) because her condition, if untreated, could cause major mental and physical disability. Id. at 1305–6. See also Prince v. Massachusetts, 321 U.S. 158, 166–67 (1944) (right to practice religion does not include liberty to expose child to communicable disease, ill health, or death).

18. See generally Myers, supra note 16.

19. Annas, G., Women as fetal containers, Hastings Center Report 1986, 16(6): 13–14.

20. See, e.g., Matter of Quackenbush, 383 A.2d 785 (N.J. Super. 1978) (ruling that competent patient with gangrene may refuse recommended leg amputation even though refusal will result in death); Lane v. Candura, 376 N.E.2d 1232 (Mass. App. 1978) (holding that irrationality of patient's refusal of amputation does not justify conclusion of incompetence and that surgery cannot be performed against patient's will); In re Melideo, 390 N.Y.S.2d 523 (N.Y. S.Ct. 1976) (Jehovah's Witness' refusal of blood transfusion upheld even though possibly necessary to save her life). These cases illustrate that courts today are likely to hold that the patient's right to privacy overrides that state's interest in preserving life.

21. See In re President and Directors of Georgetown College, Inc., 331 F.2d 1000, 1008 (D.C. Cir.), reh. denied en banc, 331 F.2d 1010, cert. denied 377 U.S. 978 (1964); Powell v. Columbian [sic] Presbyterian Medical Center, 267 N.Y.S.2d 450 (Misc. 2d 1965). Cf. In re Osborne, 294 A.2d 372 (D.C. 1972) (upholding Jehovah's Witness father's refusal of blood transfusion, noting that even if he died, his children's financial and emotional needs would be met by close relatives and the ongoing family business).

22. At least one court has held that a parent's competent decision to refuse treatment simply supersedes the state's interest in protecting children from the loss of a parent; see In re Pogue, No. M-18-74 (D.C. Nov. 11, 1974). See also In Re Jamaica Hospital (reported in the New York Law Journal, May 17, 1985, at 15) (ordering transfusion for pregnant Jehovah's Witness to save fetus, but noting that if woman, a mother of ten, were the only one whose life were at stake, she could refuse the treatment).

23. See Tribe, L., American constitutional law, Mineola, N.Y.: Foundation Press, 1978: 918.

24. Prosser, W., Keeton, W., The law of torts, 5th ed., St. Paul: West Publishing Co., 1984, §56, 376–77.

25. See, e.g., Vt. Stat. Ann. tit.12, §519(a) (1973); Minn. Stat. Ann. §604.05.01 (West Supp. 1986).

26. European countries, which generally do require rescue, exempt physically hazardous rescues. See, e.g., Code Penal, art. 63 (Fr.).

27. 10 Pa. D. & C.3d 90 (1978).

28. Id. at 92 (emphasis in original).

29. This terminology is from Judith Jarvis Thomson's famous article defending abortion on the grounds that requiring a woman to continue a pregnancy is requiring her to be a "Splendid Samaritan," a requirement not imposed on anyone else in society. See Thomson, J.J., A defense of abortion, Philosophy & Public Affairs 1971, 1(1): 47–66, 48–52.

30. Feldman, G.B., Freiman, J.A., Prophylactic Cesarean section at term?, New England Journal of Medicine 1985, 312(19): 1264–67, 1265.

31. Banta, H.D., Thacker, S.B., Assessing the costs and benefits of electronic fetal monitoring, Obstetrical and Gynecological Survey 1979, 34(8): 627–42, 628–29.

32. Id. at 629.

33. Leveno, K.J. et al., A prospective comparison of selective and universal electronic fetal monitoring in 34,995 pregnancies, New England Journal of Medicine 1986, 315(10): 615–19; Haverkamp, A.D., Orleans, M., An assessment of electronic fetal monitoring, Women & Health 1982, 7(3–4): 115–34, 116.

34. In EFM cases, there will seldom be time for more than a hasty phone call to a judge. Even when counsel is appointed for the woman, he or she often has little or no time to prepare the case. In Jefferson, Ms. Jefferson's counsel was appointed at 11 a.m. on January 23, 1981; the case was argued at noon that same day. Letter from Hugh Glidewell (July 24, 1981). In Headley, North Central Bronx Hospital was represented by Bower and Gardner, a firm specializing in health law, while the

woman was not represented at all. Telephone interview with Nancy Gold, of Bower and Gardner, who
represented North Central Bronx Hospital (Jan. 13,
1986). According to the survey by Kolder et al., in 88
percent of the cases reported to them, the court order
was obtained in six or fewer hours. See Kolder et al.,
supra note 1, at 1193.

35. People v. Stewart, No. M508197 (San Diego Mun. Ct.
Feb. 26, 1987). Developments in the *Stewart* case were
reported in several newspaper articles. See New York
Times, Oct. 9, 1986; and Feb. 27, 1987.

Justified Limits on Refusing Intervention

Frank A. Chervenak and Laurence B. McCullough

■

Respect for the autonomy of the patient is a
dominant ethical principle in the literature on
biomedical ethics, particularly in the literature
on refusal of medical intervention by competent
or apparently competent patients. There seems
to be a near uniform consensus that refusal of
surgical management of a gangrenous toe, re-
ligiously based refusal of blood products to manage shock, and refusal of cesarean delivery to
manage complete placenta previa should always
be respected. This consensus rests on the underlying view that refusal of medical intervention is
simply an instance of the general negative right
to be left alone, i.e., a negative right to noninterference in the autonomous management of the
affairs of one's life when no one else is being
harmed. We challenge this assumption and argue
that "refusal" of medical intervention, in cases
where the individual is not refusing any longer to
be a patient, is not simply refusal, but refusal
that is necessarily combined with an implicit demand for alternative medical management. That
is, refusal of medical intervention is a complex
moral phenomenon because it involves both a
negative right to noninterference and a positive
right to alternative treatment. Because a positive
right is involved, the issue of ethically justified
limits on patients' refusal of medical intervention must be addressed. We undertake that task

in this essay, focusing on the example of well-documented, complete placenta previa.[1]

Negative and Positive Rights

Refusal of medical intervention is a negative right *simpliciter* when the refusal of medical intervention takes the form of refusing any longer to be a patient. In such cases, to respect the patient's refusal, that individual's physician need only do nothing. Thus, when the competent patient, for example, discharges him- or herself from the hospital against medical advice, he or she is asserting the negative right to be left alone by his or her hospital physician.

When a patient refuses medical intervention, but does not withdraw from the role of being a patient, matters are more complex. A hospitalized patient with gangrene of a toe who refuses amputation but wants the gangrene treated on a trial basis, is (a) refusing surgery and (b) demanding the only other available alternative, namely, medical management. A Jehovah's Witness who refuses blood products in a situation when volume expanders (which need not be constituted of blood products) may be therapeutic is demanding the expanders on the grounds of religious objection to receiving blood. A pregnant woman who in the intrapartum period refuses cesarean delivery for a well-documented, complete placenta previa in favor of vaginal delivery is exercising a negative right not to have surgery and a positive right to medical management of the only other alternative, vaginal delivery. Finally, a patient with terminal disease who refuses aggressive management of the disease process but wants aggressive management of pain and suffering while he or she is dying is also exercising a combination of negative and positive rights.

A negative right is usually understood in ethics as a right of noninterference in decisionmaking and behavior. A negative right therefore generates duties on the part of others to leave the individual in question alone.[2] In law, the rights to privacy and to self-determination, both pertinent to medical decisionmaking by patients, are negative rights not to be subject to nonconsensual bodily invasion. By contrast, positive rights involve a claim on the resources of others to have some need, desire, or want met. Such rights obligate others to act in specified ways in response, as illustrated in the above examples. As a rule, positive rights are in all cases understood to be liable to limits by their very nature.[3] This feature of positive rights contrasts sharply with negative rights, for which the burden of proof is on others to establish limits (for example, on the basis of preventing serious harm to innocent others). In most cases there is no need to place limits on refusal of medical intervention that involves both negative and positive rights, because the alternative demanded by the positive right is reasonable from a clinical perspective. This will be the case when that alternative is consistent with promoting the interests of the patient construed on a beneficence model.[4]

The Beneficence Model

The beneficence model makes a peculiar claim: to interpret reliably the interests of any patient from medicine's perspective. This perspective is provided by accumulated scientific research, clinical experience, and reasoned responses to uncertainty. It is thus not a perspective peculiar or idiosyncratic to any particular physician.

On the basis of this perspective, the beneficence model identifies the goods relevant to the application of the principle of beneficence in clinical practice. These goods are those, among the many valued by human beings, that medicine is competent to seek on our behalf: the prevention of unnecessary death (death that can be prevented at reasonable rates of morbidity), and the prevention, cure, or at least management of morbidity, which can take the form of disease, injury, handicap, or unnecessary pain and suffering.

Pain and suffering become unnecessary when they do not result in achievement of the other goods of the beneficence model.

Consider the preceding examples. A patient's preference for trial of medical management of a gangrenous toe counts as reasonable because there is a not-insignificant rate of success with this modality. To be sure, medical management is not as effective in managing gangrenous infection and its serious sequelae as surgical management is. This is only to say, however, that surgical management is more effective, not that trial of medical management is ineffective altogether. Medical management is therefore reasonable to the degree that it promotes the interests of the patient, as construed from the perspective of a beneficence model. There is, therefore, no beneficence-based reason for the physician not to accept and act on the competent patient's refusal of surgical management of a gangrenous toe. The same analysis applies to the examples of refusal of blood products in favor of volume expanders and the management of terminally ill patients.

Rarely, the positive right for an alternative medical intervention is justifiably understood to be unreasonable because it is altogether inconsistent with promoting the interests of the patient as construed in the beneficence model. This occurs when the positive right is exercised on behalf of an alternative that, in Joel Feinberg's terms, "dooms" or virtually "dooms" the patient's medical interests and there is some reasonable, ready-to-hand alternative that promotes those interests. For Feinberg, to doom an interest is "to foreordain its defeat":

> To *defeat* an interest is to put it to utter rout, to conclusively and irrevocably set it back by destroying the conditions that are necessary for its fulfillment, as death can set back some interests once and for all.[5]

This would seem the case for refusal of cesarean delivery for well-documented, complete placenta previa. Vaginal delivery, with its staggering mortality rate for the fetus and very high mortality rate for the pregnant woman, would appear to doom or virtually doom the interests of both, while cesarean delivery, by contrast, unambiguously advances those interests. Vaginal delivery is therefore unreasonable from the perspective of a beneficence model.

Clinical Judgment

This conclusion can be immediately challenged, given alleged uncertainty regarding the outcome of complete placenta previa. George J. Annas, among others, has argued that clinical prognostic judgment regarding complete placenta previa is subject to uncertainty, because there apparently have been a few exceptions to the prognosis for complete placenta previa.[6] In two legal cases, complete placenta previa would appear either to have been misdiagnosed (in our view the most likely explanation) or to have spontaneously resolved. Neither of these, we want to emphasize, fits the definition of well-documented, complete placenta previa.[7]

Those who plead uncertainty make a fundamental mistake. They hold clinical prognostic judgment to a standard of truth that it can never satisfy, namely, that it never turns out to be false in an individual case. On such a standard of truth, before the outcome actually occurs, all clinical prognostic judgments must be judged possibly false and therefore disabled by uncertainty. In effect, Annas proposes an impossible epistemological standard, one that bears little relation to a reasonable test of epistemological reliability of clinical prognostic judgments. This test emphasizes the reliability with which such judgments are formed because, prospectively, knowledge of the actual outcome is unavailable.

In our view, reliability of clinical judgment involves both the process of reaching a particular clinical judgment and the data upon which that judgment is based. In the first respect, a clinical judgment is reliable when it would most likely be made again by a second competent, rigorous judger given the same data as the original judger. In the second respect, a clinical judgment is reliable when the data upon which it is based do not vary and are not expected to vary.

Assessing the reliability of prognostic clinical judgment involves several considerations. First, the clinician must identify rigorously the probability of self-limitation or spontaneous resolution of the patient's condition, specifying as precisely as possible the expected outcomes of alternative management strategies.

Second, the clinician needs to realize that prognostic clinical judgment is not about individual cases but about the natural history of a particular disease under different management strategies. Thus, if an outcome of very rare incidence happens to occur, this does not mean that the prior prognostic judgment that the most common event would be the most likely outcome was wrong. In particular, given that spontaneous resolution of well-documented, complete placenta previa diagnosed in the intrapartum period is at best an extremely rare event, the clinician who makes a recommendation for cesarean delivery on this basis is making a reliable clinical judgment. He or she is not wrong if an extremely unlikely spontaneous resolution happens to occur.

Third, to say nonetheless that clinicians can be and often are wrong in their clinical prognostic judgments only makes sense if one is employing the clinical instrument medical students fondly dub the "retrospectroscope." It has a wonderful feature: it is always crystal clear. It also has an unfortunate feature: its findings always come too late. The epistemological status of prognostic clinical judgment is not adequately captured in the two-valued logic of truth and falsehood about individual cases.

This analysis of the reliability of prognostic clinical judgment is crucial for our example

of well-documented, complete placenta previa. First, spontaneous resolution of the condition or an erroneous diagnosis are highly unlikely. Second, the outcome of vaginal delivery for the fetus is that there is a very substantial risk, approaching certainty, of death.[8] Third, the outcome of cesarean delivery for the pregnant woman vis-à-vis vaginal delivery is a dramatic reduction of risk of mortality.

Can the clinican say unconditionally that the fetus will not survive vaginal delivery? No. However, the issue for prognostic clinical judgment is its reliability, not its truth. The ethical issue regarding reliability here is this: Can any clinician competently claim to have documented evidence of a significant rate of fetal survival from vaginal delivery? No. Indeed, such a claim would properly be regarded as an irrational basis for obstetric management. Moreover, to study the question via a randomized clinical trial would be judged unethical by any IRB asked to review such a proposal, given the grave risk to fetuses in the vaginal delivery arm of such a clinical trial. The clinician is correct to conclude that the only obstetric management strategy consistent with promoting the interests of the fetus is cesarean delivery, because vaginal delivery dooms the beneficence-based interests of the fetus,[9] while cesarean delivery does the opposite.

With regard to the pregnant woman's interests, the reliability of prognostic clinical judgment here means that any clinical judgment that well-documented, complete placenta previa is most likely self-limiting and most likely to resolve spontaneously is unfounded and probably irrational. The only rational assumption to make is that vaginal delivery places the pregnant woman at grave risk for exsanguination. The gravity of such a risk is underscored by the long-standing obstetric dictum never to perform a vaginal examination on a third-trimester patient who is experiencing vaginal bleeding, because of the rapidity with which uncontrollable blood loss might result from disruption of a placenta previa.[10]

Should bleeding occur, massive blood replacement may save some women.[11] However, this intervention may not be sufficient to prevent maternal death. In addition, there are significant risks of morbidity and mortality associated with massive blood transfusion, risks that greatly exceed those of cesarean delivery. Here again, no one would seriously propose that studying this issue via a clinical trial is ethically justified, because the maternal risks are so well defined.

The upshot of this analysis of reliability is that vaginal delivery carries grave risks of maternal mortality that can only infrequently be managed successfully. By comparison, cesarean delivery, despite its morbidity and mortality risks for the woman and despite its invasiveness, unequivocally produces net medical benefit for the pregnant woman. Any clinical judgment to the contrary borders on the irrational and cannot, therefore, be consistent with promoting the beneficence-based interests of the woman. The clinician who recommends cesarean delivery to protect the pregnant woman is making a recommendation with the highest reliability that can be applied to clinical judgment: No competent, rigorous clinician will undertake her management on the basis of a clinical judgment of expected spontaneous resolution, because doing so will virtually doom the pregnant woman's beneficence-based interests.

The ethical implications of this level of reliability of clinical judgment and of refusal of cesarean delivery are the following: (1) no physician is justified in accepting such a refusal because doing so would be based on unreliable clinical judgment; and (2) the physician is justified in resisting a patient's exercise of a positive right when fulfilling that positive right contradicts the most highly reliable clinical judgment, dooms the beneficence-based interests of the fetus, and virtually dooms the beneficence-based interests of the pregnant woman. Patients do not have a positive ethical right to obligate physicians to practice medicine in ways that are patently inconsistent with the most reliable clinical judgment.[12]

Preventive Ethics

The primary response to unreasonable assertions of positive rights that are embedded in refusals of medical intervention should be the strategies of preventive ethics.[13] The goal of these strategies is to explain to the patient why the positive right is unreasonable from a clinical perspective. This is best accomplished by informed consent as an ongoing dialogue with the patient, with special attention to adequate disclosure and to the values the physician and the pregnant woman hold in common for her pregnancy. Adequate disclosure should include such information as the following: the rates of cesarean delivery in the United States for a variety of obstetric indications, both maternal and fetal, as well as the rates of cesarean delivery in the physician's own practice; the fact that a low-risk pregnancy can become a high-risk pregnancy quickly and without warning; and the fact that in high-risk pregnancies complicated decisions will be confronted, including decisions regarding cesarean delivery. The informed consent process should also invite the pregnant woman to assess this information in terms of her values and beliefs. These values in turn serve as the basis for negotiation with the pregnant woman, as well as for respectful persuasion, which takes the form of showing how a beneficence-based clinical perspective on her interests and those of her fetus is consistent with the pregnant woman's values. This process should be open to the possibility that the pregnant woman may want to seek second opinions or even consider switching physicians. In short, informed consent as an ongoing process is a crucial autonomy-enhancing clinical tool within the strategy of preventive ethics. Provided that they are utilized in a noncoercive fashion, ethics committees can also play a useful role in conflict resolution.

Court-Ordered Intervention

Strategies of preventive ethics will sometimes fail. Is it ever justified to seek court orders to override a patient's negative right not to be subjected to nonconsensual bodily invasion when this negative right is exercised in conjunction with an unreasonable positive right? Consider again the example of well-documented, complete placenta previa.

Because of their thoroughness and representativeness of the arguments of others, Nancy Rhoden's objections to court-ordered cesarean delivery must be addressed and defeated to justify limiting the refusal of cesarean delivery.[14] First, we consider Rhoden's claim that court-ordered cesarean delivery necessarily treats the pregnant woman solely as an instrument or means by which the fetus is benefitted, but by which she is not benefitted at all, being instead only placed at risk. In Rhoden's terms, court orders treat the pregnant woman as a "mere means" to benefit her fetus. To defeat this objection, we must show that forced cesarean delivery does indeed benefit the pregnant woman.

Cesarean delivery produces significant benefit for the pregnant woman (the dramatic reduction in maternal mortality risks), and significant benefit for the fetus (essentially complete elimination of risks of fetal mortality). Cesarean delivery for well-documented, complete placenta previa produces two *causally independent* effects: benefit for the pregnant woman and benefit for the fetus. Both of these promote beneficence-based interests. Thus, the pregnant woman is not a "mere means" to the benefit of the fetus, in the sense that benefit to her is not considered relevant. Instead, she is an end and is in no way

whatever reduced to being simply a "fetal container"—the dramatic but in this context totally misleading phrase of Annas.[15] The pregnant woman is, and remains throughout the procedure, a patient in her own right, a status that is never compromised, because her medical interests are promoted.

The preceding is not meant to imply that cesarean delivery is risk-free. To the contrary, because it is major abdominal surgery, it does entail risks (albeit small and usually manageable) of morbidity and rare incidence of mortality. The key feature in the present context of cesarean delivery for well-documented, complete placenta previa is that its *net effect* for the pregnant woman is to produce benefit. Because the risks involved in cesarean delivery are a means to benefit the pregnant woman, while at the same time benefiting the fetus, the pregnant woman is not a "mere means" for benefiting the fetus. By aggregating all cases of cesarean delivery—in particular fetal distress and complete placenta previa—Rhoden is prevented from identifying this unique ethical feature of cesarean delivery for well-documented, complete placenta previa.

Rhoden's next objection is that forced cesarean delivery treats pregnant women as a "means merely." That is, her autonomy, her negative right against bodily invasion, is violated without sufficient justification. This objection can be defeated by establishing that the pregnant woman is ethically obligated to accept cesarean delivery for the management of well-documented, complete placenta previa. If this is the case, her autonomy is already constrained and no new constraint is introduced by forced cesarean delivery.

We have argued elsewhere that the pregnant woman, in a pregnancy being taken to term, is ethically obligated to accept reasonable risks on behalf of the fetus in the management of her pregnancy.[16] Robertson argues for a similar legal obligation;[17] Nelson and Milliken, as well as Rhoden, accept an ethical obligation.[18] If this view is reasonable in obstetric ethics, then it is all the more reasonable to hold that the pregnant woman is ethically obligated to accept obstetric interventions that benefit the fetus *while also benefiting her*. If she is obligated to accept reasonable risks, she is surely obligated to accept well-documented benefits for herself. That is, her negative right is inherently subject to the limitation imposed by this obligation. This is different from the situation in which an unconditional negative right against nonconsensual bodily invasion exists.

The harm principle provides another justification for constraining autonomy in these cases.[19] It is a well-understood tenet of ethical theory that an individual's exercise of rights, negative and positive, can justifiably be limited to prevent virtually certain, preventable, serious, and far-reaching harm to innocent others. This justification becomes even stronger when imposing such limits also benefits the individual subject to them.

On the basis of the above analysis, it can be shown that another of Rhoden's objections fails, namely, that based on analogies to forced donation of tissue, such as bone marrow or one of a matched pair of solid organs. Just as courts have refused to order family members (more precisely, distant family members—namely, cousins) to donate tissue or organs, so too, Rhoden argues, courts should not order cesarean deliveries.

At first glance, these analogies possess a powerful intuitive appeal. On closer examination, the appeal fails in the case of well-documented, complete placenta previa. In cases of tissue and organ transplantation, the donor is subject to significant harms: the risks of morbidity and mortality of the medical procedures, of hospitalization, and—in the case of organ donation— subsequent life without the donated organ, though he or she may derive some psychological benefits from being a donor.[20] Moreover, where pediatric patients are concerned, the benefits of

transplantation are not always clearcut. In the case of bone-marrow transplantation, the benefits to the pediatric recipient are not uniformly significant, given the high failure rate of this therapy.[21] Pediatric kidney transplantation, although the preferred management of end-stage renal failure, has persistent, not insignificant rates of failure.[22] Moreover, even though independence is increased, pediatric renal transplantation can involve diminished quality of life in other respects.[23]

In contrast to organ donation and transplantation, cesarean delivery for well-documented, complete placenta previa produces clear-cut benefit for the pregnant woman (the posited analogue of the tissue or organ donor) and clear-cut benefit for the fetus (the posited analogue of the pediatric recipient of tissue or an organ). Indeed, there is no analogy in pediatric transplantation to cesarean delivery for well-documented, complete placenta previa. Hence, Rhoden's objection to interference with the pregnant woman's negative right on this score fails.

Rhoden next considers at some length differences in beliefs about outcome between pregnant women and their physicians and patients' understandable fears about major surgery. In the present context a belief on the part of the pregnant woman that vaginal delivery would be more beneficial for her or for her fetus than cesarean delivery is a matter of empirically very poorly founded belief, not a difference between two equally empirically valid opinions (as would be the case in the gangrenous toe example). Fear of the cesarean delivery is, therefore, in all likelihood, an irrational fear. False beliefs and irrational fears are properly understood in bioethics not to be an expression of autonomy, but a factor that can significantly disable autonomy.[24] Thus, neither demonstrably false belief nor irrational fear should be treated as expressions of autonomy. Rather, they should be addressed as obstacles to the exercise of autonomy via the strategies of preventive ethics. Rhoden's argument on this score would, therefore, appear to fail.

Rhoden also considers and supports religious objections to forced cesarean delivery. Here we believe that there is an analogy that defeats Rhoden's view: parents' refusal, on religious grounds, of well-documented life-saving interventions for children who are patients. Rhoden points out that one reason the courts are correct to protect patients from parental religious constraints is that no physical burden is imposed on the parents by a court order to treat their child. To be sure, cesarean delivery is invasive, major abdominal surgery. Yet in the case of well-documented, complete placenta previa invasiveness should not be the sole criterion for assessing physical burdens, because invasiveness in this case is not associated with net harm. To the contrary, it is associated with net benefit, because it dramatically reduces the risk of maternal mortality. In the pediatric cases, parents may take moral, religious, or psychological offense in being overridden, but the courts apparently do not regard this as a significant invasion of their autonomy. The same would hold true in the present instance. The net effect of cesarean delivery for this complication is to benefit the pregnant woman, not burden her. Hence, Rhoden's support of religious objections to cesarean delivery also seems to fail.

We conclude with considerable trepidation that court orders are not unjustified when strategies for preventive ethics fail to alter refusal of cesarean delivery for well-documented, complete placenta previa. We want immediately to caution that our conclusions about this clinical example should not be extended to other clinical examples of unreasonable refusal without very careful analysis and argument, especially cases in which there is only one patient. These matters are beyond the scope of this paper, the purpose of which is to put forward for serious consideration a more nuanced analysis of refusal of medical intervention and the ethical obligations of physicians in response to them.

Implications for Medical Paternalism

We close by identifying some of the implications of our argument for the issue of medical paternalism. Typically, this issue is construed in terms of the imposition of beneficence-based clinical interventions in violation of the autonomy of the patient.[25] Thus, administration of blood products rather than volume expanders to a competent Jehovah's Witness patient, over his or her express objection, is the imposition of an intervention that is life-saving (hence, beneficence-based) in violation of the patient's autonomy. That is, medical paternalism is thought to be unjustified, because, for a variety of reasons—both theoretical and practical—autonomy-based obligations override or trump beneficence-based obligations.

This construal fails to account accurately for the problem with medical paternalism in those cases—the vast majority—in which the patient rejects the physician's recommendation in favor of an alternative that is reasonable. It would be unjustified, in response, for the physician to impose the recommended management as the only management that is in the patient's interests, because the patient's preferred alternative, as reasonable, promotes his or her beneficence-based interests to some reasonable degree. The physician's mistake would be to think that, *on the grounds of beneficence,* the "best" management excludes as unreasonable all other alternatives; it cannot do so. Paternalism in such circumstances is therefore unjustified, because it is based on defective beneficence-based clinical judgment: that one management is the best, from the point of view of beneficence-based clinical judgment, does not make unacceptable those alternatives that promote the patient's interests in different ways or to a lesser, but still positive degree. It is not that autonomy-based obligations trump beneficence-

Limits on Refusing Intervention

based obligations, but that there is no compelling or controlling beneficence-based obligation to consider overriding the autonomy of the patient in the first place.

In the case of refusal of intervention necessarily coupled to a positive right to a patently unreasonable alternative, the standard construal of medical paternalism also seems inaccurate, but for a different reason. The correct analysis is the following: the negative right of the patient against nonconsensual bodily invasion is asserted against the physician's negative right against nonconsensual practice of patently unreasonable medicine, because the positive right of the patient to an unreasonable alternative threatens the physician's autonomy. Here the physician's autonomy should be understood in terms of the ethical integrity of medicine, which has been recognized by the courts and in the literature.[26]

It would seem that these (rare) cases of medical paternalism do not therefore involve a clash between beneficence and autonomy, but between autonomy and autonomy—perhaps as a side constraint of both the patient and the physician.[27] The question, How should such clashes be resolved? seems best addressed on the basis of an analysis of the harms that would ensue from the violation of the autonomy of the patient, on the one hand, and of the physician, on the other, and arguments about how those harms should be rank-ordered.

For the most part, rank-orderings in the literature strike us more as a function of public policy than of rigorous analysis and argument. Thus, for example, it is a matter of public policy in the United States, in virtue of the First Amendment and the body of law based on it, that the integrity of religious beliefs is given a protection not accorded the integrity of medicine. But this public policy is an accident of our history, not of a well-worked-out philosophical account of how harms should be ranked.

The same would seem to be the case for the near-absolute character of the legal right of self-determination, as articulated in *Schloendorff v. Society of New York Hospital*[28] and other informed consent cases. In *Schloendorff* Judge Cardozo seems unaware of the sort of analysis we suggest here. Moreover, he simply lays down the right of self-determination regarding medical decisions without argument. Neither the accidents of history nor the dicta of judges count as sustained philosophical analysis and argument. Perhaps it is time to reconsider accepted views about medical paternalism.

Notes

The authors want to thank the following individuals for their very helpful comments on earlier drafts: Thomas Bole, Baruch A. Brody, H. Tristram Engelhardt, Jr., B. Andrew Lustig, Joy H. Penticuff, Stephen Wear, and Courtney S. Campbell.

1. By well-documented, complete placenta previa we meant the following: transabdominal or transvaginal ultrasound examination is performed by individuals competent in the technique and interpretation of its results and the placenta is clearly visualized on ultrasound examination to cover the cervical os completely. To maximize reliability, ultrasound examination should be performed shortly before delivery. See William J. Ott, "Placenta Previa," in *Textbook of Ultrasound in Obstetrics and Gynecology,* ed. Frank A. Chervenak, Stuart Campbell, and Glenn Isaacson (Boston: Little, Brown, 1992); Dan Farine, Harold E. Fox, and Ilan E. Timor-Tritsch, "Placenta Previa: Transvaginal Approach," in *Textbook of Ultrasound in Obstetrics and Gynecology* (1992). The reliability of the examination varies inversely with the length of time remaining before expected date of delivery. In addition, there should be no uterine contractions and the maternal bladder should be empty, because, if these factors are not taken into account, false positive diagnosis can occur. Satisfaction of these criteria makes a false positive diagnosis of complete placenta previa highly unlikely.

2. Joel Feinberg distinguishes rights claimed against individuals from rights claimed against the state. These rights can either be claims to "noninterference in . . . private affairs" (negative rights), or claims to "assistance" and "specific services" (positive rights). See Joel

Feinberg, "Rights: Systematic Analysis," in *Encyclopedia of Bioethics,* ed. Warren T. Reich (New York: Macmillan, 1978), pp. 1508–09. See also Feinberg, *Harm to Self* (New York: Oxford University Press, 1986), p. 53.

3. See Ruth Macklin, "Rights: Rights in Bioethics," *Encyclopedia of Bioethics,* ed. Warren T. Reich (New York: Macmillan, 1978), p. 1513.

4. For a discussion of a beneficence model, see Tom L. Beauchamp and Laurence B. McCullough, *Medical Ethics: The Moral Responsibility of Physicians* (Englewood Cliffs, N.J.: Prentice Hall, 1984), especially ch. 2.

5. Joel Feinberg, *Harm to Others* (New York: Oxford University Press, 1984), pp. 54, 53.

6. George J. Annas, "Protecting the Liberty of Pregnant Patients," *NEJM* 316, no. 19 (1988): 1213–14; "Pregnant Women as Fetal Containers," *Hastings Center Report* 16, no. 6 (1986): 13–14; Sherman Elias and George J. Annas, *Reproductive Genetics and the Law* (Chicago: Year Book Medical Publishers, 1987), pp. 253–62; "Perspectives on Fetal Surgery," *American Journal of Obstetrics and Gynecology* 145, no. 7 (1983): 807–812; Lawrence J. Nelson and Nancy Milliken, "Compelled Medical Treatment of Pregnant Women: Life, Liberty, and Law in Conflict," *JAMA* 259, no. 7 (1988): 1060–66; and Committee on Ethics, American College of Obstetrics and Gynecology, "Patient Choice: Maternal-Fetal Conflict," American College of Obstetrics and Gynecology Committee Opinion Number 55, October 1987.

7. See *Jefferson v. Griffin Spalding County Hospital Authority,* 274 Ga. 86, 274 S.E. 2d 457 (1981) and *In Re Baby Jeffries,* No. 14004 (Jackson County, Mich. P. Ct. May 24, 1982).

8. Carlyle Crenshaw, D. E. Darnell Jones and Roy T. Parker, "Placenta Previa: A Survey of Twenty Years Experience with Improved Perinatal Survival by Expectant Therapy and Cesarean Delivery," *Obstetric Gynecology Survey* 28 (1973): 461–70.

9. In saying this we accept the concept of the fetus as a patient and assume that in virtue of being a patient, the fetus can correctly be said to have beneficence-based interests. See, especially, American College of Obstetricians and Gynecologists, Committee on Ethics, *Patient Choice: Maternal-Fetal Conflict* (Washington, D.C.: American College of Obstetricians and Gynecologists, 1987); American Academy of Pediatrics, Committee on Bioethics, "Fetal Therapy: Ethical Considerations," *Pediatrics* 81 (1988): 898–99. For a discussion of when the fetus is a patient and some of the ethical implications of the concept, see Frank A. Chervenak and

Laurence B. McCullough, "Does Obstetric Ethics Have Any Role in the Obstetrician's Response to the Abortion Controversy?" *American Journal of Obstetrics and Gynecology* 163, no. 5 (1990): 1425–29.

10. Jack A. Pritchard, Paul C. MacDonald, and Norman F. Gant, eds., *Williams Obstetrics,* 17th ed. (Norwalk, Conn.: Appleton-Century-Crofts, 1985), p. 409.

11. David B. Cotton, John A. Read, Richard H. Paul et al., "The Conservative Aggressive Management of Placenta Previa," *American Journal of Obstetrics and Gynecology* 137 (1980): 687–95.

12. Allen Brett and Laurence B. McCullough, "When Patients Request Specific Interventions: Defining the Limits of the Physician's Obligations," *NEJM* 315 (1986): 1347–51.

13. Frank A. Chervenak and Laurence B. McCullough, "Clinical Strategies for Preventing Ethical Conflict Between Pregnant Women and Their Physicians," *American Journal of Obstetrics and Gynecology* 162 (1990): 303–307.

14. Nancy K. Rhoden, "The Judge in the Delivery Room: The Emergence of Court-Ordered Cesareans," *California Law Review* 74, (1986): 1950–2030.

15. Annas, "Pregnant Women as Fetal Containers."

16. Frank A. Chervenak and Laurence B. McCullough, "Perinatal Ethics: A Practical Analysis of Obligations to Mother and Fetus," *Obstetrics and Gynecology* 66 (1985): 442–46.

17. John A. Robertson, "The Right to Procreate and In Utero Fetal Therapy," *Journal of Legal Medicine* 3, no. 3 (1982): 333–36; "Legal Issues in Prenatal Therapy," *Clinical Obstetrics and Gynecology* 29, no. 3 (1986): 603–11.

18. Nelson and Milliken, "Compelled Medical Treatment of Pregnant Women."

19. For a concise formulation of this principle, see Tom L. Beauchamp, "Paternalism," *Encyclopedia of Bioethics.* See also Joel Feinberg, *Harm to Others.*

20. Robert M. House and Troy L. Thompson, "Psychiatric Aspects of Organ Transplantation," *JAMA* 260, no. 4 (1988): 535–39.

21. C. Philip Steuber, "Bone-Marrow Transplantation," in *Principles and Practice of Pediatrics,* ed. Frank A. Oski et al. (Philadelphia: J. B. Lippincott, 1990), pp. 1578–79.

22. Edward C. Kohaut, "End-Stage Renal Disease," *Principles and Practice of Pediatrics,* pp. 1619–24.

23. Larry M. Gold et al., "Psychosocial Issues in Pediatric Organ Transplantation," *Pediatrics* 75, no. 5 (1986): 738–44.

24. Ruth R. Faden and Tom L. Beauchamp, *A History and Theory of Informed Consent* (New York: Oxford University Press, 1986), especially ch. 7.

25. See Tom L. Beauchamp and James F. Childress, *Principles of Biomedical Ethics,* 3d ed. (New York: Oxford University Press, 1989), pp. 209–27.

26. See, for example, *Superintendent of Belchertown v. Saikewicz* 373 Mass. 728. 370 N.E.2d 417 (1977), and *Satz v. Perlmutter,* 362 So.2d 160, affirmed 379 So2d 359 (1978); see also The Hastings Center, *Guidelines on the Termination of Life-Sustaining Treatment and the Care of the Dying* (Bloomington: Indiana University Press, 1987).

27. H. Tristram Engelhardt, Jr., *The Foundations of Bioethics* (New York: Oxford University Press, 1986).

28. *Schloendorff v. Society of New York Hospital,* 211 N.Y. 125, 105 N.E. 92 (1914).

Faith (Healing), Hope, and Charity at the FDA: The Politics of AIDS Drug Trials

George J. Annas

■

AIDS forces us to confront our mortality, the limits of modern medicine, and the contours of our compassion.[1] How we respond is a measure of our society, as well as a reflection of our values and priorities. As a fundamentally death-denying society, our response has been hampered by denial and shaped by faith that a technological fix will make the AIDS epidemic go away. Technology is our new religion, our "modern" way to deal with death. As novelist Don De-Lillo has one of his characters in *White Noise* put it to another who is worried about death: you can deny it, you can put your faith in religion, or

you could put your faith in technology. It got you here, it can get you out. This is the whole point of technology. It creates an appetite for immortality on the one hand. It threatens universal extinction on the other. . . . It's what we invented to conceal the terrible secret of our decaying bodies. But it's also life, isn't it? It prolongs life, it provides new organs for those that wear out. New devices, new techniques every day. Lasers, masers, ultrasound. Give yourself up to it. . . . They'll insert you in a gleaming tube, irradiate your body with the basic stuff of the universe. Light, energy, dreams. God's own goodness.

The less we understand about medical technology, the more we see it as magic. Nor are physicians immune from magical thinking. When medical science seems impotent to fight the claims of nature, "all kinds of senseless interventions are tried in an unconscious effort to cure the incurable magically through a 'wonder drug,' a novel surgical procedure, or a penetrating psychological interpretation."[2] In a parallel fashion, we speak of medical "miracles" in recounting techniques we cannot understand but nonetheless want to believe in. We have become modern believers in faith healing, faith based not in a Supreme Being, but in Supreme Science.

The AIDS epidemic has frightened us into "believing" that medicine will find a cure soon, and this faith in science has eroded the distinction between experimentation and therapy, has threatened to transform the U.S. Food and Drug Administration (FDA) from a consumer protection agency into a medical technology promotion agency, and has put AIDS patients, already suffering from an incurable disease, at further risk of psychological, physical, and financial exploitation by those who would sell them useless drugs. The not too subtle metamorphosis of the pre-Kessler FDA was abetted by an unusual political alliance between the antiregulation Reagan/Bush administrations and gay rights activists.

This chapter argues that the distinction between experimental and therapeutic interventions is crucial in terms of both science and individual rights; and that the FDA should continue to responsibly regulate experimental drugs and reassert its identity as a premier consumer protection agency. We should not permit the AIDS epidemic to be used as an excuse to dismantle the FDA or to put the integrity of our drugs and medical devices at risk. True compassion for AIDS patients does not involve dispensing false hope or unreasonable hype. It requires adequate funding and staffing of the National Institutes of Health (NIH) and their AIDS drug and vaccine testing programs, along with scientifically sound testing methodologies that can provide reasonable assurance that the drugs that are sold as therapies are safe and effective. To examine the politics of AIDS drug development, it is necessary to understand the purposes for the experimentation/therapy distinction in medicine, and the values that this distinction promotes and protects.

The Experimentation/Therapy Distinction

Perhaps the major source of controversy surrounding drug trials for experimental AIDS drugs is that investigators see these trials as *research,* whose purpose is to provide generalizable knowledge that may help others. On the other hand, most individuals suffering with AIDS see these trials as *therapy,* whose primary purpose is to benefit them. This confusion is not new, and a brief review of the history of human experimentation shows why it is important.

A reasonable summary of many of the major issues in human experimentation appears in Gustave Flaubert's realistic novel *Madame Bovary* (1857). Charles Bovary decides to try to make his name as a physician by curing the local stableman's club foot with experimental surgery. The experiment involved cutting the Achilles tendon and then screwing the foot and leg into "a kind of box, weighing about eight pounds, constructed by the carpenter and the locksmith, with a prodigal amount of iron, wood, sheet-iron, leather, nails and screws." The apothecary, an avid supporter of the experiment, helps convince Charles' wife, Emma: " 'What risk is there? Look!'—and he counted the 'pros' on his fingers. 'Success, practically certain. An end of suffering and disfigurement for the patient. Immediate fame for the operator.' " The stableman is urged to consent by the entire town, but the "decisive factor was that it wouldn't cost him anything."

The experiment does not go as planned, and another physician eventually must be called in to amputate the hideously painful and gangrenous leg.

Most experiments do not have such disastrous results for patients, but many share similar dangers, as well as the same motivations on the part of both physician and patient, the same inability to separate hopes from realistic appraisal of likely outcomes, and the same inability to distinguish voluntary consent from coercion. To protect subjects, rules have been developed regarding human experimentation.

The most comprehensive and authoritative legal statement on human experimentation is embodied in the Nuremberg Code. This ten-point code was articulated in a 1947 court opinion following the trial of Nazi physicians for "war crimes and crimes against humanity" committed during World War II, which included experiments designed to determine which poisons killed the fastest, how long people could live exposed to ice water and when exposed to high altitudes, and if surgically severed limbs could be reattached.[3] The Nuremberg tribunal rejected the defendant's contention that their experiments with both prisoners of war and civilians were consistent with the ethics of the medical profession as evidenced by previously published U.S., French, and British experiments on venereal disease, plague, and malaria, and U.S. prison experiments, among others. The tribunal concluded that only "certain types of medical experiments on human beings, when kept within reasonably well defined bounds, conform to the ethics of the medical profession generally."

These well-defined bounds are articulated in the ten principles of the Nuremberg Code. The basis of the code is a type of natural law reasoning. In the court's words: "All agree . . . that certain basic principles must be observed in order to satisfy moral, ethical, and legal concepts." Principle 1 of the Nuremberg Code thus requires that

the consent of the experimental subject have at least four characteristics: it must be competent, voluntary, informed, and comprehending. This is to protect the subject's rights. The other principles have primarily to do with protecting the subject's welfare: They prescribe actions that must be taken prior to seeking subject enrollment in the experiment, and actions that must be taken to protect the subject during the experiment. These include a determination that the experiment is properly designed to yield fruitful results "unprocurable by other methods"; that "anticipated results" will justify performance of the experiment; that all "unnecessary physical and mental suffering and injury" is avoided; that there is no "*a priori* reason to believe that death or disabling injury will occur"; that the project has "humanitarian importance" that outweighs the degree of risk; that "adequate preparation" is taken to "protect the experimental subject against even the remote possibilities of injury, disability, or death"; that only "scientifically qualified" persons conduct the experiment; that the subject can terminate participation at any time; and that the experimenter is prepared to terminate the experiment if "continuation is likely to result in injury, disability, or death to the experimental subject." The code has been used as the basis for other international documents, such as the Declaration of Helsinki, it is a part of international common law, and I have previously argued that it can properly be viewed as both a criminal and civil basis for liability in the United States.[4]

Today the most likely subject of medical experimentation is not the prisoner or even the soldier, but the patient with a disease. As a leading medical commentator has put it:

Volunteers for experiments will usually be influenced by hopes of obtaining better grades, earlier parole, more substantial egos, or just mundane cash. These pressures, however, are but fractional shadows of those enclosing the patient-subject. *Incapacitated and hospitalized because of illness, frightened by strange and impersonal routines, and fearful for his health and perhaps life, he is far from exercising a free power of choice* when the person to whom he anchors all his hopes asks, "say, you wouldn't mind, would you, if you joined some of the other patients on this floor and helped us to carry out some very important research we are doing?" When "informed consent" is obtained, it is not the student, the destitute bum, or the prisoner to whom, by virtue of his condition, the thumb screws of coercion are most relentlessly applied; it is *the most used and useful of all experimental subjects, the patient with disease.*[5] (emphasis added)

When the illness is fatal, pressures on both the physician-researcher and patient are much more acute, and the rules regarding research seem less relevant. Consent also seems a sham, since patients are "desperate" and are demanding to be research subjects, thinking that this is their best hope of getting "treatment" for their condition.[6] The assertion is made that patients have "nothing to lose" by engaging in all manner of experimentation, and that patients should have the "right" to be experimental subjects.[7] But it is when such political claims are made in the face of a fatal disease that consumer protection agencies like the FDA must stand firm and insist on scientific validity to those experiments that are performed. This is because, as important as informed consent is, the most important and prior question is whether the experiment should be done at all.[8] Only after this determination has been made, based on such things as prior animal and laboratory research, study design, risk/benefit analysis, and the alternatives, is it even legitimate to ask the subject to participate. And without such prior determinations, and the de-

velopment of a sound research protocol, it is extremely unlikely that experimentation will yield any useful information, but, rather, will only serve to increase suffering and exploitation of desperate patients.

The Politics of AIDS Drug Trials

AIDS politics has produced strange political allies. The antiregulation Reagan/Bush administrations and the gay community probably had only one interest in common: deregulating the drug approval process. The gay community's position is probably best summed up in a slogan used by ACT-UP (AIDS Coalition to Unleash Power): "A Drug Trial is Health Care Too." Of course, the truth is otherwise: a drug trial is research designed to test a hypothesis, not treatment meant to help individual patients. The reason for this strange alliance has little to do with shared love for those suffering with AIDS; rather, it is due to an administration composed largely of free-market advocates and the desire of drug companies for deregulation, both of whom see the AIDS epidemic as an opportunity to further their own interests. Unlike the experiment in *Madame Bovary*, experimental drugs are no longer universally delivered free, and there is tremendous pressure on the FDA to permit drug companies to sell "promising" experimental drugs to subjects. The sale of experimental drugs threatens to further erode the distinction between experimentation and therapy and makes it even more difficult for patients suffering from disease to distinguish recognized therapy from early experimentation, and false hope from reasonable expectation.

The administration's position was that drugs should be permitted to go on the market faster. President George Bush, while still Vice-President, urged the FDA to develop procedures to expedite the marketing of new drugs intended to treat AIDS and other life-threatening illnesses. In the fall of 1988, in his first debate with the Democratic presidential nominee, Michael Dukakis, Bush said that in response to his efforts FDA had "sped up bringing drugs to market that can help." He did, however, caution that, "you've got to be careful here because there's a safety factor."[9] Indeed there is, and the policy question is whether that safety factor should be ignored or radically lessened when the research subjects have a fatal illness for which there is no cure. Although the AIDS epidemic is new, this question is not. The FDA has faced it squarely before.

In the 1970s, thousands of cancer victims were traveling to Mexico and Canada to obtain laetrile, a substance derived from apricot pits. The drug was not available in the United States and was not even in experimental trials. In 1975 a group of terminally ill cancer patients and their spouses sued the federal government to enjoin it from interfering with the interstate shipment and sale of laetrile. The FDA vigorously opposed making laetrile available in the United States, even to terminally ill cancer patients, because "there were no adequate well-controlled studies of laetrile's safety or effectiveness."[10]

The United States Supreme Court upheld the FDA's position noting, among other things, that "In implementing the statutory scheme, the FDA has never made exception for drugs used by the terminally ill."[11] The Court also agreed with the FDA that effectiveness is not irrelevant simply because one is dying: "effectiveness does not necessarily denote capacity to cure. In the treatment of any illness, terminal or otherwise, a drug is effective if it fulfills, by objective indices, its sponsor's claims of prolonged life, improved physical condition, or reduced pain." Safety is also relevant to the terminally ill: "For the terminally ill, as for anyone else, a drug is unsafe if its potential for inflicting death or physical injury is not offset by the possibility of therapeutic benefit." The Court underlined that although the case involved laetrile, the logic adopted applied to all unproven drugs:

To accept the proposition that the safety and efficacy standards of the Act have no relevance for terminal patients is to deny the Commissioner's authority over all drugs, however toxic or ineffectual, for such individuals. If history is any guide, this new market would not be long overlooked. Since the turn of the century, resourceful entrepreneurs have advertised a wide variety of purportedly simple and painless cures for cancer, including liniments of turpentine, mustard, oil, eggs, and ammonia; pear moss; arrangements of colored floodlamps; pastes made from glycerin and limberger cheese; mineral tablets; and "Foundation of Youth" mixtures of spices, oil and diet. . . . Congress could reasonably have determined to protect the terminally ill, no less than other patients, from the vast range of self-styled panaceas that inventive minds can devise.

Although the breast implant controversy may have caused some reassessment, since 1979 the FDA's public position on use of unproven drugs and devices in clinical settings has been shifting. In 1985, for example, the FDA decided to encourage the use of temporary artificial hearts, even though their use in clinical settings outside of a planned research project could generate no scientifically useful information on these devices (see Chapter 16). The justification was that the FDA should not stand in the way of a physician using an unapproved medical device in an "emergency." In 1987, in response to increasing political pressure to make experimental AIDS drugs more widely available, the FDA issued new regulations that permit the treatment, use, and sale of an investigational new drug (IND) that is not otherwise approved for treatment and sale, while the drug is still in clinical trials, if:

The drug is intended to treat a serious or immediately life-threatening disease.

There is no comparable or satisfactory alternative drug or other therapy available to treat that stage of the disease in the intended patient population.

The drug is under investigation in a controlled clinical trial under an IND in effect for the trial, or all clinical trials have been completed.

The sponsor of the controlled clinical trial, or all clinical trials, is actively pursuing marketing approval of the IND with due diligence.[12]

According to the then counselor to the Undersecretary of Health and Human Services, S. Jay Plager, the purpose of these new rules was to give "desperately ill patients the opportunity to decide for themselves whether they would rather take an experimental drug or die of the disease untreated."[13] Like ACT-UP, Mr. Plager and the FDA confused experimentation with treatment and seemed so intent on denying death that they believed it could be magically prevented with unproven drugs.

No one opposes cutting "red tape" or removing regulatory hurdles that do not improve safety and efficacy. Arguably, FDA's rules are not inconsistent with *Rutherford.* But in July 1988 the former FDA commissioner took a step that clearly is inconsistent, when he announced that the FDA would permit U.S. citizens to import unapproved drugs from abroad for their personal use. In attempting to justify this policy, Commissioner Frank Young said: "There is such a degree of desperation, and people are going to die, that I'm not going to be the Commissioner that robs them of hope."[14] The reaction of the scientific community to this new FDA position was well summed up in an article in *Science:* "The new directive stunned some AIDS researchers. One official in the federal government's AIDS program went so far as to suggest that the FDA commis-

sioner had gone 'temporarily insane.' "[15] There are at least three reasons for this reaction.

First are all the arguments the FDA used in *Rutherford* to justify its central role as a consumer protection agency. All patients, particularly terminally ill patients, deserve protection from those who want to prey on their desperation for profit. People with AIDS have a lot to lose, including their health, their lives, their dignity, and their money. They can be and have been viciously exploited. Because many victims of AIDS are members of disenfranchised groups that have traditionally been rightfully suspicious of government's view of them, they may be at special risk for exploitation by those who proclaim that the government and orthodox medicine is in a conspiracy to deny them treatment. A few examples of harm to individuals from unapproved drugs illustrate the problem. The life and death of Bill Kraus frames Randy Shilts's chronicle of the politics of AIDS—*And the Band Played On* (1987). Kraus, like many other AIDS patients, including Rock Hudson (who left Paris in 1984 convinced he was cured of AIDS) traveled to Paris to be treated with HPA-23. When, in 1985, it became clear that the drug was not working, his doctor urged him to start taking another unproven medication (isoprinosine). Shilts writes: "The suggestion upset Bill because he had pinned his entire hope for survival on HPA-23. Even the possibility that it might not be a panacea enraged him, cutting to the core of his denial and bargaining with his AIDS diagnosis."[16] Almost a decade later, the efficacy of HPA-23 is still in doubt, and obviously the failure to prove or disprove its worth in France cannot be blamed on the FDA's regulations.

Suranim had been widely used to treat African sleeping sickness, and disabled HIV's ability to replicate in the test tube. When this information was made public, and the drug was touted as "promising," many patients wanted it. A subsequent trial in humans, however, found that suranim was extremely toxic in AIDS patients, worsening immune disorders and thus hastening death.[17] French researchers announced to the world that they had cured AIDS using cyclosporin. There was a clamor for the drug, and the announcement was later found to be premature hype: both patients were comatose and the drug did not improve their clinical course.[18] In late 1987 a Zairian scientist announced in a news conference that he had a possible cure for AIDS. In the aftermath of the announcement, the number of men in Zaire who believed AIDS could be cured doubled (to 57 percent), and educational efforts aimed at prevention were set back.[19] The lack of scientifically sound, carefully planned randomized clinical trials not only produces false hope but also can directly lengthen the time it will take to get a truly effective AIDS drug to those suffering from the disease.

The second reason why encouraging the use of unproven drugs is bad public policy is that denying death ultimately serves no purpose (other than providing temporary false hope). The FDA and other federal agencies (like the Centers for Disease Control) have recognized this in other aspects of the AIDS epidemic. For example, rather than continue to deny that teenagers engage in sexual activity, condom use and "safe sex" practices have been recommended to help prevent the spread of AIDS. Similarly, education about the science and epidemiology of AIDS has been used as the major weapon to fight fear and prejudice against those infected by others who would deny them education, housing, employment, and insurance. The scientific facts have been seen as the most powerful weapon against fear bred by ignorance. It is thus at least ironic that attention to scientific facts seems to have been jettisoned when it has come to research with AIDS drugs. It is not compassionate to hold out false hope to a terminally ill patient and thereby induce that patient to spend his last dollar on unproven "remedies." If anything, such a strategy seems aimed primarily at treating the guilt of a society that has done little to meet the real needs of AIDS victims by giving us the comforting illusion that we are doing something to help.

The third reason why making unproven drugs available is counterproductive public policy is that, if unproven remedies are made easily available it will be impossible to do scientifically valid trials of new drugs. Those suffering from AIDS will be unwilling to participate in randomized clinical trials, and those who are randomized to an arm of the study they do not like will take the drugs they "believe in" on the sly, making any valid finding from the study impossible.[20]

In 1988, for example, in what gay rights activists described as a "political ploy" in the midst of a presidential campaign, the FDA developed rules designed to permit the collapsing of phases II and III for certain drugs that "are intended to treat life-threatening or severely-debilitating illnesses."[21] In announcing the new rules, then FDA Commissioner Frank Young said: "I've seen a lot of folks who are suffering, and I want those people who have either cancer or AIDS to know that this agency has a heart as well as a mind."[22] These new rules, however, do little more than formalize procedures the FDA has always been able to use upon the request of the manufacturer. As the FDA noted in the comments to the rules, they essentially track the way the FDA actually went about approving zidovudine (AZT), the first, and for years the only, drug the FDA approved for the treatment of AIDS.

By mid-1992 even ACT-UP activists seemed to agree that the FDA (and its research rules) was not the real problem in drug development. One of their members, Mark Harrington, said at the Amsterdam AIDS Conference, "What is the point of streamlining access and approval when the result is merely to replace AZT with mediocre, toxic and expensive drugs?"[23] He argued that others should be encouraged to follow his example and volunteer for "experiments involving basic science." This will almost always require the painstaking work of randomized clinical trials.

Should the Rules for Research Be Changed When the Disease Is Fatal?

Randomized clinical trials (RCTs) are the "gold standard" upon which experimental treatments are judged useful, worthless, or dangerous. John McKinlay has demonstrated that in the absence of an initial well-controlled clinical trial the typical innovation in modern medicine goes through seven stages: (1) promising report; (2) professional adoption; (3) public acceptance and third-party payment; (4) standard procedure; (5) randomized clinical trial; (6) professional denunciation; and (7) discreditation.[24] He has argued forcefully that to avoid the first four and the last two stages, and the expense in terms of money and human misery that they generate, we must evaluate all newly proposed therapies at stage 5, the randomized clinical trial, before making the therapy generally available. This view is widely accepted as correct in the scientific community, and the trend has been to try to develop methods to evaluate surgery and other therapies by RCT as well, in an effort to improve the quality of care by eliminating costly therapies that provide no benefit. Although there are proposals for "community clinical trials" and to make "adjustments" in the current management of RCTs, there is no dispute that the RCT is the method most likely to produce valid results.

When Commissioner Young asserts that the FDA "has a heart as well as a mind," it is fair to ask whether the FDA's role is to provide emotional support or scientific protection to the public. The FDA may see it as compassionate to provide access to unproven remedies, but fifteen years ago it saw it as exploitative. Was it right then, or is it right today?

I think the FDA was correct on laetrile and

should continue to insist on a scientifically valid randomized clinical trial before certifying drugs safe and effective. All consumer protection legislation is to some degree paternalistic, but in this case it is also realistic. FDA certification of the safety and the efficacy of drugs recognizes that the public is in no position to judge the value or usefulness of many medications, and that many drugs are dangerous and have serious side effects (which is one reason we also license physicians and require some drugs be available only with a physician's prescription). Drug manufacturers have a distinct social role: to create and sell products. Their role is not consumer protection. Libertarians and those with extreme views of individual autonomy, and even some free marketers, object to FDA regulation, equating "pursuit of quackery" with "life, liberty, and the pursuit of happiness." True autonomy requires adequate and accurate information upon which to base decisions. This is simply impossible in the absence of responsible scientific study and properly designed clinical trials. It is appropriate to concentrate energies and resources in the time of an epidemic. It is also appropriate to assign AIDS drug testing a very high priority and to approve adequate government funding to develop and test drugs that might be effective. NIH and FDA should work together more closely and develop better dispute resolution systems when disagreements persist. But it is not ultimately helpful to AIDS sufferers to rush inadequately tested drugs to market. The thalidomide episode taught us all that lesson, and our brief fascination with suramin should have reinforced it.

The good news is that even with the "faith, hope, and charity" rhetoric of the former FDA Commissioner, with the exception of permitting the importation of quack remedies for personal use, the FDA actually stuck with its consumer protection mission. And although Commissioner David Kessler endorsed quick actions on AIDS drugs, he insisted on good science as well. The

FDA's two major rule innovations are designed primarily to speed up the bureaucratic aspects of drug testing, rather than to substantively change the rules for evaluating drugs. This is perfectly consistent with sound public policy. What would not be in the public interest is for the FDA to adopt the antiregulation agenda of the drug companies by relaxing its safety and efficacy standards.

The rhetoric has been turned up, but it is simply a repeat of the laetrile debate. A *Wall Street Journal* editorial, for example, accused the FDA of killing people with its testing procedures. It called on the FDA to accede to the demands of dying patients, rather than to insist on scientific soundness in experimentation, and to let the "patients and their families" be involved in revamping the current system for drug approval:

> Let defenders of the status quo explain to people with cancer, Alzheimer's or AIDS why redundant efficacy testing, in which half the patients get a placebo, doesn't constitute "killing" in the name of FDA-mandated medical statistics. . . . AIDS patients have driven home to the U.S. medical and political establishment what enormous risks human beings in death's grip will take to gain relief or respite.[25]

What the *Journal* does not seem to realize is that it has identified the problem—desperation—not the solution. Deregulation of the drug approval process cannot produce new drugs that don't exist. Of course, money can be made by exploiting the fear of death and desperation, and perhaps this is what the *Journal* would like to see. The profiteering pricing policy of Burroughs Wellcome in making AZT available for years only to those who could pay approximately $8,000 a year for its use, and long after the original justification for this extraordinarily high price (to recoup development costs) had been met, is a useful example of such financial exploitation.[26] No

wonder that the American Public Health Association petitioned the U.S. Department of Health and Human Services to require that mechanisms be put into place to ensure that if and when a more effective drug is developed at government institutions or with federal funding to combat AIDS that it will be made available at the lowest possible price. The quest for profit also threatens to inhibit scientific research and sharing of data concerning experimental AIDS drugs, as well as to increase the likelihood that useless drugs will be hyped in press conferences rather than evaluated at scientific meetings. This trend is much more likely to adversely affect AIDS sufferers than any FDA rule regarding clinical trials.

As a cover story in *Fortune* magazine has noted, "for the past 30 years the drug makers of the Fortune 500 have enjoyed the fattest profits in big business."[27] In the 1990 recession year, for example, drug makers "rewarded shareholders with returns on equity 50% higher than the median for Fortune's 500 industrial companies." The major reason for these profits is the lack of price competition and the marketing "muscle" of the large drug makers. In this context their pathetic cries that the FDA is somehow threatening their existence have no more credibility than a Paul Bunyon tale, and should be taken no more seriously.

Drug companies are nonetheless likely to continue to lobby Congress and the public to limit their liability for harm caused by dangerous drugs by eliminating the possibility of recovery for punitive damages when FDA standards have been followed, or by limiting liability for harm caused by vaccines. AIDS activists may be tempted to join the drug companies and the free marketers on these moves as well, at least if the drug companies promise more work on AIDS drugs and vaccines in return. But just as drug approval standards should not be driven solely by the AIDS epidemic, so policies for compensating the victims of drug injuries should not be driven by the AIDS epidemic. We should not forget why we have rules for drug safety.

The distinction between experimentation and therapy is a powerfully useful and protective one that should not be undermined. The fact that there is no cure for a fatal disease does not make experimental drugs designed for it "therapeutic," any more than a mechanical or baboon heart is therapeutic for someone with end stage heart disease. Experimental drugs are not a consumer good appropriately governed by the free market. If consumer choice was the only relevant issue, even if it was limited to terminally ill consumers, the drug of choice among most dying intravenous drug users with AIDS would likely be heroin (or other opiate derivatives such as morphine). These drugs are effective in relieving pain and anxiety in this population, and if they are delivered with clean needles in a medical setting, they can also be safe. If we really wanted to make drugs a consumer good for the terminally ill, we should begin here. The fact that we don't indicates that the political agenda at work in the AIDS context is not patient-centered.

Perhaps the fact that we don't make heroin available to terminally ill intravenous drug users is a way we have of punishing them for their illegal behavior.[28] It is equally plausible that we care so little for the victims of AIDS that we don't care if they get hurt by quack remedies imported from abroad. It has also been suggested that although we do not accept active euthanasia and look with disapproval on even terminally ill patients who want physicians to end their lives, we nonetheless believe that it is perfectly acceptable for individuals to volunteer for medical experiments that could hasten their deaths:

Our quest for a formula that will banish death seems to make it acceptable to try questionable regimens on the aged and terminally ill. . . . Those who insist on using the dying as experimental subjects . . . see death

as abnormal and dying patients as subhuman. We cast the terminally ill in modern rites of sacrifice, putting patients through experiments like the Jarvik heart that one might see as torture in the hope of postponing the inevitable.[29]

By making experimental drugs available to AIDS patients outside of organized clinical trials we are doing little, if anything, for AIDS patients. We really seem to be treating ourselves, giving ourselves the illusion that something is being done to combat death—an illusion that is more satisfying because it does not call for any additional government funding. But we will pay a high price for this comfortable illusion if it is used as an excuse to abandon the distinction between experimentation and therapy and to transform the FDA from a consumer protection agency into a drug promotion agency.

The FDA has been the focus of much criticism for not discovering a cure for AIDS. But this is not the FDA's responsibility. The FDA does not do research on, manufacture, or test new drugs; it approves drugs as "safe and effective" that are made and tested by others who seek to market them in the United States. As Commissioner Kessler has so well articulated, its role is not to further the interests of food or drug companies, but to protect the public. It does this, among other ways, by insisting on strict standards in drug testing. Shortcuts that undermine these standards risk the health of all who later use a drug that has been too hastily approved.

The excuse that patients are dying without treatment and have "nothing to lose" will not do. Terminally ill patients can be harmed, abused, and exploited. Realistic discussion of death and accurate education about the status of unproven AIDS drugs and the reason randomized clinical trials are needed is in order. It is not "compassionate" to make quack remedies easily available to those who can pay for them. Real compassion demands that we allocate the money and staff necessary to do real scientific research, and that when valid clinical trials demonstrate that a therapy is "safe and effective," we make it available to all who need it, regardless of their ability to pay. Compassion does not counsel us to supply dying patients with fabulous promises and faddish drugs.

Notes

1. This essay is based on Annas, G. J., Faith (Healing), Hope and Charity at the FDA: The Politics of AIDS Drug Trials, *Villanova L. Rev.* 34:771–797; 1989, which should be consulted for full text of notes.

2. Katz, J., *The Silent World of Doctor and Patient,* New York: Free Press, 1984, p. 151.

3. *Trials of War Criminals before the Nuremberg Military Tribunals under Control Council Law No. 10, The Medical Case,* Vols. I and II, Washington, D.C.: U.S. Gov. Print. Office, 1950.

4. Annas, G. J., Glantz, L. H. & Katz, B. F., *Informed Consent to Human Experimentation,* Cambridge, MA: Ballinger, 1977. Surprisingly, when the U.S. Supreme Court had a chance to adopt and endorse the principles of the Nuremberg Code in 1987, it failed to recognize the code as a basis to award damages in the United States military by a 5 to 4 vote. *U.S. v. Stanley,* 483 U.S. 669 (1987).

5. Ingelfinger, F., Informed (but Uneducated) Consent, *New Engl. J. Med.* 287: 465–466; 1972.

6. *Ibid. And see* Reinhold, R., Infected but Not Ill, Many Try Unproved Drugs To Stave Off AIDS, *New York Times,* May 20, 1987, p. B12.

7. For example, a French AIDS researcher experimenting with HPA-23 said of AIDS patients in 1984: "What do these people have to lose?" (Quoted in Shilts, R., *And the Band Played On,* New York: St. Martin's Press, 1987, p. 496).

8. Fletcher, J., The Evolution of the Ethics of Informed Consent (in) Berg, K. & Treanoy, K., eds., *Research Ethics,* New York: A. R. Liss, 1983, p. 211.

9. *New York Times,* Sept. 26, 1988, p. A16 (transcript of the presidential debate).

10. *U.S. v. Rutherford,* 442 U.S. 544, 1979. *See* Culbert, M., *The Fight for Laetrile Vitamin B17,* New Rochelle, NY: Arlington House, 1974, and Kittler, G. D., *Laetrile: Control for Cancer,* New York: Warner Books, 1963.

11. *Rutherford,* at p. 549. Laetrile's advocates, on the other hand, accused the government of suppressing a "cure" for cancer.

12. FDA, HHS, Investigational New Drug, Antibiotic, and Biological Drug Product Regulations; Treatment Use and Sale, 52 *Fed. Reg.* 19,465-77 (1987). *See* Young, F., Norris, J., Levitt, N., & Nightingale, S., The FDA's New Procedures for the Use of Investigational New Drugs, *JAMA* 259:2267; 1988.

13. Pear, R., U.S. To Allow Use of Trial Drugs for AIDS and Other Terminal Ills, *New York Times,* May 21, 1987, p. 1. A year later these new rules were termed a "failure" by the President's AIDS Commission. Report of the Presidential Commission on AIDS, 50 (1988).

14. Boffey, P., FDA Will Allow Patients To Import AIDS Medicines, *New York Times,* July 25, 1988, p. A15. Up to three months supply can be imported and a physician's name must be given.

15. Booth, P., An Underground Drug for AIDS, *Science,* Sept. 9, 1988, p. 1279.

16. Shilts, *supra* note 16, p. 562. "About 100 Americans were part of the AIDS exile community in Paris, making long daily treks to Percy Hospital on the edge of the city for their shots of HPA-23" (*Ibid.,* p. 563).

17. Eckholm, R., Should the Rules be Bent in an Epidemic?, *New York Times,* July 13, 1987, p. 30E.

18. Clark, M., Lerner, M. & Stadtman, N., AIDS: A Breakthrough?, *Newsweek,* Nov. 11, 1985, p. 88.

19. Brooke, J., In Zaire, AIDS Awareness vs. Prevention, *New York Times,* Oct. 10, 1988, p. B4.

20. *See, e.g.,* Kolata, G., Recruiting Problems in New York Hinder U.S. Trials of AIDS Drug, *New York Times,* Dec. 18, 1988, p. 1.

21. 53 *Fed. Reg.* 41515-24 (1988). *See also* Waldholz, M., Drug Firms Hope FDA Broadens Plan To Speed Approval of Some Medicines, *Wall St. J.,* Oct. 21, 1988, p. B3.

22. Silver, L., FDA Offers Plan To Speed Process of Drug Approval, *Boston Globe,* Oct. 20, 1988, p. 3.

23. Altman, L., At AIDS Talks Reality Weighs Down Hope, *New York Times,* July 26, 1992, p. 1.

24. McKinlay, J., From "Promising Report" to "Standard Procedure": Seven Stages in the Career of a Medical Innovation, *Milbank Mem. Fund Q.* 59:374; 1981, and sources cited therein. In an RCT trial a new drug is compared with a placebo or other drug, each being assigned at random to comparable patients. In a double blind study, neither the physician nor the patient know who is getting the new drug and who is getting the placebo.

25. New Ideas for New Drugs, *Wall St. J.,* Dec. 28, 1988,

p. A6. *See also* Waldholz, M., Drug Firms Hope FDA Broadens Plan To Speed Approval of Some Medicines, *Wall St. J.,* Oct. 21, 1988, p. B3.

26. *See, e.g.,* Editorial, Forcing Poverty on AIDS Patients, *New York Times,* Aug. 30, 1988, p. A18, stating in part, "A drug company should not unusually have to justify its profit, but AZT is a special case." *And see* Arno, P. & Feiden, K., *Against the Odds: The Story of AIDS Drug Development, Politics and Profits,* New York: Harper-Collins, 1992.

27. O'Reilly, Drug Makers Under Attack, *Fortune* 124(3): 48–63, July 29, 1991.

28. *But see* Edgar, H. & Rothman, D. J., New Rules for New Drugs: The Challenge of AIDS to the Regulatory Process, *Milbank Mem. Fund Q.* 68:111–141; 1990.

29. Brauer, R., The Promise that Failed, *New York Times Magazine,* Aug. 28, 1988, pp. 46, 76.

Case Study: The Doctor's Unproven Beliefs and the Subject's Informed Choice

Don Marquis, Ron Stephens,
Ethel S. Siris, M. Margaret Kemeny,
and Robert J. Levine

■

Mr. S, a forty-eight-year-old male, was referred to the oncology clinic with a histologically proven diagnosis of renal cell carcinoma. Lung metastases present at the time of original diagnosis have grown. Although there is a small percentage of spontaneous remission with this disease, no curative radiation therapy or chemotherapy is available. The response rate to standard progestational agents or chemotherapy is about 5 percent and those responses usually involve only modest shrinkage. Mr. S informed his physician that unless some form of treatment would improve his quality of life or extend his period of survival he would prefer to postpone treatment, particularly if a proposed therapy would risk reducing the quality of his existence.

The physician knew that a drug company was financing a randomized trial that would compare gamma-interferon to Depo-Provera, a standard progestational agent. As with almost all studies of anticancer drugs, both physicians and patients would be aware of the treatment. Two-thirds of the patients were to receive interferon; those who received Depo-Provera and did not respond to it would not be "crossed over" to interferon.

Although no interferon of any kind was then available for nonresearch uses, studies of alpha-interferon in renal cell carcinoma had indicated a 5 to 30 percent response rate. A Phase I trial of gamma-interferon designed to determine toxicity and recommended dosage level had resulted in six responses from among thirty-six patients with renal cell carcinoma at various dosage levels. No regular Phase II study had been done. On the basis of this evidence, the physician believes that gamma-interferon would be the most promising treatment she could offer Mr. S.

Should the physician ask Mr. S to participate in this study? If she does, should she make certain he understands that: (1) In her best clinical judgment, only gamma-interferon offers any real hope for his disease; (2) He has the right to withdraw from the study at any time and therefore a right to withdraw if he is randomized to Depo-Provera? Does Mr. S's agreement to participate in the study entail an obligation to accept either therapy? Finally, should the drug company have conducted a regular Phase II study of gamma-interferon before financing this randomized study?

Commentary
Don Marquis and Ron Stephens

Mr. S's physician faces a serious dilemma. She believes that gamma-interferon is the best drug available for his renal cell carcinoma. The only way for him to receive it is by participating in the clinical trial. Since physicians have an obligation to give their patients what in their judgment is the best treatment that can be obtained, it might be argued that the physician has an obligation to enroll Mr. S in the study.

Yet Mr. S is disinclined to accept ineffective treatment and the physician evidently believes that Depo-Provera is very likely to be ineffective. What, then, should she tell Mr. S? Should she enroll him in the study? One possibility is to suggest that participation is tantamount to a contract between Mr. S and the drug company: Mr. S would participate in the study even if he receives Depo-Provera in exchange for a chance to receive gamma-interferon. However, this characterization obscures the patient's right to withdraw from the study at any time.

Another possibility is to obtain Mr. S's written informed consent to participate in the study, but remain silent concerning both the supposed contract and his right to withdraw in the event of randomization to Depo-Provera. Yet since patients frequently do not read consent forms carefully and often do not understand them when they do, it is questionable whether such "consent" would be informed. If the physician is properly concerned with Mr. S's autonomy, she should explain that he can withdraw from the study at any time for any reason without his care being compromised, and make certain he understands that this provision holds even if he is randomized to receive Depo-Provera.

There are, however, substantial arguments against withdrawing the patient if he does not receive the desired therapy. If every physician adopted this alternative, the study presumably could not be completed. Further, this seems tantamount to *using* a drug company protocol to obtain experimental therapy for a patient while at the same time frustrating the purposes of the protocol.

While it might damage a physician's career in academic medicine, this last course of action is morally preferable. It is the only course of action that does not violate the physician's duty to her patient. The moral bind experienced by physicians who consider enrolling patients in the study suggests that the study itself is ethically flawed. Is this so?

This is a Phase III study of anticancer drugs designed to show that a proposed treatment regimen is better than or at least as good as, but less toxic than, standard therapy. A physician should ask her patient to participate in such a randomized study only if good evidence that one treatment is inferior to the other is not available.

Only randomized clinical trials that satisfy a condition of therapeutic equivalence should be conducted.

The physician in this case *believed* that the gamma-interferon versus Depo-Provera trial did not meet this standard, not because she was convinced that gamma-interferon was a proven therapeutic agent for metastatic renal cell carcinoma, but because she had no confidence in the "standard" therapy for the disease, Depo-Provera.

There is considerable justification for her conclusion. For some oncologists, Depo-Provera has been the drug of choice for metastatic renal cell carcinoma only because there is no other potentially effective treatment. Many would offer it to a patient only if he or she really wanted chemotherapy and then only because Depo-Provera does not have serious side effects. In addition, poorly designed studies of the efficacy of Depo-Provera have yielded mixed results. Hence the physician's belief that gamma-interferon offered Mr. S the only real hope of benefit for his disease was probably quite sound.

The trial was badly designed. A Phase III study on gamma-interferon should not have been conducted because there was no established efficacious treatment. The drug company instead should have run a regular Phase II study of gamma-interferon involving fifteen to twenty patients with renal cell carcinoma who would receive gamma-interferon at a dosage schedule suggested by the Phase I trial.

Commentary
Ethel S. Siris and M. Margaret Kemeny

One of the realities of medical practice is that there are some diseases for which no good treatments exist. The difficult question of whether to enroll a patient such as Mr. S in a clinical trial, with all of its attendant risks and uncertainties, must be faced by both the patient and the physician. Defining the roles and ethical and legal obligations of the three participants involved in the decision to enter a cancer patient into a clinical trial—the personal physician, the patient, and the clinical investigator—provides insight into the issues that arise in this setting.

The personal physician's role includes an obligation to inform the patient of the existence of the clinical trial and to give an objective opinion as to whether enrolling in the study would be in the patient's best interest. There are many considerations in deciding whether to recommend participation in a randomized trial in oncology, including possible inconvenience and considerable expense to a seriously ill patient, the loss of the primary doctor's control of treatment, and the possible risks and discomforts of untested therapies.

Unfortunately, Mr. S's doctor is not being objective about the study. Though there are only minimal data on the safety and effectiveness of gamma-interferon in treating metastatic renal cell carcinoma, she has a strong conviction that it is the treatment of choice. She may take this position in part because the results with standard treatment—Depo-Provera—are so dismal. However, she also appears to feel that gamma interferon is intrinsically a better choice, a treatment that she believes should work and be safe. Given the preliminary nature of the studies, some of which examined a different agent (alpha-interferon), her certainty seems premature. The clinical trial is being conducted to provide a more objective basis for evaluating the data.

The physician's beliefs pose a serious problem for her and her patient: She wants Mr. S to enter the study, but in light of his stated wishes concerning treatment and her strong conviction about the best therapy, she wants him to participate only if he is randomized to receive gamma-interferon. In our view this position is flawed. The physician may certainly convey her impression that gamma-interferon is promising, but she should be careful to avoid creating a situation in which her patient will suffer emotional anguish if he is randomized to the "wrong" treatment arm. Her role is not to make a judgment about which arm of a particular study she hopes her patient will receive, but to decide whether to recommend this or any appropriate study.

The patient's role in deciding whether to participate in the clinical trial also entails certain obligations. The process of obtaining informed consent should make it clear to Mr. S that he has the right to withdraw from the study at any time. This right includes the option to leave the trial solely because he is disappointed about the treatment to which he has been randomized. We would hope, however, that a patient would not enter a study with the unstated intention of leaving if he doesn't receive the treatment he wants.

It is the investigator's responsibility to be certain that the trial is designed so that it is scientifically and ethically valid, one in which all treatment arms offer equivalent risk/benefit ratios. If the patient understands this and has not been unfairly influenced by unsubstantiated opinions regarding different treatment modalities in the study, he or she should be able to accept his or her assignment in good faith. Though we strongly agree that the patient has inviolate rights, we would also argue that he or she has some obligation to remain in the study out of fairness.

The patient entering a clinical trial in oncology is typically anxious and frightened. The informed consent process, though imperfect, should convey enough information about the study and alternative management strategies to allow the patient to make a rational choice in what is invariably an emotionally turbulent setting. The researcher has the obligation to inform these individuals not only objectively, but also compassionately. All of this takes time, both the patient's and the researcher's. In fairness, Mr. S should agree to enter the study only if he reason-

ably believes that it is in his best interest to participate and is committed to fulfilling the protocol requirements in good faith.

Finally, should the drug company have performed a phase II rather than a phase III study? Both typically involve controlled trials, with phase II studies looking for a promise of efficacy of the study therapy in a small number of subjects and phase III trials seeking definitive evidence of efficacy when the experimental agent is compared with current therapies in a larger number of subjects. When a treatment arm proves significantly more effective than the control arm, the study can be stopped and the new treatment used on a wider range of patients. All new drugs eventually go through the phase II-III process, since all drugs must be compared to existing treatment regimens. There is no way to assess the efficacy of one arm over another before the clinical trial has been implemented.

The medical community's scientific obligation is to continue searching for better treatments for solid tumors and to test these treatments with an established empirical scientific method. Individual patients and their personal physicians must also recognize their responsibility to society as a whole. Without individuals who freely participate in such studies, many advances in cancer treatment modalities in such varied areas as lymphomas, testicular tumors, ovarian cancers, and some lung cancers could not have been made. Mr. S and his physician should carefully consider these issues in the context of his personal needs and wishes as they work together to do what will be best for him.

Commentary
Robert J. Levine

The authors of the two preceding commentaries agree that the drug company should have conducted a phase II rather than a phase III trial, and

I agree with them. Marquis and Stephens prefer phase II to phase III "because there was no established efficacious treatment." This point notwithstanding, as Siris and Kemeny observe, after a "promise of efficacy" has been established in phase II, "definitive evidence of efficacy" *must be* obtained by comparison with "current therapies in a larger number of subjects"; i.e., in a randomized clinical trial (RCT).

Now let us imagine that phase II has been completed and gamma-interferon seems to show substantial promise of efficacy. Should the physician advise a new Mr. S to enroll in an RCT comparing gamma-interferon with Depo-Provera? Now that phase II has been completed, the physician has substantial reinforcement for her opinion that "gamma-interferon would be the most promising therapy for Mr. S."

Preliminary data obtained from uncontrolled studies often create obstacles to the successful conduct of RCTs. Based upon such data, physicians may develop strong beliefs about the efficacy of drugs and, consequently, either refuse to cooperate in the conduct of RCTs or, as in the present case, consider taking actions, sometimes surreptitiously, to subvert their goals. This is why several commentators, most notably Thomas Chalmers, have urged randomization with the very first use of a new therapy; i.e., the first eligible patient should have a 50-50 chance of receiving either the new drug or the standard alternative drug.[1] For various practical reasons it is not, and it should not be, customary to introduce new therapies by random allocation with the very first patient.[2, pp. 187–188]

Should a physician enroll a patient in an RCT comparing two therapies when she believes one of the two is superior? Benjamin Freedman has argued persuasively that such an action may be justified if knowledge about the comparative efficacy of the two therapies is in a state of "clinical equipoise."[3] Such a state exists, for example, when

there is a split in the clinical community, with some clinicians favoring [treatment] A and others favoring B. Each side recognizes that the opposing side has evidence to support its position, yet each still thinks that overall its own view is correct. There exists (or in the case of novel therapy, there may soon exist) an honest professional disagreement among expert clinicians. . . . A clinical trial is instituted with the aim of resolving this dispute.

A state of clinical equipoise is consistent with a decided treatment preference on the part of the investigators. They must simply recognize that their less-favored treatment is preferred by colleagues whom they consider to be responsible and competent.

I agree that Mr. S should enter the study only if he "believes that it is in his best interest . . . and is committed to fulfilling the protocol in good faith." There are several persuasive reasons for limiting the freedom of subjects to withdraw from protocols.[2, pp. 113–189] Space permits mention of only one. As Lisa Newton has argued, the completely unfettered freedom to withdraw required by ethical codes and regulations "is an anomaly in ethics, since it appears to be . . . in direct conflict with [one's] ordinary duty to keep [one's] promises."[4] She recommends that future revisions of regulations should recognize that the relationship between the investigator and the subject is binding on both sides and that the regulations should "specify the circumstances that shall be taken to negate or cancel that mutual commitment."

Notes

1. Chalmers, T.C., Block, J.D., Lee, S.: Controlled Studies in Clinical Cancer Research. *New England Journal of Medicine* 287:75–78, 1972.
2. Levine, R.J.: "Ethics and Regulation of Clinical Research," Urban & Schwarzenberg, Baltimore, Second Edition, 1986.

3. Freedman, B.: Equipoise and the ethics of clinical research. *New England Journal of Medicine* 317:141–145, 1987.

4. Newton, L.H.: Agreement to participate in research: Is that a promise? *IRB: A Review of Human Subjects Research* 6 (2):7–9, March/April 1984.

3

Choices about Treatment

The final section in this part of the volume addresses both end-of-life decision making and the problem that occurs when physicians and patients (or their families) disagree about the withholding or withdrawal of treatments in what has come to be called the futility debate. This section addresses a constellation of issues so well-rehearsed in the literature that almost any combination of materials is sure to produce fruitful discussion. We have included some lesser known but excellent writings as well as some well-known ones.

In the set of readings that address end-of-life choices, Miles Edwards and Susan Tolle consider not merely moral and legal reasoning about decisions but also the emotional meaning of those decisions for all involved. Their article addresses withdrawal of treatment for a conscious patient who is clearly making an informed and autonomous decision. How might a decision to withdraw treatment from a patient who does not have, and will not regain, decisional capacity be different? Would it be harder or easier to make and carry out? What kind of responsibility do institutional medicine and its care providers bear for end-of-life treatment dilemmas? This topic recalls issues raised by some of the illness narratives and stories in parts I and II, as well as the professional socialization issues addressed in part III. Questions about language, role responsibilities, and the death-defying focus of medical training and institutions all affect the ethics of end-of-life treatment decisions.

The readings continue with a poem that has been included as a matter-of-fact alternative, in William Carlos Williams's distinctive style, to the many moving writings about patients who wish to die. Williams's grandmother is an unexpected personality—not necessarily likable, not necessarily "all there," certainly vivid and real. How should we understand what she wants? How are we to honor her wishes, or explain why we won't?

This discussion might be supplemented with readings from the extensive literatures on judging patients' decisional capacity and deciding for patients without decisional capacity. Of special note is "Fidelity," Wendell Berry's title story from one of his collections of stories about the families he calls the Port William membership (1992). It could also be useful to examine the lively debate in the bioethics and health law literatures on the role of the family in health care, or state advance directive statute(s) and the Patient Self-Determination Act, to fill out consideration of end-of-life decision-making.

Section 3 concludes with three articles on physician-assisted suicide. We include the well-known case of Diane, reported in the *New England Journal of Medicine,* which raises very effectively a wide range of pertinent issues and viewpoints for discussion. Correspondence published about it in a later issue of the journal asks a number of questions, including: Was Dr. Quill "too close" to his patient? Or is closeness required in order to assist in a patient's death? Should we be concerned that patients may want to die because palliative care and pain relief are imperfectly taught to and practiced by physicians, or because patients perceive their illnesses to be expensive and burdensome to their fam-

ilies? Should physician-assisted suicide remain illegal so that it cannot become routine but stays an unusual act, requiring courage and compassion, or should it be legalized so that patients like Diane do not need to die alone? It is also important to consider the moral similarities and differences between abating treatment and assisting suicide, from the standpoint of both patients and caregivers.

Finally, a pair of essays on the meaning of "futility" as it applies to treatment for terminal conditions acknowledges the possibility of stark conflict between the physician's authority and choices made by patients and their families, when patients and families want "everything done" in the face of permanent, grave incapacity and/or impending death. The nature and power of medical judgment is the central concern of these readings. Once again, we have chosen only a few selections from a robust and growing literature that includes cases, careful surveys and critiques of the various definitions of futility that are currently in circulation, and arguments both in favor of medical authority and deeply skeptical about its implications for patients. The futility question can be viewed as a distillation of the potential power conflict that lies at the center of every physician-patient relationship. How a society regards that conflict may well determine many of its views about all of health care. The importance of culture, ethnicity, religion, and race as factors in patients' preferences should be considered here, in order to determine whether discrimination has a place in this conflict.

The two readings present the case of Helga Wanglie, who first brought the futility issue into the public consciousness. Mrs. Wanglie's case shows how questions about who should decide are entangled with questions about what the right choice is, and begins to identify the conflicts in values that are implicated in disagreements about futile treatment.

Disconnecting a Ventilator at the Request of a Patient Who Knows He Will Then Die: The Doctor's Anguish

Miles J. Edwards and

Susan W. Tolle

■

Recently we assisted in withdrawing life support from a patient who had repeatedly asked to have his ventilator disconnected, even after being informed that he would then die. We found little in the medical literature to guide us, especially at the feeling level, so we are sharing our experience with the hope that others will find our emotional responses, reasoning, and procedures useful.

The Case

Mr. Larson was a 67-year-old, obese white man. At 23 years of age he developed poliomyelitis and "spent six weeks in an iron lung." His neurologic recovery was virtually complete, and he resumed a reasonably normal life.

In November 1990, he noted the onset of rapidly progressive dyspnea and weakness in his extremities. A month later, he was hospitalized. He was endotracheally intubated and then underwent a tracheostomy to provide continuous mechanical ventilation. Numerous attempts to wean the patient from the ventilator always failed within 1 to 2 minutes. He was alert and frustrated by his ventilator dependence and demonstrated some symptoms of situational depression. After careful pulmonologic and neurologic

evaluation, his condition was attributed to "post-polio syndrome."

When the patient asked if he would ever be able to live without the ventilator, pulmonary and neurology consultants told him that he would always be ventilator dependent. One consultant felt that he might improve enough to be taken off the ventilator during the day but that he would probably continue to need it at night. All consultants concurred that he would never become totally ventilator independent. The patient listened and, after thinking it over, asked to have ventilatory support discontinued. He stated that he realized he would die without such support.

A psychiatrist evaluated the patient and agreed that he was somewhat depressed, although not severely enough to affect his decision-making capacity. After some initial reservations, the patient's family (one grown daughter and two grown sons) showed strong support for his decision. The patient consistently made it clear that living on continuous mechanical ventilation, with the consequent inability to speak, rendered the quality of his life unacceptable. He continued to express his wish to discontinue ventilation over a 2-week period and asked to be heavily sedated in the process. Because of his unwavering request, we were called in as ethics consultants.

Ensuring That Ventilator Withdrawal Is Right for the Patient

We believe that after careful consideration in selected cases, withdrawal of the ventilator from an awake patient, allowing a natural death to occur, is the right thing to do. We object to the term "passive euthanasia"; it is not killing the patient. It is instead stepping aside and allowing the disease to take its natural course when that course is the consistent choice of a competent patient. The question then is whether that choice is ethically supportable in a particular patient. What do we need to consider before making this decision? And if we do decide to disconnect the ventilator, how can that be done with compassion to minimize or eliminate the patient's suffering?

We accept the ethical and legal principles that patients have the right to refuse medical treatment, even when they may die as a result. However, we have an obligation to verify that the refusal of life-sustaining treatment is the durable request of a mentally competent, well-informed patient. In Mr. Larson's case, we needed more information before we could respond to his request. We identify seven actions that must be addressed before such a request should be acted on.

1. Clarify the prognosis.

2. Be assured of the patient's decision-making capacity (and of the absence of a medically significant depression that might temporarily affect his or her judgment).

3. Assure durability of the patient's wish.

4. Identify any coercive influences, either personal or financial.

5. Explore concurrence of all family members.

6. Explore concurrence of all members of the health care team.

7. Consider legal mandates.

During the 1 week of our consultation, we talked repeatedly to the patient, separately to all three children, and also to some close friends of the family. One son appeared to have some misgivings, but they really represented, as further inquiry revealed, his great unhappiness about his father's condition. After coming to terms with those feelings, he agreed with his father's decision. We continued to explore the attitudes of all family members. From an ethical perspective, the patient's wishes should be respected, and unanimous agreement from the family is not necessarily required. However, we did obtain unanimous agreement from the family in support of our patient's decision.

We concluded that for Mr. Larson, withdrawal of the ventilator was both legally and ethically supportable, recognizing the right of competent, informed adults to refuse medical treatment. Then came the particularly difficult question: How could this be done with compassion and with a minimum of suffering?

Discontinuing Mechanical Ventilation in a Conscious Patient

The Patient's Right to Sedation

Discontinuing mechanical ventilation is a uniquely difficult process for the patient, the family, the physician, and other members of the health care team. Regardless of how strongly the patient may wish to have this done, the sudden feeling of suffocation that results leads to a visceral panic. This sensation constitutes the greatest of suffering. Therefore, we believe that it is mandatory to provide sedation to awake patients before ventilation is withdrawn. Any use of sedative or narcotic analgesic medication to relieve the unwanted sensations would also reduce respiratory drive; the two are inseparable. It is a physiologic reality, then, that sedating the patient probably accelerates death by some small measure of time. However, it had been determined through multiple previous attempts to wean this patient from the ventilator that death would occur anyway, so sedating the patient would not in itself cause the death.

In Mr. Larson's case, we did not advise on the types or doses of sedatives, but we did encourage adequate sedation. We suggested that the attending physician consult with an experienced pulmonologist-intensivist on the details of ventilator withdrawal, including dosing of sedation. We acknowledge that titrating sedation is difficult when the goal is relief of suffering without deliberately inducing a respiratory arrest. Marked variability in both individual needs and drug tolerance further complicates these estimates. Ideally, the patient will be heavily sedated but will continue to maintain his or her respiratory efforts.

Our Planning

We submitted our ethics consultation report to the team and were informed by the intern that the disconnection was to be done 3 days later, on 25 February 1991 at 10:00 a.m. We suggest selecting a particular time for several reasons: It allows further time to assure durability of the patient's request, and it allows the patient and family to say final good-byes, decide who will be present, arrange last rites, and so forth; in addition, selecting a time early in the day ensures that the physician and primary nurses are available in case the patient does not die right away and needs further comfort and support. A disadvantage of setting a specific time is that any delay will be a further stress for the patient and family.

Final details were planned with the patient and the health care team. The patient requested that several members of his family be present (they wanted to be there), while others would wait in an adjoining room. The primary care team discussed who would do the disconnection and decided that the pulmonary consultant and attending staff physician would administer sedatives and disconnect the ventilator. We saw our role as ethics consultants finished.

The Disconnection

Loving family had been present throughout Mr. Larson's stay, and their numbers increased as the time of disconnection approached. By 9 a.m., 25 February, 13 family members and close friends were at the patient's bedside awaiting the disconnection. All anticipated that this would lead to the patient's death. We were not in attendance. At 9:30 a.m., we received a call from a distraught intern telling us that the family was there and all were ready. However, both the pul-

monologist and the attending physician would not be available until 5 hours later, at 3 p.m. The intern felt that she alone would have to disconnect the ventilator, something she was not technically or emotionally prepared to do and had never done before. The primary care team had not verified the pulmonary consultant's availability when the disconnection was planned. The attending physician had been called away unexpectedly and had delegated this job to the intern. We believed very strongly that this would not be an appropriate procedure for the anxious intern to do alone. Although we were both technically qualified as pulmonologist-intensivist and internist to perform the disconnection, we felt that being involved this way was beyond our role as ethics consultants. (We believe that an experienced pulmonologist-intensivist should always be involved.) Nevertheless, the patient had already waited a week while we had undertaken the seven actions outlined earlier, and we felt it would be cruel for him and his family to wait any longer. So with much trepidation, we decided that we would provide sedation and disconnect the ventilator ourselves. After this experience, we conclude that the attending physician *should* be the main player, with a pulmonologist-intensivist in attendance to provide necessary technical expertise. This is not a job for interns or inexperienced physicians.

We talked with the patient again to see if he still wanted this to be done and informed him that we would be performing the disconnection. He said "yes" emphatically. The family and other members of the health care team agreed. We told the patient we could not know exactly what dose of medication would be ideal and that we might err in either direction. We explained that if we judged low in our estimate, he would suffer from dyspnea. We asked his permission to reconnect the ventilator briefly if that happened, so that we could calmly administer additional medication. We would then disconnect again. He hesitated, but agreed. We again reminded him and the family that he might not die immediately. We told them that although we did not expect it, there was a slight chance he might continue to breathe for 24 hours or more. Our tests indicated he would not be able to breathe on his own, but occasionally patients live longer than we expect. If such was the case, we planned to start an intravenous drip of morphine to ensure his comfort.

A venous line was placed. We looked into the face of an alert man who we knew would soon die. Our more rational intellects told us that his disease, not us, would be the cause of his death. Deep feelings, on the other hand, were accusing us of causing death. From deep within us, feelings were speaking to us, making accusations, "You are really killing him, practicing active euthanasia, deceptively rationalizing with your intellects that there is a difference." These were not new feelings, but they were now greatly intensified as we stood there next to the patient, preparing to use syringes containing midazolam and morphine. Both are known respiratory depressants, which at high doses would be effective in active euthanasia and even at therapeutic doses would at least cause some respiratory depression and perhaps an earlier death. Nevertheless, midazolam and morphine were medically indicated to provide comfort to withdraw the ventilator in compliance with his request. We respected his right to refuse further life dependent on the ventilator. A heavy feeling of intense emotion consumed both of us as we slowly injected midazolam and morphine, watching the patient closely so we could produce the desired level of drowsiness. He reached what we thought was the correct end point, and one of us disconnected the tube to the ventilator while the other was poised at the catheter in case more medication was necessary. We stood frozen as Mr. Larson continued to take shallow but regular breaths. We felt some relief; at least we had not sedated the patient so

heavily that this alone would cause his immediate death.

Within a minute or so, the patient turned slightly cyanotic and began to struggle. With trembling hands, we pushed more midazolam and morphine, reaching final total doses of 15 mg midazolam and 30 mg morphine sulfate. (These doses apply directly to this patient and are not recommended for anybody else; people differ greatly in their tolerances.) Mr. Larson seemed comfortable, breathing shallowly at a rate of 28/minute. He exchanged smiles with his daughter, who stood holding his hand across the bed. He appeared reasonably comfortable and relaxed. We both felt a great heaviness and deep sense of anxiety. To facilitate communication among the 13 friends and family, we requested further support by the patient advocate (who had also been involved throughout the earlier discussions). Several family members provided regular updates to family members in the adjoining room. His daughter, the primary nurse, the intern, and the two of us remained at his bedside. Mr. Larson did not struggle further. About 30 minutes passed, although it seemed like hours. The patient then gradually slipped into a coma. Forty-five minutes after the disconnection, his breathing became irregular and stopped. He was not attached to any monitors, which probably reduced the strain on the family during the final minutes. His heart continued to beat for several minutes, first regularly, then with pauses. We took turns listening and waited until we were certain that he had died. Fifty-three minutes after he was disconnected from the ventilator, we pronounced him dead.

Although we received grateful hugs from the family and thanks from the health care team, we were struck by the gravity of what we had done. Doubts kept creeping into our minds. We each experienced a wave of disquieting emotion, feelings that we had killed this patient who would have otherwise continued to live connected to the ventilator. We knew intellectually that he had the legal and ethical right to refuse this medical treatment, but the gravity of his decision and our participation haunted us. We returned to our immediate commitments of caring for other patients, one of us responding next to the need of a patient who wanted medical help for a pulmonary problem to prolong his life. Both of us remained preoccupied throughout the afternoon thinking about Mr. Larson and what we had done. Our respective medical careers have generally been devoted to responding to patient wishes to postpone death and to prolong life. We've seen our patients die of their various diseases, but now our acquiescence in allowing his death caused us much anguish. This anguish continued in both of us for several days. One of us sought counsel from a psychiatrist who reinforced our belief that we did the right thing, counteracting those deep feelings that somehow we had killed this patient. Gradually we came to terms with what had happened. We had been in a complicated situation in which technology was sustaining life artificially, and we had acted on this patient's choice to refuse that treatment. Our consciences were clear, but we were left feeling very impressed with how difficult it had been to honor this man's request.

It is beyond the usual role of ethics consultants to take over patient care responsibilities and actually perform ventilator withdrawal. We do not intend to make it our practice to do this because it is really the appropriate role of the care-providers, who should enlist the help of a pulmonary-intensivist. We appreciate what we have learned from this unusual experience. After a period of reflection, we are no longer anxious about this decision, and we believe that we did the right thing in respecting Mr. Larson's request. Having witnessed from the bedside the suffering and the determination of this patient and his family, we feel better equipped to counsel other physicians whose patient care responsibilities will require them to grapple with similar end-of-life dilemmas.

Note

The name of our patient was changed to protect patient confidentiality, and the family granted permission to share his story. The authors thank Bernard Lo, MD, Michael Garland, DScRel, Virginia Tilden, DNSc., and Sandy Poole for their thoughtful reviews of the original manuscript.

The Last Words of My

English Grandmother

William Carlos Williams

■

There were some dirty plates
and a glass of milk
beside her on a small table
near the rank, disheveled bed—

Wrinkled and nearly blind
she lay and snored
rousing with anger in her tones
to cry for food,

Gimme something to eat—
They're starving me—
I'm all right I won't go
to the hospital. No, no, no

Give me something to eat
Let me take you
to the hospital, I said
and after you are well

you can do as you please.
She smiled, Yes
you do what you please first
then I can do what I please—

Oh, oh, oh! she cried
as the ambulance men lifted
her to the stretcher—
Is this what you call

making me comfortable?
By now her mind was clear—

Oh you think you're smart
you young people,

she said, but I'll tell you
you don't know anything.
Then we started.
On the way

we passed a long row
of elms. She looked at them
awhile out of
the ambulance window and said,

What are all those
fuzzy-looking things out there?"
Trees? Well, I'm tired
of them and rolled her head away.

Death and Dignity: A Case of Individualized Decision Making

Timothy E. Quill

■

Diane was feeling tired and had a rash. A common scenario, though there was something subliminally worrisome that prompted me to check her blood count. Her hematocrit was 22, and the white-cell count was 4.3 with some metamyelocytes and unusual white cells. I wanted it to be viral, trying to deny what was staring me in the face. Perhaps in a repeated count it would disappear. I called Diane and told her it might be more serious than I had initially thought—that the test needed to be repeated and that if she felt worse, we might have to move quickly. When she pressed for the possibilities, I reluctantly opened the door to leukemia. Hearing the word seemed to make it exist. "Oh, shit!" she said. "Don't tell me that." Oh, shit! I thought, I wish I didn't have to.

Diane was no ordinary person (although no one I have ever come to know has been really ordinary). She was raised in an alcoholic family and had felt alone for much of her life. She had vaginal cancer as a young woman. Through much of her adult life, she had struggled with depression and her own alcoholism. I had come to know, respect, and admire her over the previous eight years as she confronted these problems and gradually overcame them. She was an incredibly clear, at times brutally honest, thinker and communicator. As she took control of her life, she

developed a strong sense of independence and confidence. In the previous 3½ years, her hard work had paid off. She was completely abstinent from alcohol, she had established much deeper connections with her husband, college-age son, and several friends, and her business and her artistic work were blossoming. She felt she was really living fully for the first time.

Not surprisingly, the repeated blood count was abnormal, and detailed examination of the peripheral-blood smear showed myelocytes. I advised her to come into the hospital, explaining that we needed to do a bone marrow biopsy and make some decisions relatively rapidly. She came to the hospital knowing what we would find. She was terrified, angry, and sad. Although we knew the odds, we both clung to the thread of possibility that it might be something else.

The bone marrow confirmed the worst: acute myelomonocytic leukemia. In the face of this tragedy, we looked for signs of hope. This is an area of medicine in which technological intervention has been successful, with cures 25 percent of the time—long-term cures. As I probed the costs of these cures, I heard about induction chemotherapy (three weeks in the hospital, prolonged neutropenia, probable infectious complications, and hair loss; 75 percent of patients respond, 25 percent do not). For the survivors, this is followed by consolidation chemotherapy (with similar side effects; another 25 percent die, for a net survival of 50 percent). Those still alive, to have a reasonable chance of long-term survival, then need bone marrow transplantation (hospitalization for two months and whole-body irradiation, with complete killing of the bone marrow, infectious complications, and the possibility for graft-versus-host disease—with a survival of approximately 50 percent, or 25 percent of the original group). Though hematologists may argue over the exact percentages, they don't argue about the outcome of no treatment—certain death in days, weeks, or at most a few months.

Believing that delay was dangerous, our oncologist broke the news to Diane and began making plans to insert a Hickman catheter and begin induction chemotherapy that afternoon. When I saw her shortly thereafter, she was enraged at his presumption that she would want treatment, and devastated by the finality of the diagnosis. All she wanted to do was go home and be with her family. She had no further questions about treatment and in fact had decided that she wanted none. Together we lamented her tragedy and the unfairness of life. Before she left, I felt the need to be sure that she and her husband understood that there was some risk in delay, that the problem was not going to go away, and that we needed to keep considering the options over the next several days. We agreed to meet in two days.

She returned in two days with her husband and son. They had talked extensively about the problem and the options. She remained very clear about her wish not to undergo chemotherapy and to live whatever time she had left outside the hospital. As we explored her thinking further, it became clear that she was convinced she would die during the period of treatment and would suffer unspeakably in the process (from hospitalization, from lack of control over her body, from the side effects of chemotherapy, and from pain and anguish). Although I could offer support and my best effort to minimize her suffering if she chose treatment, there was no way I could say any of this would not occur. In fact, the last four patients with acute leukemia at our hospital had died very painful deaths in the hospital during various stages of treatment (a fact I did not share with her). Her family wished she would choose treatment but sadly accepted her decision. She articulated very clearly that it was she who would be experiencing all the side effects of treatment and that odds of 25 percent were not good enough for her to undergo so toxic a course of therapy, given her expectations of chemotherapy and hospitalization and the absence of a closely matched bone marrow donor. I had her repeat her understanding of the treatment, the odds, and what to expect if there were no treatment. I clarified a few misunderstandings, but she had a remarkable grasp of the options and implications.

I have been a longtime advocate of active, informed patient choice of treatment or nontreatment, and of a patient's right to die with as much control and dignity as possible. Yet there was something about her giving up a 25 percent chance of long-term survival in favor of almost certain death that disturbed me. I had seen Diane fight and use her considerable inner resources to overcome alcoholism and depression, and I half expected her to change her mind over the next week. Since the window of time in which effective treatment can be initiated is rather narrow, we met several times that week. We obtained a second hematology consultation and talked at length about the meaning and implications of treatment and nontreatment. She talked to a psychologist she had seen in the past. I gradually understood the decision from her perspective and became convinced that it was the right decision for her. We arranged for home hospice care (although at that time Diane felt reasonably well, was active, and looked healthy), left the door open for her to change her mind, and tried to anticipate how to keep her comfortable in the time she had left.

Just as I was adjusting to her decision, she opened up another area that would stretch me profoundly. It was extraordinarily important to Diane to maintain control of herself and her own dignity during the time remaining to her. When this was no longer possible, she clearly wanted to die. As a former director of a hospice program, I know how to use pain medicines to keep patients comfortable and lessen suffering. I explained the philosophy of comfort care, which I strongly believe in. Although Diane understood and appreciated this, she had known of people lingering in what was called relative comfort, and she wanted no part of it. When the time came, she wanted to take her life in the least painful way possible. Knowing of her desire for independence and her decision to stay in control, I thought this request made perfect sense. I acknowledged and explored this wish but also thought that it was out of the realm of currently accepted medical practice and that it was more than I could offer or promise. In our discussion, it became clear that preoccupation with her fear of a lingering death would interfere with Diane's getting the most out of the time she had left until she found a safe way to ensure her death. I feared the effects of a violent death on her family, the consequences of an ineffective suicide that would leave her lingering in precisely the state she dreaded so much, and the possibility that a family member would be forced to assist her, with all the legal and personal repercussions that would follow. She discussed this at length with her family. They believed that they should respect her choice. With this in mind, I told Diane that information was available from the Hemlock Society that might be helpful to her.

A week later she phoned me with a request for barbiturates for sleep. Since I knew that this was an essential ingredient in a Hemlock Society suicide, I asked her to come to the office to talk things over. She was more than willing to protect me by participating in a superficial conversation about her insomnia, but it was important to me to know how she planned to use the drugs and to be sure that she was not in despair or overwhelmed in a way that might color her judgment. In our discussion, it was apparent that she was having trouble sleeping, but it was also evident that the security of having enough barbiturates available to commit suicide when and if the time came would leave her secure enough to live fully and concentrate on the present. It was clear that she was not despondent and that in fact she was making deep, personal connections with her family and close friends. I made sure that she knew how to use the barbiturates for sleep, and also that she knew the amount needed to commit

suicide. We agreed to meet regularly, and she promised to meet with me before taking her life, to ensure that all other avenues had been exhausted. I wrote the prescription with an uneasy feeling about the boundaries I was exploring—spiritual, legal, professional, and personal. Yet I also felt strongly that I was setting her free to get the most out of the time she had left, and to maintain dignity and control on her own terms until her death.

The next several months were very intense and important for Diane. Her son stayed home from college, and they were able to be with one another and say much that had not been said earlier. Her husband did his work at home so that he and Diane could spend more time together. She spent time with her closest friends. I had her come into the hospital for a conference with our residents, at which she illustrated in a most profound and personal way the importance of informed decision making, the right to refuse treatment, and the extraordinarily personal effects of illness and interaction with the medical system. There were emotional and physical hardships as well. She had periods of intense sadness and anger. Several times she became very weak, but she received transfusions as an outpatient and responded with marked improvement of symptoms. She had two serious infections that responded surprisingly well to empirical courses of oral antibiotics. After three tumultuous months, there were two weeks of relative calm and well-being, and fantasies of a miracle began to surface.

Unfortunately, we had no miracle. Bone pain, weakness, fatigue, and fevers began to dominate her life. Although the hospice workers, family members, and I tried our best to minimize the suffering and promote comfort, it was clear that the end was approaching. Diane's immediate future held what she feared the most—increasing discomfort, dependence, and hard choices between pain and sedation. She called up her closest friends and asked them to come over to say goodbye, telling them that she would be leaving soon. As we had agreed, she let me know as well. When we met, it was clear that she knew what she was doing, that she was sad and frightened to be leaving, but that she would be even more terrified to stay and suffer. In our tearful goodbye, she promised a reunion in the future at her favorite spot on the edge of Lake Geneva, with dragons swimming in the sunset.

Two days later her husband called to say that Diane had died. She had said her final goodbyes to her husband and son that morning, and asked them to leave her alone for an hour. After an hour, which must have seemed an eternity, they found her on the couch, lying very still and covered by her favorite shawl. There was no sign of struggle. She seemed to be at peace. They called me for advice about how to proceed. When I arrived at their house, Diane indeed seemed peaceful. Her husband and son were quiet. We talked about what a remarkable person she had been. They seemed to have no doubts about the course she had chosen or about their cooperation, although the unfairness of her illness and the finality of her death were overwhelming to us all.

I called the medical examiner to inform him that a hospice patient had died. When asked about the cause of death, I said, "acute leukemia." He said that was fine and that we should call a funeral director. Although acute leukemia was the truth, it was not the whole story. Yet any mention of suicide would have given rise to a police investigation and probably brought the arrival of an ambulance crew for resuscitation. Diane would have become a "coroner's case," and the decision to perform an autopsy would have been made at the discretion of the medical examiner. The family or I could have been subject to criminal prosecution, and I to professional review, for our roles in support of Diane's choices. Although I truly believe that the family and I gave her the best care possible, allowing her to define her limits and directions as much as possible, I am not sure the law, society, or the medi-

cal profession would agree. So I said "acute leukemia" to protect all of us, to protect Diane from an invasion into her past and her body, and to continue to shield society from the knowledge of the degree of suffering that people often undergo in the process of dying. Suffering can be lessened to some extent, but in no way eliminated or made benign, by the careful intervention of a competent, caring physician, given current social constraints.

Diane taught me about the range of help I can provide if I know people well and if I allow them to say what they really want. She taught me about life, death, and honesty and about taking charge and facing tragedy squarely when it strikes. She taught me that I can take small risks for people that I really know and care about. Although I did not assist in her suicide directly, I helped indirectly to make it possible, successful, and relatively painless. Although I know we have measures to help control pain and lessen suffering, to think that people do not suffer in the process of dying is an illusion. Prolonged dying can occasionally be peaceful, but more often the role of the physician and family is limited to lessening but not eliminating severe suffering.

I wonder how many families and physicians secretly help patients over the edge into death in the face of such severe suffering. I wonder how many severely ill or dying patients secretly take their lives, dying alone in despair. I wonder whether the image of Diane's final aloneness will persist in the minds of her family, or if they will remember more the intense, meaningful months they had together before she died. I wonder whether Diane struggled in that last hour, and whether the Hemlock Society's way of death by suicide is the most benign. I wonder why Diane, who gave so much to so many of us, had to be alone for the last hour of her life. I wonder whether I will see Diane again, on the shore of Lake Geneva at sunset, with dragons swimming on the horizon.

Informed Demand for "Non-Beneficial"

Medical Treatment

Steven H. Miles

∎

An 85-year-old woman was taken from a nursing home to Hennepin County Medical Center on January 1, 1990, for emergency treatment of dyspnea from chronic bronchiectasis. The patient, Mrs. Helga Wanglie, required emergency intubation and was placed on a respirator. She occasionally acknowledged discomfort and recognized her family but could not communicate clearly. In May, after attempts to wean her from the respirator failed, she was discharged to a chronic care hospital. One week later, her heart stopped during a weaning attempt; she was resuscitated and taken to another hospital for intensive care. She remained unconscious, and a physician suggested that it would be appropriate to consider withdrawing life support. In response, the family transferred her back to the medical center on May 31. Two weeks later, physicians concluded that she was in a persistent vegetative state as a result of severe anoxic encephalopathy. She was maintained on a respirator, with repeated courses of antibiotics, frequent airway suctioning, tube feedings, an air flotation bed, and biochemical monitoring.

In June and July of 1990, physicians suggested that life-sustaining treatment be withdrawn since it was not benefiting the patient. Her husband, daughter, and son insisted on continued treatment. They stated their view that physicians should not play God, that the patient would not be better off dead, that removing life support showed moral decay in our civilization, and that a miracle could occur. Her husband told a physician that his wife had never stated her preferences concerning life-sustaining treatment. He believed that the cardiac arrest would not have occurred if she had not been transferred from Hennepin County Medical Center in May. The family reluctantly accepted a do-not-resuscitate order based on the improbability of Mrs. Wanglie's surviving a cardiac arrest. In June, an ethics committee consultant recommended continued counseling for the family. The family declined counseling, including the counsel of their own pastor, and in late July asked that the respirator not be discussed again. In August, nurses expressed their consensus that continued life support did not seem appropriate, and I, as the newly appointed ethics consultant, counseled them.

In October 1990, a new attending physician consulted with specialists and confirmed the permanence of the patient's cerebral and pulmonary conditions. He concluded that she was at the end of her life and that the respirator was "non-beneficial," in that it could not heal her lungs, palliate her suffering, or enable this unconscious and permanently respirator-dependent woman to experience the benefit of the life afforded by respirator support. Because the respirator could prolong life, it was not characterized as "futile."[1] In November, the physician, with my concurrence, told the family that he was not willing to continue to prescribe the respirator. The husband, an attorney, rejected proposals to transfer the patient to another facility or to seek a court order mandating this unusual treatment. The hospital told the family that it would ask a court to decide whether members of its staff were obliged to continue treatment. A second conference two weeks later, after the family had hired an attorney, confirmed these positions, and the husband asserted that the patient had consistently said she wanted respirator support for such a condition.

In December, the medical director and hospital administrator asked the Hennepin County Board of Commissioners (the medical center's board of directors) to allow the hospital to go to court to resolve the dispute. In January, the county board gave permission by a 4-to-3 vote. Neither the hospital nor the county had a financial interest in terminating treatment. Medicare largely financed the $200,000 for the first hospitalization at Hennepin County; a private insurer would pay the $500,000 bill for the second. From February through May of 1991, the family and its attorney unsuccessfully searched for another health care facility that would admit Mrs. Wanglie. Facilities with empty beds cited her poor potential for rehabilitation.

The hospital chose a two-step legal procedure, first asking for the appointment of an independent conservator to decide whether the respirator was beneficial to the patient and second, if the conservator found it was not, for a second hearing on whether it was obliged to provide the respirator. The husband crossfiled, requesting to be appointed conservator. After a hearing in late May, the trial court on July 1, 1991, appointed the husband, as best able to represent the patient's interests. It noted that no request to stop treatment had been made and declined to speculate on the legality of such an order.[2] The hospital said that it would continue to provide the respirator in the light of continuing uncertainty about its legal obligation to provide it. Three days later, despite aggressive care, the patient died of multisystem organ failure resulting from septicemia. The family declined an autopsy and stated that the patient had received excellent care.

Discussion

This sad story illustrates the problem of what to do when a family demands medical treatment that the attending physician concludes cannot benefit the patient. Only 600 elderly people are treated with respirators for more than six months in the United States each year.[3] Presumably, most of these people are actually or potentially conscious. It is common practice to discontinue the use of a respirator before death when it can no longer benefit a patient.[4,5]

We do not know Mrs. Wanglie's treatment preferences. A large majority of elderly people prefer not to receive prolonged respirator support for irreversible unconsciousness.[6] Studies show that an older person's designated family proxy overestimates that person's preference for life-sustaining treatment in a hypothetical coma.[7–9] The implications of this research for clinical decision making have not been cogently analyzed.

A patient's request for a treatment does not necessarily oblige a provider or the health care system. Patients may not demand that physicians injure them (for example, by mutilation), or provide plausible but inappropriate therapies (for example, amphetamines for weight reduction), or therapies that have no value (such as laetrile for cancer). Physicians are not obliged to violate their personal moral views on medical care so long as patients' rights are served. Minnesota's Living Will law says that physicians are "legally bound to act consistently within my wishes within limits of reasonable medical practice" in acting on requests and refusals of treatment.[10] Minnesota's Bill of Patients' Rights says that patients "have the right to appropriate medical . . . care based on individual needs . . . [which is] limited where the service is not reimbursable."[11] Mrs. Wanglie also had aortic insufficiency. Had this condition worsened, a surgeon's refusal to perform a life-prolonging valve replacement as medically inappropriate would hardly occasion public controversy. As the Minneapolis *Star Tribune* said in an editorial on the eve of the trial,

> The hospital's plea is born of realism, not hubris. . . . It advances the claim that physi-

cians should not be slaves to technology—any more than patients should be its prisoners. They should be free to deliver, and act on, an honest and time-honored message: "Sorry, there's nothing more we can do."[12]

Disputes between physicians and patients about treatment plans are often handled by transferring patients to the care of other providers. In this case, every provider contacted by the hospital or the family refused to treat this patient with a respirator. These refusals occurred before and after this case became a matter of public controversy and despite the availability of third-party reimbursement. We believe they represent a medical consensus that respirator support is inappropriate in such a case.

The handling of this case is compatible with current practices regarding informed consent, respect for patients' autonomy, and the right to health care. Doctors should inform patients of all medically reasonable treatments, even those available from other providers. Patients can refuse any prescribed treatment or choose among any medical alternatives that physicians are willing to prescribe. Respect for autonomy does not empower patients to oblige physicians to prescribe treatments in ways that are fruitless or inappropriate. Previous "right to die" cases address the different situation of a patient's right to choose to be free of a prescribed therapy. This case is more about the nature of the patient's entitlement to treatment than about the patient's choice in using that entitlement.

The proposal that this family's preference for this unusual and costly treatment, which is commonly regarded as inappropriate, establishes a right to such treatment is ironic, given that preference does not create a right to other needed, efficacious, and widely desired treatments in the United States. We could not afford a universal health care system based on patients' demands. Such a system would irrationally allocate health care to socially powerful people with strong preferences for immediate treatment to the disadvantage of those with less power or less immediate needs.

After the conclusion was reached that the respirator was not benefiting the patient, the decision to seek a review of the duty to provide it was based on an ethic of "stewardship." Even though the insurer played no part in this case, physicians' discretion to prescribe requires responsible handling of requests for inappropriate treatment. Physicians exercise this stewardship by counseling against or denying such treatment or by submitting such requests to external review. This stewardship is not aimed at protecting the assets of insurance companies but rests on fairness to people who have pooled their resources to insure their collective access to appropriate health care. Several citizens complained to Hennepin County Medical Center that Mrs. Wanglie was receiving expensive treatment paid for by people who had not consented to underwrite a level of medical care whose appropriateness was defined by family demands.

Procedures for addressing this kind of dispute are at an early stage of development. Though the American Medical Association[13] and the Society of Critical Care Medicine[14] also support some decisions to withhold requested treatment, the medical center's reasoning most closely follows the guidelines of the American Thoracic Society.[15] The statements of these professional organizations do not clarify when or how a physician may legally withdraw or withhold demanded life-sustaining treatments. The request for a conservator to review the medical conclusion before considering the medical obligation was often misconstrued as implying that the husband was incompetent or ill motivated. The medical center intended to emphasize the desirability of an independent review of its medical conclusion before its obligation to provide the respirator was reviewed by the court. I believe that the grieving husband was simply mistaken about whether the respirator was benefiting his wife. A direct request to remove the respirator seems to center procedural oversight on the soundness of the medical decision making rather than on the nature of the patient's need. Clearly, the gravity of these decisions merits openness, due process, and meticulous accountability. The relative merits of various procedures need further study.

Ultimately, procedures for addressing requests for futile, marginally effective, or inappropriate therapies require a statutory framework, case law, professional standards, a social consensus, and the exercise of professional responsibility. Appropriate ends for medicine are defined by public and professional consensus. Laws can, and do, say that patients may choose only among medically appropriate options, but legislatures are ill suited to define medical appropriateness. Similarly, health-facility policies on this issue will be difficult to design and will focus on due process rather than on specific clinical situations. Public or private payers will ration according to cost and overall efficacy, a rationing that will become more onerous as therapies are misapplied in individual cases. I believe there is a social consensus that intensive care for a person as "overmastered" by disease as this woman was is inappropriate.

Each case must be evaluated individually. In this case, the husband's request seemed entirely inconsistent with what medical care could do for his wife, the standards of the community, and his fair share of resources that many people pooled for their collective medical care. This case is about limits to what can be achieved at the end of life.

Notes

1. Tomlinson, T., Brody, H. Futility and the ethics of resuscitation. JAMA 1990; 264:1276–80.
2. In re Helga Wanglie, Fourth Judicial District (Dist. Ct., Probate Ct. Div.) PX-91-283. Minnesota, Hennepin County.
3. Office of Technology Assessment Task Force. Life-sustaining technologies and the elderly. Washington, D.C.: Government Printing Office, 1987.
4. Smedira, N.G., Evans, B.H., Grais, L.S., et al. Withholding and withdrawal of life support from the critically ill. N Engl J Med 1990; 322:309–15.
5. Lantos, J.D., Singer, P.A., Walker, R.M. et al. The illusion of futility in clinical practice. Am J Med 1989; 87–81–4.
6. Emanuel, L.L., Barry, M.J., Stoeckle, J.D., Ettelson, L.M., Emanuel, E.J. Advance directives for medical care—a case for greater use. N Engl J Med 1991; 324:889–95.
7. Zweibel, N.R., Cassel, C.K. Treatment choices at the end of life: a comparison of decisions by older patients and their physician-selected proxies. Gerontologist 1989; 29:615–21.
8. Tomlinson, T., Howe, K., Notman, M., Rossmiller, D. An empirical study of proxy consent for elderly persons. Gerontologist 1990; 30:54–64.
9. Danis, M., Southerland, L.I., Garrett, J.M. et al. A prospective study of advance directives for life-sustaining care. N Engl J Med 1991; 324:882–8.
10. Minnesota Statutes. Adult Health Care Decisions Act. 145b.04.
11. Minnesota Statutes. Patients and residents of health care facilities; Bill of rights. 144.651:Subd. 6.
12. Helga Wanglie's life. Minneapolis Star Tribune. May 26, 1991:18A.
13. Council on Ethical and Judicial Affairs, American Medical Association. Guidelines for the appropriate use of do-not-resuscitate orders. JAMA 1991; 265:1868–71.
14. Task Force on Ethics of the Society of Critical Care Medicine. Consensus report on the ethics of foregoing life-sustaining treatments in the critically ill. Crit Care Med 1990; 18:1435–9.
15. American Thoracic Society. Withholding and withdrawing life-sustaining therapy. Am Rev Respir Dis 1992.

The Case of Helga Wanglie:

A New Kind of "Right to Die" Case

Marcia Angell

■

Helga Wanglie, an 86-year-old Minneapolis woman, died of sepsis on July 4 after being in a persistent vegetative state for over a year. She was the focus of an extremely important controversy over the right to die that culminated in a court decision just three days before her death.[1] The controversy pitted her husband and children, who wanted her life maintained on a respirator, against doctors at the Hennepin County Medical Center, who wanted her removed from the respirator because they regarded the treatment as inappropriate. The judge decided in favor of Mr. Wanglie, and Helga Wanglie died still supported by the respirator.

The Wanglie case differed in a crucial way from earlier right-to-die cases, beginning with the case of Karen Quinlan 16 years ago. In the earlier cases, the families wished to withhold life-sustaining treatment and the institutions had misgivings. Here it was the reverse; the family wanted to continue life-sustaining treatment, not to stop it, and the institution argued for the right to die. Mr. Wanglie believed that life should be maintained as long as possible, no matter what the circumstances, and he asserted that his wife shared this belief.

In one sense, the court's opinion in the Wanglie case would seem to be at odds with most of the earlier opinions in that it resulted in con-tinued treatment of a patient in a persistent vegetative state. In another sense, however, the opinion was quite consistent, because it affirmed the right of the family to make decisions about life-sustaining treatment when the patient was no longer able to do so. By granting guardianship of Mrs. Wanglie to her husband, the judge indicated that the most important consideration was who made the decision, not what the decision was. I believe that this was wise; any other decision by the court would have been inimical to patient autonomy and would have undermined the consensus on the right to die that has been carefully crafted since the Quinlan case.

What are the elements of that consensus and how should they be applied to the Wanglie case and others like it? There is general agreement that competent adults may refuse any recommended medical care. This right, based on principles of self-determination, has repeatedly been buttressed by the courts. When patients are no longer mentally competent, families are to act in accordance with what the patient would wish (a principle known as substituted judgment).[2–4] Disputes have arisen, however, when the patient had not, while competent, clearly expressed his or her preferences. This was the situation in the Wanglie case, as it was thought to be in the Cruzan case.[5]

To avoid these disputes, there is a growing movement to encourage all adults to prepare a document that would provide guidance, if necessary, for their families and doctors.[6] Such documents include living wills, durable powers of attorney, and other instruments that have been specially devised for the purpose. Congress recently mandated that as of December 1991, all health care facilities must provide an opportunity for patients to prepare such a document on admission.

We are still left with the problem of deciding for those who have nevertheless provided no guidance, including those who were unable to do so, such as children or profoundly retarded adults. In these cases as well, families usually make decisions on behalf of the patient, but since the patient's wishes are unknown, the consensus holds that the family's decision must be consistent with the patient's best interests.[2–4] A decision consistent with best interests is usually defined as a choice that reasonable adults might make if faced with the problem. This is a vague but useful standard that, by definition, restricts the range of permissible decisions. It can, however, allow for more than one possible choice. For example, the decision to withdraw the respirator from Karen Quinlan was thought by the New Jersey Supreme Court to be consistent with her best interests, but her father was given the latitude to decide either way.[7]

The well-publicized legal disputes involving the right to die—such as the Quinlan case, the Brophy case in Massachusetts,[8] and the Cruzan case in Missouri—have reached the courts either because the institution believed it improper to withhold life-sustaining treatment at the family's request or because the institution wanted legal immunity before doing so. Until the Wanglie case, there was only one well-publicized case of the reverse situation—that is, of a family wishing to persist in treatment over the objections of the institution. This was the poignant case of Baby L, described last year in the *Journal*.[9] The case involved a two-year-old child, profoundly retarded and completely immobile, who required repeated cardiopulmonary resuscitation for survival. Baby L's mother insisted that this be done as often as necessary, despite the fact that there was no hope of recovery. Representatives of the hospital challenged her decision in court on the grounds that the continued treatment caused great suffering to the child and thus violated its best interests. Before the court reached a decision, however, the mother transferred the child to a hospital that agreed to continue the treatment, and the case became legally moot.

Unlike the case of Baby L, the Wanglie case did not involve a course that would cause the patient great suffering. Because she was in a persistent vegetative state, Mrs. Wanglie was incapable of suffering. Therefore, a compelling case could not be made that her best interests were being violated by continued use of the respirator. Instead, representatives of the institution invoked Mrs. Wanglie's best interests to make a weaker case: that the use of the respirator failed to serve Mrs. Wanglie's best interests and should therefore not be continued. It was suggested that a victory for Mr. Wanglie would mean that patients or their families could demand whatever treatment they wished, regardless of its efficacy. Many commentators also emphasized the enormous expense of maintaining a patient on life support when those resources are needed to care for people who would clearly benefit. In the previous essay, Steven H. Miles, M.D., the ethics committee consultant at the Hennepin County Medical Center who was the petitioner in the Wanglie case, presents the arguments of the institution.[10] They are strong arguments that deserve to be examined, but I believe that they are on balance not persuasive.

It is generally agreed, as Miles points out, that patients or their surrogates do not have the right to demand any medical treatment they choose.[11,12] For example, a patient cannot insist that his doctor give him penicillin for a head cold. Patients' rights on this score are limited to refusing treatment or to choosing among effective ones. In the case of Helga Wanglie, the institution saw the respirator as "non-beneficial" because it would not restore her to consciousness. In the family's view, however, merely maintaining life was a worthy goal, and the respirator was not only effective toward that end, but essential.

Public opinion polls indicate that most people would not want their lives maintained in a persistent vegetative state. Many consider life in this state to be an indignity, and care givers often find caring for such patients demoralizing. It is important, however, to acknowledge that not everyone agrees with this view and it is a highly personal issue. For the decision to rest with the family is the most sensitive and workable approach, and it is the generally accepted one. Furthermore, a system in which life-sustaining treatment is discontinued over the objections of those who love the patient, on a case-by-case basis, would be callous. It can be argued on medical grounds that the definition of brain death should be legally extended to include a persistent vegetative state, but unless that is done universally we have no principled basis on which to override a family's decision in this kind of case. It is dismaying, of course, that resources are spent sustaining the lives of patients who will never be sentient, but we as a society would be on the slipperiest of slopes if we permitted ourselves to withdraw life support from a patient simply because it would save money.

Since the Quinlan case it has gradually been accepted that the particular decision is less important than a clear understanding of who should make it, and the Wanglie case underscores this approach. When self-determination is impossible or an unambiguous proxy decision is unavailable, the consensus is that the family should make the decision. To be meaningful, this approach requires that we be willing to accept decisions with which we disagree. Only if a decision appears to violate the best interests of a patient who left no guidance or could provide none, as in the case of Baby L, should it be challenged by the institution. Thus, the sources of decisions about refusing medical treatment are, in order of precedence, the patient, the patient's prior directives or designated proxy, and the patient's family. Decisions from each of these sources should reflect the following standards, respectively: immediate self-determination, self-determination exercised earlier, and the best interests of the patient. Institutions lie outside this hierarchy of decision making and should intervene by going to court only if they believe a decision violates these standards. Although I am sympathetic with the view of the doctors at the Hennepin County Medical Center, I agree with the court that they were wrong to try to impose it on the Wanglie family.

Notes

1. In re Helga Wanglie, Fourth Judicial District (Dist. Ct., Probate Ct. Div.) PX-91-283. Minnesota, Hennepin County.
2. Society for the Right to Die. The physician and the hopelessly ill patient: legal, medical and ethical guidelines. New York: Society for the Right to Die, 1985.
3. Guidelines on the termination of life-sustaining treatment and the care of the dying: a report by the Hastings Center. Briarcliff Manor, N.Y.: Hastings Center, 1987.
4. President's Commission for the Study of Ethical Problems in Medicine and Biomedical and Behavioral Research. Deciding to forego life-sustaining treatment: a report on the ethical, medical, and legal issues in treatment decisions. Washington, D.C.: Government Printing Office, 1983.
5. Cruzan v. Harmon, 760 S.W.2d 408 (1988).
6. Annas, G.J. The health care proxy and the living will. N Engl J Med 1991; 324:1210–3.
7. In re Quinlan, 70 NJ 10, 355 A.2d 647 (1976).
8. Brophy v. New England Sinai Hospital, Inc., (Mass. Probate County Ct., Oct. 21, Nov. 29, 1985) 85E0009-G1.
9. Paris, J.J., Crone, R.K., Reardon F. Physicians' refusal of requested treatment: the case of Baby L. N Engl J Med 1990; 322:1012–5.
10. Miles, S.H. Informed demand for "non-beneficial" medical treatment. N Engl J Med 1991; 325:512–5.
11. Brett, A.S., McCullough, L.B. When patients request specific interventions: defining the limits of the physician's obligation. N Engl J Med 1986; 315:1347–51.
12. Blackhall, L.J. Must we always use CPR? N Engl J Med 1987; 317:1281–5.

PART V

Medical Care Financing, Rationing,

and Managed Care

This part of the *Social Medicine Reader* deals with three areas that are closely related: the financing of medical care, the rationing of health services, and the physician's role in managed care. Each area serves as context for the others. For example, the dilemmas of rationing are sharpened by understanding the history of health care financing in the United States, and by considering the new duties of physicians under managed care.

The lead essay is Donald Madison's "Paying for Medical Care in America," which includes a glossary of key terms for the first section, on medical care financing. The remaining two areas also have their specialized terminology and complex history, which are discussed in this introduction.

Rationing may be defined as the equitable distribution of a scarce good according to a central plan. This is the standard dictionary definition, and it is illustrated by food or gasoline rationing in wartime, in which the goods received are called "rations." Under this definition, it is clear that health care rationing does not occur in the United States. There is no central plan for the distribution of health services, and equity of distribution exists only as an ideal. Yet there are other meanings and uses of this term. The economist Victor Fuchs, for example, says that warnings about future rationing are "nonsense because the United States has always rationed medical care. . . . [N]o nation can provide 'presidential medicine' for all its citizens" (Fuchs 1984, 1572). The chief method of rationing medical goods and services in the United States is through the market, by means of price rationing, and in this respect the United States stands alone among developed nations. Other modern industrial democracies collectively finance and regulate the distribution of health services, with the goal of providing access to some level of services to all citizens. By contrast, Americans have a tradition of allowing access to be a function of individual purchasing power. Those with high incomes or employer-sponsored health insurance have relatively prompt and steady access, while those without money or insurance have limited and sporadic access and rely chiefly on charity. This is an inevitable effect of market forces in health care, and accounts for the large and growing number of uninsured and underserved persons. Roughly 40 million Americans are uninsured and underserved for health care. Another 30 million are seriously underinsured and would be financially ruined by a major illness. These numbers are occasionally a source of national embarrassment and calls for change, as in 1991 and 1992, when general anxiety about access to health care helped to decide senatorial and presidential elections. Yet this anxiety has not been sufficiently deep or sustained to alter the status quo of markets and private modes of distribution rather than more collective and equitable ones.

Lester Thurow says that in matters of medical care Americans are both egalitarians and capitalists (Thurow 1984). We believe that no one should be turned away from needed health services for lack of money, but we also believe that those who can afford it should be able to spend as much as they like for medical care. These beliefs are incompatible. A system that aims for equity in access cannot rely primarily on market forces,

and any system that allows the costs of medical services to be driven by consumer demands will inevitably "price out" those who are poor or have expensive illnesses. This contradictory set of beliefs about health care is one of the reasons that the rationing of health care has been addressed infrequently, and when it is addressed, is so vexing for Americans.

Another key question in the rationing debate is whether it should be done implicitly or explicitly. Rationing decisions are by definition difficult; they involve denying some persons the care that they need and want. One of the potentially attractive features of the market (to some) is that it works implicitly, without any explicit decisions ever being made, or often even put forward. Those who like the market system consider it unfortunate that the working poor, for example, have no coverage and receive few services. Yet, they argue, no explicit decision was made to exclude the poor; it's their lack of money (or insurance) that keeps them away from needed care. In a market system, lacking as it does a central distributional authority, no one is directly responsible for bad outcomes (Churchill 1987). Whether this displacement of explicit decision making and responsibility is considered an asset or a liability is widely debated.

One line of reasoning in support of explicit rationing begins with the premise that medical services are not comparable to other consumer items, like color televisions and cars (Walzer 1983). Medical services also differ from other necessities, like food, since the need for them can be unpredictable. No one wakes up needing $10,000 worth of food, but it is not unusual for persons to find themselves in immediate need of $10,000 in medical care (Carmenisch 1979). Advocates of explicit rationing argue that since health services are an essential part of modern life, the processes by which care is allocated should not remain hidden in the workings of the market but be openly debated, as befits democratic processes. Only then can the trade-offs among different uses of scarce resources be recognized. The state of Oregon has undertaken just such an open and explicit process for deciding which services will be included in its Medicaid expenditures.

Questions about rationing are fundamentally questions about how to allocate scarce resources fairly; they ask what factors are morally relevant to allocation choices. For example, should age be a factor? Should first access be given to persons who have maintained a healthy life-style? Who should be served when not all can be served fully? Who (or what) can be justifiably excluded? These debates are always difficult because there is a vast array of procedures and interventions that fall under the category "health services," from facelifts to inoculations, from preventive services to heart transplants. Moreover, health services are not only valued differently by different people, but valued differently by each of us at different times. Inevitably, they are valued more when we are ill or injured, and perhaps also when we are older.

In seeking to devise a fair system of distribution, most of us tend to fall into one or more of three categories for thinking about fairness: libertarian, egalitarian, and utilitarian.

Libertarians, as the name suggests, value liberty and noninterference from others. A fair allocation system maximizes and protects the freedoms of all concerned. Justice, in libertarian terms, means respecting the freedoms of others and keeping hands off their property. Libertarians are typically opposed to the notion that we have a "right to health care," since they see it as coercive—forcing citizens to pay higher taxes to support care for the uninsured, forcing physicians to train in specialties or practice in geographic areas they might not choose (to achieve adequate distribution of personnel), and forcing patients to receive services in regulated ways (Sade 1971). The current U.S. health care system is largely libertarian in orientation, distributing medical goods and services to those who can afford and access it, emphasizing "consumer choice" and physician prerogatives to select their patients. Libertarians see the resulting inequities in access as unfortunate but not unfair, and the remedy—because it would compromise liberty—as worse than the problem.

Egalitarians, by contrast, emphasize the similarities and commonalities among persons, which they believe should lead to more equitable policies. They point to the equal vulnerability of people to disease, disability, and death, despite obvious differences in age, income, or health status. Egalitarians often express their commitment in terms of a right to health care, or a right to equitable access to basic health services. Norman Daniels, for example, argues that equitable distribution of medical and health resources is necessary in order to provide a fair "equality of opportunity," thereby putting equal access to health care on a par with equal access to jobs, income, and other goods and rewards open to persons in a democracy (Daniels 1985).

While both libertarians and egalitarians focus on goods that have intrinsic value (liberty or equality), utilitarians avoid intrinsic standards and focus simply on the consequences. Good actions are the ones that achieve the best balance of good over evil, measured in terms of the happiness of the greatest number of people (Mill 1957). Fairness, for utilitarians, is a measurable outcome, a matter of the aggregate happiness or well-being. It is not what makes me as an individual happy, but what makes for the greatest happiness when everyone is considered. One way to measure happiness in health care is in terms of health status, so that a just or fair allocation system would be the one that produced the highest overall health status for a population. Utilitarians are interested in comparing different kinds of treatment to find out which ones most improve patients' health status, and in comparing outcomes in the U.S. system, which relies on the market, with Canadian or European outcomes, which rely on regulation and social insurance programs.

These sketches of theories of justice, or ideals of fairness, are precisely that—outlines of alternative ways of thinking. They are intended to stimulate and orient conversations about fair choices in rationing. The readings of section 2 will focus this discussion in a more concrete way.

Section 3 examines managed care and the physician's changing role in this new environment. "Managed care" is a loose term used to describe a wide variety of practices. Until recently this term referred to a system that integrated financing and delivery in order to provide comprehensive services to enrolled members. The typical managed care organization (MCO) was a nonprofit, prepaid, group practice health maintenance organization (HMO), enrolling members for a monthly, capitated fee, and providing most needed services and coordinating the provision of those not directly provided. Kaiser Permanente and Group Health Cooperative of Puget Sound are examples of this more traditional type of MCO. More recently, however, "managed care" has expanded to include more loosely affiliated physician networks, such as preferred provider organizations (PPOs) and independent practice associations (IPAs), who contract with insurers to provide services at a volume discount and assume varying degrees of the financial risk. Even indemnity insurance plans with utilization review (which cover policyholders for their indemnity, or financial loss, in paying for medical care) now claim they are offering managed care. Such indemnity plans hope to associate themselves with the record of quality and savings established by HMOs, even though they offer none of the comprehensive care or coordinating services of HMOs and frequently operate as for-profit, investor-owned enterprises (Starr 1994).

The chief aim of managed care is to control costs, and this immediately raises the question in the minds of both physicians and patients of whether the price of cost control is a reduction in quality. It has become customary, therefore, to hear a litany of reassurances about quality from MCOs. Such assurances are necessary in part because, to the public, more care is almost always thought to be better care, and because for the past several decades we have been schooled to believe that once we have paid our health insurance premiums we have purchased anything we might need or want. These popular beliefs are not easily changed, and the cost-effective practices of managed care run directly counter to them. If, however, well-insured Americans run a greater risk from overtreatment than from undertreatment (as some claim), some parsimony in services may be a real benefit, and thus managed care—if it is *well managed*—may present no ethical problems in terms of the aggregate quality of care provided. At least one study of managed care practices during the period from 1980 to 1994 indicated that when physicians adhere to managed care guidelines, health outcomes compare favorably with those of traditional financing and delivery systems (Miller and Luft 1994).

The ethical tensions of managed care for physicians have a different source. Ethical tensions arise with the recognition that even in the best managed care system a small number of patients will be placed at some (hopefully small) additional risk in order to benefit others covered by the plan, and to keep the plan itself solvent. This happens by design, not by accident, and must be acknowledged even by those who believe that well-insured Americans, generally, are more likely to suffer from too many interventions rather than too few. Managed care guidelines for diagnosis and treatment are population-based norms, and as such they reflect an implicit obligation of both the organization and the physician to the health of a population, in addition to the health of any given individual patient. Moreover, physicians who work in managed care environments are given a financial incentive to practice in this more cost-effective way. Their incomes are increased or reduced based on the cost implications of their clinical choices, and on the MCO's overall record in meeting target budgets or profit expectations. Traditional medical ethics expresses a single allegiance to the patient, and none to the patient population (Veatch 1981). The new dual set of obligations, to the old ethics and the new standards of managed care, can become divided obligations, or conflicting obligations, and this complicates the physician's ethical role.

For example, when a patient requires a diagnostic CT scan for a suspicious series of headaches, there is a choice in dyes between an inexpensive high-osmolality contrast agent and a far more costly low-osmolality contrast agent. A small percentage of patients will have greater discomfort, and a very few will have severe reactions to the less expensive dye. The new evidence-based, population-oriented system will call for the less expensive alternative, unless there are specific contraindications, while the system that is geared to the individual patient (to patient choice) could easily lead in the opposite direction (Fleck and Squier 1995). The doctor can be thorough in taking down the patient's history, and so reduce some of the risk of discomfort or a severe reaction, but the only way to eliminate it entirely would be to use the more expensive dye. Far more problematic are situations in which patients seek a procedure still classified as "experimental" and not included in the managed care plan's clinical guidelines, such as bone marrow transplantation for some forms of breast cancer.

In brief, the fear is that managed care may not be something the physician does *for* the patient, but something the physician does *to* the patient, to benefit herself or himself and the MCO. If pa-

tients are denied care they think they need, they will seek reassurance that they are being told "no" for reasons that relate to their well-being, and not to the financial interests of the physician or the MCO. Reassuring patients on this question may be more difficult if the plan is the product of an investor-owned, for-profit organization expected to produce dividends for its stockholders. To respond to these issues, physicians and bioethicists have been busy developing ethical guidelines. The content and rationale for such ethical guidelines are discussed in detail in the final section.

The American health care system is in the midst of major changes, and it is unclear at what point and in what form a stasis will be achieved. Primary care has taken on increasing importance, chiefly because managed care requires primary care physicians to be gatekeepers for specialty care and hospitalization. The gatekeeping role creates new burdens of competence on primary care physicians, who must now take responsibility for treating a wider range of illnesses and referring with greater parsimony, but also appropriately. This creates tensions, not only between physicians and patients, as discussed above, but also among primary care physicians and their specialty colleagues, who must depend on the gatekeepers for access to patients. In terms of the future, it is unclear whether Americans will choose to finance medical care on a private consumer model or a social insurance model, that is, whether capitalistic or egalitarian values will dominate. A closely related question is whether the uninsured and underinsured will find a voice in the ongoing health policy debates.

Larry R. Churchill

Medical Care

Financing

Paying for Medical Care

in America

Donald L. Madison

∎

In its simplest terms, the financing of medical care is about how doctors and hospitals are paid for their services. From the patient's perspective this is typically an issue of what services are covered and how much must be paid out of pocket. The readings in this section demand a larger perspective; they examine the workings of medical care financing as indicators of historical processes and cultural and political values. Donald Madison's essay is a brief history of medical care financing in the United States, providing an understanding of why we have the system we do, how it developed and the past efforts to change it. The essay is threaded with a glossary of basic organizational and financing terms. Uwe Reinhardt's article surveys alternative approaches by which advanced industrial nations seek to cope with the chief problems all nations face: how to increase access to needed medical services while controlling costs. Reinhardt stresses that each nation's financing methods reflect distinct cultural and political values; still, he envisions a convergence of financing methods within the next decade. Together these two essays provide the basis for grasping the complex issues of rationing and the promise and hazards of managed care, which are the subjects of the last two sections of the book.

A Word of Explanation

This essay is an introduction to the world of health insurance, managed care, health care "reform," and related matters. It is a primer, intended for medical students and other beginners. Ideally, students should learn health care financing in its proper context as one piece of the much larger subject of medical care organization. In this chapter, however, I mention only in passing such other major topics in medical care as the hospital—the most prominent of our medical care institutions—or the organized medical profession, the pharmaceutical industry, medical practice organization, regulation of health care and the policymaking process. Much later, as a practicing physician, you will need to know a good deal more about these other topics of medical care organization. This primer on payment should help you get started.

Medical care organization is not, unfortunately, a jargon-free field. To explicate certain concepts that may be unfamiliar and to clarify some words and phrases that will be familiar but are often misunderstood, I have scattered GLOSSARY entries throughout the essay.

In order to understand the current situation, you must know something of how it developed. Therefore, I have organized the material around a chronological history of medical care financing in the United States. Where terms and concepts need explaining I have tried to explain them as nearly as possible within their historical context.

Any chronology must inevitably reach the interface between present and future. During the years 1993 to 1996 two payment issues—"health care reform" and the "preservation" of Medicare—made the national political agenda. At the end of the essay I have attempted to summarize, very briefly (and tentatively) some of the recent political debate on these issues, without attempting to predict what may happen next.

Glossary: *Medical Care Organization*—The study of organized arrangements for the financing, delivery, and regulation of personal health services.

The Basis of Health Insurance

Medical care is, among other things, a service for sale. It costs something to produce it and to purchase it. How the money flows is the stuff of medical care financing.

Once upon a time paying for medical care was a simple matter. Doctors treated patients and in return patients paid the doctor's fee *at the time of illness.* That's all there was to it. The fee covered nearly everything. Hospitals were not a part of the picture. Pharmacies were, but not nearly as much nor as often as now. There were not diagnostic centers nor commercial laboratories. If the patient ran short of funds to pay the doctor, barter was often acceptable since the doctor's costs consisted mostly of his time and household expenses. (The office, with no staff beyond the doctor and his or her spouse, was usually part of the home.) No longer. Office lease, malpractice insurance, equipment purchase and maintenance, corporate taxes, medical supplies, continuing education, automobile depreciation, professional society dues, reference lab fees, staff salaries with social security payments and other fringe benefits, debt service, and so on, ad infinitum, must all now be paid as the necessary costs of carrying on a medical practice. A chicken, a bushel of apples, or a new fence in lieu of a fee doesn't help much in meeting these kinds of costs.

Still, the physician's side of medical care financing is actually simple compared to the patient's. Hospital costs now consume nearly half of the medical care dollar. In addition to the basic charge, usually calculated as for a hotel on a perday basis, payments must be made for lab, X-ray, and electrocardiogram charges (including the fees of the medical specialists who interpret each of these three technological forms of diagnosis), procedures of all sorts, emergency room fees, operating room charges, anesthesiologist's fees, medical consultations, drugs, supplies, and appliances. (The average total charge now exceeds $1,500 per day in many urban hospitals.) Then there are the costs of prescription drugs, nursing homes, home care, and so on. And this doesn't consider the *indirect* costs to the patient (such as transportation or child care) or the *opportunity* costs (such as income foregone due to time away from work).

Obviously, even a moderately severe episode of sickness today would leave any but the most wealthy patient unable to pay *at the time the medical care is needed.* Actually, that has been true for a long time, and it is why the old method of paying at the time of illness had to be replaced by the idea of collective financing—the regular collection of small amounts of money from everyone to pay for the care of people who are sick. In this way, people could be protected (insured) from financial ruin caused by the unpredictability of illness. They absorbed a *small certain loss* (the known amount of the premium) to avoid a *large uncertain loss* (the unknown but probably large outlay for medical and hospital care, if and when it should ever be required).

There are two main kinds of health insurance at work in the United States: *social insurance* and *private insurance.* Most of this primer will explain the evolution and some of the features of these two types of insurance. Social insurance came first in the evolution.

Glossary: *Social Insurance*—The distinctive characteristic of social insurance as compared to private insurance is its compulsory nature. The government requires coverage by law. It may provide the insurance itself, or it may require (or allow) people to obtain it in the private sector. The best known American example of social insurance is the federal Old-Age, Survivors, Disability and Health Insurance, usually called, simply, Social Security. It includes a social *health* insurance program, Medicare. At the state level, the most familiar example of social insurance (with indirect health care benefits) is the liability insurance that automobile owners are required to purchase.

Social Insurance versus Public Assistance— Social insurance is distinguished from public assistance by the payment of premiums that bear some relation to benefits—the majority of social insurance in the United States is financed through equal employer and employee contributions held in the Social Security Trust Fund—and by the principle that benefits are given to the recipients as a matter of right, not as a matter of charity. Public Assistance is *not* insurance; it is paid for out of general tax revenue to people found to be in need, regardless of how much if anything they paid in taxes. Of the two major government medical care financing programs, one, Medicare, is social insurance; the other, Medicaid, is public assistance. A large number of government programs provide health benefits, but only two (Medicare and Workmen's Compensation) are social insurance.

Social Insurance: Bismarck (1883)

Insurance for the *indirect costs of illness* came into being well before insurance for the *direct costs of medical care*. Before the twentieth cen-

tury, few hospitals charged the patient anything. There were no expensive diagnostic tests. Physicians charged fees, of course, but except for surgical operations, they were usually modest. The doctor wouldn't have been able to collect otherwise. But when a workman fell ill his family faced a financial problem—the loss of his income. There was no such thing then as unemployment insurance or sick leave.

To meet this problem, workers organized mutual benefit funds, usually through their social clubs, lodges, or "friendly societies." These workers' clubs collected small, regular payments from each member. Then, when a member fell ill and was unable to work, the fund helped out. The other time when a friendly society helped was when the worker died. The family received a modest cash benefit to help with the expense of the burial.

Workers' mutual benefit societies had been active in Europe since the thirteenth century, but they grew rapidly during the last half of the nineteenth century, when the industrial revolution and accompanying urbanization produced both a greater concentration of workers and greater risk of illness and injury. Along with urban industrialization came labor unrest, which led to political agitation.

In the new nation-state of Germany, Prince Otto Eduard Leopold von Bismarck, the "Iron Chancellor," was in firm control. Bismarck was disturbed, however, by the rapid gains the socialists were making among the German industrial workers. Despite his suppressive anti-socialism law of 1878, the popularity of socialism as an idea continued to grow. So, in 1883 Bismarck changed tactics. He reasoned that a generous, paternalistic state might win the workers' loyalties, or at least mollify those who were the most discontented. That was why he proposed a social insurance program that would be operated and financed directly by the state. He wanted it closely identified with his government.

But Bismarck hadn't counted on the strength of the mutual benefit societies. By 1883 there were many of these sickness funds—called, in German, *Krankenkassen*—and the workers had a vested interest in them. And this, combined with a certain distaste for Prussian-style government administration that was shared by workers and employers alike, convinced Bismarck that it would be politically expedient to alter his original plan. So instead of getting the state-run program he had wanted, Bismarck settled for a state-*mandated* system in which the German government would require all industrial workers to join one of these employment-based (operated either by the workers or the employer) *private* sickness funds.

The 1883 German social insurance program was the world's first. Soon other European nations began following Bismarck's example, although usually not for the same political reasons.

Social Insurance: Lloyd George (1911)

Great Britain was one of the nations to follow the German example. Under the leadership of David Lloyd George, the Chancellor of the Exchequer (the British name for Secretary of the Treasury), a national program of social insurance was enacted in 1911. Lloyd George preferred the term "health insurance" to "sickness insurance," and so it was called the National *Health* Insurance Act. The British program was also based on the "friendly societies" movement, which was particularly strong in the United Kingdom. And like Bismarck's program, it covered manual workers only, and not their dependents.

Glossary: *National Health Insurance*—A national program of social insurance that finances medical care for all or part of the population. Usually the term "national health insurance" refers to programs that cover *most* of a country's population (for example, 64% in the Netherlands, 85% in Belgium, 89% in Germany, 97% in Canada). It is not any longer, as it was in Lloyd George's day,

used to describe compulsory social insurance programs that cover only industrial workers or some other minority of the citizens of the country (for example, Americans aged 65 and older who are covered by Medicare). Under national health insurance, the government, either directly or through private sector agents, makes payments to physicians, hospitals, pharmacies, laboratories, etc., which themselves operate privately. However, in order to participate (be paid by the program) these private entities must meet the standards that have been set by the national insurance plan.

Both the German and the British health insurance programs (and those of other countries enacted during the same period) primarily paid cash benefits at the time of sickness and a burial benefit at death. It is true that they also paid for physicians' services, but this was, at least in the beginning, less important.

The practice of paying for physicians' services by mutual benefit societies came about gradually. Originally these societies' sickness funds didn't involve doctors at all. But before long the age-old question arose: how could a friendly society be certain that the beneficiary was actually sick and deserving of the cash benefit, and not merely malingering or drunk? That's when doctors entered the picture. For a sum that varied with the size of the friendly society (so much per member per year) a doctor would agree to examine and certify each case of illness. The main reason for paying the doctor by "capitation" instead of some other method—fee-for-service, for example—was that it was easier for these small, worker-run funds to administer.

Then, since it was obviously in the interest of the friendly society to restore the sick member to health as rapidly as possible, so as to minimize the drain on the fund, *treatment* was added to the doctor's original job of *certifying*. And the doctor usually also contracted to furnish whatever medicine the sick member might need. So by the time of the early national health insurance laws, physicians' services—in the office and in the homes of patients—were already among the benefits that most German *Krankenkassen* and British friendly societies were providing their members.

Bismarck's program was extended little by little until by the 1920s it covered virtually everyone. By contrast, British national health insurance was never extended beyond its original target, the industrial workers, not even to their dependents. Universal coverage for Britons came only after World War II when a new Labor government in 1948 replaced Lloyd George's national health insurance with a *national health service*.

Glossary: *National Health Service*—A national program of health care in which the government controls *both* financing *and* delivery of services for all or a large majority of the population. In a health service the government employs the physicians as well as the other health personnel, and operates the clinics and hospitals. This arrangement is often modified, as in the United Kingdom, where the medical specialists are government employees but the general practitioners are not. (Although almost all of them are exclusive contractors with the British National Health Service, GPs in the United Kingdom are actually in private practice.) The Scandinavian countries and Finland have both a national health service and a national health insurance program. In these countries local government operates the hospitals and health centers and employs most of the physicians (those not in private practice), but the national government also operates a health insurance scheme, which helps pay for the care delivered by the government-operated centers and hospitals as well as that delivered by the private practitioners.

Social Insurance: The AALL Episode (1912–1920)

The year after Lloyd George's British program was enacted, a group of American social welfare activists began planning a similar sickness insurance program for industrial workers in this country. The American Association for Labor Legislation (AALL) had already led a successful effort to enact workmen's compensation laws. When it turned its attention to health insurance, the group followed the same strategy it had used with workmen's compensation: first, draft a model law, and then try to get it enacted by as many state legislatures as possible.

In 1916, the AALL gained an important ally when the American Medical Association lent its support to the campaign, even appointing one of its staff to work full-time in the AALL's New York headquarters.

Ultimately, this first American campaign for social health insurance went nowhere. It fell victim to World War I. The war marked a watershed in American political opinion: The Progressive Era had passed; states were less interested in progressive legislation; and social insurance, which had after all been a German invention, fell out of favor. Yet, the AALL health insurance plan may have been doomed anyway, since both big business and most of organized labor opposed it. Like Lloyd George's British program, the American proposal would have required employers to insure industrial workers for sick leave and the costs of physicians' services. And it would also have paid a small burial benefit, a feature that especially raised the ire of the life insurance companies.

Although the leadership of the AMA had generally favored health insurance, the Association's grass roots membership, which was ambivalent at best, turned adamantly against it after the war. Speaking to a county medical society meeting in 1919, one New York physician called the AALL plan "Un-American, Unsafe, Uneconomic, Unscientific, Unfair and Unscrupulous . . . ," the invention of "Paid Professional Philanthropists, busybody Social Workers, Misguided Clergymen, and Hysterical women."[1] In 1920 the AMA House of Delegates made a dramatic and permanent about face, repudiating those of its leaders who had supported the AALL's health insurance proposal and declaring its opposition to "any plan embodying the system of compulsory contributory insurance against illness, or any other plan . . . provided, controlled, or regulated by any state or the Federal Government."[2]

The AMA's leaders made an important discovery in 1920. They discovered the Association's membership base—what it stood for and, especially, what it stood against. To use a metaphor from immunology, the AALL episode had an antigenic effect on the AMA. Afterwards, every time a government-sponsored or even a local, consumer-sponsored health plan was suggested, organized medicine's antibody titer rose sharply.

Health insurance as a public issue went into hibernation in the United States during the 1920s. It would not be raised again seriously until the 1940s. This isn't to say that nothing of significance happened in American medical care during this time. Actually, quite a lot happened. In 1921 Congress enacted the first *federal grant program* to assist the delivery of public health services, the Sheppard-Towner Act.

Glossary: *Federal Grant Programs*—Mechanisms by which the federal government provides funds for special purposes, including health purposes. For example, federal grants to the states support local public health services. Some of these are financed through "formula grants" (matching grants given to each state by a formula that considers the size of the population, the relative income level of the state's citizens, and other indicators of need) and some are "project" grants (given in response to competitive proposals that may be submitted by a state or local government, a university, or some other non-profit community organization). Today, the federal government finances medical research, residency training in primary care, community health centers in underserved rural and urban communities and a wide variety of other services and resources through project grant programs.]

Sheppard-Towner gave matching money to the states for health instruction and preventive care for mothers and children from poor families, and it helped purchase milk for babies. Passage of Sheppard-Towner was a result of the nineteenth (suffrage) amendment (1920). Congressmen feared the women's vote. The AMA, with its antibody titer still running high in the wake of the AALL episode, opposed the Sheppard-Towner Act when it was introduced and throughout the 1920s. Finally, in 1929, the AMA's lobbying paid off. When the authorization had to be extended, Congress and President Hoover allowed Sheppard-Towner to expire.

No Insurance: Paying Hospitals and Doctors (the 1920s)

Before the twentieth century people usually didn't go to hospitals if they could be cared for at home. And when they were hospitalized they usually weren't charged anything, since the hospitals were seen by the public—and saw themselves—as charities. Gradually that changed. Hospitals became more essential to medical practice, more complex, and more expensive to operate, until by the early 1920s most of them were charging any patient who could pay. This change brought a new social problem for which there appeared to be no easy solution: A family's financial resources were now endangered not only by the unpredictable indirect costs of *sickness,* but also by the unpredictable expenses of *medical care.*

The medical care cost issue had two parts: one was the hospital charge; the other was the doctor's charge. Too many doctors' fees seemed excessively high, and with no apparent justification. The problem related to the way doctors set their fees. Medical writers on this topic agreed that each doctor should be left to determine the proper fee for his service and that it ought to be based on three considerations:

1. *The relative skill and standing of the physi-*

cian. Established physicians, like established lawyers, could justifiably charge more than novices and those with less standing in the community. Also, those who called themselves specialists could charge more.[3]

2. *The nature of the service.* Not only did surgery obviously require a certain technical proficiency, it could also demonstrate a rather immediate and dramatic result. Moreover, it carried some risk. Accordingly operations should command high fees.

3. *The ability of the patient to pay.* The physician's ability to judge the economic standing of his patient was still in the 1920s considered part of the art of medical practice. The 1922 "Crowning Edition" of the leading textbook on practice economics, Cathell's *Book on the Physician Himself,* advised physicians that "while the grocer may charge every customer the same for a pound of sugar, the physician cannot do this and must have a sliding scale of charges according to the class of society to which the patient belongs . . ." A problem that writers in the popular press complained about throughout the '20s was that physicians often erred in judging the class of society to which the patient belonged, and that their "sliding scale of charges" seemed always to be sliding up.

Fee-for-service is one of three traditional ways in which physicians are remunerated. The other two are *capitation* and *salary.* All three are as old as the profession itself, and each has variations and combinations. For example, one very *old* variation of fee-for-service is *case-payment* (the physician receives a fixed sum for giving a patient all necessary care for a particular illness or condition, e.g., pregnancy). A relatively *new* variation on the salary method is "formula share of income," which is mostly restricted to physicians in private group practices.

It is important when thinking about remuneration to separate how the *patient* pays (and thus how the *practice* is financed) from how the *individual physician* is paid. Note in this respect the two-part definitions below for "capitation" and "fee-for-service."

Glossary: *Capitation*—(1) A method of financing medical practice. The practice receives—from an insurance company, health maintenance organization, employer, membership association, university, or government—a fixed amount for each person (a "per capita" amount) who is enrolled, subscribed, registered, or otherwise entitled to receive medical care from the practice. This fixed amount is paid regardless of whether or not the person ever actually uses the service or of how much service she uses. The amount of the capitation payment is negotiated in advance between the practice and some health care financing agency. In the United States, a medical practice that is financed *entirely* by capitation will virtually always be a multispecialty group practice (see the section on HMOs). (2) A method of remunerating physicians. This method, nearly as old as fee-for-service and salary, does not exist in its pure form in the United States. (Note that medical groups receiving capitation payments do not compensate their individual physician members by this method. Also, those primary care physicians who are paid by managed care organizations on a capitation basis see most of their other patients on a fee-for-service basis.) A good example of capitation as a means of remunerating individual physicians is the British National Health Service, where those general practitioners who do not practice in groups receive a fixed amount for each person on their "list." (Specialists in the British National Health Service are salaried, while most larger groups of GPs now receive a budget payment from the NHS sufficient to operate the practice and purchase specialty care for the patients on the group's list.) General practitioners in several other European countries also receive much of their remuneration in the form of capitation payments. In the United States primary care physicians in some IPA-type HMOs may agree to be individually responsible not just for providing primary medical care themselves but also for purchasing or selecting whatever additional care (specialists' services, diagnostic laboratory services, hospitalization) the enrollee might require. In this case the HMO pays the participating primary care physician a capitation payment for each patient who is an HMO member and who selects that physician as "personal" doctor (see the discussion of "*gatekeeper*" *IPA HMOs*).

Salary—A common method of paying physicians (and the most common method of paying other workers). The level of the physician's salary may be fixed relative to training, specialty, seniority, merit, time spent in the practice, or any number of other considerations, but it is *not directly* related to the amount of money the physician generates or the number of patients served. Note again: the *physician* may be paid via fixed salary regardless of whether the *practice* is financed by fee-for-service, capitation, contract, budget appropriation, or any other method.

Fee-for-Service—(1) A method of financing medical practice. Services (visits, procedures, lab tests, etc.) are sold to patients, who pay (or have paid on their behalf) a fee for each individual "service" supplied or provided. (2) A method of remunerating physicians. The physician is paid with (or in proportion to) the fees he or she generates. NOTE: Physicians who work in "fee-for-service" practices may or may not be remunerated themselves on a fee-for-service basis, but may instead receive a fixed salary, formula share of income, or even (rarely) a per capita amount as the basis of their compensation. In other words, fee-for-service *financing* is distinct from fee-for-service *remuneration*.

Each of these three methods for paying physicians has its protagonists and critics.

Capitation is most popular among those who must pay the bills. When the amount of money that will change hands is fixed and known in advance, fiscal planning and the control of expenditures are easier. Also, when the physician's

responsibility for providing the patient's care is absolute, and not discretionary, he or she is much more likely to act according to the patient's need for care, instead of according to the physician's ability to collect the fee or the patient's ability to pay it. In fact, one of the more important advantages claimed for capitation is that the physician need never worry about the patient's ability to pay for whatever care is needed, since it is in effect already paid for. "Whatever care is needed" includes, of course, sending the patient to other physicians for referrals and consultations, something fee-for-service physicians have at times been reluctant to do for fear of losing patients to competitors.

The critics of capitation say that the physician who is remunerated in this way has an incentive to do as little as possible for the patient since the amount of payment will be the same no matter what. Capitation's defenders reply that such scrimping, if done very often, would offend the patient, who would then change his "enrollment" to another practice (or another "plan") and perhaps persuade others to do likewise, thus causing, ultimately, a far greater loss of income to the offending physician.

Salary, it is claimed by its detractors, best suits the physician who is lazy, since there is no financial incentive toward either individual productivity or quality. Its defenders reply to the contrary that the salaried physician's disincentives to skimp or cut corners are in fact great, since under salary it is not one's volume of fees (as with fee-for-service) or the size of one's practice (as with capitation) that may be jeopardized by poor performance, but one's very employment. Further, they point out that some of the most reputable and prestigious practice organizations— private, academic, and governmental—remunerate their physicians by salary.

Fee-for-service can deliver, at least potentially, the largest income to the physician, and this may partially explain its popularity among the medical profession. (It may also yield, potentially, the lowest income.) Moreover, its defenders say, the fee-for-service method of payment rewards the physician who works hardest. As with any other piecework method, those who work the most (ergo, who presumably are the most deserving) are remunerated with the most. There is evidence that office-based doctors work longer hours and see more patients when they are paid on a fee-for-service basis than when they are on salary.

There has also been much criticism of fee-for-service. Virtually all of it is directed in one way or another to the basic incentive that is at work whenever physicians sell their services in exchange for fees. George Bernard Shaw said it this way: "That any sane nation, having observed that you could provide for the supply of bread by giving bakers a pecuniary interest in baking for you, should go on to give a surgeon a pecuniary interest in cutting off your leg, is enough to make one despair of political humanity. But that is precisely what we have done. And the more appalling the mutilation, the more the mutilator is paid. He who corrects the ingrowing toe-nail receives a few shillings; he who cuts your inside out receives hundreds of guineas."[4]

Shaw's surgical examples, especially his fascination with surgical "mutilation," may seem old-fashioned to us now, but the principle he cites applies still. Fee-for-service is indeed an inducement for the physician to favor the more highly remunerative procedures over the lower paying services (such as listening and explaining). There is very good evidence that the incentive for the physician to do a "greater" service when a higher fee is linked to it works very well.

Private doctors in the United States have generally believed that fee-for-service is the most advantageous for them, amenable to their control, and the most difficult for government or private purchasers of care to manipulate. However, health care planners and financing sources (including employers, unions, managed care firms, and government) dislike the open-endedness of fee-for-service and the difficulty it presents for controlling expenditures. Yet, because the two payment methods that are fixed (capitation and salary) allow such "third parties" greater potential control over the amount of physicians' future remuneration, private doctors are wary of these methods. They believe, no doubt correctly, that in the event of a fiscal crisis such control would be used. On the other hand, some observers believe that the greatest threat to the fiscal stability of the "third parties" is the lack of control over expenditures that has long been associated with fee-for-service. Indeed, in recent years private payers, pushed by escalating costs, have found new ways of controlling expenditures under fee-for-service, as well (see *managed care*).

Private Insurance: The CCMC Report (1932)

Heightened concern over the inability of many people to pay hospital and physician charges led a small group of social scientists and physicians in 1927 to form the Committee on the Costs of Medical Care. Funded by private foundations, the CCMC represented the first major effort in health services research. The staff was guided by a blue-ribbon panel of 50 members who constituted a veritable who's who of American health care policy. The Committee published over 30 separate studies of the main problems of American medical care and of some of the more interesting experiments that were going on at the time.

The final report, which came out in November of 1932, emphasized two main findings: The first was that Americans, especially middle-class Americans, needed health insurance of some kind. The report didn't specify what form it should ultimately take—whether it should be public or private, voluntary or compulsory—

although the majority of the Committee preferred to begin with a voluntary approach. The second finding was that medical practice needed to be organized more rationally. The report called for "community medical centers," which would be quasi-group practice organizations based at or from community hospitals. Since these medical groups were to be linked to insurance, the Committee seemed to have in mind what would later be called direct service plans or, in today's terminology, HMOs, although the report didn't describe in any detail how the "community medical centers" were to be organized.

There was also a minority report, drafted and promoted by some of the AMA officers and staff who were on the Committee. It took issue with the findings of the majority and found neither insurance nor group practice desirable. An editorial in the following week's issue of the *Journal of the American Medical Association* used harsher language, calling the proposed hospital-based group practices "medical soviets."

The Committee on the Costs of Medical Care had attempted to draw the public's attention to a new innovation in medical care financing—private insurance for hospital care and medical services. In 1932, the first examples were barely visible.

Private Insurance: Indemnity Insurance and Blue Cross (the 1930s)

Historically, there have been *three main types* of private health insurance in the United States: (1) *indemnity insurance,* (2) *service benefit plans,* and (3) *direct service plans.* All of our present-day health care financing mechanisms are derived from these three.

Only one of these three types—indemnity insurance—is true insurance by the traditional meaning of that term.

Glossary: *Indemnity Insurance*—The insurance principle holds that in exchange for regular payment of the premium, the insurance company will compensate the insured the amount of a loss ("indemnification"). This is easy to understand if the loss was caused by theft or fire or death, since these "indemnities" are easy to recognize, and the amount of each of them is known (it was stated in the policy in advance). In the case of health insurance, however, the exact nature and therefore the amount of the "indemnity" isn't so clear. Who is to say what is an illness? And who is to say how much or what kind of medical attention is necessary? In fact, for a long time most commercial insurance companies refused to write policies against the cost of medical care because it was so unpredictable. When they finally did begin selling health insurance on a larger scale in the late 1930s, the commercial insurers placed strict limits on the amounts they would pay, and they demanded to see the bill (the amount the patient was charged by the doctor or the hospital) as proof that the policy holder did indeed have an "indemnity" before they would pay (in the amount of the bill up to the limit stated in the policy). Since indemnity insurance is strictly a matter between the insurance company and the policy holder, the doctor and the hospital are able to charge the patient whatever they wish. The patient pays the bill; then the patient submits the claim; then the patient receives the check back from the insurance company; meanwhile the doctor does nothing. This series of events explains why indemnity insurance has long been favored by the medical profession: in its pure form it doesn't involve doctors at all. Nor does it place any restrictions on patients, such as telling them which doctors they may or may not use.

The private health insurance industry began during the Depression, when people had little money to pay hospitals, leaving the private hospitals with unpaid bills and empty beds (public hospitals were operating at full capacity). In 1929 a private hospital in Dallas, Texas, came up with what it hoped would be a solution to its financial jeopardy. The Baylor University Hospital approached the Dallas public school teachers with a proposal. If the teachers would agree to have a small amount (50 cents) deducted from their monthly paychecks, to be paid over to the Baylor Hospital, the Hospital in return would provide up to twenty-one days of hospitalization each year for any teacher who needed it. The teachers consented to this novel plan, which worked so well that other hospitals in Dallas, and soon elsewhere around the country, began imitating it.

In 1932, the three major hospitals in the Sacramento, California, area agreed on a joint hospitalization plan which they then offered to local employee groups. Not only did this community-wide plan make its sponsoring hospitals happy by paying some of their patients' bills, it also avoided the inter-hospital competition that was inevitable whenever a single hospital plan, like the one in Dallas, offered itself to employee groups. The Sacramento plan gave the patients a choice of any of the local hospitals (and, thus, their choice of doctors as well). Community-wide "hospital service plans" soon spread throughout the country. Later they consolidated into state-wide or metropolitan area-wide plans. In 1934 one of them adopted a logo with a blue cross on it, and soon that's what they called themselves.

The new "Blue Cross" hospital service plans offered something they called *service benefits*.

Glossary: *Service Benefit Plans*—Unlike indemnity insurance, service benefit plans pay doctors and hospitals directly. The Blue Cross plans did not originally consider themselves "insurance companies" in the usual sense. Although most of them do now provide traditional insurance products, their hospital "service benefit" tradition is strong. Listen to the television commercials for Blue Cross or look at its ads in the paper. You will never hear or read the word "insurance." This is because the Blue Cross plans were not set up to compensate the insured for a loss; instead, their purpose was to pay "service benefits." Patients didn't submit claims to Blue Cross, hospitals did. This difference was a very important one to Blue Cross. But it was an equally important issue for the organized medical profession, since the doctors feared the control that being paid directly by an "insurance" plan would bring or implied might come.

The commercial insurance companies had watched the beginnings of Blue Cross with skepticism. They had been reluctant to offer health insurance themselves, because they saw so many problems with it—the high expenses of paying commissions to a force of sales agents, the expense of collecting the premium each month, the issue of how to control abuse (the question, again, of exactly what is the "indemnity" in health care) and, especially, the fear that those who purchased health insurance would do so because they were already sick or likely to become sick (the insurance companies called this problem "adverse selection"). Yet, contrary to the insurance industry's expectation that Blue Cross would fail, it grew rapidly—so rapidly that by the late-1930s, the commercial carriers also began offering hospitalization coverage to employee groups. (Blue Cross had by then demonstrated that group coverage could largely eliminate the "adverse selection" problem.) Unlike the Blue Cross policies, which paid service benefits, the hospitalization coverage of the commercial carriers was in the form of traditional indemnity insurance.

During this time the American Medical Association was watching the new Blue Cross plans warily. It warned them to stick to covering hospital expenses and not try branching out to include medical services. The AMA objected to doctors' being paid by a plan—any plan. It would be alright, the AMA said, if cash benefits were paid "directly to the individual plan member . . .

[since that] will not disturb the relations of patients [and] physicians . . . ," but the doctors should not be involved. In other words, indemnity plans, but not service benefit plans, could cover medical services. Soon the commercial insurance companies began covering surgeons' fees in their group policies.

Later, the AMA changed its position and said that service benefits might be acceptable, but only if medical societies controlled the plans. So medical society-sponsored plans, which covered surgical and medical services during hospitalization, were established during the 1940s. They called themselves "Blue Shield." Blue Cross helped many of them get started and even provided their administrative staffs. There was a good reason why Blue Cross was so willing to lend assistance. By offering Blue Cross and Blue Shield benefits in a single package, Blue Cross could maintain the competitive edge that its older "service benefit" plans enjoyed over the younger, but rapidly growing commercial "indemnity" plans.

Social Insurance: The Social Security Act (1935)

The 1932 CCMC report had again raised the AMA's antibody titer against health insurance—this time to such a high level that when President Roosevelt appointed a cabinet committee in 1934 to study social insurance (it was chaired by the Secretary of Labor, Francis Perkins) the AMA was already prepared for battle.

The Perkins committee's charge was to study unemployment insurance, old-age pensions, and health insurance. Although its subcommittee on health insurance recommended that a compulsory, state by state program be incorporated into the social security bill, President Roosevelt excluded it from the final version. When he considered the strength of the doctors' opposition, the President guessed that the health insurance pro-

vision would be an albatross that could sink the entire bill.

But while the Social Security Act of 1935 didn't include health insurance, it did other things in health care, like reviving (and expanding) the maternal and child care provisions of the old Sheppard-Towner Act. It also gave federal grants to the states that put public health departments on a sound basis; and it established the crippled children's program.

The main feature of the Act was, of course, its old age pension provision. And in this respect the United States broke with the pattern that the European countries had generally followed.

In most countries the order of social security enactment had been, first, *protection against industrial accidents* (workmen's compensation). Here America followed suit. Second came *protection against the costs of illness* (sickness insurance in the form of cash payments for time lost from work), followed by *protection against the costs of medical and hospital bills* (health insurance). Only after these social insurance programs were in place did most of the European nations enact *protection against the inability to earn a living in old age* (old age pensions) and *protection against loss of income due to losing one's job* (unemployment insurance).

In the United States health insurance had been next after workmen's compensation on the social reformers' agenda. Even though the AALL campaign had failed, health insurance was still going to be the next item, as the work of the CCMC made clear.

But then came the Depression, which not only put millions of people out of work, it also stirred up a political movement for old-age pensions. The consequence was that in America unemployment insurance came second—the states began enacting it in 1932—and following close behind came the old-age pensions in the Social Security Act of 1935.

Health insurance was never part of President Roosevelt's legislative program. In fact, he backed away from it again, in 1938, when his National Health Conference recommended the same proposal the health insurance subcommittee of the Perkins Committee had advanced back in 1934. FDR was apparently hoping to push health insurance in the wake of the 1938 conference; but World War II began the next year, and social insurance for health care once more dropped off the American agenda.

Social Insurance: The Truman Program (1945–1950)

It reappeared after the war when President Truman gave his support to the second Wagner-Murray-Dingell bill. When someone asked how he'd pay for it, Truman replied that he thought the American people could afford to spend more than the 4 percent of *gross domestic product* (GDP) that the nation was then spending on health care. In 1945 escalation of health care costs was not a problem.

Glossary: Gross Domestic Product (GDP)—The value of all goods and services produced in the nation. The rate at which the GDP moves is a measure of the nation's economic health: during recessions it lags; in good times it grows. But since it can never grow larger than 100 percent, knowing the percentage of GDP that is occupied by any particular sector of the economy tells how much is left for everything else people need or want—individually or collectively. For example, if we had to spend 30 percent of our total national wealth on food, we would have only 70 percent left for national defense, college tuition, shoes, interest on the national debt, housing, repairing roads and bridges, church offerings, movie tickets, medical care, and everything else we must have or would like to have.

When President Truman made national health insurance an issue in the 1948 presidential campaign, the AMA was concerned, but not overly so—its antibody titer rose only slightly. The doctors believed, along with nearly everyone else, that the President would be defeated in the fall election, and that would be the end of that. But Truman was elected, and so was, again, a Democratic Congress.

When the election results were known, organized medicine panicked and launched a massive national publicity campaign that capitalized on the anti-Communist hysteria then permeating the air. The AMA called the Truman plan *socialized medicine,* unashamedly equated it with Communism, and raised the specter of enslaved doctors operating on unwilling patients. That kind of propaganda was highly effective in 1949.

Glossary: Socialized Medicine—A term without specific meaning. It is used mostly by those who are unable or do not wish to be more precise. Physicians have often used it pejoratively when referring to some greater degree of organization of and/or control over medical practice than already exists. "Socialized medicine" has, therefore, been applied at various times to Blue Cross, salaried employment of physicians by hospitals, well baby clinics in public health departments, medical faculty practice plans, Medicare, the medical care system of the former Soviet Union, the British National Health Service, neighborhood health centers for the poor, publicly administered mass immunization for polio, Veterans Administration hospitals, public campaigns against venereal disease, government payment for medical services under the "Crippled Children" program, HMOs, PPOs, and student health infirmaries at universities. Politicians and public relations consultants have also used the term whenever the connotation of socialism served their purpose.

Yet, even without the AMA's opposition, the Truman plan had little chance politically. The forces aligned against it were too powerful: Big business and the Republican Party both opposed national health insurance and so did most of the Southern Congressional Democrats, who not only chaired the key committees but with the Republicans made up a conservative majority in both houses.

But the main reason the Truman health insurance plan failed wasn't the strength of the opposition but rather the rapid growth of private insurance. In 1940, only about seven percent of Americans had any health insurance coverage of any kind. By 1975, only 35 years later, nearly everyone was covered. The most rapid period of growth, however, came during the Truman years, between the end of the war and 1950. So it is understandable that in 1949 the most effective argument against the Truman plan was that social health insurance wasn't needed, because soon everyone would be covered by voluntary, private health insurance.

Private Insurance: Fragmentation of the Risk Pool (1942–1957)

The prodigious growth in private health insurance coverage had been effectively stimulated by two important decisions. The first came in 1942. At the beginning of the war a huge army of workers, many from rural areas, migrated to take jobs in the defense industry. Even so, industry faced a labor shortage. In order to compete for workers employers had to offer something, but because of the controls that the government had enacted to combat wartime inflation, they couldn't raise wages. The War Labor Board ruled, however, that while wage increases would be inflationary, a reasonable expansion of fringe benefits—including health benefits—would not be.

The second decision came soon after the war ended. Ever since passage of the Wagner Act in 1935,[5] unions and employers had argued over the meaning of a phrase in the Act. Did the rights of unions to bargain collectively "for wages and conditions of employment" include the right to bargain for employee benefits? The unions said

"yes"; the employers said "no." Finally, in 1947, the Supreme Court handed down its decision: employee health benefits were "conditions of work" and could indeed be bargained for under the Wagner Act.

Over the next six years the number of workers and dependents covered by the health plans that had been negotiated by workers and management more than quadrupled, which meant also that many non-union employers would eventually have to match what the unions had won for their members through collective bargaining.

The result of these two decisions, one during the war and one after, was that instead of a system of universal entitlement to health care like those that other high-income, industrialized nations already had or were well on the way to enacting, the United States would stay with an employment-based system of private health insurance.

The commercial insurance companies were successful in capturing a large share of this new employment-based health insurance market. Much of the reason for their success had to do with the important concepts of *community rating* and *experience rating.*

Glossary: *Community Rating*—A method used by insurance companies to set the amount of premium. In community rating, the entire population of an area is charged one rate, regardless of their risk as individuals of becoming ill. Therefore, people who are more likely to become sick are actually being subsidized by people who are more likely to remain healthy. Yet the sickness-prone people don't pay any more than the others, even though the first group will use doctors and hospitals the most.

Experience Rating—A method used by insurance companies to set the amount of premium. In experience rating, each group (usually the employees of a company) in the population is charged a different rate, reflecting how much the members are likely to use doctors and hospitals.

In this way, insurance companies charge lower rates to healthy people and higher rates to those who are sick or who have been sick in the past, and to high risk groups such as the poor and the elderly. Since the actuaries can predict that these groups are likely to use more medical care, they must pay a higher insurance premium.

The essential difference between community rating and experience rating is in how the risk is pooled. If either rating method were to be applied to the entire population, the effects would be dramatic.

One way to understand this is to consider how things would be under what we might call the socialist ideal, or Christian ideal (depending on your view—both groups claim original authorship of the idea but neither has yet demonstrated its full implementation). Those most able to give would be required to *give* the most, and those with the greatest need would be permitted to *take* the most. Thus, the poor and sick would give little but take a lot, while the most wealthy and healthy would give much but take little.

By contrast, one's *ability* to give is not a consideration under either community rating or experience rating. Community rating demands that everyone pay the same; but those who are least healthy may take more, while the most healthy would naturally take less. Under experience rating, the most healthy people would again take the least, but they could also get by with paying the least; on the other hand, the least healthy would take the most but in return would also have to pay the most.

Social health insurance programs like Germany's and Great Britain's had always charged coal miners, carpenters, and railway ticket clerks the same premium for health insurance. So had the Blue Cross plans, which began as community-wide hospital service associations charging everyone the same "community rate." But the commercial insurance companies *were* willing to isolate workers, and everyone else, by

risk. For them, experience rating for health insurance was no different than what they had always done in their life insurance business, charging more for older people near the end of life, or in their casualty insurance business, quoting a lower fire insurance premium for the house next door to the fire station.

Active workers are on average young and healthy, and therefore likely to use less medical care (unless they are in high-risk occupations like coal-mining). So if the insurance actuary can isolate the experience of the typical large groups of workers from that of the rest of the community, the insurance company should be able to quote them a lower premium. Using their extensive experience of insuring people having various characteristics, the commercial companies were able to predict how much each new group of workers would use medical care. With this knowledge they could set the premium as low as possible and still make a predictable profit from each group.

When they discovered that their group health risk was below that of the community as a whole, employers and unions alike wanted rates that reflected this more favorable experience. Soon, the commercial companies began to overtake the Blues in writing group health insurance. And soon, the Blues realized that they, too, would have to use experience rating if they expected to compete for the large employment-based group insurance market.

Social Insurance: The Road to Medicare (1958–1965)

Here is a principle: the more fragmented the risk pool becomes the more difficult it is for those left in the common pool to find affordable health insurance. Throughout the 1950s, as unions and employers purchased health plans that used experience rating, they left behind a community risk pool that included a greater proportion of the poor and marginally employed, the sick and disabled, and, especially, the elderly. When the most attractive members of society from a risk standpoint are covered under an experience rating system, the average risk of illness among the "community" left behind rises. Since the experience of the healthiest group is no longer being factored into the community rate, the premium for those who remain in the community pool—the residue—also rises until, finally, they find themselves priced out of the private health insurance market. That's what happened to the elderly during the 1950s.

In 1958 a Rhode Island Congressman named Aime Forand introduced a bill to correct this problem. His bill would have insured the elderly for hospitalization under Social Security. President Eisenhower opposed it. However, presidential candidate Kennedy supported the idea. In fact, social health insurance for the elderly became a minor issue in the 1960 presidential campaign between Kennedy and Nixon. Kennedy favored the King-Anderson Bill (successor to the Forand Bill), while Nixon supported another plan (Kerr-Mills) by which the federal government would help the states to provide additional public assistance (welfare) to the elderly poor to help them pay hospital bills.

After Kennedy became President he tried to get King-Anderson passed, but there wasn't enough Congressional support. The AMA vigorously opposed it, and at that time the AMA, with about 175,000 doctor members, had the second largest political lobbying organization in Washington, second only to the AFL-CIO, which in the early 1960s represented nearly sixteen *million* labor union members.

After the 1964 election the necessary Congressional support was there, and President Johnson signed the Medicare bill into law the following year—1965. The new law also included a federally subsidized, but state operated public assistance program for the poor, called Medicaid.

It was not President Johnson, however, but a popular grass-roots campaign by the nation's elderly that really forced the issue. The AMA, of course, lobbied, advertised, and even sent doctors' wives anti-Medicare phonograph records and tapes to play for their neighbors. (They called their program "Operation Coffee Cup.") But this time, organized medicine's antibody titer against social insurance wasn't high enough to defeat it. Before long, the doctors liked Medicare well enough. It sent their incomes soaring.

After Medicare it appeared that the United States had put in place a satisfactory system of medical care financing, consisting of voluntary private health insurance for employed people, welfare medical care for the poor and marginally employed, and social health insurance for the elderly and disabled.

Social Insurance: Cost Crisis (1966–1980)

But soon a new problem arose, one that has preoccupied both government and private employers ever since. The problem of inflation of medical care costs had been building ever since the implementation of Medicare (which went into effect on July 1, 1966). By 1969 the apparent uncontrollability of the costs of Medicare and Medicaid had become the number one health care policy issue for the federal government.

That was when President Nixon declared that American health care was in a "state of massive crisis." Opinion polls showed that 75% of Americans agreed with him. Not only did costs appear to be out of control, but lack of access for the poor and maldistribution of physicians—by specialty and by location—were also seen as serious problems in need of solution. At the time, the nation's total health care expenditures amounted to $60 billion, or 7.3 percent of GDP.

The main political response to the crisis was a proposal for universal, compulsory health insurance, the first such proposal in more than 20 years. Congressional Democrats, led by Senator Edward Kennedy, called for a *single payer* national health insurance plan in which costs would be more strictly controlled than they had been with Medicare. The Republican President countered by calling for an *employer mandate* for private insurance. Although their methods differed, both sides agreed on the same goal. At least they did for the moment. But the moment passed.

Glossary: Single Payer versus Multiple Payer— The two alternative organizational frameworks for social health insurance. Either government (or its appointed agent) collects the premiums and pays the benefits (single payer), or government permits multiple plans (public and/ or private) to participate. There are numerous precedents in this country and elsewhere for both alternatives. Medicare, for example, is a single payer plan. The federal government collects the premium through the Internal Revenue Service, places it in a Medicare trust fund, and pays the benefits via its agents, called "intermediaries," which are typically state-wide Blue Cross plans. Since the 1930s, most of the American proposals for national health insurance have called for single payer plans. Several other countries have successful single payer plans—for example, Canada, Sweden, Denmark, Norway, Finland, and New Zealand. And just as many have successful multi-payer plans—for example, The Netherlands, Germany, France, Japan, Australia, and Switzerland. The main disadvantage of multi-payer is its greater bureaucratic complexity and higher administrative costs. Single payer is simpler and cheaper. However, it also raises the almost uniquely American question of how to limit government's role in society (this has rarely been so cherished a goal for other nations). The majority of national health insurance plans proposed for the United States during the early 1990s envisioned the participation of many *private* plans. This reflected the situation already in place, and it partially avoided the issue of a major new tax.

Employer and Individual Mandates—A legal requirement that employers help pay for their workers' coverage, or that individuals pay for their own coverage. National health insurance (universal coverage) requires either a major new tax, a major increase in an existing tax, or a mandate. The mandate may be imposed on employers, individuals, or both.

Between 1910 and 1920 most states enacted employer mandates to provide workmen's compensation insurance. States also impose individual mandates on automobile owners to purchase automobile liability insurance. Note from these examples that the fact of a mandate doesn't necessarily mean that the payments must go toward a government-operated program like Medicare or Social Security. The mandate may instead, as in worker's compensation and automobile liability insurance, permit the employer or automobile owner to purchase the required insurance from any carrier that sells it.

President Nixon's interest in health insurance flagged after his reelection in 1972. Although his plan might have passed Congress had he pursued it more vigorously, he didn't; soon he was totally preoccupied with his own survival—Watergate was one problem, OPEC was the other. The price of oil went through the ceiling—which led to general price inflation in the country, which increased the deficit, which scared fiscal conservatives away from the health care issue, which convinced President Ford to delay any action.

President Carter ultimately took the same position as President Ford. Carter said that he wanted to postpone action until health care costs came under control, something that presumably would happen during his second term. But he never had a second term. Nor did health care costs ever come under control.

Private Insurance: Terms and Conditions (1950s–1990s)

Meanwhile the private insurance industry continued its steady growth.[6] During the 1970s and '80s, however, health insurance products also became more complex, branching out well beyond the traditional indemnity insurance and service benefit plans. Moreover, the differences between the Blues and the commercial companies narrowed; their distinguishing characteristics faded. Not only did the Blues talk of turning themselves into investor-owned, profit-making corporations, they sold coverage that looked just like indemnity insurance. And because large employers demanded more aggressive cost control from their insurance carriers, some of the commercial companies began selling a product that resembled service benefit coverage. More unlikely still, during the 1970s both the Blues and the commercial insurance companies initiated their own direct service plans (HMOs). By the late 1980s, they were offering an identical range of what were by then being called "managed care" products. Some of this change represented an adjustment by private insurance to the demands of its best customers—the large employers. But virtually all of it was driven by the imperative to contain costs.

Over the last 50 years, the health insurance industry has devised a set of methods for limiting its risks and maximizing its profits. Below are some common health insurance terms. They are important for understanding how traditional private health insurance works.

Glossary: Group versus Individual Policies—
Group policies are generally offered through an employer as a benefit of employment. Everyone who works for the employer is eligible to participate and all employees are treated the same regardless of their age or medical history (subject to the terms of the policy, which may contain "exclusions"). Individual policies, unlike group policies, are usually purchased through an outside salesman ("insurance agent"). They typically require a qualifying physical exam in advance of coverage and usually exclude "pre-existing conditions." Moreover, they are *always* more expensive (for the same amount of coverage) than group

policies, for three main reasons: (1) In a group plan enough healthy employees will be enrolled to dilute the effect of the few who might constitute "adverse risks" (for example, a worker with a daughter who is a juvenile diabetic, or an obese husband who smokes and has high blood pressure). (2) The collection of premiums is done automatically by the employer in a group plan and therefore inexpensively (there is no need for the insurance company to mail out monthly or quarterly statements as there would be for an individual policy). (3) Most group policies are not sold through independent agents, which means there are no commissions to pay. For these reasons, individual policies often are *so* much more expensive than group policies as to be virtually prohibitive for many people. However, for the self-employed, and those who work for employers who offer little in the way of fringe benefits (a description of much of rural America and, increasingly, much of young America), an individual policy may be the only choice available.

*Co-insurance—*A provision in many health insurance policies whereby the insured person pays part of the medical or hospital bill, usually a fixed percentage. For example, the insured person may be required to pay co-insurance in the amount of 20% of all charges up to a limit of $10,000 per year. The insurance company pays the rest. The purpose of co-insurance is to make the insured individual think twice before using the policy.

*Deductibles—*A provision in many health insurance policies whereby the insured person pays the *first* part of the medical or hospital bill. For example, the insured person may be required to pay a deductible of $500 (of physician, pharmacy, and hospital charges) before the insurance company will pay anything at all. Deductibles have the same purpose as co-insurance. They are supposed to deter the insured person from using the policy.

*Exclusions—*Services and conditions listed in a

clause in the insurance contract for which the policy will not pay. For example, the policy may pay for visits to physicians only for a *diagnosed illness* (meaning that preventive services are excluded). There may also be exclusions for mental and emotional illness, and for "pre-existing conditions" (diseases and health problems the patient had before the policy went into effect). If a person is temporarily laid off or goes on unpaid leave and during this time develops a new condition requiring medical care, this condition may also be ruled "pre-existing" and thus be excluded from coverage after the employment-based policy resumes. Again, the purpose of exclusions is to keep insurance costs down, since the insurance company knows that each such exclusion represents large expenses that it would otherwise have to pay.

Limited Conversion Privileges—
A barrier erected by the insurance company to prevent people enrolled in a group plan from keeping their group insurance coverage when they leave the group (quit their jobs or are laid off). The policy holder may be allowed to "convert" the group policy to an individual policy, but in doing so certain benefits of the group policy may be "limited" (removed) and, of course, the premium is sure to rise.

"Creaming," "Cherry Picking," or "Selection of Least Risks"—Still another means of protecting the insurance company. By identifying which workers must not be included in an employer's group health insurance plan—most often the part-time, seasonal, aged, and laid-off workers—the insurance company is able to "select" those most capable of being insured, primarily younger workers with a good employment record, who are also less likely to use the policy. Insurance companies also try to "redline" certain kinds of employers (those in which employees have a greater risk of injury), locations where racial minorities and low income people reside (groups more likely to be in poor health), and certain occupational

groups known for their high use of services (e.g., physicians), or a tendency to induce litigation (e.g., lawyers), or those at higher risk of contracting dread disease (male interior decorators and hairdressers). Insurers believe they have to "cream skim" to gain a competitive edge. As a Blue Cross executive told a Congressional committee: "On average, only 4 per cent of insured individuals generate 50 per cent of claims expenses, while 20 per cent of enrollees generate 80 per cent of claims. Clearly, the insurer that can avoid the 4 per cent or a significant share of the 20 per cent will have the more competitive premiums."

Private Insurance: Direct Service Plans (1929–1969)

Although service benefit plans and indemnity insurance dominated the industry from the 1940s to the 1980s, direct service plans are actually the oldest of the three kinds of private health insurance in the United States. They started well before service benefit and indemnity plans but grew much more slowly—until recently. Now, they are the fastest growing form of private health insurance.

Glossary: Direct Service Plans—In contrast with traditional indemnity insurance, which compensates the patient for a loss, and service benefit plans, which pay "costs" incurred by hospitals or agreed upon fees to physicians, direct service plans actually see to it that the needed service is delivered to the patient. They pay their benefits not in the form of money—to either patient or provider—but in the form of direct services. The reason they can do this is that they either employ, or contract with, or own all of the service resources—physicians, hospitals, laboratories, etc.—their enrolled members are likely to need. The huge cash reserves that are required of indemnity insurance companies and Blue Cross aren't necessary for direct service plans, since the benefits are not paid as cash disbursements, but rather as entitled services from hospitals and doctors whose service delivery capacity has been "reserved" for the plan's members. So in a sense, these plans aren't selling insurance at all, but "assurance." Of course, the members may not use any but the plan's own doctors and hospitals, and the medical work will naturally be monitored closely by the plan. For these two reasons, the organized medical profession has seldom held a favorable opinion of direct service plans.

The earliest direct service plans were almost all based on simple geography. Extractive industries are usually in non-urban locations. Yet, these are also intensive industries, requiring a large workforce. The companies needed a healthy workforce in order to have a productive workforce. Since there weren't enough doctors in these places, the industrial employers who located there had to find ways of attracting them. The company did this by guaranteeing the doctors a clientele consisting of the workers, who would then pay the doctors in advance through a "check-off" system (a regular amount deducted from their paychecks). Sometimes the company contracted with the doctors; sometimes it employed them. Direct service plans were operated from the late nineteenth century until well after World War II by mines, railroads, lumber companies, and by the large construction firms that built the dams and aqueducts in the far West.

Enrollment in virtually all of these early direct service plans was limited to the sponsoring company's own employees and sometimes their dependents—until 1929. In that year (the same year the Baylor University Hospital started its prepaid hospitalization plan) two new direct service plans started, both organized around group practices. One was operated by the Ross-Loos Medical Group of Los Angeles; the other was a Farmer's Union-sponsored cooperative hospital in Elk City, Oklahoma. In spite of harassment by organized medicine—the physicians in both groups

were expelled from their county medical societies, resulting in, among other things, an inability to purchase malpractice insurance—they both succeeded.

Unlike early Blue Cross, which covered only hospital services, these new group practice plans provided both hospitalization and medical services. Although a few more direct service plans opened during the 1930s, "prepaid group practice," as these plans later called themselves, grew hardly at all until just after World War II, when the Kaiser-Permanente Health Plans on the West Coast, the Group Health Cooperative of Puget Sound in Seattle, and the Health Insurance Plan of Greater New York began enrolling the general public—especially members of labor unions—in direct competition with the Blues and the commercial carriers.

One problem that the direct service plans faced wherever they opened was opposition from the local medical profession (see *"Free Choice" or "Expanded Choice"* below). Another problem was the huge capital expenditures that were required to start a new multi-specialty group practice from scratch. On the other hand, the direct service, prepaid group practice plans held a major advantage over the commercial indemnity plans and the Blues; they could deliver care of as high or higher quality at lower cost, even though, like the Blues, they used community rating. Research reports documenting this advantage began appearing in the 1950s; but it wasn't until the early 1970s, after the federal government discovered a medical care cost crisis, that their cost advantage translated into a national policy favoring direct service plans.

Private Insurance: HMOs, IPAs, PPOs (1970–1992)

The Nixon administration began promoting direct service plans as a way of curbing the rapidly escalating costs of medical care. It also gave them a new name: *Health Maintenance Organizations* or *HMOs*.

Glossary: *Health Maintenance Organization (HMO)* A direct service plan with certain general features. The vagueness of that statement should tell you that I think the best definition of this term is a description. HMOs fall into two major types with variations under each type. The two types are actually very different, and this has led to confusion. However, all HMOs share two principles in common: (1) They accept the responsibility for *delivering* a comprehensive scope of medical care to their "members" or "enrollees" (in other words, HMOs are direct service plans); and (2) The members enroll voluntarily and pay a fixed amount periodically, regardless of the amount of services they actually receive (in other words, HMOs are prepayment plans).

The rapid growth of HMOs in recent years is primarily because of their potential for cost containment, which in turn is due to a difference in the providers' (particularly the physicians') incentive. It works as follows.

Since the HMO obtains a fixed sum of money from each enrolled member, and since it accepts the responsibility to provide *all* the medical care each member will need (primary physician office visits, specialty physician office visits, laboratory, X-ray, drugs, hospitalization) within that fixed revenue constraint, the HMO providers, especially the physicians, must be concerned not only with the quality of the care they deliver but also with its total cost. This incentive differs markedly from that of traditional indemnity or service benefit insurance, especially with regard to hospitalization. If, for example, a patient in a traditional plan is well-insured for hospitalization, then neither she nor her physician need be concerned with hospital costs. This may be fortunate for the individual patient, but it is disastrous for the aggregate. When costs can be disregarded, they escalate for everyone. On the

other hand, physicians in an HMO have a strong incentive to provide the necessary care in the most efficient and economical way possible. There are at least three ways to do this: (1) by reducing the length of the hospital stay; (2) by performing more tests and procedures on an outpatient basis, thus reducing the number of hospital admissions; and (3) by stressing preventive services, especially early detection of disease. Physicians in an HMO could, of course, also decide to cut costs by cutting services. Although this and other potential dangers cannot be ignored, a large body of evidence from well-established group practice-type HMOs shows that they provide high quality medical care at lower costs than the conventional system. This evidence, in the face of the rapid rise in health costs generally, and those borne by the federal government in particular, generated the national interest in HMOs beginning in the early 1970s.

HMOs fall under two main organizational types: (1) *group practice,* and (2) *independent practice.*

Group Practice HMOs (traditionally termed "prepaid group practice") are the original prototype HMOs. For a long time they were the only type. The largest and best known example is the Kaiser Permanente Health Plan, which was established in California in the 1940s and now operates in fifteen states. A few other large group practice HMOs began in the 1940s, '50s, and '60s, and many more have formed within the last 20 years. Most major metropolitan areas in the United States now have at least one. Some, like Kaiser and the Group Health Cooperative of Puget Sound, are nonprofit; but some major commercial insurance companies and other for-profit firms have also entered the group practice HMO field.

The participating physicians in group practice HMOs are full-time members of a multi-specialty group and are remunerated as individuals either with a fixed salary or a formula share of the group's income. The group practice is paid a certain amount per capita for serving the HMO's members. There are two main varieties of group practice HMOs: (1) *staff model,* and (2) *group model.*

Glossary: *Staff Model*—A variety of group practice HMO in which the physicians in the group work directly as the employees (or exclusive contractors) of the HMO and therefore serve only its enrolled members. In other words, the HMO and the group practice are essentially one and the same organization.

Group Model—A variety of group practice HMO in which the HMO is affiliated with a multi-specialty group practice that is large enough to provide all or nearly all of the medical services required by the enrolled members. The medical group (which is ordinarily owned by its practicing physician staff) usually continues to serve other, fee-for-service clients alongside its prepaid HMO clients. The HMO and the group practice are closely affiliated and bound by contract, but they are still separate, independent organizations. The HMO pays the group a pre-negotiated, per capita amount for the care of the HMO members. If the group's costs exceed this amount, the group loses; if its costs stay under this amount, it enjoys a surplus. What the group does with the surplus or how it manages the loss is its own affair. (A variation on the group model is the "network model" where several separate multi-specialty or primary care-based group practices within the same metropolitan area affiliate with an HMO to care for its members. The enrollees in the HMO may then elect to receive their medical care from any one of these affiliated groups.)

It is important to remember that while many HMOs are of the group practice type, not every direct service plan based on group practice can meet the definition of an HMO: for example, a student health service at a large university, although usually organized as a group practice

and financed by capitation-based pre-payment (through student fees), does not serve people who enrolled *voluntarily;* that is, when students matriculate at the university they are not ordinarily given their choice of the student health service or some other health plan. Therefore, although the student health service is indeed a direct service plan, it does not fully meet the definition of an HMO.

Independent Practice HMOs are those in which the affiliated physicians remain in their solo or other independent practice settings (including group practice). Usually the physicians organize themselves into what are called *Independent Practice Associations (IPAs).* The IPA may actually operate the HMO, or it may contract with the HMO to provide the medical services. In addition, when the IPA and the HMO are separate entities, especially in places like urban California where there are many HMOs, an IPA may be "married"—having an exclusive relationship with one HMO for which it becomes, essentially, that HMO's "physician division"; or it may be "single"—playing the field and having relationships with several different HMOs. Unlike the physicians in staff and group model HMOs, most IPA-affiliated physicians will know that the members of a particular HMO constitute a minority, sometimes a very small minority, of these physicians' total patients. The physicians in an IPA-type HMO are remunerated for the care they provide to HMO members either on a controlled fee-for-service basis or by capitation. These two methods of payment also tend to correspond to the two main varieties of IPAs: (1) "*traditional*" and (2) "*gatekeeper.*"

Glossary: "*Traditional*" IPA HMO—A variety of IPA-HMO in which the participating physicians are paid by a controlled fee-for-service method, as follows: Part of the physician's fee (for providing a service to an HMO member) is held back by the HMO in a reserve account; the remaining (larger) portion is paid to the physician. The money kept in reserve is later distributed back to the physicians whose work generated it if the HMO's overall costs stay within some previously agreed upon limit. If, however, that limit is exceeded, the reserve will not be returned to the physicians, since it will be needed to meet the cost overrun. Should the costs run so high that even the reserve account is inadequate to meet them, then the portion of the fee kept in reserve is increased. In a "traditional" IPA HMO, the incentive to contain costs is based on this fee reduction/reserve fund mechanism. This incentive is not, however, terribly strong when, as is usually the case, the number of physicians participating in the IPA is very large and the percentage of an individual physician's practice consisting of HMO members is very small. Under these conditions the overall penalty for generating excessive costs will not be felt severely by any single physician. "Traditional" IPAs have usually been sponsored by local and state medical societies, and they have usually been open to participation by all physicians in an area, regardless of specialty. The main source of their appeal to the physicians who join them (and to the medical societies who sponsor them) has been as an answer to the threat of competition from (loss of patients to) the more aggressive group practice HMOs and the "gatekeeper" IPA HMOs.

"Gatekeeper" IPA HMO—A variety of IPA usually open *only* to primary care physicians, who are most often paid by a modified capitation method instead of by fee-for-service. "Gatekeeper" IPA HMOs tend to be sponsored by insurance carriers, although some have been formed as public companies whose stock is traded on Wall Street. They are seldom sponsored by practicing physicians and never by medical societies. The reason for the modified capitation method of payment is that it is a more powerful incentive to control costs than modified fee-for-service. In a "gatekeeper" IPA, the independent primary care physician is placed at risk in much the same way as the group practice is at risk in a group practice type HMO. It works like

this: Each IPA physician is paid a fixed amount for each HMO member who selects that physician as her regular primary physician. Using the capitation payment, the physician not only provides primary care for the enrollee (patient), but also selects and pays for any specialist care the patient needs, any diagnostic laboratory work, and so on. Should hospitalization be necessary, its cost is debited against the primary physician's HMO hospitalization "account," the size of which at year's end determines in part whether the physician receives a bonus. Likewise, a record of fewer diagnostic tests and less (or less expensive) specialist care would mean less drain on the primary care physician's own capitation income. The primary care physician has an incentive, therefore, to be judicious in the use of diagnostic tests, specialist consultations, and hospitals.

Another recent organizational mechanism for cost control is the *Preferred Provider Organization (PPO).*

Glossary: *Preferred Provider Organization (PPO)*— An arrangement for price discounting that requires an agreement between (1) a group of individual providers (hospitals and/or physicians) and (2) one or more insurance companies or self-insured employers. The "preferred" providers agree to accept discounted prices for the services they provide to people who hold policies with the insurance company. In return, the insurance company agrees to pass on some of the savings to its policy holders by reducing their out-of-pocket costs, *so long as* they use one of the designated physicians or hospitals. The individual policy holder is not *obligated* to select from among this list of "preferred providers." The insurance is still good regardless of where or from whom the medical service is received, but the policy pays less when the patient uses the services of a provider not on the list. However, when patients *do* select from the "preferred list," the insurance company may "forgive" all or part of the deductible, or the co-insurance, or both. Patients and providers both have incentives to participate in the PPO—patients because they stand to pay less, providers because they stand to attract (or at least not lose) patients from among the presumably large number of people who would welcome the opportunity of paying less.

Any one of the parties in a PPO—doctors, hospitals, insurance company, or employers—might have taken the lead in organizing it, since all of them would have had something to gain by participating. The employers and the insurance companies would have been interested in the PPO as a way to reduce costs and, in the case of a commercial insurance company, as a marketing ploy, the opportunity for introducing a new product. (The insurance company is seen as offering an optional, lower cost plan to its policy holders who will agree to limit their choice of physicians and/or hospitals to those that are "preferred" by the insurance company, preferred because they will accept discounted rates.) NOTE: There is no enrollment of members in PPOs, nor is there any assumed responsibility on the part of providers to deliver services to a group of people (and thus no financial risk). PPOs, therefore, are not HMOs.

Since PPOs offer the patient an option of using a provider *not* on the approved list, a decision that need not be exercised in advance but may be made at the time the service is received (at the point of service), PPOs have become known as *"Point-of-Service" plans.*

Glossary: "Point-of-Service" Plan—
A plan in which the patient is given the option of either selecting a provider on an approved list (and thus being covered in the usual way) or using a provider not on the list (and paying extra for the privilege). The choice is not between two different plans (say a traditional fee-for-service indemnity plan with complete freedom of choice of

provider and a closed-panel HMO). Rather, it is exercised *within* a plan at the "point of service." PPOs are one example of a point-of-service plan, but the point-of-service option can also be added to HMOs.

Social and Private Insurance: Preoccupation with Cost Control (the 1980s)

During the 1980s, the problem of *inaccess* to medical care virtually dropped off the public policy agenda. Cost control dominated. As the cost crisis worsened, government, industry, the insurance industry, and the health care providers responded with new or changed financing mechanisms.

One new device designed to curb costs, put into effect by a change in the Medicare law, was the "prospective payment" of hospitals according to Diagnosis Related Groups (DRGs). Prior to prospective payment, Medicare paid hospitals, just as the service benefit plans of Blue Cross did, on a "cost" basis. A hospital examined its total institutional costs and calculated the average daily cost of caring for a patient. Medicare then paid the hospital this amount. The problem for the Medicare program was that two perverse incentives were at work: (1) for the hospital to spend more, since all expenditures would ultimately be recouped in its higher average daily cost figure; and (2) for the hospital to keep the patient an extra day or two, since a longer stay meant more money; a shorter stay less money.

Since 1984, the Medicare program has paid hospitals on a "fee-for-case" basis, according to an established schedule that reflects the average cost of a hospital stay for each type of case, or to be precise, for each "Diagnosis Related Group" of cases. Hospital care is thus no longer paid according to what the hospital's actual cost is for providing the care. Payment by Medicare is instead "prospective." The total is known as soon as the diagnosis is known. For example, the hospital care of a patient undergoing an elective surgical repair of an inguinal hernia now costs the Medicare program whatever the DRG book says it costs—no more, no less. (Before DRGs it would have cost whatever that particular hospital calculated its average daily cost per patient to be times the number of days the patient ended up staying in the hospital plus the hospital's per hour charge for use of the operating room times the number of hours it was used plus the charge for each test ordered from the laboratory and X-ray departments plus each medication ordered from the pharmacy, and so on.) If the total amount of hospital care required for a particular "case" ends up costing more than the amount listed in the book for that kind of "case," the hospital (not the Medicare program) must absorb the difference. If it costs less, then the hospital stands to gain by the amount of the difference. In this way the Medicare program has placed an incentive for hospital administrators to control the costs of hospital care. The introduction of DRGs did not, however, prevent managers from "gaming" the system. It was still sometimes possible for the hospital to collect more by "documenting" complications in treatment, or in the case of an imprecise diagnosis to classify the case within the DRG that paid a larger amount. A hospital could also direct a patient requiring expensive diagnostic tests to its outpatient department where the DRG system doesn't apply.

By the end of the 1980s, a new term had appeared at the top of the *private* policy agenda—*managed care.*

Glossary: *Managed Care*—A generic term, implying active participation by the financing agency in monitoring the cost and quality of the service. Managed care means that regardless of what payment method is used by the insurance carrier, payment won't be automatic; that is, the doctors and hospitals won't be paid whatever amount they bill with no questions asked, which was the way that Blue Cross, the commercial insurance companies, and most of the government programs operated in the past. Instead, someone will be monitoring costs and quality of the care, and setting incentives for providers and patients that influence how much the care costs and how it is delivered. The easiest definition of "managed care" is a negative one: it includes everything *except* traditional indemnity insurance. Exactly how the "managing" is done depends on the type of mechanism used. HMOs and PPOs are both examples of "managed care," since both contain the mechanism of administrative oversight plus budgeting and bargaining for controlling costs. But the most common example of a "managed care" plan—although it is rapidly losing ground to the HMOs and point-of-service plans—is modified indemnity insurance. Here, just as with traditional indemnity insurance, the insured person may visit any physician (or hospital); but the insurance company that once asked no questions of that physician will now conduct a review of the physician's "utilization" and at a minimum will require pre-authorization before payment is allowed for hospitalization, surgery, expensive diagnostic procedures, or further consultations by specialists.

Managed care plans are unquestionably more effective in controlling costs than traditional indemnity insurance. However, not all managed care plans are equal. Not only are some less expensive, they also vary widely in the amount of premium that is returned to the enrollees in the form of benefits. For example, a 1994 study by the California Medical Association found Kaiser, a non-profit, staff-model HMO, to be highly efficient, spending all but 5 cents of its premium dollar on benefits. On the other hand, Wellpoint Health Networks, a for-profit, IPA-type HMO, spent only 69 cents of every premium dollar on benefits; the rest went to pay for administrative costs and profit to the stockholders.

Since a large and growing majority of employment-based health insurance consists of managed care of one kind or another, most private physicians have become involved in managed care. In 1993, the typical office-based physician participated in at least four different managed care plans. This means that the physician's office must deal with many more insurance company "managers of care." So much dealing with so many managers means that a small medical practice (of one to four physicians) must now have insurance "managers" of its own.

In another recent development, large employers, formerly the best customers of the commercial insurance companies and Blue Cross, stopped using them for the traditional, fundamental insurance function of risk-bearing. These employers instead began taking on the risk themselves.

There has never been any reason why an employer, if it is large enough, could not "self-insure" its employees' health coverage. Indeed, that's what the early industry-sponsored direct service plans did. During the 1980s, as the expense of purchasing health benefits escalated ever higher, many large employers went to *self-insurance,* because it cost them less.

Glossary: *Self-Insurance*—A way for an employer to provide health benefits to employees without purchasing insurance. The employer collects the employees' contributions by the usual payroll deduction method, but instead of turning the funds (both the employee's and employer's shares) over to Blue Cross or a commercial insurance company, it keeps them in a reserve account and either pays its employees' claims directly or contracts with its former health benefits supplier to process the claims. Since the employer is providing health benefits directly to its own employees and not selling insurance in the open market, its self-insurance plan is not subject to the same sort of regulation by the state insurance commission as would apply to a private insurance company (for example, regulation of rate-setting, requirements on cash reserves, and rules against changing benefits in mid-stream, even after someone is ill and receiving treatment). To protect itself against the possibility of its employees' claims temporarily draining the self-insurance fund, the self-insuring employer purchases what is called "reinsurance" from a large insurance company. Approximately half of all medical bills covered by employer-based health plans are now paid through self-insurance.

As employers assumed the risk of health insurance, some of the companies that had previously been these employers' insurance carriers became instead their managers of "managed care." They in effect turned managed care into a large new service industry that relies primarily on the self-insurance of the large employers and, conceivably in the future, on government-guaranteed private health insurance. The five largest commercial health insurance carriers—Travelers, MetLife, CIGNA, Prudential, and Aetna—left the Health Insurance Association of America in the early 1990s to form their own new organization devoted to managed care.

A consequence of self-insurance is that when the larger employers pull out of the private insurers' risk pool, they leave only smaller employee groups and unaffiliated, self-employed people. When the insurance companies insured very large groups, they found it difficult to "cherry pick." Cherry picking is much easier with smaller groups. Further, the insurers insist on higher premiums for these smaller groups to cover the presumed larger risk when even one member of the group has a serious illness. This makes the cost of good insurance much higher for small businesses, a circumstance that has led many of them to drop their employee health benefits, thus adding to the number of uninsured. Also, the smaller the employee group the more likely that enrollees will be given policies with very high deductibles and multiple exclusions, thus adding to the number of *under*insured. Again, we see the principle of the fragmented risk pool at work: the more fragmented the risk pool becomes, the more difficult it is for the people left in the pool to find insurance.

Social and Private Insurance: The Road to Reform (1981–1992)

There was good reason why cost control should have dominated the health care agenda of the 1980s. The percentage of GDP that the nation was spending on health care had been rising at the rate of a full percentage point every 35 months ever since 1971. By 1980 it had reached 9 percent; during 1990 it passed 12 percent.

Meanwhile, the private health insurance that had once seemed so satisfactory to Americans was in effect shrinking, covering fewer people for less of their health care expenses and, ironically, costing much more. The 66 percent of working Americans who in 1979 were receiving health insurance through their employment was down to 61 percent in 1992 and falling.

During the 1980s the talk among policymakers turned once again to a universal program of social insurance for health care. Without it, said the advocates, costs would never come under control. *Cost-shifting* (the practice by hospitals of making up from the insured what they lose by caring for the uninsured and underinsured) was driving up the price of private insurance at more than twice the rate of general inflation.

In the 1970s, Presidents Ford and Carter had said that they supported some form of government-guaranteed health coverage but wanted to wait until costs were under control.

President Reagan, however, opposed national health insurance on ideological grounds. So did President Bush—at least he did until late 1991, when Harris Wofford overcame a 40 point deficit

in the polls to defeat Bush's attorney general, Richard Thornburgh, in a special Senatorial election in Pennsylvania. Senator Wofford's winning issue was health care, which Thornburgh—and Bush—had ignored. It was clear from that moment that whichever candidate the Democratic Party nominated to oppose George Bush in 1992 would raise the health care issue more prominently than it had been raised in any previous Presidential campaign.

President Clinton saw universal health insurance not just as an access issue but an economic issue was well. The argument shifted away from Ford's and Carter's position. They had argued, "Wait until costs are controlled so we can afford it." The new argument said, "Not only will we be unable to control costs *until* we have universal entitlement, we won't even be able to keep what we already have." In other words, for Clinton the key to cost control was universal entitlement. This was a radically different formulation.

By 1992, new problems in health care financing were attracting the attention of politicians and students of public policy. Among these were "*cost-shifting*," "*job-lock,*" and "*restricted choice.*"

Glossary: *Cost-Shifting*—A process of health care financing through which insured people subsidize the health care of the uninsured and underinsured. As the price of health services and health insurance coverage escalated during the late 1980s and early 1990s, hospitals found themselves caring for more and more people who were uninsured. Although many of these people attempted to pay, they compensated the hospitals on average only 20 percent of the costs of the care they used. The hospitals recouped the remainder by raising their prices, thus charging people with private insurance an average of 130 percent of the costs they incurred. The insurance plans, who paid the hospitals these higher charges, raised their premiums, whereupon the employers, who paid the largest share of these raised premiums, recouped their costs by increasing the employee's share, by switching to insurance plans with higher deductibles, and in some cases by dropping their employee insurance benefits altogether, thus adding to the number of people who are uninsured and unable to pay, and adding momentum to the process. The process also gains acceleration each time Congress in its attempt to reduce federal spending attempts to cut Medicare and, especially, the federal share of Medicaid (thus leaving the states to bear a larger share of the burden). Yet another force behind cost-shifting is the banding together of large self-insured employers to obtain discounts, sometimes by offering exclusive contracts to the hospital that gives them the best deal for some special service, like oncology or cardiology and heart surgery. Managed care plans also use this same ploy. The hospitals then try to recoup this reduction in income by increasing their prices to the other (more passive) insurance payers. Health economists call this kind of process a "death spiral." Students of pathophysiology will recognize it by another name: "vicious cycle."

Job-Lock—The unwillingness of workers to leave their jobs because of the loss of health benefits. By the early 1990s, people in jobs that provided health insurance could no longer assume that the next job would also provide health insurance. Therefore, those who were unhappy in their present jobs, or wished to move to another location, or hoped for an early retirement, were afraid to leave. People who had been diagnosed with a chronic condition of some kind—for example, arthritis, emphysema, breast cancer, diabetes—could not afford to accept a better job because the new health plan would be likely to exclude this "pre-existing condition."

Restricted Choice—The inability of an insured patient to select any doctor or hospital and still be covered by the insurance plan. As managed care replaced indemnity insurance as the most favored health benefits vehicle for employers, choice of provider was increasingly restricted for the employee. IPA-type HMOs tend to select their panels of physicians according to the size of the enrollment, and they prefer to have only a relatively small number of each kind of specialist on the panel—physicians whom the plan can rely on to carry out its quality and cost control procedures. When employers found they could save by restricting the number of alternative plans offered to their employees, they began replacing "multiple choice" of plans with a single, least expensive, plan. By 1994, 84% of all U.S. firms were offering a single choice to their employees (although half of the firms with over 1,000 employees offered at least three plans). See also *"Free Choice" or "Expanded Choice"* below.

In 1984, 88 percent of Americans had some form of health coverage (through employment or through government); by 1994 that percentage had slipped to 83%. The slippage was disproportionately among those who worked for small employers. Insured people were also, however, feeling less secure. Further, as the size of deductibles and number of limitations in most private insurance policies increased, non-insured, "out-of-pocket" medical expenses continued to increase—they grew by 600% between 1975 and 1992—until they were consuming a full 10 percent of average household income, and this at a time when Americans were experiencing a *decline* in median family income (from $39,000 in 1989 to $37,000 in 1992). It was not surprising, then, that the inability to pay medical bills was being called the leading cause of personal bankruptcy.

Recent Agendas for Reform (1993–1996)

At nearly 15 percent of the GDP, the cost of health care either delayed or removed other competing economic choices from the agendas of individuals, businesses, and government. Because of health care cost inflation, workers had to forego pay raises. Businesses deferred investing in new equipment. Governors were unable to fulfill their campaign promises as Medicaid grew to become the second largest item—after education—in state budgets. And the President and the Congress were unable to repair the nation's infrastructure, reform the welfare system, or reduce the size of the federal deficit as rapidly as they wished.

This assortment of problems led to a plethora of proposed solutions, all captured under the rubric of "reform." The 1993–1994 debate over President Clinton's Health Security plan and the 1995–1996 debate over "cutting" versus "preserving" Medicare added to the jargon of health care financing. Here is an attempt at defining two of the more significant of these terms and slogans.

Glossary: *Managed Competition*—An administrative and regulatory arrangement by which private insurance and managed care plans compete to provide health benefits to people who might otherwise be priced out of the market. A government-sponsored or government-sanctioned agency enrolls individuals and/or multiple small employers and employee groups who desire to purchase health insurance at lower rates and from a wider selection of plans. The agency does this by gathering these individuals and small groups into large purchasing pools—sometimes called "*health insurance purchasing cooperatives,*" "*regional health care alliances,*" or something similar—that are independent of these enrollees' work affiliations. Since the purchasing pool contains many more people than the total employees of any small firm, it can curtail "experience rating" and obviate many of the exclusions that small groups and individuals must bear when they attempt to purchase insurance on their own. Acting on behalf of its members, the purchasing agency solicits and reviews bids and bargains with insurance carriers over rates. Beyond this minimum

function, the agency may also take on the tasks of approving the participation of the competing plans, monitoring their performance, collecting and disseminating performance data to the public, even collecting premiums from employers and employees. Although President Clinton's proposed federal program based on managed competition was not enacted during 1993–1994, several states did set up regulated health insurance purchasing pools or cooperatives. NOTE: Some people understandably confuse the terms "managed" care and "managed" competition. One refers to a particular type of health plan. The other refers to an arrangement or mechanism by which all health plans of whatever type can compete fairly for everyone's business.

"Free Choice" or "Expanded Choice"—This slogan was first used by the AMA and state and county medical societies in the mid-1930s to combat prepaid group practice plans or "contract practice" as they were called then. A prepaid group practice plan naturally limited the patient's choice of physician to members of the staff of the group practice. Medical societies objected since people enrolling in the group practice plan were effectively removing themselves from being customers of the other doctors in the community. In 1959, the AMA made peace with the prepaid group practice plans, changed its policy, and proclaimed that free choice among plans could substitute for free choice among physicians. The "free choice" slogan was used again by opponents of President Clinton's Health Security plan of 1993, which would have encouraged the use of managed care plans, which tend to restrict choice of physician. The Clinton plan would, however, have mandated multiple choice of plans at a time when take-it-or-leave-it, single choice was fast becoming the rule rather than the exception for employment-based health coverage. More recently, the "free choice" slogan was used against Medicare, which has always permitted patients to choose virtually any physician and

hospital in America. But Medicare has generally not included the choice of a managed care plan and never a medical savings account. Interestingly, many of the same politicians who in 1993 and 1994 condemned the narrowed choices inherent in most managed care plans and who discounted the increased choice of plans that the Clinton program would have mandated, were quick to endorse the "expanded choice" of managed care for Medicare. Although it has proven to be a versatile and effective slogan for politicians and organized medicine, "free choice" for the patient is usually a fiction. This is because the choice of which physician the patient will actually see is usually made by another physician and for hospitalized patients is usually limited to physicians who are on the staff of that particular hospital. While this may make for a wise choice, it is not really a "free choice."

The two principal goals of reform are to contain costs and expand access by increasing (or preserving) coverage. The political debate over each of these goals is many-sided. It can, however, be reduced to a few essential points:

Containing Costs

All nations with universal coverage also have cost controls of some kind, usually relying on "global budgets" or "targets" set by government. In a multi-payer system based in the private sector and financed mostly with contributions from employees and employers, "global budgets" (with sub-budgets for each hospital and negotiated fee schedules for physicians) are far more difficult to implement than they are in a tax-financed, single-payer system. Some politicians and other interested parties—including the private insurers—believe that a "reformed" market (meaning competition among health plans, managed by government or by large private purchasers of care or by both) will lead to cost-containment naturally and therefore that no cost

control legislation is necessary. Others would agree to government-imposed cost controls but only as "standby" measures in case the market doesn't behave like it is supposed to. Still others oppose virtually all government controls on ideological grounds, especially when such controls are targeted at private insurance plans. These same politicians see little problem, however, in imposing financing ceilings or cut-offs when the target of cost control is a public, single-payer plan like, for example, Medicare.

Expanding Access

There are two ways to assure *universal* financial access: either through (1) a national health service, or (2) a national program of social insurance. Americans have never generated a groundswell of political support for a national health service, which explains why all of the past proposals centered on social insurance. There are also only two ways of funding social insurance: either through (1) taxes, or (2) mandates. Since American politicians abhor the prospect of openly taxing for anything, and since many of them also believe as an article of faith that any collective financing scheme will remain unpolluted only to the extent that it can be made to bypass government, mandates to purchase private insurance have received the most attention. Although this recent shift of opinion—every serious proposal in the past, from the AALL program to Medicare, envisioned the flow of money going through government—is far from a consensus, single payer proposals have been losing favor in recent decades. (The move by Congressional Republicans to change Medicare from a single payer plan to a multiple choice option is the most recent case in point.) If universal coverage were to be based largely on mandates (presumably with tax-supported subsidies for low-income people and/or small employers), the next question would be whether the mandate should be imposed on the employer, the individual, or both, and in what combination?

This, however, must remain a second order question so long as the political majority prefers to avoid the issue of universal coverage altogether. The view that ultimately prevailed in the debate of 1993–94—and that was ratified in the 1994 mid-term Congressional election—was that expansion of social insurance is neither necessary nor desirable, since *private* insurance will reform itself in ways that should make it "accessible" (affordable) to many of those not now covered. The market competition that has already enhanced the bottom line of employers will ultimately benefit everyone. Although it won the political contest, this argument's validity is questionable. Certainly, managed care plans have curbed the inflation in employer-paid health benefits. But this has come at a cost to employees of increased out-of-pocket payments, less choice, and a transfer of money away from actual payment for health care into the greater administrative burden represented by the new managed care industry. Nor do lower prices paid for employment-linked health benefits necessarily translate into increased access for the American public. The number of uninsured and underinsured continues to rise even as growth and competition in the managed care industry increases.

Two Final Observations

I will end this primer with two historical observations on health reform. The first is that, except following full-scale political revolution or major political changes imposed in the wake of war, no nation has ever enacted a program of social insurance for health care that did not build on the incomplete private system that was already in place. As we have seen, this was true of the programs enacted by Bismarck and Lloyd George. And it was true in this country in the case of Medicare, which built on the Blue Cross sys-

tem of hospital payment and the private indemnity insurance system of paying physicians. The American private system of medical care financing has changed dramatically since 1965 and is continuing to change rapidly. It is dominated by an aggressive, highly competitive private sector that responds hardly at all, except defensively, to political pressure and is forceful, even vicious in implementing its new forms of corporate-style "integrated" delivery systems. Whether or not this is a desirable direction for reform is a matter of opinion. We should, however, expect that any future program of universal coverage will build on the private system that is evolving from these current changes.

My second observation is merely a reminder that there have been several unsuccessful attempts to enact compulsory health insurance in the United States in the 20th century. On each occasion the popular expectations exceeded the results. The outcome of the 1993–94 debate certainly followed this course. Although it is possible that the critical link between health care and the broader economy—a connection that is more evident now than in the past—could yet force a different outcome, the historical record advises a guarded prognosis.

Notes

1. John J. A. O'Reilly to the Medical Society of the County of Kings, New York, October 21, 1919. Quoted in Ronald L. Numbers, *Almost Persuaded: American Physicians and Compulsory Health Insurance, 1912–1920* (Baltimore: Johns Hopkins University Press, 1978), p. 93.
2. Minutes of the House of Delegates, *Journal of the American Medical Association* 74 (May 8, 1920): 1319.
3. At the end of the 1920s only two specialties—ophthalmology and otolaryngology—had formal specialty boards. However, many physicians considered themselves specialists in virtually all the branches of medical practice that would later be recognized as formal specialties.
4. From the "Preface on Doctors," *The Doctor's Dilemma* (New York: Brentano's, 1913).

5. Known officially as the National Labor Relations Act, the Wagner Act guaranteed workers the right to join unions and bargain collectively with their employers.

6. By 1993 private health insurance was being financed through 69 separate Blue Cross and Blue Shield agencies, more than 1,200 different commercial health insurance companies, and an unknown number of self-insured employers.

Reforming the Health Care

System: The Universal

Dilemma

Uwe E. Reinhardt

■

I. Introduction

The human condition surrounding the delivery of health care is the same everywhere in the world: the providers of health care seek to give their patients the maximum feasible degree of physical relief, but they also aspire to a healthy slice of the gross national product ("GNP") as a reward for their efforts. Patients seek from health care providers the maximum feasible degree of physical relief, but, collectively, they also seek to minimize the slice of the GNP that they must cede to providers as the price for that care.

In other words, while there typically is a meeting of the minds between patients and providers on the *clinical* side of the health care transaction, there very often is conflict on the *economic* front. It has always been so, since time immemorial, and it will always be so. It is part of the human condition. Health insurance does not lessen this perennial economic conflict; it merely transfers it from the patient's bedside to the desk of some private or public bureaucrat who is charged with guarding a collective insurance treasury.

However, health insurance does realign the parties to the economic fray. Because insurance shields patients from the cost of their medical treatments at the point of service, it tends to move them squarely into the providers' corner when they are sick. Usually, in that corner, patients rail, with little chance of success, against the heartless bureaucrats who refuse to finance procedures. On the other hand, when patients are healthy and faced with mounting taxes or insurance premiums, they are typically found in the bureaucrats' corner. In that corner, patients rail against health care providers' voracious financial appetite and holler for cost controls.

In this essay, I explore how different nations approach the universal twin problems of modern health care: the provisions of access to health care on equitable terms and the control of health care costs. It is true that there is a rich variety of alternative approaches to these twin problems. It is also true that virtually every developed nation is now dissatisfied with its health care system and seeks to reform it. Unfortunately, there does not seem to be a single *ideal* solution.

II. Controlling the Transfer of GNP to Providers

Society can control the total annual transfer of GNP to health care providers through the demand side of the health care market, the supply side, or both. Nations differ substantially in the mix of approaches they use. Their choice of cost-control policies hinges crucially on the social role that they ascribe to health care. The two extremes of the spectrum of views on this issue are:

1. Health care is essentially a *private consumption good,* whose financing is the responsibility of its individual recipient.

2. Health care is a *social good* that should be collectively financed and available to all citizens who need health care, regardless of the individual recipient's ability to pay for that care.

Canadians and Europeans have long since reached a broad social consensus that health care is a social good. Although their health systems exhibit distinct, national idiosyncrasies, they share an obedience to that overarching, ethical precept.

Americans have never been able to reach a similarly broad political consensus regarding the point at which they would like their health care system to sit on the ideological spectrum that is defined by these two extreme views. Instead, American health policy has meandered back and forth between the two views, in step with the ideological temper of the time. During the 1960s and 1970s, the American health care system moved toward the social good end of the spectrum. On the other hand, during the 1980s, a concerted effort was made to move the system in the opposite direction. This meandering between distinct, ethical precepts has produced contradictions between professed principles and actual practice that confuse and frustrate even the initiated in the United States.

Table 1 presents a menu of alternative approaches to financing and organizing health care. It makes explicit distinctions between the ownership of the health insurance mechanism and the production of health care. Almost all health care systems in the world fit into this grid, and most extend over more than one cell in the grid.

For example, the health systems of the United Kingdom and Sweden occupy primarily Cell A in Table 1, though private medical practices in the United Kingdom occupy Cell C. One may think of Cell A as socialized medicine in its purest sense because the production of health care is substantially owned by the government. Clearly, the health care system of the United States Department of Veterans Affairs also resides in Cell A, as does the bulk of the health care system for the United States armed forces.

The Canadian health care system occupies primarily Cells A, B, and C, as does the American federal Medicare program and the federal-state Medicaid program. Systems falling into Cells A, B, and C represent *government-run health insurance,* not *socialized medicine,* because the delivery system is largely in private hands. This distinction between *socialized insurance* and *socialized medicine* is often lost on American critics of foreign health care systems.

Table 1. Alternative Mixes of Health Insurance and Health Care Delivery

| Production and Delivery | Collectivized (Socialized) Financing of Health Care | | | Direct Financing |
| | Government-Financed Insurance | Private Health Insurance[a] | | Out-of-Pocket by Patients at Point of Service |
		within a statutory framework	within an unregulated market	
Purely Government-Owned	A	D	G	J
Private Not-for-Profit Entities	B	E	H	K
Private For-Profit Entities	C	F	I	L
	The Canadian health system	The West German health system	The private portion of the American system	

[a] Note: Technically, whenever the receipt of health care is paid for by a third party rather than the recipient at point of service, it is financed out of a *collective* pool and is, thus, "socialized" financing. In this sense, private health insurance is just as "collectivist" or "socialized" as government-provided health insurance. Both forms of financing destroy the normal workings of a market because both eliminate the individual benefit-cost calculus that is the *sine qua non* of a proper market.

Germany's health care system is best described by Cells D, E, and F. Health insurance in Germany is provided by a structured system of not-for-profit sickness funds that are privately administered, albeit within a federal statute that tightly regulates their conduct.[1] This statutory health insurance system has evolved gradually over the span of 100 years and now covers eighty-eight percent of the population.[2] The remainder is covered by private, commercial insurers more akin to commercial insurers in the United States.[3] On the other hand, Germany's health care delivery system is a mixture of private and public, for-profit and not-for-profit, providers that is similar to the mix of providers found in the United States. In other words, the German health care system also does not represent socialized medicine, but socialized insurance.

As noted above, parts of the American health system fall squarely into Cell A. Others fall into Cells A, B, and C. Together, Cells A through C accounted for about forty-four percent of national health care spending in 1991.[4] The rest of the system, its private sector, is spread from Cells G to L. As part of the impending reform of the American health care system, this private sector is likely to slide toward either Cells D, E, and F, or even toward Cells A, B, and C. The concept of "managed competition," for example, fits into Cells D, E, and F, as would an "all-payer" system, under which multiple private insurance carriers would be subject to common fee schedules. On the other hand, if Congress legislated a single-payer system based on the Canadian model—or "Medicare For All"—the American system would rest in Cells A, B, and C.

A. The Approaches Used in Canada and Europe

As noted, Canadians and Europeans typically view health care as a social good. In these countries, it is anathema to link an individual household's health care financing contribution to the health status of that household's members. Health care in these countries is collectively financed, with taxes or premiums based on the individual household's ability to pay.[5] Only a small, well-to-do minority—so far, less than ten percent of the population—opts out of collective social insurance in favor of privately insured or privately financed health care.[6] Nevertheless, nearly ninety percent of the population typically shares one common level of quality and amenities in health care.

Control of health care costs in these countries is exercised partly by controlling the physical capacity of the supply side. The chief instrument for this purpose is formal regional health planning.[7] Planning enables policymakers to limit the number of hospital beds, big-ticket technology (such as CT scanners or lithotripters), and sometimes even the number of physicians who are issued billing numbers under these nations' health insurance systems.

However, regulatory limits on the capacity of the health care system inevitably create monopolies on the supply side. To make sure that these artificially created monopolies do not exploit their economic power, these countries generally couple health planning on the supply side with stiff price and budgetary controls imposed on the demand side. Sometimes, price controls alone are deemed sufficient to control overall health spending. However, where the intent of price controls has been thwarted through rapid increases in the volume of health services rendered, these countries have imposed strictly limited global budgets on the health care systems as a whole, or upon particular segments (e.g., hospitals and doctors). Canada, for example, has long compensated its hospitals through pre-set global budgets. Similarly, West Germany now operates strict, state-wide expenditure caps for all physicians who practice within a state under the nation's Statutory Health Insurance system. The United Kingdom and the Nordic countries budget virtually their entire health systems.[8]

To implement their price and budget controls, Canada and the European countries tend to struc-ture their health insurance systems so that money flows from third-party payers to health care providers through only one or a few large money-pipes. The "money-pipe" throughput is then controlled through formal negotiations between regional or national associations of third-party payers and associations of providers. The negotiated prices in these countries are usually binding on providers, who may not bill patients for extra charges above these prices. Although France permits extra billing within limits, most of these countries perceive unrestrained extra billing as a violation of the spirit of health insurance.[9]

Remarkably, and in sharp contrast with the United States, Canada and Europe typically do not look to the individual patient as an agent of cost control. Usually, there is no significant flow of money from patient to provider at the time health services are received. Instead, most of these countries provide patients with comprehensive, universal *first-dollar* coverage for a wide range of services, including drugs (Canada covers drugs only for the poor). France does have co-payments at the point of service for all ambulatory care and hospital care, but not for certain high-cost illnesses.[10] Furthermore, many French patients have supplemental private insurance to cover any co-payments.[11]

One should not assume that Canada and the European nations eclipse patients from cost control because these nations' health policy analysts and policymakers lack the savvy of their American colleagues. American debates on health policy tend to characterize patients as "consumers" who are expected to shop around for cost-effective health care. One suspects that Canadians and Europeans are inclined to perceive patients as, for the most part, "sick persons" who should be treated as such. Table 2 suggests why that perception may be a valid one. As Table 2 illustrates, the distribution of health expenditures across a population tends to be highly skewed. In the United States, for example, only

Table 2. Distribution of Health Expenditures for the U.S. Population, by Magnitude of Expenditures, Selected Years, 1928—1987

Percent of U.S. population ranked by expenditures	1928	1963	1970	1977	1980	1987
Top 1 percent	—	17%	26%	27%	29%	30%
Top 2 percent	—	—	35	38	39	41
Top 5 percent	52%	43	50	55	55	58
Top 10 percent	—	59	66	70	70	72
Top 30 percent	93	—	88	90	90	91
Top 50 percent	—	95	96	97	96	97
Bottom 50 percent	—	5	4	3	4	3

Source: Marc L. Berk and Alan C. Monheit "*Data Watch: The Concentration of Health Expenditures: An Update,*" Health Aff., Winter 1992, at 145, 146.

five percent of the population accounts for about half of all national health expenditures in any given year, and ten percent account for about seventy percent. The distribution of health expenditures in other countries is apt to present a similar pattern.

One must wonder whether the few individuals who account for the bulk of health care expenditures in any given year can actually act like regular "consumers" who shop around for cost-effective health care. Although cost sharing by patients can be shown to have some constraining effect on utilization for mild to semi-serious illness,[12] it is unlikely to play a major role in the serious cases that appear to account for the bulk of national health care expenditures.

Where price and ability to pay cannot ration health care, something else must. Usually, in Canada and Europe, that non-price rationing device is a queue for elective medical procedures. At the extreme, some high-tech medical interventions, such as renal dialysis or certain organ transplantations, are simply unavailable to particular patients if the attending physician judges the likely benefits of intervention to be low. High-tech innovations are introduced rather cautiously in these nations, and only after intensive

benefit-cost analysis. Therefore, at any given time, these nations' health care systems are likely to lag behind that in the United States in the degree to which a new medical technology has been adopted.[13]

Finally, the tight control on overall outlays for health care tends to preclude the often luxurious settings in which health care is dispensed to well-insured patients in the United States. Atriums and gourmet dining in hospitals, or physician offices with plush carpets, are not common in Canada or Europe.

B. The Entrepreneurial American Approach

Americans have traditionally looked askance at regulation. To be sure, some regulatory controls of the supply side of health care have been attempted at various times in a number of states (e.g., through Certificate-of-Need laws). There have also been occasional flirtations with price controls (e.g., under Richard Nixon's presidency, or in states that regulate hospital rates).[14] For the most part, however, Americans have always viewed the supply side of their health sector as an open economic frontier in which any and all profit-seeking entrepreneurs may gain economic fortunes. Indeed, traditionally, Americans have seen the very openness of their health system to profit-seeking entrepreneurship as the main driving force that has made the American health care system, in their own eyes, the best in the world.[15]

American physicians, for example, have always prided themselves on their status as staunch "free-enterprisers," and have vigorously, although not entirely successfully, defended that status against inroads by third-party payers. Furthermore, as historian Rosemary Stevens has shown convincingly in *In Sickness and in Wealth: A History of the American Hospital in the Twentieth Century,* even the nation's so-called not-for-profit hospitals have typically run their enterprises very much like businesses.[16] Normally, they have booked profits, though they do not distribute them to outside owners.

In contrast to Canadians and Europeans, who tightly control the supply side of their health sectors, Americans have generally[17] freely opened theirs to fortune seekers. The American belief is that the GNP transfer that health care providers can extract from the rest of society can easily be controlled through the demand side of the sector—primarily by forcing patients to behave like regular consumers.

The traditional instrument of demand-side cost control in the United States has been cost sharing by patients. As shown in Table 3, on average, American patients are not nearly as well insured as is sometimes supposed—not even considering the heyday of the Great Society—though there is a wide dispersion around this average. Some Americans have no health insurance at all, others have very shallow insurance, and some receive from their employers generous coverage that approximates the comprehensive, first-dollar coverage available to Canadians and Europeans. Typical among the latter insured are unionized workers in the Northern rust belt.

Even the relatively high degree of cost sharing

by American patients, however, has not been able to contain the growth of national health care expenditures.[18] For that reason, additional forms of demand-side controls have been implemented in recent years, namely: (1) ex-post utilization control, (2) prospective and concurrent utilization review by third-party payers (otherwise known as "managed care"), and (3) the so-called Preferred Provider Organizations ("PPOs").[19]

A uniquely American form of cost control, aimed more at the supply side of the health care market, is the Health Maintenance Organization ("HMO"). Basically, the HMO is an insurance contract under which a network of providers is prepaid an annual lump sum capitation per insured in return for the obligation to furnish the insured

Table 3. Cost Sharing by American Patients 1987[*]

Category of Expenditure	Mean Annual Spending Per Person With That Expense	Mean Percentage of Expenditure Paid Out of Pocket
All Health Services	$1,804	24%
All inpatient services	$7,120	8%
Inpatient physician services	$1,976	16%
Ambulatory physician services	$ 470	26%
Ambulatory non-physician services	$ 422	29%
Outpatient prescribed medicines	$ 162	57%
Dental services	$ 295	56%

[*] As of 1993, this is the most recent year for which national survey data are available.

Source: B. Hahn & D. Lefkowitz, Annual Expenses and Sources of Payment for Health Care Services (Agency for Health Care Policy and Research, Pub. No. 93-0007, 1992) (Tables 1 to 7).

with all medically necessary care during the contract period. The contract is designed to make providers hold their use of resources in treating patients to the medically necessary minimum. Usually, the HMO contract leads to lower hospitalization rates, other things being equal, and to relatively lower average per capita health care costs.[20] Drawbacks include limiting patient choice among providers and underserving patients.

III. The Economic Footprints of These Approaches

It is generally agreed, both here and abroad, that the American entrepreneurial approach to health care has begotten one of the most luxurious, dynamic, clinically and organizationally innovative, and technically sophisticated health care systems in the world. At its best, the system has few rivals anywhere, though many health care systems abroad also have facets of genuine excellence. At its worst, however, it has few rivals as well.

A. The Cost of Health Care

Unfortunately, but perfectly predictably, the open-ended supply side of the American health care system, coupled with a financing system that looks to sick human beings (patients) as major agents of cost control, has led to perennial excess capacity in most parts of the country, and to large and rapidly growing costs. With the exception of New York City and a few states—in which capacity has been tightly controlled through health planning—the average hospital occupancy ratio in the United States is now between sixty and seventy percent.[21] It is below fifty percent in some cities.[22] American physicians, for their part, have long deplored a growing physician surplus.[23]

This enormous and excess capacity comes at a stiff price. In 1992, the United States spent close to fourteen percent of its GNP on health care, up from 9.1 percent in 1980.[24] Current forecasts project a ratio of eighteen percent for the year 2000.[25] By contrast, none of the other industrialized nations currently spends more than ten percent of its GNP on health care, and some (the United Kingdom and Japan) spend less than seven percent.

It is fair to assert that the high cost of American health care has contributed to a major ethical problem faced by the system. So expensive has American health care become that the nation's middle- and upper-income classes now seem increasingly unwilling to share the blessings of their health care system with their millions of low-income, uninsured fellow citizens. The gentleness and kindness for which Americans had come to be known after World War II has, thus, literally been priced out of the nation's soul. By international standards, American health policy toward the poor—particularly toward poor children—now appears rather callous.

B. The Uninsured

At this time, some thirty-seven million Americans,[26] over sixty percent of them full-time employees and their dependents,[27] and more than one-quarter of them children,[28] have no health insurance coverage of any type. Most of these American families have incomes below $20,000 per year.[29] However, for such healthy families, an individually purchased commercial insurance policy with considerable cost sharing can run as high as $4,000 per year.[30] Some insurance companies have ceased to offer the policies even at these prices because they are unprofitable. If such families have chronically ill members, however, a private health insurance policy may not be available to them at all.

Such enormous gaps in health insurance coverage do not occur anywhere else in the industrialized world. As noted above, the other member nations in the Organization for Economic

Cooperation and Development ("OECD") offer their citizenry universal health insurance coverage for a comprehensive set of health services and supplies, which typically includes dental care and prescription drugs (with the exception of Canada, where these items are covered only for low-income families).[31]

Traditionally, the American health care system has dealt with the uninsured in the following way: for mild to semi-serious illness, care has been effectively rationed on the basis of price and ability to pay. For critically serious illness, however, care has been made available through hospital emergency rooms, which then shift the cost of such charity care (including necessary inpatient care) to paying patients, notably those insured by the business sector.

Unfortunately, in recent years, this source of charity care has begun to disappear. The profit margins of hospitals are squeezed by a combination of excess capacity and downward price pressure by both public and private sector payers. On average, an uninsured, low-income American now receives only about fifty to seventy percent of the health care that an identical, regularly insured American receives.[32]

C. Styles of Rationing

The myth that, unlike other nations, America does not ration health care is just that, a myth. Americans do ration health care by price and ability to pay, sometimes in rather disturbing ways.[33] Nations differ from one another not in whether they ration health care—all of them do somehow and in varying degrees—but in their style of rationing and their definition of that very term.

One rationing style is to limit physical capacity and use triage, based on medical judgment and the queue, to determine the allocation of artificially scarce resources among the population.[34] That style of rationing is sometimes referred to as *implicit rationing.* The other style is

to ration *explicitly* by price and ability to pay.[35] It is the natural by-product of the so-called "market approach" to health care.

Implicit rationing predominates outside of the United States. In principle, the approach is thought to allocate health care strictly on the basis of medical need, as perceived and ranked by physicians. It is not known whether other variables, such as the patient's social status, ultimately enter the allocation decision as well. For example, one wonders whether a gas station attendant in the United Kingdom has the same degree of access to limited resources as a barrister or university professor who may be able to use social connections to jump the queue.

Many Americans believe that health care is not currently rationed in the United States. That belief seems warranted for well-insured patients who are covered by traditional, open-ended indemnity insurance and living in areas with excess capacity. For many of these patients, there seems to be virtually no limit to the use of real resources in attempts to preserve life or gain certainty in diagnosis.

On the other hand, persons who are less well-insured, uninsured, or covered by managed-care plans (including HMOs) do occasionally experience the withholding of health care resources strictly for economic reasons. In fact, in a recent cross-national survey, some 7.5 percent of the American respondents (the equivalent of eighteen million Americans) claimed that they had been denied health care for financial reasons.[36] In Canada and the United Kingdom, fewer than one percent of the survey respondents made that claim.[37]

Remarkably, the defenders of the American system, who are typically also vehement detractors of all foreign health systems, generally define rationing as only the withholding of health care from people who would have been able and willing to pay for such care with their own money. It is the nightmare of the well-to-do. Apparently, denial of health care to needy, uninsured patients

Table 4. Competing Objectives in Health Care: Basic Prototypical Systems that Span the Set of Actual Systems

	—DESIDERATA—		
Egalitarian Distribution	Freedom From Government Interference in Pricing and in the Practice of Medicine	Budgetary and Cost Control	Prototypical System
Yes	Yes	No	The Health Care Provider's Dream World
Yes	No*	Yes	A National Health Insurance System with Fee Schedules and Other Utilization Review (e.g., Canada, West Germany)
No*	Yes	Yes	A Price-Competitive Market System

* Trade-off

who are unable to pay for that care is not viewed as rationing by these commentators because they have long countenanced it. How else can one explain these commentators' warnings that health care in, for example, the Canadian model would lead to rationing of health care, as if no American were ever denied needed or wanted health care?

It seems easier to implement the *implicit,* supply-side rationing practiced in most other countries than to use the *explicit* American approach to rationing. For some reason, both physicians and patients appear to accept with greater equanimity the verdict that the necessary capacity is simply not available, rather than the verdict that available, idle capacity will not be made available because some budget has run out.[38] No one likes to see monetary factors enter medical decisions quite so blatantly as explicit rationing requires, yet a nation using the market approach to health care ultimately cannot escape consideration of these factors.

D. Summary of the Economic Footsteps

There appears to be a trade-off in the organization of health care that simply cannot be avoided. It is a trade-off among three distinct desiderata in health care, namely: (1) the freedom granted health care providers to organize the production of health care and price their products and services as they see fit; (2) the degree of control over total health care expenditures; and (3) the degree of equity attained in the distribution of health care. Table 4 illustrates this trade-off schematically.

IV. The Convergence of Health Care Systems

If one wished to paint with a very broad brush the evolution of health care policy during the past four decades in the industrialized world, one might describe it as a gradual shift from *expenditure-driven financing of health care* to *budget-driven delivery of health care.*

Under expenditure-driven financing, health care providers were allowed to do for patients whatever they saw fit and send the rest of society a bill at prices that seemed "reasonable." Typically, those presented with that bill paid without reservation. If they had reservations, they paid the bill nevertheless because they lacked the countervailing power present in normal markets without third-party payment. Naturally, under this open-ended approach, the supply side of the health sector became a rich economic frontier that attracted both the genius of private entrepreneurship and its relentless search for revenues.

Technological innovation flourished under this approach as the health sector stood an old adage on its head: instead of necessity being the mother of invention, invention became the mother of necessity. Once a technological innovation was at hand, its application was quickly deemed a "medical necessity" as long as it promised any additional benefits at all to the patient.[39] Benefit-cost ratios played no role in this world because the denominator of that ratio—cost—was deemed irrelevant. Indeed, even to consider cost was deemed ethically unacceptable because that consideration might lead to the "rationing" of health care, which was deemed unacceptable on its face.

Under the second approach, budget-driven health care delivery, society establishes some sort of prospective budget for health care and tells providers to do the best they can within that budget. Typically, the establishment of the overall budget has been rather arbitrary in practice, in the sense that the budget is tied to some arbitrary criterion—such as a fixed percentage of the GNP or a fixed annual growth rate.[40] Ideally, this approach should lead policymakers to explore what additional benefits might be gained through incremental budget expansions, and to set the ultimate budget limits accordingly. In any event, however, the application of new medical technologies in this world will typically be subjected to rigorous benefit-cost analysis before payment for such technologies will be made out of the fixed budget. Merely demonstrating promised benefits is no longer sufficient and will not be accepted by those who would stand to lose from applications of novel technology within the given budget constraints.

As noted earlier, most of the industrialized world has already gone a long way toward budget-driven health care delivery, some (England and Sweden, for example) completely. The United States is the odd one out because it is only just beginning to move in that direction. For the most part, both government and private sector payers in the United States are able to figure out what they have spent on health care in any given year with only a lag of a year or so. In fact, the announcement of total national health spending in recent years has lagged behind actual spending by almost two years. The announcement is eagerly anticipated by all concerned, and the actual numbers never cease to surprise.

There seems little doubt, however, that the 1980s represented the last decade of the completely open economic health care frontier in the United States. There is wide agreement in both the public and private sectors that health spending in the United States is out of control and needs to be reigned in by means other than the free market.

Several recent health reform proposals—including the proposal put forth by President Clinton during his campaign, and one by the prestigious American College of Physicians—have called for a global national health care budget.[41] A national board of stakeholders, somewhat akin to Germany's *Konzertierte Aktion,* determines that budget.[42] At this time, of course, the United States lacks the organizational infrastructure for setting such a budget and apportioning it to the local level. Establishing that infrastructure alone will take over half a decade.

Furthermore, there is already widespread, open hostility toward the very idea of global budgets in the United States, not only among those who define "health care spending" as "health care income." Opponents of global budgeting in the United States offer the strategy of managed competition/managed care as an alternative.[43] Some proponents of that approach market it as the "last hurrah" of the free market, though, in fact, the approach is inherently regulatory in nature.

"Managed competition" is frequently confused with "managed care," but these terms relate to entirely different concepts. Managed care refers to the external monitoring and co-managing of an ongoing doctor-patient relationship to ensure that the attending physician prescribes only "appropriate" interventions. The term "appropriate" excludes procedures with no proven medical benefit, but may also eventually exclude beneficial procedures with a low benefit-cost ratio.

Managed competition, on the other hand, refers to a highly structured and highly regulated framework that forces vertically integrated, income-seeking managed care systems to compete for patients on the basis of prepaid capitation premiums and quality; the latter is to be measured by clinical outcomes and the satisfaction of patients. In other words, the central idea is to put competing managed care systems into transparent, statistical "medico-fishbowls" that can be compared by both patients and those who pay on behalf of patients—for example, government agencies or business firms procuring health insurance coverage for their employees.

At this time, the contrast between the current Canadian/European approach to resource allocation in health care and this newly emerging American approach is stark. Canadians and Europeans still appear to believe that the best way to control overall health spending is to: (1) constrain the physical capacity of the health system, (2) control prices, and, for good measure, (3) impose something as close as possible to global monetary budgets on the entire system. Within these constraints, however, they allow doctors and their patients considerable clinical freedom. In this way, the system will tend to maximize the benefits that are wrung out of the constrained set of real and financial resources. In other words, there is considerable trust in the medical establishment's willingness and ability to use the resources made available to it properly, without the need for day-to-day supervision. Direct co-managing of an ongoing patient-doctor relationship in the American model is still rather rare in Canada and Europe.

In contrast, the American proponents of managed competition believe that, by paying for everything that is beneficial, but denying payment for everything else, the nation can avoid setting an arbitrary global budget and will, in the end, devote the "right" percentage of GNP to health care.[44] These proponents have considerable faith in the ability of ordinary consumers to choose wisely among the alternative cost-quality combinations that competing managed-care systems in the health care market offer. On the other hand, they have little faith in the ability or willingness of the individual physician to use scarce resources wisely in the treatment of patients; therefore, they would subject each doctor to constant statistical monitoring and hands-on supervision.[45]

A huge health services research industry has already been busily working on constructing the statistical "fishbowls" that managed competition will require. Whether the American automobile industry will grow in the 1990s is an open question, but the growth of the health services research industry by leaps and bounds seems assured. By the end of the decade, clinical freedom—which older American physicians once knew and loved—will be all but dead. The physicians' daily activities, their successes and failures, will become highly visible blips on sundry computer screens.

V. Conclusion

And what of the twenty-first century? How will the health care systems of Canada and Europe compare with the American health care system?

It is my thesis that the current differences between the systems will vanish over time. Most likely, Americans will learn that a managed care/managed competition approach will do many wondrous things, but it will not be able to stop the medical arms race that characterizes the American health system. The proponents of managed competition probably oversell the importance of price in consumers' choices concerning health care. To be sure, price does matter much among low-income households. Nevertheless, it is a safe bet that the competing managed care systems will beckon higher-income households, not chiefly with lower premiums, but with promises of ever-new and abundant medical technology that these elevated economic classes will find irresistible. To deny the well-to-do such novel technology in the American context is very difficult. In the end, those who would be forced to deny it will seek comfortable refuge behind some larger constraint—something like a global national or regional budget. Therefore, the United States health system will eventually envelop the competing medico-fishbowls by a global national budget imposed from the top.

At the same time, however, one must wonder whether countries that could not resist McDonald's hamburgers and Apple computers will be able to resist the magnificent statistical medico-fishbowls now being manufactured all over the United States. There will continue to be top-down budgeting in these countries, but there is apt to be less faith in the ability or willingness of the delivery system to use these budgets and without hands-on supervision. Would it not be nice, and eminently proper, to inquire as to exactly what the little "medico-fish" in the health system actually do with all of the dollars, francs, marks, and pounds poured into these health care systems, particularly when such information is easily retrieved and structured? Should there not be better accountability, by individual doctors and hospitals, for their spending, their clinical outcomes, and the satisfaction they achieve among patients?

Thus, it is my bet that, around the year 2005, the health care systems of Canada and Europe will also be a combination of budgets and statistical medico-fishbowls, and that there will be a brisk commerce of ideas among health services researchers and health care managers across the globe regarding the best ways to construct these medico-fishbowls, behold them, and direct the busy medico-fish within them toward desirable ends. In short, our health systems will converge substantially, bound together by the imperative to constrain the share of GNP allocated to health care, and the awesome capacity of new information technology to extract accountability, even from the hitherto impenetrable health care delivery system.

Notes

1. *See* Uwe E. Reinhardt, *West Germany's Health-Care and Health-Insurance System: Combining Universal Access with Cost Control, in* U.S. BIPARTISAN COMM'N ON COMPREHENSIVE HEALTH CARE (THE PEPPER COMMISSION), A CALL FOR ACTION, 3, 7–9 (Supp. 1990); John K. Iglehart, *Germany's Health Care System,* 324 NEW ENG. J. MED. 503, 503 (1991) (first of two parts).

2. Reinhardt, *supra* note 1, at 7; Iglehart, *supra* note 1, at 503, 504; *see also* Craig R. Whitney, *Paying for Health the German Way,* N.Y. TIMES, Jan. 23, 1993, at 1, 4.

3. *See* Reinhardt, *supra* note 1, at 10–11; Iglehart, *supra* note 1, at 504. The private carriers in Germany are also subject to considerable federal regulations—among them a government-imposed fee schedule for physicians.

4. Suzanne W. Letsch, *National Health Care Spending in 1991,* HEALTH AFF., Spring 1993, at 94, 101.

5. Jeremy W. Hurst, *Reforming Health Care in Seven European Nations,* HEALTH AFF., Fall 1991, at 9 (reporting results of a study of recent reforms to the health care systems of seven Organization for Economic Cooperation and Development [OECD] countries: Belgium, France, Germany, Ireland, the Netherlands, Spain, and the United Kingdom).

6. *See* Reinhardt, *supra* note 1, at 10. *See also* Iglehart, *supra* note 1, at 507 ("Some 6.3 million Germans—affluent people and many childless couples—purchase comprehensive private insurance."). In Canada, "[p]rivate insurance may cover additional services but duplication of the public coverage is proscribed." Steffie Woolhandler & David U. Himmelstein, *The Deteriorating Administrative Efficiency of the U.S. Health Care System,* 324 NEW ENG. J. MED. 1253, 1253 (1991).

7. *See* Hurst, *supra* note 5, at 12; Eugene Vayda & Raisa B.

Deber, *The Canadian Health Care System: A Developmental Overview, in* CANADIAN HEALTH CARE AND THE STATE 125–26 (1992).

8. Hurst, *supra* note 5, at 13–14.

9. *Id.* at 10.

10. GENERAL ACCOUNTING OFFICE, HEALTH CARE SPENDING CONTROL: THE EXPERIENCE OF FRANCE, GERMANY AND JAPAN 32 (1991).

11. Hurst, *supra* note 5, at 10.

12. *See* Willard G. Manning et al., *Health Insurance and the Demand for Medical Care,* AM. ECON. REV. 251 (1987) (reporting results of the Rand Health Insurance Experiment).

13. *See* Dale A. Rublee, *Medical Technology In Canada, Germany, and the United States,* HEALTH AFF., Fall 1989, at 178, 180 ("American physicians, with a universe of modern technology at their fingertips, are the envy of the world's physicians.").

14. *See* Stuart H. Altman & Marc A. Rodwin, *Halfway Competitive Markets and Ineffective Regulation: The American Health Care System,* 13 J. HEALTH POL., POL'Y & L. 323, 334 (1988). For a discussion of state efforts to control costs, *see* GEORGE J. ANNAS ET AL., AMERICAN HEALTH LAW 219 (1990).

15. *See* Arnold S. Relman & Uwe E. Reinhardt, *Debating For-Profit Health Care and the Ethics of Physicians,* HEALTH AFF., Summer 1986, at 5, 12. For a general discussion of physician entrepreneurs, see COMMITTEE ON IMPLICATIONS OF FOR-PROFIT ENTERPRISE IN HEALTH CARE, INSTITUTE OF MEDICINE, *Physicians and Entrepreneurism in Health Care, in* FOR-PROFIT ENTERPRISE IN HEALTH CARE 151–70 (Bradford H. Gray ed., 1986).

16. ROSEMARY STEVENS, IN SICKNESS AND IN WEALTH: A HISTORY OF THE AMERICAN HOSPITAL IN THE TWENTIETH CENTURY 359–61 (1989).

17. As already noted, some states in the United States control certain segments of their health sector through formal planning—for example, through Certificates-of-Need for hospital beds or hospital-based, high-tech equipment. *See supra* Section II.B. These strictures, however, have generally been of limited effectiveness. Where hospitals have been prohibited from acquiring certain high-tech equipment, for example, physicians have been able to acquire and operate it in close proximity to the hospital without regulatory control.

18. As Table 2 suggests, perhaps that particular donkey is just too weak to carry much of a cost-containment load.

19. PPOs are networks of fee-for-service providers that have agreed to grant large, third-party payers price discounts in return for insurance contracts that steer the insured toward these "preferred" providers through specially tailored forms of cost sharing. *See* ANNAS ET AL., *supra* note 14, at 775.

20. *See, e.g.,* Julie Kosterlitz, *Managing Medicaid,* 24 NAT'L L.J. 1111 (1992) (describing how HMOs have lower per capita health care costs than does Medicaid in Ohio).

21. Edmund F. Haislmaier, *Why Global Budgets and Price Controls Will Not Curb Health Costs,* HERITAGE FOUND. REP., Mar. 8, 1993, *available in* LEXIS, Nexis Library, Omni File.

22. *See* George D. Pillari, *Those Pliable Occupancy Rates,* MOD. HEALTHCARE, May 20, 1991, at 26, 27 (listing 1990's median occupancy rate for 5600 U.S. hospitals at 48.85%).

23. Kevin Grumbach & Philip Lee, *How Many Physicians Can We Afford,* 265 JAMA 2369, 2369 (1991).

24. *See* Erik Eckholm, *Those Who Pay Health Costs Think About Drawing Lines,* N.Y. TIMES, Mar. 28, 1993, § 4, at 1.

25. CONGRESSIONAL BUDGET OFFICE, PROJECTION OF NATIONAL HEALTH EXPENDITURES 1 (1992); *see also* Dana Priest, *Health Care Price Caps Considered,* WASH. POST, Feb. 14, 1993, at A1.

26. Glenn Kessler, *Bitter Medicine: Reform Is Coming—And This Could Be Painful,* NEWSDAY, Apr. 11, 1993, at 11.

27. BNA, *Number of Uninsured Persons Increased to 36.6 Million in 1991,* DAILY LABOR REP., Jan. 12, 1993, *available in* LEXIS, Nexis Library, Omni file (reporting results of the Employee Benefit Research Institute Study).

28. M. Susan Marquis & Stephen H. Long, *Uninsured Children and National Health Reform,* 268 JAMA 3473, 3473 (1992).

29. BNA, *supra* note 27; *see also* David U. Himmelstein et al., *The Vanishing Health Care Safety Net: New Data on Uninsured Americans,* 22 INT'L J. HEALTH SVCS. 381, 387 (1992).

30. *See, e.g.,* Susan Dentzer, *Health Care Gridlock,* U.S. NEWS & WORLD REP., Jan. 20, 1992, at 22; Lynn Wagner, *Health Economist Trashes Reform Plans of Both Bush and Clinton,* MOD. HEALTHCARE, Oct. 12, 1992, at 10.

31. *See* Raisa B. Deber, *Canadian Medicare: Can It Work in the United States? Will It Survive in Canada?,* 19 AM. J. L. & MED. 75, 79 (1993). For a discussion about Canada's funding drugs for low-income families, see *supra* Section II.A.

32. *See* U.S. BIPARTISAN COMM'N ON COMPREHENSIVE HEALTH CARE (THE PEPPER COMMISSION), A CALL FOR ACTION 34–35 (1990).

33. For example, "(o)ne obstetrician . . . said she doesn't inform pregnant Medicaid patients that they are entitled to a pain killing epidural while in labor [because] Medicaid reimbursements to anesthesiologists are so low, they balk at taking her patients." Kinsey Wilson, *Nobody Likes the R-Word: Rationing of Care Is Unpopular, But It's Happening Just the Same,* NEWSDAY, Apr. 22, 1993, at 23.

34. *See, e.g.,* Richard E. Brown, *From Advocacy to Allocation: The Evolving American Health Care System,* 316 NEW ENG. J. MED. 169 (1987).

35. *See, e.g.,* David Kirkpatrick, *Practicing Medicine Above and Below the 49th Parallel; One Physician's Experience: The Fiction, The Facts,* 151 ARCH. INTERN. MED. 2150, 2152 (1991).

36. Robert J. Blendon, *Views on Health Care: Public Opinion in Three Nations,* HEALTH AFF., Spring 1989, at 151, 156.

37. *Id.*

38. In this regard, see the fascinating analysis of this facet of British health care in HENRY J. AARON & WILLIAM B. SCHWARTZ, THE PAINFUL PRESCRIPTION: RATIONING HOSPITAL CARE (1984).

39. For a discussion of the "career" of a medical technology innovation, see John B. McKinlay, *From "Promising Report" to "Standard Procedure": Seven Stages in the Career of a Medical Innovation,* 59 MILBANK MEM. FUND Q. 374 (1981).

40. For example, Germany's health care spending limit is tied to the growth of workers' salaries and wages. *See* John K. Iglehart, *Germany's Health Care System,* 324 NEW ENG. J. MED. 1750, 1751 (1991) (second of two parts).

41. For a description of this aspect of the Clinton proposal, see Uwe E. Reinhardt, *Commentary: Politics and the Health Care System,* 327 NEW ENG. J. MED. 809, 811 (1992). The American College of Physicians's proposal was first outlined in American College of Physicians, *Universal Insurance For American Health Care,* 117 ANN. INTERN. MED. 511 (1992).

42. *Konzertierte Aktion,* or the Concerted Action Conference, is a group that recommends the annual aggregate increases in providers' fees and suppliers' prices. Iglehart, *supra* note 40, at 1752.

43. *See, e.g.,* Alain C. Enthoven, *Commentary: Measuring The Candidates On Health Care,* 327 NEW ENG. J. MED. 807 (1992). For a discussion of one of Enthoven's proposal, see John B. Judis, *Whose Managed Competition?,* NEW REPUBLIC, Mar. 29, 1993, at 22–23. For a critical review of the concept of managed competition, see Uwe E. Reinhardt, *Comment on the Jackson Hole Initiatives for a Twenty-First Century American Health Care System,* HEALTH ECON., Apr. 1993, at 7.

44. *See* Alain C. Enthoven, *The History and Principles of Managed Competition,* HEALTH AFF., Supp. 1993, at 24, 29.

45. Alan L. Hillman et al., *Safeguarding Quality in Managed Competition,* HEALTH AFF., Supp. 1993, at 110 (discussing strategies for implementing a system of quality assurance under managed competition).

2

Rationing: The Dilemmas of

Fair Distribution

No modern society has devised a way to meet all the medical needs of its citizens. This means that some of the health needs of some of the people will go unmet. So the debates about rationing are not, as Victor Fuchs points out in this section, whether it can be avoided, but how to do it fairly. What counts as fair, of course, is shaped by the dominant moral and political values in each society. Still, the ethical question remains: How should any society measure fairness in allocating its scarce medical resources? This section of part V is designed to explore this question, and to do so in both a national and international context.

George Annas, for example, explores the assets and liabilities of different ways of allocating access to solid organ transplantation, examining market approaches, a lottery, and social worth criteria. The essays by Jafna Cox, and Sharon Redmayne and Rudolf Klein, indicate how other societies are approaching the issue of fair allocation. Queuing for coronary artery bypass surgery seems to work relatively well for Canadians, whereas market forces dictate access in the United States. How can these differences be accounted for? These essays also raise the further question of whether coronary artery bypass should be allocated in one way, and in vitro fertilization services in another. Are some services more basic, or more important than others, so that different methods of allocation are appropriate for different services? Should the importance of a medical service be decided by the population served, or by health and medical experts? Problems of allocation and rationing indicate how medical judgments are inextricably tied to social and ethical ones.

The "Rationing" of Medical Care

Victor R. Fuchs

■

"The United States will soon have to begin rationing medical care." Although we hear this warning with increasing frequency,[1] taken literally the statement is sheer nonsense. It is nonsense because the United States has always rationed medical care, just as every country always has and always will ration care. No nation is wealthy enough to supply all the care that is technically feasible and desirable; no nation can provide "presidential medicine" for all its citizens. Moreover, medical care is hardly unique in this respect. The United States "rations" automobiles, houses, restaurant meals—all the goods and services that make up our standard of living.

The dictionary says that to ration is to apportion or to distribute. The suggestion that until now this country has not apportioned or distributed medical care can hardly be taken seriously. What, then, is all the fuss about? Is anything changing? Indeed, there are changes under way—not from no rationing to rationing, but rather in the way rationing takes place—who does the rationing and who is affected by it.

The basic method of rationing goods and services in this country is through the market. The willingness and ability of consumers to pay for goods and services, and of producers to supply them, determine how they are apportioned or distributed. As recently as 20 years ago, more than half of all personal health-care expenditures were paid for directly by patients. Did this ration care? Of course it did. Consider, for instance, surgery rates among urban whites 65 years of age and over before the introduction of Medicare. In 1963 the rate was 66 operations per 1000 for persons with below-average incomes and 86 per 1000 for those whose incomes were above average. It is not likely that the poorer elderly were less in need of surgery than their wealthier counterparts. The "system" was rationing care even though individual physicians may not have been. Medicare changed this distribution dramatically. By 1970 the rate for persons with below-average incomes was up to 85 per 1000, whereas the rate for those with above-average incomes had actually fallen to 80 per 1000.[2]

The growth of federal insurance programs substantially diminished the role of income as a rationing device, but large differences in the availability of care remain, frequently as a result of geographic location. For instance, in short-term-care hospitals in Massachusetts there is one registered nurse for every patient, but in Arkansas there is only one for every two patients. In the average American community there are 2 physicians to care for every 1000 persons, but in San Francisco there are approximately 5. Thus, even with widespread third-party payment, the amount and kind of care that physicians provide is still constrained by how busy they are, what facilities, equipment, and auxiliary personnel are available, how much training the physicians have had, and the informal messages that they receive from peers about what constitutes "appropriate" care in any particular situation.

To the extent that the spread of private and public insurance has relieved the economic pressure on patients and physicians, it has also been a major factor in the expansion of expenditures. Now, questions are being raised about the benefits of the additional care relative to its cost. In the American economic system, expenditures for most goods and services are determined by consumers, who balance the benefits expected from an additional purchase against the additional cost. By and large, this balancing results in a reasonably efficient allocation of resources, given the distribution of income and the preferences of consumers.

Expenditures for medical care are different. Because most Americans want to be insured against large medical bills and most do not want to see the poor dying for lack of care, the bulk of medical care is paid for by third parties, private or public. But when a third party is paying, the patient will want additional care and the conscientious physician will provide it, even though its cost to society exceeds the benefit to the patient.

This divergence between what is good for the patient (given insurance) and what is efficient for society as a whole is a key element in current concerns over health-care spending. Deductibles and coinsurance can reduce this divergence a little, but the basic problem remains: how to provide insurance without pushing the use of resources to the point at which the additional cost far exceeds the additional benefit.

Increasingly, physicians are being asked to resolve this problem; that is one reason why the issue of "rationing" takes on a new urgency. The pressure to be more economical in the provision of care will force physicians to make decisions that are contrary to the best interests of individual patients, even though these decisions may make a great deal of sense from the viewpoint of society as a whole. Moreover, pressure to control costs will raise explicitly the question of who gets how much care. In the past this question was often answered implicitly by where the patient lived and whether he could pay. In the future, in the interest of maintaining equity while controlling costs, it may be necessary to withhold care from patients who have ample income or complete insurance and who therefore believe that they are entitled to "everything possible." Reim-

bursement methods, such as Medicare's Prospective Payment System plan, that pay a uniform amount for each admission in a diagnosis-related group will tend to redistribute resources away from hospitals that have been providing a great deal of care to those that have been providing less.

A major concern is whether attempts to control the use of health-care resources will affect the health of the population. Opinions differ concerning this question, and no one knows the answer with certainty. Some health experts contend that it is possible to cut expenditures substantially without seriously affecting health. They claim that some care—say, 10 per cent—is actually harmful to patients, that they would be better off without it. It is not difficult to believe that another 10 per cent has a relatively low yield even though there may be a slight benefit. Thus, *if* cuts were concentrated on the 20 per cent that had a negative or low yield, the overall effect on health would be small. But that is a big "if." Two major problems stand in the way of such an outcome. First, much of medical practice lacks a firm, quantified, scientific base; therefore, no one can be certain just which care should be cut. Second, even as clinical experience and systematic research reveal which hospital admissions, operations, x-ray procedures, prescriptions, and the like can be foregone without harm (or even possible benefit) to patients, there is no guarantee that medical practice will be modified accordingly. Media hype, irrational patient preferences, distortional insurance coverage, and perverse incentives for health-care professionals and institutions may result in a pattern of care that is far different from the ideal.

What needs to be done? First, the nation's practitioners, hospitals, and academic medical centers must launch a major effort to identify the benefits that patients receive from the various components of the $400 billion that is spent annually for health care. Second, experts on health-care policy need to continue to press for reforms in organization and finance that will lead patients to want, and health professionals to deliver, more cost-effective care.

Even with more knowledge and better incentives, however, limitation of resources will eventually mean worse health for some patients, even if it changes the probability of complications or survival by only a small fraction. "Low-yield" medicine is not "no-yield" medicine. For physicians to have to face these trade-offs explicitly every day is to assign to them an unreasonable and undesirable burden. The commitment of the individual physician to the individual patient is one of the most valuable features of American medical care. It would therefore be a great mistake to turn each physician into an explicit maximizer of the social-benefit/social-cost ratio in his or her daily practice.

But the trade-offs must be made. Usually the best time for making such decisions is during the evaluation of the costs and benefits of new facilities, the development and diffusion of new technologies, and the training of personnel. As I suggested at the beginning of this essay, physicians have always practiced within constraints, but as long as the "rationing" is implicit, it is tolerable.

In the past, the "system" produced the constraints without a great deal of analysis or a conscious policy choice. In the future, there will be considerably more systematic analyses regarding the location of facilities, investment in equipment, training of specialists, and designing of screening programs and treatment protocols. Health-plan managers, hospital administrators, insurance-company executives, and government officials will use these analyses to help them make difficult decisions about the allocation of scarce resources. This shift in the locus of decision making will inevitably reduce the power of practicing physicians. To the extent that these decisions set the constraints within which individual practitioners function, however, there will be less need for them to ration care to their patients explicitly.

Notes

1. Schwartz, W.B., Aaron, H.J. Rationing hospital care: lessons from Britain. N Engl J Med 1984; 310:52–6.
2. Bombardier, C., Fuchs, V.R., Lillard, L.A., Warner, K.E. Socioeconomic factors affecting the utilization of surgical operations. N Engl J Med 1977; 297:699–705.

The Prostitute, the Playboy, and the Poet: Rationing Schemes for Organ Transplantation

George J. Annas

∎

In the public debate about the availability of heart and liver transplants, the issue of rationing on a massive scale has been credibly raised for the first time in United States medical care. In an era of scarce resources, the eventual arrival of such a discussion was, of course, inevitable.[1] Unless we decide to ban heart and liver transplantation, or make them available to everyone, some rationing scheme must be used to choose among potential transplant candidates. The debate has existed throughout the history of medical ethics. Traditionally it has been stated as a choice between saving one of two patients, both of whom require the immediate assistance of the only available physician to survive.

National attention was focused on decisions regarding the rationing of kidney dialysis machines when they were first used on a limited basis in the late 1960s. As one commentator described the debate within the medical profession:

"Shall machines or organs go to the sickest, or to the ones with most promise of recovery; on a first-come, first-served basis; to the most 'valuable' patient (based on wealth, education, position, what?); to the one with the most dependents; to women and children first; to those who can pay; to whom? Or should lots be cast, impersonally and uncritically?"[2]

In Seattle, Washington, an anonymous screening committee was set up to pick who among competing candidates would receive the life-saving technology. One lay member of the screening committee is quoted as saying:

"The choice were hard . . . I remember voting against a young woman who was a known prostitute. I found I couldn't vote for her, rather than another candidate, a young wife and mother. I also voted against a young man who, until he learned he had renal failure, had been a ne'er do-well, a real playboy. He promised he would reform his character, go back to school, and so on, if only he were selected for treatment. But I felt I'd lived long enough to know that a person like that won't really do what he was promising at the time."[3]

When the biases and selection criteria of the committee were made public, there was a general negative reaction against this type of arbitrary device. Two experts reacted to the "numbing accounts of how close to the surface lie the prejudices and mindless cliches that pollute the committee's deliberations," by concluding that the committee was "measuring persons in accordance with its own middle-class values." The committee process, they noted, ruled out "creative nonconformists" and made the Pacific Northwest "no place for a Henry David Thoreau with bad kidneys."[4]

To avoid having to make such explicit, arbitrary, "social worth" determinations, the Congress, in 1972, enacted legislation that provided federal funds for virtually all kidney dialysis and kidney transplantation procedures in the United States.[5] This decision, however, simply served to postpone the time when identical decisions will have to be made about candidates for heart and liver transplantation in a society that does not provide sufficient financial and medical resources to provide all "suitable" candidates with the operation.

There are four major approaches to rationing scarce medical resources: the market approach; the selection committee approach; the lottery approach; and the "customary" approach.[1]

The Market Approach

The market approach would provide an organ to everyone who could pay for it with their own funds or private insurance. It puts a very high value on individual rights, and a very low value on equality and fairness. It has properly been criticized on a number of bases, including that the transplant technologies have been developed and are supported with public funds, that medical resources used for transplantation will not be available for higher priority care, and that financial success alone is an insufficient justification for demanding a medical procedure. Most telling is its complete lack of concern for fairness and equity.[6]

A "bake sale" or charity approach that requires the less financially fortunate to make public appeals for funding is demeaning to the individuals involved, and to society as a whole. Rationing by financial ability says we do not believe in equality, but believe that a price can and should be placed on human life and that it should be paid by the individual whose life is at stake. Neither belief is tolerable in a society in which income is inequitably distributed.

The Committee Selection Process

The Seattle Selection Committee is a model of the committee process. Ethics Committees set up in some hospitals to decide whether or not certain handicapped newborn infants should be given medical care may represent another.[7]

These committees have developed because it was seen as unworkable or unwise to explicitly set forth the criteria on which selection decisions would be made. But only two results are possible, as Professor Guido Calabresi has pointed out: either a pattern of decision-making will develop or it will not. If a pattern does develop (e.g., in Seattle, the imposition of middle-class values), then it can be articulated and those decision "rules" codified and used directly, without resort to the committee. If a pattern does not develop, the committee is vulnerable to the charge that it is acting arbitrarily, or dishonestly, and therefore cannot be permitted to continue to make such important decisions.[1]

In the end, public designation of a committee to make selection decisions on vague criteria will fail because it too closely involves the state and all members of society in explicitly preferring specific individuals over others, and in devaluing the interests those others have in living. It thus directly undermines, as surely as the market system does, society's view of equality and the value of human life.

The Lottery Approach

The lottery approach is the ultimate equalizer which puts equality ahead of every other value. This makes it extremely attractive, since all comers have an equal chance at selection regardless of race, color, creed, or financial status. On the other hand, it offends our notions of efficiency and fairness since it makes *no* distinctions among such things as the strength of the desires of the candidates, their potential survival, and their quality of life. In this sense it is a mindless method of trying to solve society's dilemma which is caused by its unwillingness or inability to spend enough resources to make a lottery unnecessary. By making this macro spending decision evident to all, it also undermines society's view of the pricelessness of human life. A first-come, first-served system is a type of natural lottery since referral to a transplant program is generally random in time. Nonetheless, higher income groups have quicker access to referral networks and thus have an inherent advantage over the poor in a strict first-come, first-served system.[8,9]

The Customary Approach

Society has traditionally attempted to avoid explicitly recognizing that we are making a choice not to save individual lives because it is too expensive to do so. As long as such decisions are not explicitly acknowledged, they can be tolerated by society. For example, until recently there was said to be a general understanding among general practitioners in Britain that individuals over age 55 suffering from end-stage kidney disease not be referred for dialysis or transplant. In 1984, however, this unwritten practice became highly publicized, with figures that showed a rate of new cases of end-stage kidney disease treated in Britain at 40 per million (versus the US figure of 80 per million) resulting in 1500–3000 "unnecessary deaths" annually.[10] This has, predictably, led to movements to enlarge the National Health Service budget to expand dialysis services to meet this need, a more socially acceptable solution than permitting the now publicly recognized situation to continue.

In the US, the customary approach permits individual physicians to select their patients on the basis of medical criteria or clinical suitability. This, however, contains much hidden social worth criteria. For example, one criterion, common in the transplant literature, requires an individual to have sufficient family support for successful aftercare. This discriminates against individuals without families and those who have become alienated from their families. The criterion may be relevant, but it is hardly medical.

Similar observations can be made about medical criteria that include IQ, mental illness, criminal records, employment, indigency, alcoholism, drug addiction, or geographical location. Age is perhaps more difficult, since it may be impressionistically related to outcome. But it is not medically logical to assume that an individual who is 49 years old is necessarily a better medical candidate for a transplant than one who is 50 years old. Unless specific examination of the characteristics of older persons that make them less desirable candidates is undertaken, such a cut off is arbitrary, and thus devalues the lives of older citizens. The same can be said of blanket exclusions of alcoholics and drug addicts.

In short, the customary approach has one great advantage for society and one great disadvantage: it gives us the illusion that we do not have to make choices; but the cost is mass deception, and when this deception is uncovered, we must deal with it either by universal entitlement or by choosing another method of patient selection.

A Combination of Approaches

A socially acceptable approach must be fair, efficient, and reflective of important social values. The most important values at stake in organ transplantation are fairness itself, equity in the sense of equality, and the value of life. To promote efficiency, it is important that no one receive a transplant unless they want one and are likely to obtain significant benefit from it in the sense of years of life at a reasonable level of functioning.

Accordingly, it is appropriate for there to be an initial screening process that is based *exclusively* on medical criteria designed to measure the probability of a successful transplant, i.e., one in which the patient survives for at least a number of years and is rehabilitated. There is room in medical criteria for social worth judgments, but there is probably no way to avoid this completely. For example, it has been noted that "in many respects social and medical criteria are inextricably intertwined" and that therefore medical criteria might "exclude the poor and disadvantaged because health and socioeconomic status are highly interdependent."[11] Roger Evans gives an example. In the End Stage Renal Disease Program, "those of lower socioeconomic status are likely to have multiple comorbid health conditions such as diabetes, hepatitis, and hypertension" making them both less desirable candidates and more expensive to treat.[11]

To prevent the gulf between the haves and have nots from widening, we must make every reasonable attempt to develop medical criteria that are objective and independent of social worth categories. One minimal way to approach this is to require that medical screening be reviewed and approved by an ethics committee with significant public representation, filed with a public agency, and made readily available to the public for comment. In the event that more than one hospital in a state or region is offering a particular transplant service, it would be most fair and efficient for the individual hospitals to perform the initial medical screening themselves (based on the uniform, objective criteria), but to have all subsequent nonmedical selection done by a method approved by a single selection committee composed of representatives of all hospitals engaged in a particular transplant procedure, as well as significant representation of the public at large.

As this implies, after the medical screening is performed, there may be more acceptable candidates in the "pool" than there are organs or surgical teams to go around. Selection among waiting candidates will then be necessary. This situation occurs now in kidney transplantation, but since the organ matching is much more sophisticated than in hearts and livers (permitting much more precise matching of organ and recipient), and since dialysis permits individuals to wait almost indefinitely for an organ without risking death,

the situations are not close enough to permit use of the same matching criteria. On the other hand, to the extent that organs are specifically tissue- and size-matched and fairly distributed to the best matched candidate, the organ distribution system itself will resemble a natural lottery.

When a pool of acceptable candidates is developed, a decision about who gets the next available, suitable organ must be made. We must choose between using a conscious, value-laden, social worth selection criterion (including a committee to make the actual choice), or some type of random device. In view of the unacceptability and arbitrariness of social worth criteria being applied, implicitly or explicitly, by committee, this method is neither viable nor proper. On the other hand, strict adherence to a lottery might create a situation where an individual who has only a one-in-four chance of living five years with a transplant (but who could survive another six months without one) would get an organ before an individual who could survive as long or longer, but who will die within days or hours if he or she is not immediately transplanted. Accordingly, the most reasonable approach seems to be to allocate organs on a first-come, first-served basis to members of the pool but permit individuals to "jump" the queue if the second level selection committee believes they are in immediate danger of death (but still have a reasonable prospect for long-term survival with a transplant) and the person who would otherwise get the organ can survive long enough to be reasonably assured that he or she will be able to get another organ.

The first-come, first-served method of basic selection (after a medical screen) seems the preferred method because it most closely approximates the randomness of a straight lottery without the obviousness of making equity the only promoted value. Some unfairness is introduced by the fact that the more wealthy and medically astute will likely get into the pool first, and thus be ahead in line, but this advantage should decrease sharply as public awareness of the system grows. The possibility of unfairness is also inherent in permitting individuals to jump the queue, but some flexibility needs to be retained in the system to permit it to respond to reasonable contingencies.

We will have to face the fact that should the resources devoted to organ transplantation be limited (as they are now and are likely to be in the future), at some point it is likely that significant numbers of individuals will die in the pool waiting for a transplant. Three things can be done to avoid this: (1) medical criteria can be made stricter, perhaps by adding a more rigorous notion of "quality" of life to longevity and prospects for rehabilitation; (2) resources devoted to transplantation and organ procurement can be increased; or (3) individuals can be persuaded not to attempt to join the pool.

Of these three options, only the third has the promise of both conserving resources and promoting autonomy. While most persons medically eligible for a transplant would probably want one, some would not—at least if they understood all that was involved, including the need for a lifetime commitment to daily immunosuppression medications, and periodic medical monitoring for rejection symptoms. Accordingly, it makes public policy sense to publicize the risks and side effects of transplantation, and to require careful explanations of the procedure be given to prospective patients *before* they undergo medical screening. It is likely that by the time patients come to the transplant center they have made up their minds and would do almost anything to get the transplant. Nonetheless, if there are patients who, when confronted with all the facts, would voluntarily elect not to proceed, we enhance both their own freedom and the efficiency and cost-effectiveness of the transplantation system by screening them out as early as possible.

Conclusion

Choices among patients that seem to condemn some to death and give others an opportunity to survive will always be tragic. Society has developed a number of mechanisms to make such decisions more acceptable by camouflaging them. In an era of scarce resources and conscious cost containment, such mechanisms will become public, and they will be usable only if they are fair and efficient. If they are not so perceived, we will shift from one mechanism to another in an effort to continue the illusion that tragic choices really don't have to be made, and that we can simultaneously move toward equity of access, quality of services, and cost containment without any challenges to our values. Along with the prostitute, the playboy, and the poet, we all need to be involved in the development of an access model to extreme and expensive medical technologies with which we can live.

Notes

1. Calabresi, G., Bobbitt, P. *Tragic Choices.* New York: Norton, 1978.
2. Fletcher, J. Our shameful waste of human tissue. *In: Cutler* DR (ed): The Religious Situation. Boston: Beacon Press, 1969; 223–252.
3. Quoted in Fox, R., Swazey, J. *The Courage to Fail.* Chicago: Univ of Chicago Press, 1974; 232.
4. Sanders & Dukeminier: Medical advance and legal lag: hemodialysis and kidney transplantation. UCLA L Rev 1968; 15:357.
5. Rettig, R.A. The policy debate on patient care financing for victims of end stage renal disease. Law & Contemporary Problems 1976; 40:196.
6. President's Commission for the Study of Ethical Problems in Medicine: *Securing Access to Health Care.* US Govt Printing Office, 1983; 25.
7. Annas, G.J. Ethics committees on neonatal care: substantive protection or procedural diversion? Am J Public Health 1984; 74:843–845.
8. Bayer, R. Justice and health care in an era of cost containment: allocating scarce medical resources. Soc Responsibility 1984; 9:37–52.
9. Annas, G.J. Allocation of artificial hearts in the year

2002: *Minerva v National Health Agency.* Am J Law
Med 1977; 3:59–76.

10. Commentary: UK's poor record in treatment of renal
failure. Lancet July 7, 1984; 53.

11. Evans, R. Health care technology and the inevitability
of resource allocation and rationing decisions, Part II.
JAMA 1983; 249:2208, 2217.

Ethics of Queuing for Coronary Artery Bypass Grafting in Canada

Jafna L. Cox

■

The primary objective of Canadian health care policy is "to facilitate reasonable access to health services without financial or other barriers."[1] However, Canada's assets are finite. Limits on health care funding have resulted in rationing by queue when fixed medical resources have not met demand. Although a policy of managed delay is preferable to one of restricted access, there are major concerns about patient safety and justice. Furthermore, rationing engenders a conflict between a physician's traditional responsibility to the individual patient and the exigencies of medical practice in the universal health care system, wherein a broader responsibility to society is required. This conflict cannot be reconciled at the bedside.

The process currently used to queue patients for coronary artery bypass grafting (CABG) in Canada provides an ideal paradigm for reviewing these issues. It follows explicit, physician-established guidelines based on medical need and includes peer review to ensure their just application. This strategy allows rational selection of patients with low vital risk and, I will argue, an ethical solution to the dilemma of competing physician responsibilities to individual patients and to society.

Limits on Access to CABG in Canada

In 1988–89, a dramatic increase in referrals for CABG in Canada overtook caseload growth.[2] Patients across the country waited a mean of 22.6 weeks for elective surgery,[3] and some died. Although government provided funding to augment surgical capacity[4] a mismatch between CABG demand and supply persisted.

Canadian physicians endeavoured to obtain timely surgery for their patients. However, approaches to queuing patients were inconsistent.[4] In Toronto, interhospital differences in mean wait times were as great as 8 weeks. In the hospital with the shortest queues, patients referred by offsite cardiologists waited twice as long as similar ones referred by their onsite colleagues.[5] Similarly, in British Columbia analysts noted an "impressive lack" of coordinated patient referral.[6]

Panacea of Increased Funding

Canadian physicians would prefer not to have to queue their patients. A theoretically attractive expedient is yet more spending to expand surgical facilities. But bypass surgery is costly, ranging from $10,982 to $33,676 with a mean of $14,328 in 1988 Canadian dollars,[7] and health care is only one of many competing social programs that government must finance.

Waste and poor management exist. However, more efficient management is unlikely, by itself, to obviate the need for rationing:[8] the Canadian health care system is expensive despite efficient management (administrative fees being half those in the United States[9]), yet queues persist.

More important, increased medical spending to expand services does not inevitably result in better health. Greater availability of revascularization facilities leads to increased service use despite unclear survival benefit.[10,11] Indeed, revascularization facilities and procedures in Can-

ada are few only by comparison with those in the United States.[12]

Solution of Patient Prioritization

Canadian physicians dealt with CABG queues by developing a more efficient referral process, including a rational system of assessing patient priority. This evolved, with regional modifications, from triage guidelines published in 1990 by a consensus panel.[13] In general, patients are referred, and an urgency ranking based on explicit clinical and diagnostic criteria is requested. A conference of cardiovascular specialists uses these same guidelines to review the suitability and relative urgency of surgery among all patients referred and hence ensures appropriate order in the queue. Although the process may have improved, concerns persist about its safety and fairness.

Safety of Queuing Patients for CABG

Highly publicized anecdotal accounts of patients dying while awaiting surgery neglect the immediate and delayed risks of the procedure itself.[6] In California hundreds of excess deaths result from readily available CABG at low-volume (hence high-risk) centres, and Wikler[14] questions whether in Canada the number of excess deaths due to queuing is greater.

Appropriately applied guidelines can distinguish between patients requiring immediate care and those at lower risk.[15–17] The vital risk of a 6-week wait in a patient with mild to moderate stable angina, three-vessel disease and impaired left ventricular function is approximately 0.25%.[18] This is also the average risk of death from medical negligence during hospitalization, as documented in the Harvard-New York State Medical Practice Study.[18]

Indeed, the true clinical impact of the queue is unlikely to show up as excess patient deaths or major complications.[15–16] Rather, what need to be assessed are the effects on patients of persistent symptoms and the frustration and anxiety associated with waiting, as well as the hidden social and economic costs of ongoing (often intensive) medical care, lost work days and sick benefits.[4] Anxiety could be lessened through broader appreciation that most CABG is palliative, that the vital risk associated with waiting is consequently small, and that ongoing stable symptoms need not relate to prognosis.[19]

Justice of Queuing Patients for CABG

Although CABG queues have gained particular notoriety, access to health care has always been circumscribed.[4,20] Financial factors impede access in the United States, where some 58 million people were without medical insurance at some time in 1992.[21] In Canada, implicit nonfinancial rationing in the form of queues exists instead.[22]

There is nothing inherently wrong with rationing, especially by means of queues that delay but do not deny access altogether.[22] However, the process must be safe, fair and justifiable not simply economically but also medically and ethically.[23] The law does not proscribe selection by preset, explicit allocation criteria that are rational and nondiscriminatory.[24]

Physicians tend to allocate scarce health care resources according to medical need.[25–28] Ethicists may argue whether this is the most reasonable precept to follow, but it is legally and ethically sound if the medical judgements are defensible.[27–31] According to Sulmasy,[30] physicians may be wrong in their judgements, but unless culpably ignorant they cannot be held to be acting unjustly. To ensure procedural justice and hence equal treatment of similar patients, guidelines should preferably be set and administered at higher levels of social organization (e.g., by a committee of peers).[29–31] The efficacy of a given therapy for a given patient is another morally relevant criterion.[32] The appropriate balance of urgency (patient need) and efficacy (likelihood of therapeutic success) is a critical issue for any allocation system.

When medical utility and the probability of success are roughly equal among candidates, rationing systems generally use length of wait as the fairest way to make the final selection.[33] Although imperfect, this rule of "first come, first served" has legal and ethical sanction.[31,34,35] Criticism that the process does not compensate for such impediments as distance from and ease of travel to a medical centre, which might influence one's position on the queue,[36] is less compelling in Canada, where regionalization of cardiovascular surgical services minimizes such potential inequities in access.

Principles of medical utility and of "first come, first served" are used to build the CABG queue in Canada. All medically deserving patients are considered equally, but the sickest—for whom the procedure can make the greatest difference—receive precedence.

Challenges to Queuing for CABG

Most commonly, challenges to queuing arise from patients or their physicians seeking shorter wait times. Patients have sought to jump the queue on the basis of personal connections, professional courtesy and social merit, the latter having been proposed as a possible criterion for allocating scarce resources.[31] However, decisions based on social merit are difficult to justify given the lack of an acceptable method for assessing relative social worth. By arbitrarily prolonging the anxiety and frustration of patients passed over as well as increasing the risk associated with extended waiting, queue jumping on the basis of personal connections or professional courtesy is indefensible.

Some argue that by providing patients with therapy at different times queuing is unfair. An egalitarian theory of justice in the distribution of health care has been proposed by Rawls[37] and by Young[35] and Daniels.[36] In its most radical form, this theory holds that any deviation from absolute equality in distribution, including differences in wait time for therapy, is unjust. However, Kluge[38] offers a compelling rebuttal that emphasizes "equity rather than equality," since the provision of equal health care services to patients with unequal needs only perpetuates an unjustified inequity. Furthermore, the Canada Health Act promises "reasonable" and not "equal" access.

A different challenge comes from those willing to pay for prompt surgery. Libertarians argue that economic and social benefits should be allotted in proportion to a person's contribution to those benefits, and they support the distribution of health care services according to ability to pay.[26,39] However, this view runs counter to Canadian health care policy, which strives to eliminate financial barriers in access to health care.[1,22,40] Recent work suggests that the ability to pay led to queue jumping and hence unjust access to heart and liver transplantation in the United States in the late 1980s.[41]

Ultimately, the challenge to queuing comes from patients' demands for a right to specific and prompt treatment or from demands by physicians for a right to manage patients how and when they see fit. These individual rights may conflict with the rights of other individuals needing medical care, with the professionals involved in distributing that care or with society as a whole.[25] Indeed, to the extent that maximizing the care of an individual either restricts the resources available to others or drives up costs for others, there will be a conflict between that individual and society, which is itself a collection of individuals with their own perceived rights.[42] Comparative justice demands a fair share, not an excessive one.[26] Physicians invoking a right to manage patients as they see fit are faced with

David Eddy's[43] question: "Who gave physicians that right?"

Ethical Dilemma: Physicians and Queuing

Physicians in a universal health care system face an ethical dilemma arising out of conflicting responsibilities to the individual patient and to society. A fiduciary relationship compels physicians to advocate on behalf of their patients, and many clinicians consider unethical any intrusion of economic considerations. However, whether costs are interpreted as a financial or other kind of sacrifice, the investment of resources on one patient comes at the expense of another. To ignore this cost imposed on another individual is itself unethical.[44] Moreover, competition between individual physicians advocating on behalf of individual patients in a constrained health care system can be detrimental, as highlighted by the discrepant referral practices that exacerbated the CABG crisis in the late 1980s.

Analogous to the traditional doctor-patient relationship, there is a public health model under which physicians have obligations to people who are not their patients.[28] Moreover, physicians cannot simultaneously be advocates of their patients and also serve as financial guardians of society without incurring divided loyalties and ethical peril.[28,30,35,45]

Indeed, the traditional ethic of the physician's responsibility to the patient cannot be adequately reconciled with the countervailing demands of social justice in a health care system promising universal access to limited resources. Hence, the conference of specialists is important as a gatekeeper, a forum for debating which priority should prevail. When physicians disagree in matters of clinical judgement but agree on the principle of mobilizing resources for the good of each patient according to need, unequal treatment of similar patients may occur without injustice.[27,28] This does not imply that choosing one patient over another should be easy or free from guilt. However, peer review permits impartial assessment and broader opinion, and it safeguards equal treatment of similar patients; at the same time more efficient patient processing results in decreased illness and death among those on waiting lists. Consensus judgement additionally provides a legal defence for triage decisions.

The health care system in Canada has promised its consumers reasonable access to all appropriate services. As stakeholders, physicians should work in concert with their colleagues to uphold that ideal. This does not imply that physicians should become agents of public or economic policy with cost-effectiveness as the only relevant consideration. Rather, they should continue to design guidelines for the just distribution of scarce health care resources, since it is through the efficient and effective management of medical services that benefits to both the individual and society can be maximized.

Because any universal system must allow for variation in individual perceptions of need, in that different values are placed on each disability or condition, physicians must remain patients' advocates. They can thereby ensure that guidelines are relevant to the specific needs of patients and, moreover, that such guidelines have been fairly applied. Appropriate physician advocacy on behalf of patients, together with a committee of physicians acting as gatekeepers in accordance with explicit guidelines, will provide an ethical mechanism for balancing competing claims to limited resources. Thus, within the constraints on health resource availability physicians remain free to promote the interests of their patients. At the same time, consensus guidelines and peer review, through the committee, protect the interests of society by imposing reasonable limits on what might be done and when. Although this represents some loss of physician autonomy over the management of the individual

patient there is a corresponding broadening of responsibility toward society.[43]

Finally, as much as they must restrain demagogic attitudes and inflammatory responses to allocation problems, physicians should avoid the trap of becoming silent queue managers. Queuing can be performed fairly and at low risk given an adequate level of medical services. There is a danger, however, that government may withhold the funds needed to maintain or expand such services on the mistaken assumption that current triage efforts will continue to be effective. Physicians and their patients must determine how much of a given medical service is adequate in terms of minimizing patient risk and discomfort; guidelines should be modified accordingly. They are duty bound to speak up when resources are so restricted that queues put patients at risk or make their discomfort intolerable.

Conclusion

Queues provide an imperfect but practical solution whenever fixed resources cannot meet demand. They are defensible if considered a temporary delay in the delivery of a service and if there is no significant adverse effect on patient health. Indeed, a policy of managed delay has advantages over systems of financial rationing, which may deny access altogether. Rationing decisions are difficult, but queuing is ethical if based on medical need and if patients understand the process, its rationale and the low associated risk. Competing responsibilities to patients and society may present physicians with an ethical dilemma. However, although their primary obligation is to their patients, their collective responsibility is to establish and follow guidelines that ensure an appropriate level of care as well as efficient and equitable allocation of available resources. Since increased funding is doubtful, physician cooperation in the rational distribution of scarce health commodities will be needed to preserve the ideal of a universal health care system. Nevertheless, rather than simply manage queues physicians must remain vigilant against cuts in medical services that would unacceptably put patients at risk.

Notes

I am indebted to Dr. C. David Naylor and Professor Arthur Schafer for reviewing the manuscript and providing helpful comments. However, the views expressed are mine, and responsibility for them rests solely with me.

1. *Canada Health Act,* RSC 1985, c6, s3
2. Ugnat, A.M., Naylor, C.D. Trends in coronary artery bypass grafting in Ontario from 1981 to 1989. *Can Med Assoc J* 1993; 148: 569–575
3. Higginson, L.A.J., Cairns, J.A., Keon, W.J. et al. Rates of cardiac catheterization, coronary angioplasty and open-heart surgery in adults in Canada. *Can Med Assoc J* 1992; 146: 921–925
4. Naylor, C.D. A different view of queues in Ontario. *Health Aff (Millwood)* 1991; 10: 110–128
5. Naylor, C.D., Levinton, C.M., Wheeler, S.M. et al. Queuing for coronary surgery during severe supply–demand mismatch in a Canadian referral centre: a case study of implicit rationing. *Soc Sci Med* 1993; 37(1): 61–67
6. Katz, S.I., Mizgala, H.F., Welch, G. British Columbia sends patients to Seattle for coronary artery surgery: bypassing the queue in Canada. *JAMA* 1991; 266: 1108–1111
7. Krueger, H., Goncalves, J.L., Caruth, F.M. et al. Coronary artery bypass grafting: How much does it cost? *Can Med Assoc J* 1992; 146: 163–168
8. Brook, R.H., Lohr, K.N.G. Will we need to ration effective health care? *Issues Sci Technol* 1986; 3: 68–77
9. Woolhandler, S., Himmelstein, D.U. The deteriorating administrative efficiency of the US health care system. *N Engl J Med* 1991; 324: 1253–1258
10. Every, N.R., Larson, E.B., Litwin, P.E. et al. The association between on-site cardiac catheterization facilities and the use of coronary angiography after acute myocardial infarction. *N Engl J Med* 1993; 329: 546–551
11. Cox, J.L., Chen, C., Naylor, C.D. Revascularization after acute myocardial infarction: Impact of hospital teaching status and on-site invasive facilities. *J Gen Int Med* 1994.
12. Collins-Nakai, R.L., Huysmans, H.A., Scully, H.E. Access to cardiovascular care: an international comparison. *J Am Coll Cardiol* 1992; 19: 1477–1485
13. Naylor, C.D., Baigrie, R.S., Goldman, B.S. et al. Revascularisation Panel and Consensus Methods Group: Assessment of priority for coronary revascularisation procedures. *Lancet* 1990; 335: 1070–1073
14. Wikler, D. Ethics and rationing: "Whether", "how", or "how much"? *J Am Geriatr Soc* 1992; 40: 398–403
15. Cox, J.L., Petrie, J.F., Pollak, P.T. et al. Is queuing for coronary artery bypass surgery safe? A Canadian perspective. [abstract] *Circulation* 1993; 88(4 pt 2): I-10
16. Naylor, G.D., Morgan, C.D., Levinton, C.M. et al. Waiting for coronary revascularization in Toronto: 2 years' experience with a regional referral office. *Can Med Assoc J* 1993; 149: 955–962
17. Morris, A.L., Roos, L.L., Brazauskas, R. et al. Managing scarce services: a waiting list approach to cardiac catheterization. *Med Care* 1990; 28: 784–792
18. Rachlis, M.M., Olak, J., Naylor, C.D. The vital risk of delayed coronary surgery: lessons from the randomized trials. *Iatrogenics* 1991; 1: 103–111
19. Cox, J., Naylor, C.D. The Canadian Cardiovascular Society grading scale for angina of effort: Is it time for refinements? *Ann Intern Med* 1992; 117: 677–683
20. Blank, R.H. Rationing medicine: hard choices in the 1990s. *Am J Gastroenterol* 1992; 87: 1076–1084
21. Swartz, K. Dynamics of people without health insurance: Don't let the numbers fool you. *JAMA* 1994; 271: 64–66
22. Naylor, C.D. The Canadian health care system: A model for America to emulate? *Health Economics* 1992; 1: 19–37
23. Relman, A.S. The trouble with rationing. *N Engl J Med* 1990; 323: 911–913
24. Sanders, D., Jesse, D. Jr. Medical advance and legal lag. Hemodialysis and kidney transplantation. *UCLA Law Review* 1968; 15: 366–380
25. Horvath, D.G. The ethics of resource allocation. *Med J Aust* 1990; 153: 437–438
26. Beauchamp, T.L., Childress, J.F. *Principles of Biomedical Ethics,* 3rd ed, Oxford University Press, New York, 1989: 256–306
27. Ashley, B.M., O'Rourke, K.D. *Health Care Ethics: a Theological Analysis,* Catholic Association of the United States, St Louis, Mo, 1982: 239–242
28. Macklin, R. *Mortal choices: Ethical Dilemmas in Modern Medicine,* Houghton Mifflin Company, Boston, 1987: 149–181
29. Edwards, R.B., Graber, G.C. *Bio-Ethics,* Harcourt Brace Jovanovich, Publishers, San Diego, 1988: 699–713

30. Sulmasy, D.P. Physicians, cost control, and ethics. *Ann Intern Med* 1992; 116: 920–926

31. Rescher, N. The allocation of exotic medical lifesaving therapy. *Ethics* 1969; 79: 173–186

32. Kilner, J.F. *Who Lives? Who Dies? Ethical Criteria and Patient Selection.* Yale University Press, New Haven, Conn, 1990

33. Task Force on Organ Transplantation: *Organ Transplantation: Issues and Recommendations,* US Department of Health and Human Services, Apr 1986

34. Childress, J.F. Who shall live when not all can live? *Soundings* 1970; 53: 339–355

35. Young, R. Some criteria for making decisions concerning the distribution of scarce medical resources. *Theory and Decision* 1975; 6: 439–455

36. Daniels, N. *Just Health Care,* Cambridge University Press, Cambridge, England, 1985

37. Rawls, J. *A Theory of Justice,* Harvard University Press, Cambridge, Mass, 1971

38. Kluge, E.-H.W. *Biomedical Ethics in a Canadian Context,* Prentice-Hall, Scarborough, Ont, 1992: 206–235

39. Sade, R.M. Medical care as a right: a refutation. *N Engl J Med* 1971; 285: 1288–1292

40. Evans, R.G. The real issues. *J Health Polit Policy Law* 1992; 17: 739–762

41. Ozminkowski, R.J., Friedman, B., Taylor, Z. Access to heart and liver transplantation in the late 1980s. *Med Care* 1993; 31: 1027–1042

42. Eddy, D.M. The individual vs society: Is there a conflict? *JAMA* 1991; 265: 1446, 1449–1450

43 Eddy, D.M. Broadening the responsibilities of practitioners: the team approach. *JAMA* 1993; 269: 1849–1855

44. Williams, A. Cost-effectiveness analysis: is it ethical? *J Med Ethics* 1992; 18: 7–11

45. Pellegrino, E.D. Rationing health care: the ethics of medical gatekeeping. *J Contemp Health Law Policy* 1986; 2: 23–45

Rationing in Practice:
The Case of In Vitro Fertilisation
Sharon Redmayne and Rudolf Klein

■

Explicit decisions by purchasers to stop offering specific forms of treatment, on the Oregon model,[1] are still very much the exception in the National Health Service. For the most part rationing takes the traditional, less visible, form of limiting the resources that are available for particular services and leaving it to doctors to determine priorities between different procedures and patients. There are, however, exceptions. One such is in vitro fertilisation. Analysis of 114 purchasing plans for 1992–3 found six authorities which explicitly stated that they would not be buying any in vitro fertilisation or gamete intrafallopian transfer treatment for their populations.[2] At the same time, other purchasers were continuing to buy in vitro fertilisation and, some were even planning to put extra money into the service.

The case of in vitro fertilisation therefore provides an intriguing, and rare, opportunity to explore the way in which such explicit rationing decisions are reached. In vitro fertilisation produces results, although there is some debate about its success rate and about the circumstances in which its use is appropriate.[3] In contrast to procedures like tattoo removal (struck off the National Health Service menu by seven purchasing authorities), it cannot be seen as a response to a self inflicted injury or as a tribute to vanity. Furthermore, the use of in vitro fertilisation is widespread in Europe: in France its use is reimbursed by the social security system, and in Belgium, Denmark, and Norway the state will bear most or all of the cost.[4]

Why, then, do purchasers disagree about the desirability of buying this procedure? What evidence and arguments were used in coming to these decisions? What local circumstances or pressures influenced the decision to buy or not to buy? And can any general insights into the dilemmas and problems of rationing be derived from this specific case?

To answer these questions, we compare three purchasing authorities which decided not to buy in vitro fertilisation with three others which took the opposite decision. In each case our account is based on the documents produced by the authorities and informed by the views of relevant health authority officials, who were either interviewed or contacted by letter. These are in no sense a sample. Apart from anything else, we do not know how many purchasers have quietly decided not to offer in vitro fertilisation without making their views explicit. All six authorities are gainers, if to differing degrees, under the weighted capitation formula. The differences between them cannot therefore be explained by variations in resource constraints.

Non-Purchasers of In Vitro Fertilisation

Health Authority A

This first health authority provides a subfertility service but not in vitro fertilisation or gamete intrafallopian transfer. The scope of the infertility service was one of the issues discussed at the authority's "choices for health day," which brought together a range of interested professionals to rank a list of bids for development money. They decided that in vitro fertilisation

would not be offered because of its cost: the health authority, it was argued, should not spend so much money on people who were not "ill." The view was not unanimous: the women were generally more sympathetic to the case for in vitro fertilisation than the men. They argued that the mental distress of being infertile should be taken into account and that the people of the district should have the choice available to them.

The health authority decided that while people on the waiting list for in vitro fertilisation in 1992–3 should still be seen the treatment would thereafter be provided only as an extra contractual referral. In practice, however the authority has been turning down such extracontractual referrals. Several factors have influenced the authority in this stance, quite apart from the views of the "choices for health day" meeting. The general practitioners are happy with current service provision and are not exerting any pressure to extend it. Neighbouring health authorities do not provide in vitro fertilisation either. There is also a general feeling that, since the district is relatively affluent, people can afford to be treated privately.

Health Authority B

As part of its assisted conception services the second health authority provides donor insemination and intrauterine insemination but no in vitro fertilisation or gamete intrafallopian transfer. It has deliberately decided against purchasing in vitro fertilisation because of cost. The nearest provider unit charges about £2000 per cycle. In contrast, donor insemination costs £70 per cycle. Instead of buying in vitro fertilisation, the authority has therefore decided to strengthen its donor insemination services. Requests for in vitro fertilisation under the extra contractual referral procedure are turned down.

The authority's reasoning is that equity demands that any service provided should give everyone requiring treatment a fair chance of getting it. To buy only a few cycles of in vitro fertilisation is therefore unfair. Also, the authority does not consider that in vitro fertilisation represents good value for money. Although the success rate of in vitro fertilisation is actually better than for donor insemination in terms of babies produced, the cost per birth is higher. Moreover, for every cycle of in vitro fertilisation, which has a one in four chance of success, a new hip can be bought.

So far, the authority's decision about in vitro fertilisation has brought no backlash from the local community. There does not appear to be either a community or a professional lobby pressing for the purchase of in vitro fertilisation. If there were a groundswell of opinion the authority would reconsider its position.

Authority C

Authority C differs from the previous two in that it did not decide explicitly against providing in vitro fertilisation but simply gave it a low priority. It was originally included in the list of purchasing developments for 1992–3, but it was not high enough on the list of priorities to justify additional funds. In vitro fertilisation is thus excluded from the authority's contracts, although it can be made available through extra contractual referrals. In effect in vitro fertilisation has become a casualty of the competitive battle for resources.

Not surprisingly, given this decision making process, there has been no extensive discussion or assessment of in vitro fertilisation in this district. The authority has largely drawn on the results of national research and appears to have been strongly influenced by the director of public health's view that the clinical effectiveness of in vitro fertilisation treatment is generally low.

Purchasers of In Vitro Fertilisation

Authority D

Authority D decided to buy in vitro fertilisation as part of a whole range of fertility services. It calculated that it would cost £280 000 per year to provide subfertility treatment for all the residents who might present, but it could afford to put only £150 000 into the service. So it decided to fund 20 in vitro fertilisation cycles, agreeing with the providers on the criteria to be used in choosing the beneficiaries. It also agreed with the provider on the number of embryos to be used in order to limit the number of multiple births and the pressure on maternity services.

Local circumstances clearly influenced this decision. A local provider of in vitro fertilisation is already in place, and the unit is highly regarded and has strong support among clinicians. The consultant in charge of the infertility service is also an effective lobbyist.

Members of the authority played an active role in the decision, examining the evidence about the extent of infertility problems in the community and the medical evidence about the effectiveness of in vitro fertilisation. Four considerations appear to have determined their views.

Firstly, they concluded that infertility can cause psychological harm as well as marital difficulties. Secondly, they attached much importance to the role of the family. Thirdly, they saw themselves as having a moral obligation to put more money into their subfertility package for in vitro fertilisation since, at the other end of the scale, they purchase abortions, sterilisations, and contraception services. To spend additional money preventing babies being born without also doing likewise to help the infertile was felt to be ethically unjustifiable. Fourthly, they believed that it would breach the National Health Service's principle of equality of access to deny in vitro fertilisation treatment of local women when it is available in other districts.

Authority E

Authority E came into being only in April 1993, as the result of the amalgamation of three districts, and decided to purchase about 62 cycles of in vitro fertilisation in 1993–4. There are 24 in vitro fertilisation centres within acceptable travelling distance, whose costs range from £498 to £2546, excluding drugs, so the authority is inviting tenders from these providers. Each centre has been asked to supply information on outcomes, numbers of treatment cycles, and patient selection to help the authority in choosing the most cost effective options.

This authority's decision reflects its view that subfertility is a health care problem with very definite physiological, psychological, and social implications. It also differs from the decisions made by other authorities in that it was based on an elaborate needs assessment exercise carried out by the public health department.

The report that emerged from this exercise integrated epidemiological evidence, the results of a survey of consultants in obstetrics and gynecology, and information from local in vitro fertilisation centres. It estimated, on the basis of a survey of the evidence by the *Effective Health Care Bulletin*,[3] that about 333 women a year would need in vitro fertilisation or gamete intrafallopian transfer but recommended that only in vitro fertilisation should be bought. The report argued that gamete intrafallopian transfer did not have in vitro fertilisation's advantage of detecting poor fertilisation and bypassing tubal damage.

The authority subsequently carried out a survey of consultants to establish local need and decided to buy 62 cycles of in vitro fertilisation. This still left the question of how those limited resources should be allocated—for example, what rationing principles should be used. Here

the decision has been to use two criteria: age and family size. Women over 40 will be excluded because the success of in vitro fertilisation decreases with age, and only couples who have no children or only one child will be considered. The final selection will be made by the consultant in charge, and there will be a maximum of two cycles per patient. In addition, purchasers and providers are to produce shared protocols for general practitioners, consultants, and the specialist centres to improve the investigation and treatment of subfertility.

Authority F

The last authority decided to fund in vitro fertilisation and gamete intrafallopian transfer for the first time ever in 1993–4, although it has not yet fixed the budgetary allocation. Previously it had refused to provide funding because of doubts about effectiveness in the early pioneering years, concern about possible side effects, and the belief that the treatments, as new technologies, should be developed and tested more centrally.

The decision to change policy reflects the influence of two factors. Firstly, local pressure groups have been vociferous in pressing the authority to fund in vitro fertilisation and gamete intrafallopian transfer. Secondly, a policy review carried out by the authority's public health departments dispelled some of the earlier doubts about effectiveness.

The policy review estimated that about 270 couples a year would require subfertility services, of whom some 50 might benefit from in vitro fertilisation. It also recognised, however, that the high Asian population in the area may make the demand on the service greater. As in authority E, demand is therefore likely to exceed supply, thus raising, once again, the question of selection. No formal criteria for in vitro fertilisation treatment have yet been laid down. But current discussions suggest that criteria for selection are likely to include primary versus secondary infertility, and prognosis. In addition, a local protocol for managing subfertility has been developed with general practitioners and obstetricians in the hope that this will save money by reducing unnecessary and repeated investigations.

The Dynamics of Rationing

Our six cameo case studies do not purport to illustrate the whole range of decision making among purchasers. But they do identify some of the main issues. Firstly, they suggest the importance of local champions for any given service or procedure. In vitro fertilisation is more likely to be purchased in those authorities where there is a local provider and, thus, a local constituency of support. Pressure from general practitioners and the community is another factor that influences purchasing authorities. Such influence may work both positively and negatively: if there is no pressure authorities may conclude that there is no demand.

Secondly, the case studies also indicate the importance of public health departments, both as the interpreters of the evidence about effectiveness and value for money and as assessors of need.

Thirdly, however, the case studies show some differences of opinion about what should count as a need when it comes to allocating resources—for example, where the frontiers of the National Health Service's responsibilities should be drawn. This issue is also raised by decisions not to buy various cosmetic procedures. Thus authority A was not prepared to spend money on individuals who were not perceived to be really "ill." In contrast, the purchasers of in vitro fertilisation believed that there was a health need which had to be addressed. They were convinced by the arguments of the Royal College of Obstetricians and Gynaecologists[5] and others[6] that the inability to have children can cause psy-

chological distress and damage—that the "pain of childlessness is every bit as great as that of osteoarthritis of the hip."[7]

Effectiveness

Fourthly, those authorities which accept that infertility does represent a legitimate claim on National Health Service resources then had to ask whether in vitro fertilisation was the best way of meeting that need. In considering this question the authorities had to address questions of effectiveness. A recent *Effective Health Care Bulletin* on the management of subfertility concluded that techniques such as in vitro fertilisation are quite effective, although this is often offset by poor organisation of the service.[3] Success rates have increased over the past few years,[8] and one study concluded that in couples where the woman was under 40 and the man had normal sperm a pregnancy rate of 30% per cycle had been achieved by 1991.[9]

Fifthly, however, showing that a treatment is effective—in the sense of producing results—does not necessarily demonstrate that it should be purchased. Inevitably such decisions merge with questions of value for money, and this involves comparison with other claims on resources. Questions also arise about whether such comparisons should be made solely in terms of the relative cost-effectiveness of different treatments within the same field (in vitro fertilisation or donor insemination?) or whether they should be made between treatments in different fields (in vitro fertilisation or hips?). Whichever sort of comparison is done it seems to demand a rough and ready assessment of the relative health gains produced by different interventions. The case studies suggest that authorities do not make such systematic comparisons—no doubt because the required information is not available. Quality adjusted life years-style analyses were conspicuous by their absence.

Sixthly, the case studies illustrate two quite different types of rationing decisions. On the one hand, there are decisions about how much to allocate to a particular type of activity. On the other hand, having decided to support a particular type of activity an authority then has to decide who to treat when supply falls short of demand. Even authorities which are buying in vitro fertilisation have to make the second type of decision. Interestingly, too, the case studies suggest that—in the case of in vitro fertilisation at least—authorities are beginning to become involved in devising criteria and protocols for allocating treatment to individual patients. This trend can be expected to become more general.

Equity

Lastly, the case studies raise some fundamental questions for the National Health Service. Does the principle of equity of access require that everyone should have an equal chance of treatment irrespective of where he or she lives? Both authority B and authority D assumed that it did, though they drew diametrically opposed conclusions. And if equity does demand an equal chance of treatment (at least once a treatment has passed the experimental stage) does this mean, in turn, that rationing decisions should be made nationally, since it cannot be left to individual purchasers to determine what services should or should not be available? Again, in determining priorities, how legitimate is it for health authorities to take into account the availability of services in the private sector? Does not the fact that an estimated 90% of births achieved through in vitro fertilisation in the United Kingdom (though not all in United Kingdom nationals) are the result of private treatment[10] offend against the principle of equity? And if so, are we not once again left with the uncomfortable conclusion that equity demands that a service should be provided either universally—at least in the sense of giving everyone the same statistical chance of access—or not at all?

These questions, to which the answers are far from self evident, are prompted by the case of in vitro fertilisation. They demonstrate, however, that the issues raised by in vitro fertilisation range far beyond this particular treatment and need to be addressed in the context of the National Health Service as a whole.

Notes

The research on which this essay draws is funded by the Nuffield Provincial Hospitals Trust.

1. Klein, R. Warning signals from Oregon. *BMJ* 1992; 304:1457–8.
2. Klein, R., Redmayne, S. *Patterns of priorities*. Birmingham: NAHAT, 1992.
3. *The management of subfertility*. Leeds: School of Public Health, Leeds University, 1992 (*Effective Health Care Bulletin* No 3).
4. Gunning, J. *Human IVF, embryo research, fetal tissue for research and treatment, and abortion: international information*. London: HMSO, 1990.
5. Fertility Committee, Royal College of Obstetricians and Gynaecologists. *Infertility: guidelines for practice*. London: RCOG Press, 1992.
6. Mazor, M.D. Emotional reactions to infertility. In: Mazor, M.D., Simons, H.F., eds. *Infertility: medical, emotional, and social considerations*. New York: Human Sciences Press Inc, 1984:29–39.
7. Pain of childlessness. *BMJ* 1991;302:1345.
8. Human Fertilisation and Embryology Authority. *Annual report*. London: HMSO, 1992.
9. Hull, M.G.R., Eddowes, H.A., Fahy, U., Abuzeid, M.I., Mills, M.S., Cahill, D.J. et al. Expectations of assisted conception for infertility. *BMJ* 1992;304:1465–9.
10. Hunt, L. Infertility units face struggle for survival. *Independent*, 1992; 2 Nov:4, cols 1–7.

Managed Care and the

Physician's Changing Role

the potential for conflict and which forms diminish it? What ethical guidelines are needed to deal with the inevitable problems that arise when physicians strive to benefit a population of subscribers to a health care plan as well as serve the needs of particular patients? And how will managed care alter the relationships among physicians themselves, especially those between primary care physicians and specialists?

Managed care (more completely defined in the introductory essay for part V and in Donald Madison's essay, which opens it) changes the traditional basis of medical practice based on indemnity and fee-for-service by integrating the financing and delivery of medical services, with the aim of controlling costs and improving quality. Managed care changes and complicates the doctor's role by adding new responsibilities—for the patient population as a group and for the managed care organization—to his or her traditional responsibility for individual patients. There are monetary incentives for the physician who follows efficient and costworthy practices.

All the readings in this section examine the conflicts that arise as doctors sort out these multiple loyalties. Gail Povar and Jonathan Moreno, while they recognize risks, are optimistic about the possibility of retaining a traditional medical ethic in an HMO setting. Arnold Relman, by contrast, sees great dangers in the business norms evident in many current cost containment strategies. Ezekiel Emanuel and Nancy Neveloff Dubler present an "ideal conception of the physician-patient relationship," and analyze how managed care can both diminish and enhance the potential for such ideal relationships.

At least three questions of special importance remain: Which forms of managed care heighten

Hippocrates and the Health Maintenance Organization: A Discussion of Ethical Issues

Gail Povar and Jonathan Moreno

■

Since the Health Maintenance Organization (HMO) Act of 1973 provided HMOs with both financial and regulatory support, these organizations have enjoyed a broad spectrum of political advocacy. Three important assumptions underlie this support.

First, HMOs can control costs. Studies over the last 20 years, spanning various regions and different populations, have found that HMOs can provide care for 25% less than the fee-for-service system (1). Although HMOs may find it difficult to maintain this differential, such cost savings are achieved primarily by reducing patient hospitalization (2–4), elective surgery, and elective medical admissions (5).

The salaried or capitated relation to providers typical of many HMOs may alter some of the incentives in the fee-for-service system (2, 6, 7). One study found that internists in several large fee-for-service groups were doing 50% more electrocardiograms and 40% more chest roentgenograms in uncomplicated hypertensive patients than internists in two HMOs. The authors conclude, albeit tentatively, that the group practice physicians' beliefs about profitability of the tests, given existing reimbursement mechanisms, may have influenced their decisions (8).

Second, HMOs reduce barriers to outpatient care. Because HMO benefits do not ordinarily include significant deductibles or copayments for outpatient care, and because they do not distinguish between cognitive and technologic services from the patient's point of view, there are few or no financial deterrents to seek early and frequent care. Early planners of HMOs hoped that patients would pursue care earlier in the disease process and that practitioners would pursue preventive medicine, for instance, emphasizing more frequent outpatient visits for the diabetic patient to prevent hospitalization.

The degree to which these hopes have been realized is unclear. One complication is that an HMO must retain a specific population for a relatively long period to benefit from preventive strategies. The transient nature of our society undermines such efforts. Furthermore, patients may fail to seek care for other than financial reasons (9). Busy phone lines, for instance, can discourage some persons from making an appointment. For both patients and practitioners, the time investment required for education and implementation may seem excessive in the face of other demands.

Third, inappropriate underutilization is avoidable. A reasonable concern about HMOs is that quality of care will be reduced along with costs. Bonus packages for physicians, in many cases tied to decreased testing, fewer hospital days, and other factors, may create incentives to underserve. The HMO advocates argue that professional training and socialization, fear of liability, and in-house peer and quality assurance review can and do prevent such abuses. Although the question has not been settled, many papers have reported the quality of care in HMOs to be comparable with that in the fee-for-service system (10–13). Furthermore, some persons might argue that the latter sector is flawed by overutilization: unnecessary surgery, risky and wasteful tests, and excessively frequent or prolonged hospitalizations (14, 15). Against that background, a reduction in use would represent an improvement in quality of care.

Proponents of HMOs assert that these institutions have incentives to provide a cost-effective, equitable, and high-quality alternative health care system. From an ethical standpoint, these "ideal characteristics" of HMOs promote both the principles of beneficence, or taking positive action to do good, and justice, understood as the equitable distribution of social goods, on behalf of enrolled members. Furthermore, HMOs may prove morally superior to fee-for-service medicine in one respect: The lack of incentives to overtreat promotes the goal for nonmaleficence, the avoidance of needless pain and suffering. For many persons, the most troubling characteristic of HMO practice lies in its gatekeeping function, raising the image of bedside cost-benefit analysis and resource allocation (16, 17). One reason for this discomfort is that an HMO is more than an insurance company that pays for care. Rather, it not only pays for, but contracts to provide care. The HMO promises good quality care, and takes responsibility as the patient's agent for arranging care and assuring that the physicians it employs (contracts with), the laboratories it uses, and so forth can fulfill that promise. In short, it has a fiduciary relation with its enrollees. Therefore, the HMO meets the criteria for what Pellegrino (18, 19) has called a "moral agent" in health care, sharing the obligations of the traditional moral agent, the physician.

Three obligations, paraphrased here from Pellegrino and Thomasma (20), are especially worth examining within the context of the HMO: a duty to a level of skill (that is, competence); a duty to make that skill maximally available to the patient (even at some personal cost); and a duty to act as the patient's advocate. As a moral agent, the HMO incurs these obligations as well. We examine whether the HMO meets these duties, or

at least does not constrain its physicians from meeting them.

The duty to a level of skill. Like any institution, the HMO can insist that its member practitioners be trained by accredited institutions, be board certified, and so on. But to meet the obligation to a level of skill, must an institution go further and make specialty care available whenever the patient requests it? Does the existence of a checkpoint (the primary care physician) to the patient's desire to see a specialist constitute a default on the obligation to a level of skill?

The decline in primary care physicians and the rise of specialty care have led the American public to a unique pattern of self-referral to specialists (6). Whether for skin or stomach, Americans tend to identify specialty care with optimal care. Arguably, the specialist does represent the "gold standard" for that group of problems within his or her purview. Nevertheless, HMOs assert that the primary care physician can deliver approximately equivalent care for certain medical problems for which the patient might have seen specialists in the past. According to HMOs, the gatekeeping doctor, not the patient, is the good and fair judge of when a referral is necessary.

Specialists' care must be subject to critical evaluation; such physicians do not necessarily offer the best outcomes nor may they be appropriately discriminatory in their use of tests. Nevertheless, the burden lies with HMOs and their primary care physicians to show that, for a given set of complaints, the care they provide approximates that of a competent, parsimonious specialist in terms of appropriateness of evaluation, and length and severity of morbidity, and mortality. Any differences must be exceedingly small. Training in the primary care specialties will therefore have to include extensive exposure to and training in the common problems of ophthalmology, gynecology, orthopedics, otolaryngology, and others. Many programs already of-

fer such training, but training alone is insufficient. The HMOs that hire physicians trained
specifically in primary care must evaluate and
certify that these physicians can provide approximately equivalent care and exercise prudent
judgment concerning referrals. Should the HMO
hire physicians from traditional programs, it has
an obligation to provide additional training in
deficient areas, and perhaps to relieve those physicians temporarily of gatekeeping responsibilities in those areas.

To the extent that HMOs do not acknowledge a
decrease in quality of care as being concomitant
with lower premiums, they must achieve the
standard of approximate equivalence. This concern is financial as well as ethical, for the poorly
trained doctor will generate unnecessary consultations as well as fail to meet the duty to an
acceptable level of skill. If HMOs do meet this obligation, the patient's demands to see a specialist
will not constitute a moral claim unless the referral is truly medically necessary (21).

*The duty to make that skill maximally avail-
able to the patient.* We will assume that this category of obligation includes the technologies to
which the physician controls access as well as
his or her own abilities as a practitioner. The diagnostic test is a good illustration because it frequently involves high technology and it represents the "skills" of the health care system.

Physicians and patients tend to have somewhat different interpretations of the process of
test ordering. Physicians' estimations of appropriateness should involve risk-benefit calculations weighing the chance for a false-positive result that can trigger a cascade of unnecessary
further tests against the odds of overlooking actual disease. "Maximum" quality of care can
mean a great investment in technology, or none
at all. However, because patients cannot analyze
test results or rank diagnoses, they usually substitute quantity of care for quality of care (22).

The doctor who orders more tests is the better
doctor; at least that doctor is "doing something."
Surgical procedures may be an exception, but because many tests pose little or no physical threat,
more information becomes a proxy for better
information.

The traditional fee-for-service physician has
reasons to order the so-called marginal test, especially if it is as relatively risk free as, for instance,
the computed tomography scan for headache or
the abdominal sonogram for nondescript belly
pain. Because such "large ticket" tests are usually paid for by a third-party insurer, the costs
are external and imperceptible to both doctor
and patient, and some information could be obtained, even if only a confirmation of normalcy.
Should the patient's coverage be inadequate, the
physician's charges may still be passed on to the
patient. In this case, the physician, protected
from cost considerations, may set the agenda,
while the patient, anxious for certainty, follows
along even at some financial hazard. If the neurologist happens to own the scanner or the gas-
troenterologist owns the sonographic device,
then other incentives to test are added to the
strictly diagnostic ones. In any event, in this system the patient's and physician's desire to maximize certainty are not in conflict.

In an HMO, the physician may think twice
about ordering the same test. Even without the
financial bonus, HMO physicians are probably a
self-selected group who may be inclined to restrict testing (3, 23, 24). In addition, and again
without considerations of personal gain, cost
may be an intrinsic element in medical decision
making within the medical sub-culture of the
HMO (3, 23). These factors would then make the
marginal test unattractive. The value of redun-
dant information is assessed as zero. The cost of
the test is not externalized, and is therefore a
negative. In addition, a false-positive result will
not only generate needless anxiety, but also the

necessity for additional tests, and hence expenditures. But the patient, still operating on the principle that absence of risk means that the test should be done, might regard the doctor's unwillingness to order it as a default on the duty to make skill maximally available.

A perception alone does not generate a moral obligation; there must also be valid grounds for the claim (21). The patient's belief that a test, if risk free, is necessary is not tantamount to an obligation to do it. Instead, a legitimate ground would be the reasonable prospect that the patient could benefit medically from the test results.

By definition, the marginal test is unlikely to alter the medical outcome. There is, however, a benefit from testing that is not strictly medical, but that can affect the doctor-patient relation and the well-being of the patient: the extent to which the patient feels comforted by positive action (the test) or by the confirmation received from test results. We believe this sort of benefit should be taken seriously. In lieu of testing, the HMO doctor must find other, more creative ways to provide comfort. Most often, the cost is time instead of money. The physician must explore the patient's residual fears, explain the basis for his or her advice in detail, and achieve reassurance by conversation rather than technology.

The deeper problem here is deciding what constitutes marginally indifferent information: that additional information that is unlikely to change the diagnosis or treatment, but has a remote chance of doing so (21, 25). The meaning of the terms "unlikely" and "remote" is of critical importance. Because traditional third-party coverage tends to encourage increased testing and treating at the margin, fee-for-service physicians may do the additional test that will discover the 1 case in 1000 that would otherwise have been missed. However, they will also do many tests on healthy persons to find that case, risking false-positive results. In the HMO the incentives are

such that the physician is likely to avoid unnecessary tests on healthy persons, but may risk missing the 1 in a 1000 case to save testing the other 999 patients.

The ethical issue is broader than the choice between two forms of health care reimbursement. It raises questions of how many "missed diagnoses" our society can tolerate, at what cost, and on the basis of whose criteria. Limitless testing generates medical problems as well as financial ones by creating false-positive results. Limited testing will overlook people with disease. Americans seem ambivalent on the subject, "deeply disturbed by sharply rising prices," yet not wishing to limit their own options (26).

Whatever the answer to the larger social question is, the HMO environment creates special constraints on the physician's duty to make his or her skills maximally available to the patient. One constraint arises because the person who chooses an HMO does so in part because he or she is price sensitive. Thus the HMO incurs some obligation not to spend its resources casually and to hold premiums down. But the public may be unaware that, to meet this obligation, the HMO physician will make marginally different choices than a fee-for-service physician. This difference places two more burdens on the HMO: It must fully disclose the conditions under which it operates, and it must educate its public about the risk-benefit/ cost-benefit dilemma and discuss "how much is enough." The view that the quality of medical care is the same or better in HMOs compared with fee-for-service medicine, because fewer tests and procedures result in fewer risks, will require explanation to a skeptical public who suspects that the physician who does not do a cardiac catheterization is "just trying to save money."

The duty to patient advocacy. The red flag of conflict of interest has often been waved before HMOs, but it can easily fly in front of all doctors' offices. Physicians have always profited from their patient's miseries. Indeed, American physicians for at least 100 years have behaved distinctly like small businessmen (27).

However, HMOs have been lightning rods for the worry about conflict of interest in medicine. One reason lies in our society's reluctance to acknowledge explicitly that it will forego the discovery of even one case of cancer for economic reasons. Thus we are dubious about the physician who, weighing the odds of detection against the cost of the procedure, advises us against colonoscopy (especially when not doing the procedures is in his or her own economic interest).

In addition, individual resource allocation decisions are often idiosyncratic and inequitable. Ramsey (28) and others have commented on physicians' tendency to mix sociologic and economic factors into apparently medical discussions of prognosis and treatment. Such confusion of medical and social considerations is more dangerous when there is institutional pressure to save money. The patient may be unaware of what has been left unoffered. And the language and knowledge differences between physician and patient make it possible for the physician to mask a resource allocation argument in medical terms. In the worst case, the physician may not even realize what he or she has done.

Several years ago, two distinguished commentators observed that "The physician is not a policymaker. . . . Physicians are to do all they can for their patients without counting society's resources and without taking into account the kinds of factors—such as statistical lives and the cost of medical research—that policymakers rightly should consider" (29). That discussion of microallocation, like many others, addressed rationing in terms of extreme conditions, such as the allocation of funds for costly programs to develop artificial organs or the distribution of resources in crises that require various forms of triage. Under extreme conditions, some patients must lose for the sake of some greater good. The well-being of the individual is placed at odds with that of the community.

Under routine conditions of microallocation there is usually not such a stark confrontation between the patient's good and the social good. Thus an analysis of ethical obligations under emergency conditions is of limited value, and may even be misleading when it comes to routine rationing. It need not be the case that an individual's interest must be incompatible with the social interest; in fact, they may dovetail. The social benefit of keeping costs down in a group health plan may be entirely consistent with protecting a particular patient from the stress, discomfort, inconvenience, and even risk associated with marginal tests, treatments, or procedures.

The HMOs do seek to create a cost-conscious milieu. The physicians' incomes, ultimately even their jobs, may be contingent on the degree to which they are good bureaucrats. To borrow from Friedson (30), in the HMO the doctor is expected to obstruct the patient to a degree, whether in access to specialists or to marginal tests. Society has assumed that the professional integrity of physicians would prevent them from accepting financial gain at their patient's expense, that their status as "double agents" would not cloud physicians' medical judgment. Unfortunately, such faith is not universally deserved. The scalpel-happy surgeon in fee-for-service practice and the HMO internist who protects his income by limiting the cancer work-up in an elderly person both abuse our faith.

What then of patient advocacy? Will cost constraints force physicians to attend as much to the needs of the institution as to the needs of the individual? Probably so, and perhaps they ought to. An ethic of community has long undergirded public health campaigns, both in disease prevention and intervention (31). The required preschool immunization and air pollution legislation set the concerns and desires of individuals behind the need for group immunity from infectious disease in the former, or for respiratory safety of the community in the latter. A similar ethic may play a role in other phases of health care. It is not unreasonable to argue that the institution and its physicians have an obligation to act as advocates for the community of patients who participate in the program, and not only for the individual patient. Granted the obligation is coincident with self-interest, but we have shown that an analagous situation exists in fee-for-service practice.

Our argument states that HMOs' incentive systems are justifiable if the cost-savings reflect an obligation to just use of resources on behalf of a community—the enrollees. Although we cannot fully address the complex issue of the role of profits in health care, our equity-based arguments will be insufficient by themselves to support overt physician incentives to save money in for-profit HMOs. Cost-containment for profit rather than equity shifts the doctor's advocacy not only away from the individual patient, but from the group of patients as well. In for-profit contexts, the potentially problematic incentive structure no longer directly preserves the benefit package or reduces premiums, but satisfies parties whose interests are not the health care mission of the HMO per se. Such parties are outside the community on which we have grounded our claim to justice.

Assuring Quality

How can the conflict between individual and group claims be resolved so that the duties to advocacy, quality, and equity are preserved? The 1973 federal legislation that established support for HMOs foresaw such questions. It requires all federally assisted and certified HMOs to maintain quality assurance programs, charged with keeping a close eye on medical care (32).

In many respects, the staff model, and some group model HMOs are ideal sites for monitoring. The practice is closed and geographically linked. Records are accessible and comparable. The practitioners have the opportunity to meet and establish standards of care and algorithms that are in accord with high-quality care, reflecting current knowledge about the cost-effectiveness and risk-benefit profiles of different interventions. Such protocols reduce the risk for bedside financial management by encouraging generally cost-effective care. Furthermore, the quality assurance program can then act as the ultimate patient advocate, seeking evidence of compliance with such standards.

It is in this area that the traditional system, now beleaguered even by indemnity carriers, may ultimately default more on the obligation to patient advocacy than HMOs. Not only quality, but also equity in treatment of patients is more likely to be assured by required review and discussion of like cases across and within physician practices. Practically, it is far more difficult to monitor care in settings that differ markedly in organization, record keeping, computerization, and so on Furthermore, the development of a high-quality, cost-conscious culture is inhibited by lack of geographic proximity or consistent group interaction. Therefore, HMOs based in group practices, staff model, or other, are at an advantage. On a day-to-day basis, the routine guarantor of HMO ethics could be an emergent HMO ethos, but the ultimate guarantor, short of the courts, is the quality assurance program.

However, the quality assurance mechanism cannot work if, under an insensitive administration, it is a thinly disguised office of utilization review. In addition, patients will have to get used to a system that asserts that it is defending their interests even as it restricts the individual's freedom to direct certain elements of his or her own care. Defensible criteria, openness, a good track record, on-going education, consensus-building, and accountability to the community of patients are critical to the achievement of this goal. It can be helpful to have patient representatives serve on the HMO's quality assurance committees.

Thus quality assurance represents one way the HMO can satisfy the duties of quality, equity, and advocacy. The HMO, as it acknowledges its potential for cost-savings, must make a specific effort to identify underservice. In addition, the HMO must spearhead the open discussion of marginal choices in health care, a subject that will ultimately emerge in all medical practices. Finally, in exchange for limiting patients' opportunity to direct their care, HMOs will have to become particularly aggressive in evaluating and promoting the competency of the gatekeeper physician. Given the unique structure of staff model HMOs, we feel they have a special opportunity to promote the duties to competence, skill, and advocacy.

Independent Practice Associations and Staff Models

We have referred to problems inherent in all HMOs and to solutions unique to the "staff model" in particular. It is important to appreciate that two dominant forms of HMO, the staff model and the independent practice association, diverge in some basic respects and raise separate moral questions.

In the staff model, the client pays a premium to the institution, which in turn maintains a staff to provide care, usually in a facility owned or operated by the HMO. In general, practitioners in these settings see only or mostly HMO clients (3, 33). The physicians typically receive a salary and a bonus variably tied to measurements of performance.

In the independent practice association, individual physicians in separate office locations agree to see the HMO's patients, who, in return for their premium, pay no individual fees (except occasional copayments or deductibles), regardless of utilization. Member physicians may be paid on a capitation basis, fee-for-service, or in other ways, but almost all will have some portion of their income tied to either individual performance or to that of the organization as a whole. A solo practitioner or group might join several competing independent practice associations and maintain a fee-for-service practice (3, 33).

These different models share two important features. Both depend to some extent on gatekeepers; referrals are often covered only to the extent that they are initiated by the primary care doctor. And both use economic incentives to encourage the gatekeeper to be cost-efficient. Physicians benefit or lose economically depending on their own utilization experience, that of the organization, or both (34–36).

Although this feature has generated the most heated debate, we have tried to show that much of the concern is misplaced or can be ameliorated. However, we would like to identify some ethical problems raised uniquely by the independent practice association model. Several of these issues have been widely recognized; others have not.

Many physicians who participate in independent practice associations also see fee-for-service patients. This mix of patients raises questions of equity within a given practice, especially between patients with "high option" fee-for-service coverage and patients in prepaid plans. The former may have different access to tests or procedures than the latter, depending on differentials in coverage. The physician's ability or willingness to maintain an equal standard of care with regard to need, notwithstanding such differentials, is critical (3, 37). Fee-for-service patients may also elect to use any consultant they or their physician choose. The HMO patients may enjoy broader general coverage, but may be limited to consultants approved by the association, who may be neither the primary physician's nor the patient's first choice.

Other inequities may surface as well. Patients who have prepaid may be more demanding of services, and the physician may feel underpaid for seeing them (38). These individuals then become "problem patients." Finally, such "mixed panels" have engendered a new creature: the physician as insurance broker. Both patients and their physicians may find it economically advantageous to "game the system." The physician will move patients in and out of different insurance packages as particular medical and economic issues arise (37). If the movement benefits both physician and patient, such activities may be laudable. If it serves the physician, and puts the patient at risk, it is not.

Another particular concern regarding independent practice associations is that although they use incentives to underserve, their decentralized nature, reflecting the traditional organization of medicine, makes it especially difficult for a quality assurance program to monitor practice patterns. There is no clear external balance to the potential of serious underservice.

Independent practice associations may be attractive to many physicians because they appear to preserve independent practice (34, 39). But a geographically distinct small office practice is not the same as an independent practice, and the illusion that they are the same has dangers. Construing independent practice associations as representative of the generic strengths and weaknesses of an HMO risks devaluing potential significant advantages of HMOs. At the same time, these entities create unique ethical quandaries for the previously independent practitioner. Because the two HMO models differ considerably, our discussion of gatekeeping in HMOs can therefore be applied only with considerable caution to independent practice associations.

Conclusion

The HMOs are moral agents with attendant ethical duties that are analogous to duties of the physician. The potential for HMOs to default on the duty to skill, to a level of competence, and to

patient advocacy exists, but remedies for these dangers are not difficult to identify. Careful attention must be paid, however, to the significant differences between independent practice associations and staff or group model HMOs with regard to the ethical issues they raise. For both, the problem of testing and treating at the margin will prove especially vexing. It is a topic that has received inadequate attention, not only within HMOs, but within medicine and society at large.

Perhaps the greatest menace to the ethical legitimacy of HMOs comes from their achievements in reducing the costs of health care delivery. For-profit enterprises are rapidly entering the HMO industry. Competition is so fierce, that some suggest that only seven major chains, for profit and non-profit, will survive the century (40). One must be concerned about the potential for confusion between a form of organization that began with an ethic of cost-savings on beneficent ethical grounds and a form of organization that saves money to pay dividends. Insofar as HMOs behave cost-effectively to hold down premiums and reduce the costs in the medical commons, the potential for conflict of interest was a conflict between two salutory moral ends: individual care and social well-being. The ethical justification for cost-savings at the margin is harder to sustain if the difference mainly boosts stock prices. As is the case elsewhere in medicine, the profit motive raises issues that no single institution, HMO or otherwise, can address or solve. However, the ethical legitimacy of the entire HMO industry is clearly at stake.

Notes

The authors thank the Kellogg National Fellowship Program, Robert Berenson, and Bradford Gray.

1. Stern, L., Rossiter, L.F., Wilensky, G.R. Ethics, health care, and the Enthoven proposal. *Health Aff (Millwood).* 1982;1:48–63.
2. Moore, S. Cost containment through risk-sharing by primary-care physicians. *N Engl J Med.* 1979;300: 1359–62.

3. Luft, H. Health maintenance organizations and the rationing of medical care. In: *Securing Access to Health Care: A Report on the Ethical Implications of Differences in the Availability of Health Services.* Vol. 3: Washington, DC: President's Commission for the Study of Ethical Problems in Medicine and Biomedical and Behavioral Research; 1983:313–37.

4. Welch, W.P. Health care utilization in HMOs: results from two national samples. *J Health Econ.* 1984;4:293–308.

5. Siu, A.L., Brook, R.H., Liebowitz, A., Goldman, N.S., Lurie, N., Newhouse, P. How does one health maintenance organization reduce hospital admissions? In: *Abstract Reprints.* Philadelphia: Society for Research and Education in Primary Care; 1986.

6. Somers, A.R. And who shall be the gatekeeper? The role of the primary care physician in the health care delivery system. *Inquiry.* 1983;20:301–13.

7. Moore, S.H. An HMO with private family physicians coordinating care and controlling costs. *J Fam Pract.* 1981;13:508–12.

8. Epstein, A.M., Begg, C.B., McNeil, B.J. The use of ambulatory testing in prepaid and fee-for-service group practices. *N Engl J Med.* 1986;314:1089–94.

9. Lurie, N., Manning, W.G., Peterson, C., Goldberg, G.A., Phelps, C.A., Lillard, L. Preventive care: do we practice what we preach? *Am J Public Health.* 1987;77:801–4.

10. Yelin, E.H., Shearn, M.A., Epstein, W.V. Health outcomes for a chronic disease in prepaid group practice and fee-for-service settings: the case of rheumatoid arthritis. *Med Care.* 1986;24:236–47.

11. Wright, C.H., Gardin, T.H., Wright, C.L. Obstetric care in a health maintenance organization and a private fee-for-service practice: a comparative analysis. *Am J Obstet Gynecol.* 1984;149:848–56.

12. Roemer, M.I. Sickness absenteeism in members of health maintenance organizations and open market insurance plans. *Med Care.* 1982;20:1140–6.

13. Quick, J.D., Greenlick, M.R., Roghmann, K.J. Prenatal care and pregnancy outcome in an HMO and general population: a multivariate cohort analysis. *Am J Public Health.* 1981;71:381–90.

14. Siu, A.L., Sonnenberg, F.A., Manning, W.G. et al. Inappropriate use of hospitals in a randomized trial of health insurance plans. *N Engl J Med.* 1986;315:1259–66.

15. Wennberg, J.E. On patient need, equity, supplier-induced demand, and the need to assess the outcome of common medical practices. *Med Care.* 1985;23:512–20.

16. Morreim, E.H. The MD and the DRG. *Hastings Cent Rep.* 1985;15:30–8.

17. Veatch, R., Cohen, M.F. The HMO physician's duty to cut costs. *Hastings Cent Rep.* 1985;15:13–5.

18. Pelligrino, E.D. Rationing health care: the ethics of medical gatekeeping. *Journal Contemp Health Law Policy.* 1986;2:23–45.

19. Pellegrino, E.D. *Humanism and the Physician.* Knoxville: University of Tennessee Press; 1979:145–50.

20. Pellegrino, E.D., Thomasma, D.C. *A Philosophical Basis of Medical Practice.* New York: Oxford University Press; 1981:207–19.

21. Brett, A.S., McCullough, L.B. When patients request specific interventions: defining the limits of the physician's obligation. *N Engl J Med.* 1986;315:1347–51.

22. Ginsberg, E. The monetarization of medical care. *N Engl J Med.* 1984;310:1162–5.

23. Eisenberg, J.M. The internist as gatekeeper: preparing the general internist for a new role. *Ann Intern Med.* 1985;102:537–43.

24. Eisenberg, J.M. Sociologic influences on decision-making by clinicians. *Ann Intern Med.* 1979;90:957–64.

25. Begley, C.E. Physicians and cost control. In: Agich, G.J., Begley, C.E., eds. *The Price of Health.* Boston: Reidel; 1986:227–44.

26. Blendon, R.J., Altman, D.E. Public attitudes about health-care costs: a lesson in national schizophrenia. *N Engl J Med.* 1984;311:613–6.

27. Starr, P. *The Social Transformation of American Medicine.* New York: Basic Books; 1982:79–92, 225–34, 270–89.

28. Ramsey, P. *Ethics at the Edges of Life: Medical and Legal Intersections.* New Haven: Yale University Press; 1978:201–3.

29. Beauchamp, T.L., Childress, J.F. *Principles of Biomedical Ethics.* Oxford: Oxford University Press; 1983:213.

30. Friedson, E. Prepaid group practice and the new "demanding" patient. *Milbank Mem Fund Q Health Soc.* 1973;51:473–88.

31. Beauchamp, D.E. Community: the neglected tradition of public health. *Hastings Cent Rep.* 1985;15:28–36.

32. Public Health Service Act, title 13 (Health Maintenance Act of 1973). Washington, DC: U.S. Government Printing Office, 1976.

33. Blue, J.W. PPOs, HMOs, IPAs—understanding their concepts. *Radiology Management.* 1985;17:15–9.

34. Kircher, M. Can IPAs save small practices? *Med Econ.* 1985;62:176–88.

35. Tobias, J.J. An IPA organizer tells why and how. *Patient Care.* 1981;15:182–90.

36. Moore, S.H., Martin, D.P., Richardson, W.C. Does the primary care gatekeeper control the costs of health care? Lessons from the Safeco experience. *N Engl J Med.* 1982;309:1400–4.

37. Berenson, R.A. Capitation and conflict of interest. *Health Aff (Millwood).* 1986;5:141–6.

38. Schroeder, J.L., Clarke, J.T., Webster, J.R. Jr. Prepaid entitlements: a new challenge for physician-patient relationships. *JAMA.* 1985;254:3080–2.

39. Freund, D.A., Allen, K.S. Factors affecting physicians' choice to practice in a fee-for-service setting versus an individual practice association. *Med Care.* 1985; 23:799–808.

40. Petty, R. HMO's: it ain't what you do but the way you do it. *Health Med.* 1985;3:24–9.

Physicians and

Business Managers:

A Clash of Cultures

Arnold S. Relman

■

As this is being written, it is still not clear whether a health-reform bill will be enacted in this session of Congress or what its provisions will be. For the purposes of the present essay, however, that does not really matter. This piece is about relations between physicians and health-care managers, and the tensions between professional values and business imperatives. These problems appeared in the private sector with the advent of managed care. They will persist, regardless of federal legislation, as long as employers press the use of managed-care plans to control the costs of their employees' medical insurance.

Although universal coverage was the Clinton administration's avowed major objective in their proposal for healthcare reform, containment of costs was in fact the prime consideration. The administration's policymakers understood very clearly that expanded coverage would not be affordable without control of costs. They were also acutely aware that reduction of the federal deficit would require some moderation of the runaway costs of Medicare and Medicaid. Employers were even more explicit in their determination to control rising medical costs, which had begun to threaten the profitability of their businesses. Not surprisingly, they did not wait for federal legislation but initiated their own efforts at cost control. It was largely in response to these pressures from employers that the managed-care revolution began.

Cost control sounds like it ought to be a task for economists and business managers, but their expertise has only limited applicability to the medical-care system. Most economists (but fortunately not all) tend to think of the health system as a market not fundamentally different from others, in which prices and expenditures are determined by supply and demand. As a result, their recommendations for cost control usually rely on market forces and the manipulation of tax incentives. For their part, business managers are inclined to look at medical care as just another business, best managed according to the principles they learned in business school. But market theory and business principles do not sit comfortably in the health-care system. In fact, they often clash with deeply held societal views about health care and the personal value of medical services. The industrial model of health care, so widely accepted in current discussions of reform, overlooks the unique nature of medical services and the many ways our health-care system differs from the rest of the U.S. economy.

One of the most important of these differences is the special role of physicians. Physicians are not simply skilled workers or technicians providing the services that consumers can choose to buy in a free market for health care. They are autonomous professionals, prepared through long and arduous education and empowered by law to assume primary responsibility for the care of the sick. Based on their professional assessment of the medical need in each patient's case, physicians, not consumers, make most of the decisions about the use of health-care resources. Of course, patients are consulted in the decision-making process and, whenever possible, give their informed consent. But patients must rely largely on the advice of their physicians, especially when they are sick, and it is the physician who assesses the medical problem and directs the strategy for diagnosis and treatment.

Medicine is a profession in which physicians act as agents, fiduciaries and counselors for their patients. Regardless of how they are paid, they are expected to put their patients' interests above all other considerations. Physicians are trained to focus more on quality of medical care and their patients' medical needs than on the costs of the services they provide or recommend. The growth of third-party payment was, of course, a major factor in creating this relative indifference to costs, but a commitment to do the best for the patient, regardless of cost, is deeply ingrained in the traditions of the medical profession and has long been part of the de facto contract between the profession and society. This feature of the contract may be about to change, because private insurers are now demanding that physicians take costs into consideration when making clinical decisions, and medical education has begun to pay more attention to this subject. However, regardless of the future emphasis that may be given to costs when bedside decisions are made, physicians will—and should—insist on being responsible for those decisions. The law, public expectations and the ethical canons of their profession will continue to hold them accountable for the medical management of their patients.

In the traditional fee-for-service system that dominated medical care for the first half of this century, physicians were free to exercise this responsibility as they saw fit. In so doing, they were in a position of conflict of interest because, in effect, they controlled the demand for their own services. Nevertheless, fee-for-service worked relatively well (at least in the sense that it was affordable) until the last few decades, when third-party payment began to dominate the system and costs started to rise steeply. The advent of managed care and the resurgence of capitated prepayment of providers was a direct consequence of the revolt of employers, who were threatened by seemingly uncontrollable inflation of medical costs and refused to allow the insurers simply to pass along in the form of higher premiums the steadily rising bills from the providers. Under managed care, insurers changed from being passive third-party payers to managers of costs.

Managed care and capitated prepayment of providers are now sweeping the private health-insurance market and are making inroads into Medicare and Medicaid as well. If one counts only health-maintenance organizations (HMOs) with primary-care gatekeepers (which would include group- and staff-model HMOs as well as independent-practice associations (IPAs)), nearly 50 million subscribers are now enrolled, mostly through their employers. If one adds preferred-provider organizations (PPOs), self-insured businesses and indemnity fee-for-service insurance plans that have strong cost-control and utilization-review programs, the total number of lives now covered by managed-care plans of some type probably exceeds half the population. The premiums collected in this vast insurance system (or, in the case of self-insured businesses, the total costs to the employers) can only be approximated, but I would estimate them to be in the order of $400 billion this year. Not surprisingly, this market is enormously attractive to entrepreneurs, and hundreds of new companies, large and small, are now staking their claims to a share of these revenues. Managed care has become a huge and rapidly growing industry. The consequences of this revolution, yet to be fully played out, are already changing the practice of medicine and are likely to have profound effects on our health care.

The most important fact about the managed-care insurance system is that it is largely profit-oriented. The great majority of existing and newly formed HMOs and other kinds of managed-

care plans are investor-owned, and a growing number are publicly traded. To those who believe in a private market solution to health-care reform, the good news about this arrangement is that it provides the necessary risk capital to start up new competing health plans without requiring additional public funds or tax revenues. Of course, without public monies these new managed-care plans could not be expected to enroll the poor and the uninsured. Whatever its patient mix, however, the managed-care system has powerful economic incentives to control medical costs—and that is also part of the good news for those committed to the private market. To those who, like me, believe that health care is a social service, not a purely economic commodity, the bad news is that it replaces the old conflict of interest in fee-for-service private practice with a new conflict of interest between the economic objectives of investors and the medical needs of patients. In the new world of investor-owned managed care, expenditures on the care of patients become "medical losses" for the company, whose executives and managers are striving to keep their "medical loss ratio" as low as possible so that the company's financial statement will look attractive to investors. Even more worrisome, the responsibility of physicians for the management of their patients' medical problems is attenuated by the cost-containment policies of the company. In short, investor-owned managed care raises the possibility—even the likelihood—of a confrontation between two cultures: the investor-owned business corporation and the medical profession.

The economic arrangements for physicians in managed-care systems vary with the nature of the plan. These variations notwithstanding, all managed-care plans constrain the traditional freedom of physicians to make decisions for their patients, some of them in ways that have aroused considerable professional ire. It is difficult to make generalizations, but my impression is that professional dissatisfaction is least among physicians who have joined group- and staff-model HMOs and greatest among office-based private practitioners who have contractual relations with one or more managed-care plans. The reasons are obvious. In group- and staff-model HMOs, each physician has voluntarily chosen to practice as a salaried member of a group. In most cases, management of medical costs is the responsibility of the group's physicians, thus permitting them to establish acceptable guidelines for the use of diagnostic and therapeutic resources and for the conduct of office practice. When this does not occur—that is, when there is intrusive management of medical practice by business administrators—the medical staff is usually restive.

Another reason that physicians may be more content in group- and staff-model HMOs than in IPAs and other forms of managed care may lie in the fact that many of the largest group- and staff-model HMOs are not-for-profit and do not have the same managerial philosophy as the investor-owned IPAs and PPOs. Most of the latter are managed by non-physicians whose primary concern is with financial performance and whose primary allegiance is to owners and investors. They tend to view physicians simply as expensive contractors and pieceworkers, whose costs must be kept in line. Those investor-owned plans that employ physicians as cost managers and involve them in developing cost- and quality-control policies, have been the most successful in winning the cooperation of their participating physicians.

No one wants to be taken care of by an angry or demoralized physician, so managers risk the success of their plans if they ignore the morale and professional concerns of their doctors. However, in sections of the country where IPAs and PPOs have a large share of the market, their business managers seem to have the upper hand in dealing with individual private practitioners. Worried about their economic futures and dependent on the patients supplied through the plans, practitioners feel they have no recourse but to sign contracts and accept the arrangements offered by the managed-care plans.

What about the quality of patient care in such a system? The owners and managers of managed-care plans insist that their first concern is the quality of the care their subscribers receive. They claim that in a competitive market they must provide good care or go out of business. Some of them point with pride to the measures of their quality, such as childhood immunization rates and screening programs for breast cancer, hypertension, hyperlipidemia and prostate cancer. Some also display impressive statistics on patient-satisfaction questionnaires and membership turnover.

While such data are useful, they hardly scratch the surface. The satisfaction of patients, which is heavily influenced by the courtesy with which they are treated by the support staff and the promptness with which they gain access to care, is not a reliable criterion of the basic quality of medical care. Many corners can be cut that may risk or even damage health without attracting the patient's notice. Despite the growing use of outcomes reporting, the science of quality assessment is still in its infancy. There are at present no reliable ways to measure the overall quality of medical care provided by managed-care plans. The best definition of quality care, in my view, is "that care which is provided by competent, well-informed and compassionate physicians who have no incentive to do more or less than is medically appropriate for each patient, and who practice in facilities with adequate resources and good management."

Most physicians are willing to practice within fixed but reasonable financial limits and will work with managers to improve the cost-effectiveness of the services they provide, as long as the following conditions are met:

—Physicians should have the responsibility for all medical decisions, with the understanding that the quality of their performance will be subject to peer review.

—Overall financial limits and clinical guidelines for the use of scarce or expensive resources in individual cases should be established and agreed in advance.

—Physicians and business managers should work together in a collegial way toward agreed-upon common objectives of quality care and cost control.

—Physicians should be compensated in ways that encourage neither over- nor under-use of resources. In my opinion, that means salaries based on professional performance and contribution to the goals of the organization, as judged by one's professional peers.

The advent of the investor-owned managed-care industry may well impede the achievement of these objectives because the imperatives of investor-owned businesses inevitably compete with the traditions of the medical profession. For-profit managed-care corporations have their own agendas. The economic stakes are high, and financial considerations are likely to dominate policy decisions. Too often in these corporations, business managers are in charge of the physicians. Maybe such corporations will prove to be responsible custodians for the health care of their subscribers. Maybe they will be able to control rising costs while promoting quality of care and encouraging the professional values and autonomy of their physicians. Maybe, but I remain to be convinced. More likely, in my opinion, the investor-owned managed-care industry ultimately will need to be closely regulated, like a public utility, or largely replaced by a new system of not-for-profit, community-based organizations of physicians and hospitals.

Preserving the Physician-Patient Relationship in the Era of Managed Care

Ezekiel J. Emanuel and
Nancy Neveloff Dubler

■

Major health care system reform legislation died—or was killed—in the last Congress. Yet changes in our health care system are continuing, even accelerating. The most obvious change is the ever-expanding use of managed care, especially to control rising health care costs. The debate over managed care has tended to focus on whether—and how—it can control costs.[1-3] No one doubts that this is a fundamental issue. Nevertheless, the tremendous changes brought about by the widespread implementation of managed care will extend beyond health care costs. While some have raised questions about the effect of managed care on use of technology and patient satisfaction, there has been woefully little discussion of other probable and important consequences, such as restrictions on clinical research, the probable reduced funding for physician training programs, and the closing of hospitals in rural areas and small communities.[4,5] In addition, little attention has been paid to how managed care might affect the physician-patient relationship. Yet, the public outcry over choice of physician in the recent debates about health care system reform has made clear that this is a major concern for the vast majority of citizens, whose interaction with the health care system is principally, if not exclusively, as patients. Thus, one of the fundamental questions for most Americans about the changes fostered by managed care is, How will managed care affect my relationship with my physician?

The Ideal Physician-Patient Relationship

To evaluate the effects of managed care, we need to delineate an ideal conception of the physician-patient relationship.[6] This ideal establishes the normative standard for assessing the effect of the current health care system as well as changes in the system. Although patients receive health care from a diverse number of providers, and the use of nonphysician providers, such as nurse practitioners, physician assistants, and nurse midwives, is likely to increase with more emphasis on primary care and managed care, we chose to concentrate on the physician-patient relationship. The reasons for this focus are many: physicians outnumber nonphysician providers; most Americans continue to receive their health care from physicians rather than nonphysician providers; there have been many more years, indeed, centuries, for reflection on the elements that constitute the ideal physician-patient relationship, while the ethical guidelines and legal rulings on nonphysician provider–patient relationships are more recent and have not been as exhaustively developed; and there is substantially more empirical research on the physician-patient relationship with which to formulate educated projections. Where relevant, we explore how relationships between physicians and nonphysician providers might affect interactions with patients. Americans have intuitions about what they consider to be an ideal physician-patient relationship. These intuitions are personified in books, television programs, and other media through the portrayals of physicians, such as Marcus Welby. In addition, much has been written by physicians, ethicists, and lawyers about what constitutes the ideal physician-

patient relationship.[7-19] In characterizing the many facets of the ideal physician-patient relationship, we try to specify and organize these intuitions and then refine them by comparing them with the ideal explicitly defined in the literature and by the standards of practice embodied in ethical guidelines, legal rulings, and health care policies.[20-22] No characterization of this ideal will receive universal assent; physicians, ethicists, and lawyers disagree among themselves about how to articulate the ideal physician-patient relationship. Often these disagreements are a result of emphasizing different aspects of the relationship rather than unbridgeable philosophical differences. Despite these differences, we believe it is possible to elucidate core understandings that are widely, if not uniformly, shared.

It is also important to recognize that this ideal evolves over time. Traits admired decades ago may no longer be revered, while other traits have become more prominent. For instance, paternalism might have been the accepted norm previously, but today respect for patient autonomy is widely agreed to be a core facet of the ideal physician-patient relationship. In addition, the ideal may not describe actual physician-patient relationships.[6,9] Physicians may not recognize or may fail to fulfill their duties, or adverse practice conditions may interfere with the realization of the ideal. Nevertheless, the fundamental elements of the ideal physician-patient relationship seem to be enduring and define the goal toward which we aspire. We measure our achievement by the ideal even when we fall short.

We suggest that the fundamental elements of the ideal physician-patient relationship that are embodied in our intuitions and common to ethical analyses and legal standards can be expressed as six C's: choice, competence, communication, compassion, continuity, and (no) conflict of interest. While many people emphasize the importance of trust in the physician-patient relationship, we believe trust is the culmination of realizing these six C's, not an independent element.

Choice

As became clear in the debate over President Clinton's health care system reform proposal, many Americans consider choice to be a critical dimension of the ideal physician-patient relationship.[23-25] Four critical dimensions of this choice are (1) choice of practice type and setting, (2) choice of primary care physician, (3) choice of a specialist or special facility in an emergency or for a special condition, and (4) choice among treatment alternatives.[7,12,14,17,18] Patients want to be able to choose whether to receive their care from an independent practitioner or in an integrated health care system. More important, they also want to be able to choose who provides them with routine health care, to find a person with whom they have a rapport and to whom they can entrust their secrets and confidences. They fear being forced to receive care from a physician with whom they do not get along. If they confront a serious threat to their health, such as requiring major surgery or being diagnosed with cancer, patients want to be sure they can choose to go to "the best." For many Americans, choice of the best is a critical element in feeling that "no stone will be left unturned" when a major illness arises.[23,24] Finally, when there are several appropriate treatment options for a condition, such as mastectomy or breast-conserving therapy for breast cancer, Americans want to be able to choose for themselves which one to receive. This is the element of choice embodied in informed consent.[12,14,16-18] The tremendous emphasis Americans place on choice can sometimes appear as a fetish,[26,27] but we value it as one component of self-determination, a central ideal of American culture.[7,8,12,14-16,20,24]

Competence

Patients expect their physicians to be competent. While technical proficiency may not be sufficient, it is a necessary precondition for having a good physician-patient relationship; physicians who lack technical expertise cannot meet the ideal. Competence entails four elements. Physicians must possess (1) a good fund of knowledge that is kept current with developing practices; (2) good technical skills to perform diagnostic and therapeutic procedures; (3) good clinical judgment to differentiate important signs and symptoms from secondary ones, to know what diagnostic tests to utilize in what order, and to select the most appropriate therapies; and (4) an understanding of their own limitations and a willingness to consult specialists or other health care providers as required by the situation.[8,9,13,17,18]

Communication

An ideal physician-patient relationship requires good communication. First, good communication means that physicians listen to and understand the patient and communicate their understanding. This entails understanding the patient's symptoms, the patient's values, the effect of the disease on the patient's life, family, job, and other pursuits, and any other health-related concerns the patient deems important.[7-14,16-19] In addition, patients should be able to tell their physicians what kind of information they want and do not want to know. For example, some patients with cancer prefer not to know their prognosis or a detailed delineation of the side effects of treatment alternatives. In circumstances where patients, especially children and adolescents, may not be especially articulate or may be confronting new experiences that they have difficulty characterizing, physicians must be able to help patients explicate their experiences, values, and feelings.[9–12,14,16,19]

Good communication skills also mean that physicians are capable of explaining to patients, in clear and comprehensible language, the nature of their disease, the diagnostic and therapeutic treatment alternatives available, and how these alternatives are likely to fulfill or undermine the patients' values. In this sense, physicians offer advice and direction that guide their patients through the issues raised by their illness and possible treatments.[7,9,10,12,14,16,17] For example, the physician can help patients with arthritis assess how alternative treatment options will help achieve their goals of functional independence and freedom from pain.

By strengthening the bond between patients and physicians, good communication prevents arguments, misunderstandings, and disputes.[28–30] When communication is good, patients are less likely to misinterpret the information they receive, more willing to ask for clarification when information is unclear, quicker to call if symptoms fail to resolve. Good communication thus can mitigate the occurrence of negative events that lead to malpractice litigation.[31,32]

Compassion

Patients not only want technically proficient physicians, they also want empathic physicians.[33] Empathy from their physician enables patients to feel supported during times of great stress. This may be especially important for adolescents, whose health problems may also cause strains in their family. This is not to suggest that compassionate physicians simply reaffirm whatever values, feelings, and experiences patients have.[9,10,16,19,33] Sometimes physicians see the need to help patients reconsider and revise their values, overcome their feelings, and place their experiences in a larger perspective. But these efforts are all undertaken with the intention of demonstrating compassion for the patient.[9,10,16,19,33]

Continuity

Once established, a patient's relationship with a competent and compassionate physician who is providing most of his or her care should endure over time.[7–10,12,13,16,17,19,24] The establishment of an ideal physician-patient relationship requires a significant investment of time. Patients frequently must search to identify a physician whom they consider competent and with whom they can communicate. It also takes time for physicians to understand and empathize with patients' values and feelings and to be able to help patients identify and utilize health care services that are appropriate for their condition and life situation.

Trusting relationships ensure that in times of stress patients can rely on their physicians secure in the knowledge that their history, attachments, values, and feelings are understood. If patients are frequently forced to change physicians, it is hard for them to develop a deep and understanding relationship. An ongoing relationship is particularly important for patients who have chronic conditions such as arthritis, diabetes, or cancer and require repeated medical interventions over time. It may also be important for younger patients for whom choices by the patient or the patient's parents can profoundly affect future life prospects. Decisions to adopt healthy habits, to stop smoking to spare a child from passive smoke, or to bear painful but efficacious therapies are more likely to be made if recommended by a trusted physician in the context of an ongoing relationship.

Relationships that endure over time may be more efficient. Knowing a patient means that a physician more easily identifies therapies appropriate for the personality and capabilities of the patient. The physician will know what support services the patient can draw on. Similarly, patients are more likely to accept recommendations to "wait and see" or to delay expensive diagnostic testing from a physician in whom they have confidence by virtue of having established a trusting relationship.

(No) Conflict of Interest

We expect that a physician's primary concern will be his or her patient's well-being, even though physicians may have obligations that conflict. Attending to the well-being of one patient may conflict with caring for another patient.[34] Similarly, it is well recognized that caring for a patient may conflict with—and even be superseded by—the need to protect the interests of a third party.[7,12,14,17,35,36] Nevertheless, we do expect that the physician's care of a patient and concern for the patient's well-being will take precedence over the physician's own personal interests, especially financial interests.[7,12,13,15,17,18] This means that in a fee-for-service environment physicians should not order procedures merely for their personal financial enrichment.[37] Conversely, in a capitated system, physicians should not withhold appropriate medical services to increase their own financial rewards. These expectations inform the rules restricting conflict of interest.[38–41]

The Physician-Patient Relationship in the Current Health Care System

Uninsured Patients

At any one time, approximately 37 million Americans are uninsured, almost 25% of whom are children, and it is estimated that fully 63 million Americans go without insurance for at least 1 month during each 28-month period.[42] For these uninsured people without a regular physician, the current system precludes the possi-

bility of having an ideal physician-patient relationship. Without health insurance or significant financial resources, the uninsured do not have any meaningful choice of health care setting or of a primary care physician.[43] They are often forced to forgo regular care or to receive their regular health care from emergency departments, public hospitals, or similar institutions that provide care to the uninsured.[23] Many physicians who work in these institutions are highly trained professionals, dedicated to serving the poor and to providing high-quality care to the uninsured. Yet in such settings, the uninsured will often see a different physician at each visit, in a rushed atmosphere where overworked staff tend to proceed at a frenzied pace. And the frequent changes in health insurance coverage, going from insured to uninsured and back to insured over a few years, disrupt continuity of care. Health care provided under these conditions precludes good communication or continuity. Even if the health care providers are individually competent, compassionate, and dedicated and have no financial conflicts of interest, it appears that uninsured patients do have worse health outcomes, which casts doubt on the competence of the total care they receive and highlights that outcomes depend on more than the qualities of health care providers.[44,45] While competence and compassion are essential elements of an ideal physician-patient relationship, they are insufficient without patient choice, good communication, and continuity. Thus, for millions of uninsured Americans, impersonal care has all but displaced caring and enduring physician-patient relationships.

Insured Patients

Many Americans with health insurance—or, rarely, with independent financial means—have been able to choose a physician they believe to be competent and caring and with whom they can communicate about their health care. More than two thirds of Americans have maintained such a relationship over many years.[23,24] In some instances the physician has become as much a family friend as a provider of medical services. As the statistics on high patient satisfaction with their current physician demonstrate, many Americans believe their relationship with their physician is close to the ideal.[23,24] But even for them some of the characteristics of the current system jeopardize that good relationship.

There are many ways in which choice of physician and choice of procedures are currently limited even for insured Americans. Insurance companies and managed care plans may discourage utilization of or exclude coverage for certain physicians, procedures, and treatments, or may prohibit patients from going to specialty hospitals for treatment.[24,46,47] Utilization review, preapprovals, and other practice oversights may serve to overrule informed patient and physician choices. And finally, many health insurance programs fail to cover many services, especially preventive services, limiting the patient's choice and utilization of those services, even when they are efficacious and cost-effective.

A second flaw of the current system is that it lacks a systematic mechanism for assessing and informing patients about the competence of their health care delivery system and personal physician. There are few reliable and validated measures of physician and health care quality.[48,49] Medical licensure is only an indicator of minimum standards of proficiency. Specialty board examinations indicate attainment of specialized knowledge and skills beyond those required for safe practice[50]; they do not, however, provide an assessment of competence over time.[51] Hospital staff privileges are subject to review by peers and regulatory bodies. Unfortunately, their decisions tend to be influenced by politics as much as competence. Further, information about a physician's performance is not easily available to patients. Appointments to a medical faculty provide an informal system for evaluating competence, but the criteria for these appointments emphasize research, publications, and other factors not necessarily associated with clinical competence. Personal recommendations and reviews of physicians in the popular press are based more on word of mouth by nonprofessionals than on reliable standards of competence. While most US physicians have a good fund of knowledge and sound clinical judgment, the system fails to provide an assurance of competence. Thus, even for the best-insured Americans, the current system fails to provide reliable assessments of physician competence. Patients are left to rely on subjective impressions and reputations, neither of which are adequate.

Third, the current system contains and perpetuates threats to good communication and compassionate care. The emphasis on specialization and technical expertise and the limited training in humanistic care, communication skills, and ethical considerations tend to produce physicians limited in communication skills.[52–54] Under the threat of malpractice litigation, physicians may be inclined to order more interventions than they think are warranted.[55–57] Financial incentives in the current system encourage physicians to offer high-technology procedures rather than primary and preventive care. There are disincentives to talking with patients. Indeed, this is the paradigm of nonreimbursable care. In addition, bureaucratic demands for preprocedure permission, postprocedure justification, multiple reimbursement forms, and other administrative requirements take up significant physician time that might otherwise be spent discussing present and future care plans with patients.[58] Physicians may be forced to see more patients and shorten each visit so they can cover the mounting administrative personnel costs created by the explosion of paperwork.

When companies require their employees to

select physicians from a restricted list, workers may be forced to change their physician.[23] Similarly, annual shifts in the cheapest managed care plan offered by a company can create a dilemma for workers as to whether continuity of care with a specific physician is worth the extra price. One recent survey found that 40% of patients in health maintenance organizations (HMOs) had to change doctors when they joined the HMO.[23] Another study found that almost half of all patients in HMOs had been with their physician for fewer than 4 years and patients in HMOs had been with their physician for a shorter period of time than patients in fee-for-service settings.[24] Thus, even for the insured American, choice and continuity of care may be, or become, an elusive ideal.

Finally, there is significant potential, if not actual, conflict of interest in the current system.[38,39,59] Physicians who practice in a fee-for-service setting and who invest in radiological or other service centers often gain financially by ordering tests and performing procedures that may not always be in the patient's best interest.[32,39,60] Conversely, physicians who practice in managed care settings may gain financially by ordering fewer tests and performing fewer procedures than is appropriate.[39,40] While the current system has implemented some rules to reduce this financial conflict of interest,[37] these rules have many defects and do not ensure no conflict of interest.[38–41]

The Physician-Patient Relationship in the Era of Managed Care

Despite the lack of comprehensive health care system reform legislation, significant changes are occurring without legislative and governmental regulation, driven predominantly by the increased efforts of employers to reduce health care costs. These changes include more managed care, increased use of primary care physicians and generalists rather than specialists, increased use of nonphysician providers, emphasis on preventive measures, greater commitment to the care of children, and intensive quality assessment.[61,62] Although it is impossible to predict the precise concrete manifestations and effects of all these changes, it is possible to provide some educated reflections on their probable implications for the physician-patient relationship (Table 1). Because the health care system is so complex, the changes may not always tend in a coherent direction; some aspects may enhance a particular element of the physician-patient relationship while others undermine it. It is often difficult to know which tendency will dominate in practice, and so we try to outline the potential trends in both directions.

Admittedly, these predictions are speculative. But they are no more speculative than projections on the cost of certain changes or on the economic consequences of particular managed care programs.[63] And just as economic projections, with uncertainty, are essential in evaluating health care proposals, so too we hope these predictions will provide a basis for planning and promoting those parts of the trend toward managed care that enhance the ideal physician-patient relationship, anticipating threats to the ideal posed by managed care, and acting to mitigate the ill effects.

Potential Improvements

With some expansion of managed care, the range of choice for many insured Americans could also increase. Americans who live in regions without significant managed care penetration, such as the South, will soon have the option of care in a managed care setting. In addition, other Americans could now have several managed care plans as well as fee-for-service options to choose from. However, if managed care expands too much, it may threaten to eliminate fee-for-service practi-

Table 1. The Effects of Managed Care on the Physician-Patient Relationship

Potential Improvements	Potential Threats
Choice	
• Expanded choice of managed care plans, particularly in areas with low managed care penetration • Expanded choice of preventive and pediatric services	• "Cherry picking" increasing the number of uninsured Americans • Employers restricting patients' choice of managed care plans and physicians • Price competition forcing patients to choose between continuing with their current physicians or switching to a cheaper plan • Financial failures of managed care plans forcing change in managed care plan without choice • Restrictions by managed care plans of choice of specialists and particular services
Competence	
• Development and use of measures to assess quality of physicians and managed care plans • Greater use of preventive medical care	• Underutilization of specialists and specialized facilities • Unreliable and non–risk-adjusted quality measures providing a distorted view of competence
Communication	
• Increased number of generalists and primary care providers • Creation of physician–nonphysician provider teams to provide a broader range of providers knowledgeable about the patient's condition	• Productivity requirements creating shorter office visits, reduced telephone access, and other access barriers to physicians • Advertising creating inflated patient expectations
Compassion	
. . .	• Less time for interaction with patients during stressful decisions
Continuity	
. . .	• Price competition forcing patient choice of continuity at a higher price vs the cheapest plan • "Deselection" of physicians disrupting existing physician-patient relations • Frequent changes by employer of managed care plans forcing changes of physician
(No) Conflict of Interest	
. . .	• Linking physician salary incentives and bonuses to reduced use of tests and procedures for patients

tioners in a region altogether, as it appears to be doing in northern California and Minnesota. Under such circumstances, patients' choice of practice setting, even for well-insured Americans, could be effectively reduced.

Managed care may also provide the insured with a wider range of treatment alternatives. For example, by removing financial barriers, managed care plans should give enrollees more effective choice over utilizing preventive interventions, such as screening tests. Indeed, studies consistently demonstrate greater use of preventive tests and procedures among managed care enrollees.[64-66] In addition, many managed care plans contain benefits packages that include services not currently covered by many insurance programs. Indeed, pediatric patients may significantly benefit from the coverage of vaccinations, small co-payments for well-child visits, and coverage of dental and visual services for children.

Managed care plans are increasingly attempting to develop quality measures; they are trying to use these quality measures for routine assessments of performance and to provide the public with the performance results based on these quality indicators. While such extensive efforts at quality assessment in medicine have never before been undertaken and there is skepticism that these measures will be reliable and valid, if this effort is successful, many Americans will have a rigorous and systematic mechanism to evaluate the competence of their health plans and physicians.[48,49]

Besides closer monitoring of quality, other changes could improve physicians' competence and their communication with patients. The pressure created by cost controls, the resource-based relative value scale, and managed care has resulted in trends to improve reimbursement for primary care and to train more generalists. Although these initiatives are untested, they could increase the number of generalists, prompt the

retraining of specialists in general medicine, and decrease the excessive reliance on specialists with their tendency toward higher use of diagnostic tests and technical interventions without notable effect on traditional health status measures.[67,68] In addition, managed care's increased emphasis on primary care will accelerate the trend toward greater use of nurse practitioners, physician assistants, and midwives and teams composed of physicians and nonphysician providers. While the transition to such a team approach could not be accomplished instantaneously, and while it would require changing habits and increased communications among health care providers, research demonstrates that, when it is well implemented, it can improve patient care, communication, and satisfaction.[69-71] With such multidisciplinary teams, several providers are knowledgeable about the patient's condition and available to the patient, enhancing communication and continuity of care.[69,70] By increasing the number of providers for a patient, this team approach may increase the chances that patients with different cultural backgrounds might establish rapport and understanding with a provider.[69,70]

Potential Threats

There are aspects of managed care, especially under significant cost controls and price competition, with the potential to undermine, or preclude the realization of, the ideal physician-patient relationship. The spread of managed care is being promoted by big employers and corporations; it is closely linked to price competition—if not outright managed competition—which has ramifications for almost every facet of the ideal physician-patient interaction.

First, to hold down costs, many insurance companies and managed care organizations may try to select enrollees who are likely to use fewer and cheaper services ("cherry pick") through selective marketing, increased use of exclusions, modifications of benefits offered, and other techniques. In the absence of significant health insurance regulatory reform legislation or universal coverage, such techniques could mean that more Americans will be unable to afford health insurance or effectively barred from coverage. Indeed, recent statistics suggest that the ranks of the uninsured are growing.[72] In turn, this deprives more Americans of the ideal physician-patient relationship. In addition, without insurance reform legislation to ensure transportability of health coverage when people change jobs, a significant number of Americans could be forced either to forgo coverage for periods of time or to change managed care plans with each job change. Given that 7 million Americans change jobs or become employed each month, there could be significant disruption of choice, communication, and continuity.

Second, to restrain costs, a growing number of employers are restricting patient choice in all its facets.[23,73–76] An increasing number of employers are offering only one health care plan; other employers are requiring their workers to enroll in a particular managed care plan or select a physician from a precertified list; still others are requiring their workers to enroll in a particular managed care plan or select a physician from a precertified list; still others are requiring their workers to pay substantially more for the opportunity to see a physician of their choosing outside their managed care panel; and still others are discouraging workers from selecting higher priced health plans. Some employers are even reverting to an old practice of hiring their own "company" physicians.[76] Through these and other techniques, a growing, albeit unknown, number of insured Americans are having their choice limited mainly by employers.[23] These practices may seriously disrupt, or require patients to abandon, long-standing relationships with physicians. In addition, in some instances, especially in man-

aged care settings, patient choice of specialists, specialty facilities, and particular treatments is being eroded.[24]

Increasingly, managed care plans will compete for employers' contracts and subscribers on the basis of price. Yet there is no guarantee that the cheapest plan this year will be the cheapest plan during the next enrollment period. Indeed, if price competition is effective, the cheapest plan should change from year to year.[77] In such a price-competitive marketplace, employers may switch health care plans from year to year and patients may be forced to choose between continuing with their current physician and managed care plan at a higher price or switching to the cheaper plan. While patients may appear to opt for discontinuous care rather than pay more, the cost pressures—which fall disproportionately on those with lower incomes—hardly make such choices voluntary.[78–80] A recent study demonstrates a direct linear relationship between a lower family income and willingness to switch to cheaper health care plans.[23] The importance of such decisions lies in the reason for change of physician.[77] Change is harmful if it is imposed on patients explicitly or implicitly by financial incentives and interrupts continuity. When the patient, however, decides to switch physicians, continuity of care has been outweighed in the patient's mind by other factors, such as competence or communication. Consequently, significant price competition, while not engendered by managed care, is certainly exacerbated by it and could have an adverse effect on both patient choice of practice type and physician and continuity of care.[23,77]

A third threat to choice in the physician-patient relationship comes from the potential financial failure of managed care plans. If price competition is effective, inefficient plans will lose in the marketplace and close. Plan failure could pose a serious threat to patient choice and continuity of care, especially if the collapse happens between enrollment periods. Under such conditions, patients may be randomly assigned to other managed care plans. Or, their former physician may become affiliated with a plan that they are unable to join. Another threat to the physician-patient relationship may occur when managed care plans "deselect" a physician. In such circumstances, patients cannot choose that physician unless they are willing to go out of the plan. More important, patients who have been receiving care from that physician may be forced to switch to another physician in the managed care panel, again undermining patient choice and continuity of care.

Managed care also poses potential threats to competence. Its greater emphasis on the provision of primary care could adversely affect competence. Since specialists are more expensive than generalists, cost considerations foster a tendency to have generalists or even nonphysicians manage conditions that are best handled by specialists. For example, follow-up of cancer patients may be shifted from oncologists to primary care physicians. And there is some suggestion that these changes lead to fewer follow-up visits and less monitoring of the progress of disease in the managed care setting.[81] In addition, since time spent with specialists is expensive, there may be a tendency to use medications or other less expensive interventions in place of consultations with specialists.[82] Similarly, given the current shortage of generalists, there is already a movement to retrain specialist physicians as generalists. Since there are no standards for the amount and type of education needed for retraining, these retrained specialists may lack the breadth of knowledge, skills, and experience necessary to be competent primary care providers. Assessments of quality outcomes may be insensitive to these threats to competence.[83]

There are worries about the development of quality indicators. We lack quality indicators for most aspects of medical care. In addition, many quality indicators require risk adjustments for severity of illness that cannot be, or currently are not being, performed.[83,84] It will take significant time and resources to develop reliable and validated quality indicators and risk adjustors for medical procedures. Yet the demand for these indicators could result in a rush to implementation without proper pretesting and validation. Mistakes related to the imperative to release of Medicare hospital mortality data as a quality measure before they were properly adjusted may be repeated on an even larger scale.[85-88] Use of faulty quality information could damage attempts to improve the competence of physicians, undermine patient trust, and cause patients to switch physicians unnecessarily.

Communication in the physician-patient relationship could be undermined by practice efficiencies necessitated by intensified price competition and financial pressures on managed care plans. Productivity requirements may translate into pressure on physicians to see more patients in shorter time periods, reducing the time to discuss patient values, alternative treatments, or the impact of a therapy on the patient's overall life.[89,90] Such changes have been tried by managed care plans in the competitive Boston, Mass, health care market.[91] Compressing physician-patient interactions into short time periods in the name of productivity could curtail, if not eliminate, productive communication and compassion. A recent survey of patients in managed care plans showed that the physician spent less time with the patient and offered less explanation of care compared with those in traditional fee-for-service settings.[24] Similarly, to reduce costs, managed care plans might restrict telephone calls to the patient's primary care physician. Currently some plans limit patients' calls to their physicians to 1-hour time periods in the day. In addition, incentives might be put into place to encourage patients to talk with or see physicians or nonphysician providers with whom they are unfamiliar or who are not of their choosing.[82,90] All of these cost-saving mechanisms could easily inhibit physician-patient communication and continuity of care.

A further problem may arise in the competition among managed care plans to lure subscribers. They are likely to use advertising with implicit if not explicit promises of higher quality or more wide-ranging services. Such advertisements could easily create high expectations on the part of patients.[92-94] Simultaneously, however, to control costs plans will require physicians to be efficient in their personal time allocation as well as in their ordering of tests and use of other services. This could easily create a conflict between patient expectations and physician restrictions, undermining good communication, compassion, and trust.

Finally, while there has been significant attention on conflict of interest in fee-for-service practice,[39] there has been much less effort to investigate and address conflict of interest in managed care. Physician decision making may account for as much as 75% of health care costs. In the setting of significant price competition, managed care plans trying to reduce costs will therefore try to influence physician decision making, especially to reduce the use of medical services.[89] Managed care plans have already tried various mechanisms to try to reduce physician use of health care resources for their patients, including providing bonuses to physicians who order few tests and basing a percentage of physicians' salaries on volume and test ordering standards.[39,40,89] Such conflicts of interest may proliferate with increased price competition, the need for managed care plans to reduce costs, and the absence of governmental regulation.

Conclusions

The physician-patient relationship is the cornerstone for achieving, maintaining, and improving health. The structure of financing and regulation should be designed to foster and support an ideal relationship between the physician and the patient. Clearly, the current system incompletely realizes this ideal even for many well-insured Americans, and trends within the current system threaten to make this ideal even more elusive.

Managed care offers some advantages in realizing the ideal physician-patient relationship. For many Americans, increased use of managed care may secure choice, especially for preventive services, possibly expand continuity in their relationship with physicians, and implement a systematic assessment of quality and competence. But the expansion of managed care, in an environment that encourages competition and makes financial pressures intense and omnipresent, could promote serious impediments to realizing the ideal physician-patient relationship. Some practical steps that might diminish these impediments include (1) using global budgets instead of price competition among managed care plans for cost control; (2) prohibiting all schemes that use salary incentives or bonuses tied to physician test ordering patterns; (3) restricting expensive advertising by managed care plans by capping their promotion budgets; (4) requiring managed care plans to have a board of patients and physicians to approve policies regarding length of office visits and telephone calls; (5) creating an independent review board to assess the reliability and validity of all quality indicators before they are approved or required for use by managed care plans; (6) implementing insurance reform legislation to ensure mobility of insurance with job changes and purchasing of coverage by individuals; and (7) providing universal coverage to enable otherwise uninsured patients to have an opportunity for an ideal physician-patient relationship. As changes in our health care system develop, we must find ways, such as these, to encourage fiscal prudence without undermining the fundamental elements of the ideal physician-patient relationship.

Notes

The authors thank Patricia Rieker, PhD, for her review of the manuscript.

1. Miller, R.H., Luft, H.S. Managed care plan performance since 1980. *JAMA*. 1994;271:1512–1519.

2. Schwartz, W.B., Mendelson, D.N. Why managed care cannot contain hospital costs—without rationing. *Health Aff (Millwood)*. 1992;11:100–107.

3. Moran, D.W., Wolfe, P.R. Can managed care control costs? *Health Aff (Millwood)*. 1991;10:120–128.

4. Fox, P.D., Wasserman, J. Academic medical centers and managed care. *Health Aff (Millwood)*. 1993;12:85–93.

5. Eckholm, E. A town loses its hospital in the name of cost control. *New York Times*. September 26, 1994:A1.

6. Weber, M. The fundamental concepts of sociology. In: Parsons, T., ed. *The Theory of Social and Economic Organizations*. New York, NY: The Free Press; 1947: 87–157.

7. Macklin, R. *Enemies of Patients*. New York, NY: Oxford University Press Inc; 1993:chaps 1, 5, 7, 11.

8. Brody, H. *The Healer's Power*. New Haven, Conn: Yale University Press; 1992:chaps 4–8.

9. Emanuel, E.J., Emanuel, L.L. Four models of the physician-patient relationship. *JAMA*. 1992;267:2221–2226.

10. Brock, D. The ideal of shared decision-making between physicians and patients. *Kennedy Inst J Ethics*. 1991; 1:28–47.

11. Campbell, J.D., Mauksch, H.O., Meikirk, H.J., Hosokawa, M.C. Collaborative practice and provider styles of delivering health care. *Soc Sci Med*. 1990;30:1359–1385.

12. Beauchamp, T., Childress, J. *Principles of Biomedical Ethics*. 3rd ed. New York, NY: Oxford University Press; 1989:chaps 3–5, 7.

13. Kass, L.R. *Toward a More Natural Science*. New York, NY: The Free Press; 1988:chaps 6–9.

14. Appelbaum, P.S., Lidz, C., Meisel, A. *Informed Consent: Legal Theory and Clinical Practice*. New York, NY: Oxford University Press Inc; 1987.

15. Siegler, M. The profession of medicine: from physician paternalism to patient autonomy to bureaucratic parsimony. *Arch Intern Med*. 1985;145:713–715.

16. Katz, J. *The Silent World of Doctor and Patient*. New York, NY: The Free Press; 1984.

17. *Making Health Care Decisions*. Washington, DC: President's Commission for the Study of Ethical Problems in Medicine and Biomedical and Behavioral Research; 1982.

18. Veatch, R.M. *A Theory of Medical Ethics*. New York, NY: Basic Books Inc Publishers; 1980:pts 2 and 3.

19. Szasz, T.S., Hollender, M.H. The basic models of the doctor-patient relationship. *Arch Intern Med*. 1956; 97:585–592.

20. Rawls, J. *Political Liberalism*. New York, NY: Columbia University Press; 1993:pt 1.

21. Dworkin, R. *Taking Rights Seriously*. Cambridge, Mass: Harvard University Press; 1977:chaps 2–4.

22. Emanuel, E.J. *The Ends of Human Life: Medical Ethics in a Liberal Polity*. Cambridge, Mass: Harvard University Press; 1991:chap 1.

23. The Kaiser/Commonwealth Fund Second National Health Insurance Survey. November 10, 1993.

24. Blendon, R.J., Knox, R.A., Brodie, M., Benson, J.M., Chervinsky, G. Americans compare managed care, Medicare, and fee for service. *J Am Health Policy*. 1994;4:42–47.

25. Sofaer, S. Informing and protecting consumers under managed competition. *Health Aff (Millwood)*. 1993; 12(suppl):76–86.

26. Ingelfinger, F.J. Arrogance. *N Engl J Med*. 1980;304: 1507.

27. Marzuk, P.M. The right kind of paternalism. *N Engl J Med*. 1985;313:1474–1476.

28. Applegate, W.B. Physician management of patients with adverse outcomes. *Arch Intern Med*. 1986;146: 2249–2252.

29. Ware, J., Snyder, M. Dimensions of patient attitudes regarding doctors and medical care services. *Med Care*. 1975;13:669–682.

30. Woolley, F.R., Kane, R.L., Hughes, C.C., Wright, D.D. The effects of doctor-patient communication on satisfaction and outcome of care. *Soc Sci Med*. 1978; 12:123–128.

31. Hickson, G.B., Clayton, E.W., Githens, P.B., Sloan, F.A. Factors that prompted families to file medical malpractice claims following perinatal injuries. *JAMA*. 1992;267:1359–1363.

32. Feilich, B. The death of a baby: neither forgiven nor forgotten. *JAMA*. 1992;268:1413–1414.

33. Spiro, H., McCrea-Curnen, M.G., Peschel, I., St. James, D., eds. *Empathy and the Practice of Medicine*. New Haven, Conn: Yale University Press; 1993:chaps 1–3, 8, 9, 13–16.

34. Jonsen, A. *The New Medicine and the Old Ethics*. Cambridge, Mass: Harvard University Press; 1990.

35. *Tarasoff v Regents of the University of California et al*, 131 Cal Rptr 14 (1976).

36. *McIntosh v Milano*, 168 NJ 466 (1979).

37. Council on Ethical and Judicial Affairs, American Medical Association. Conflict of interest: physician ownership of medical facilities. *JAMA*. 1992;267: 2366–2369.

38. Thompson, D. Understanding financial conflicts of interest. *N Engl J Med*. 1993;329:573–576.

39. Rodwin, M. *Medicine, Money, and Morals*. New York, NY: Oxford University Press Inc; 1993.

40. Hillman, A.L., Pauly, M.V., Kerstein, J.J. How do financial incentives affect physicians' clinical decisions and the financial performance of health maintenance organizations? *N Engl J Med*. 1989;321:86–92.

41. Relman, A.S. Dealing with conflicts of interest. *N Engl J Med*. 1985;313:749–751.

42. Nelson, C., Short, K. *Health Insurance Coverage, 1986–88*. Washington, DC: US Bureau of the Census; 1990.

43. Lewin-Epstein, N. Determinants of regular source of health care in black, Mexican, Puerto Rican, and non-Hispanic white populations. *Med Care*. 1991;29:543–557.

44. Hadley, J., Steinberg, E.P., Feder, J. Comparison of uninsured and privately insured hospital patients: condition on admission, resource use, and outcome. *JAMA*. 1991;265:374–379.

45. Burstin, H.R., Lipsitz, S.R., Brennan, T.A. Socioeconomic status and risk for substandard medical care. *JAMA*. 1992;268:2383–2387.

46. Iglehart, J.K. The American health care system: teaching hospitals. *N Engl J Med*. 1993;329:1052–1056.

47. Hoch S. Tsongas's case. *New York Times*. February 20, 1992:A23.

48. Laffel, G., Berwick, D.M. Quality in health care. *JAMA*. 1992;268:407–409.

49. Kritchevsky, S.B., Simmons, B.P. Continuous quality improvement: concepts and applications for physician care. *JAMA*. 1991;266:1817–1823.

50. Ramsey, P.G., Carline, J.D., Inui, T.S., Larson, E.B., LoGerfo, J.P., Wenrich, M.D. Predictive validity of certification by the American Board of Internal Medicine. *Ann Intern Med*. 1989;110:719–726.

51. Benson, J.A. Certification and recertification: one approach to professional accountability. *Ann Intern Med*. 1991;114:238–242.

52. Merkel, W.T., Margolis, R.B., Smith, R.C. Teaching humanistic and psychosocial aspects of care. *J Gen Intern Med*. 1990;5:34–41.

53. Beckman, H., Frankel, R., Kihm, J., Kulesza, G., Geheb, M. Measurement and improvement of humanistic skills in first year trainees. *J Gen Intern Med*. 1990; 5:42–45.

54. Levinson, W., Roter, D. The effects of two continuing medical education programs on communication skills of practicing primary care physicians. *J Gen Intern Med*. 1993;8:318–324.

55. Perkins, H.S., Bauer, R.L., Hazuda, H.P. Schoolfield, J.D. Impact of legal liability, family wishes, and other 'external factors' on physicians' life support decisions. *Am J Med*. 1990;89:185–194.

56. Localio, A.R., Lawthers, A.G., Bengtson, J.M. et al. Relationship between malpractice claims and cesarean delivery. *JAMA*. 1993;269:366–373.

57. Rosenbach, M.L., Stone, A.G. Malpractice insurance costs and physician practice 1983–1986. *Health Aff (Millwood)*. 1990;9:176–185.

58. Woolhandler, S., Himmelstein, D. The deteriorating administrative efficiency of the U.S. health care system. *N Engl J Med*. 1991;324:1253–1258.

59. Gray, B. *The Profit Motive and Patient Care*. Cambridge, Mass: Harvard University Press; 1991:chaps 5–8, 10, 11.

60. Mitchell, J.M., Scott, E. Physician ownership of physical therapy services: effects on charges, utilization, profits, and service characteristics. *JAMA*. 1992;268: 2055–2059.

61. Igelhart, J.K. The struggle between managed care and fee for service practice. *N Engl J Med*. 1994;331:63–67.

62. *Effects of Managed Care: An Update*. Washington, DC: Congressional Budget Office; 1994.

63. *Managed Health Care: Effects on Employers' Costs Difficult to Measure*. Washington, DC: US General Accounting Office; 1993.

64. Bernstein, A.B., Thompson, G.B., Harlan, L.C. Differences in rates of cancer screening by usual source of medical care: data from the 1987 National Health Interview Survey. *Med Care*. 1991;29:196–209.

65. Retchin, S.M., Brown, B. The quality of ambulatory care in Medicare health maintenance organizations. *Am J Public Health*. 1990;80:411–415.

66. Udvarhelyi, I.S., Jennison, K., Phillips, R.S., Epstein, A.M. Comparison of the quality of ambulatory care for fee-for-service and prepaid patients. *Ann Intern Med*. 1991;327:424–429.

67. Greenfield, S., Nelson, E.C., Zubkoff, M. et al. Variations in resource utilization among medical specialties and systems of care. *JAMA*. 1992;267:1624–1630.

68. Schroeder, S.A., Sandy, L.G. Specialty distribution of U.S. physicians—the invisible driver of health care costs. *N Engl J Med*. 1993;328:961–963.

69. *Nurse Practitioners, Physicians' Assistants, and Certified Nurse Midwives: Policy Analysis.* Washington, DC: Office of Technology Assessment; 1986.

70. Freund, C. Research in support of nurse practitioners. In: Mezey, M., McGivern, D., eds. *Nurses and Nurse Practitioners: The Evolution to Advanced Practice.* New York, NY: Springer Publishing Co Inc; 1993.

71. Kavesh, W. Physician and nurse-practitioner relationships. In: Mezey, M., McGivern, D., eds. *Nurses and Nurse Practitioners: The Evolution to Advanced Practice.* New York, NY: Springer Publishing Co Inc; 1993.

72. Pear, R. Health insurance percentage is lowest in four Sun Belt states. *New York Times.* October 6, 1994:A16.

73. Lewis, D.E. Coping without coverage. *Boston Globe.* May 5, 1993:45.

74. Lewis, D.E. Union oks Boston gas accord. *Boston Globe.* May 21, 1993:53.

75. Seitz, R. The political tea leaves point to medical networks. *New York Times.* December 20, 1992:D10.

76. Pasternak, J. In-house doctors give some firms a health care remedy. *Los Angeles Times.* July 11, 1993:A1.

77. Emanuel, E.J., Brett, A.S. Managed competition and the patient-physician relationship. *N Engl J Med.* 1993; 329:879–882.

78. Travis, M.R., Russell, G., Cronin, S. Determinants of voluntary disenrollment. *J Health Care Marketing.* 1989;9:75–76.

79. Hennelly, V.D., Boxerman, S.B. Out-of-plan use and disenrollment: outgrowths of dissatisfaction with a prepaid group plan. *Med Care.* 1983;21:348–359.

80. Sorenson, A.A., Wersinger, R.P. Factors influencing disenrollment from an HMO. *Med Care.* 1981; 19:766–773.

81. Clement, D.G., Retchin, S.M., Brown, R.S., Stegall, M.H. Access and outcomes of elderly patients enrolled in managed care. *JAMA.* 1994;271:1487–1492.

82. Henneberger, M. Managed care changing practice of psychotherapy. *New York Times.* October 9, 1994:A1, A50.

83. Salem-Schatz, S., Moore, G., Rucker, M., Pearson, S.D. The case for case-mix adjustment in practice profiling: when good apples look bad. *JAMA.* 1994;272:871–874.

84. McNeil, B.J., Pederson, S.H., Gatsonis, C. Current issues in profiling quality of care. *Inquiry.* 1992;29:298–307.

85. Green, J., Passman, L.J., Wintfield, N. Analyzing hospital mortality: the consequences of diversity in patient mix. *JAMA.* 1991;265:1849–1853.

86. Burke, M. HCFA's Medicare mortality data: the controversy continues. *Hospitals.* 1992:118, 120, 122.

87. Greenfield, S., Aronow, H.U., Elashoff, R.M., Wantanabe, D. Flaws in mortality data: the hazards of ignoring comorbid disease. *JAMA.* 1988;260:2253–2255.

88. Robinson, M.L. Limitations of mortality data confirmed: studies. *Hospitals.* 1988;62:23–24.

89. Baker, L.C., Cantor, J.C. Physician satisfaction under managed care. *Health Aff (Millwood).* 1993; 12(suppl): 258–270.

90. Jellinek, M.S., Nurcombe, B. Two wrongs don't make a right: managed care, mental health, and the marketplace. *JAMA.* 1993;270:1737–1739.

91. Knox, R.A., Stein, C. HMO doctors want boss out in dispute on patient load. *Boston Globe.* November 21, 1991:1, 27.

92. Freidson, E. Prepaid group practice and the new 'demanding patients.' *Milbank Mem Fund Q.* 1973;51: 473–488.

93. Schroeder, J.L., Clarke, J.T., Webster, J.R. Prepaid entitlements: a new challenge for physician-patient relationships. *JAMA.* 1985;254:3080–3082.

94. Brett, A.S. The case against persuasive advertising by health maintenance organizations. *N Engl J Med.* 1992;326:1253–1257.

Bibliography

The references listed below are cited in the introduction to the volume, the introductions to each of the five parts of the volume, and the notes that appear at the openings of each section. References particular to the selections are given at the ends of each selection.

Antonovsky, Aaron, and Judith Bernstein. 1977. Social class and infant mortality. *Social Science and Medicine* 11:453–70.

Aristotle. 1941. Nichomachean ethics. In *Basic Works,* edited by Richard McKeon. New York: Random House.

Arras, John D., and Bonnie Steinbock. 1995. Moral reasoning in the medical context. Introduction to *Ethical Issues in Modern Medicine.* 4th ed. Mountain View, Calif.: Mayfield Publishing.

Beauchamp, Tom L., and James Childress. 1994. *Principles of Medical Ethics.* 4th ed. New York: Oxford University Press.

Becker, Howard S., et al. 1961. *Boys in White: Student Culture in Medical School.* Chicago: University of Chicago Press.

Berkman, Lisa F., and S. Leonard Syme. 1979. Social networks, host resistance, and mortality: A nine-year follow-up study of Alameda County residents. *American Journal of Epidemiology* 109:186–204.

Berry, Wendell. 1992. *Fidelity.* New York: Pantheon.

Bickel, Nina A., et al. 1992. Referral patterns for coronary artery disease treatment: gender bias or good clinical judgment? *Annals of Internal Medicine* 116:791–97.

Bloom, Samuel. 1963. *The Doctor and His Patient—A Sociological Interpretation.* New York: Russell Sage Foundation.

Blythe, Ronald. 1979. *The View in Winter.* New York: Harcourt, Brace, Jovanovich.

Brandt, Allan. 1985. *No Magic Bullet: A Social History of Venereal Disease in the United States Since 1800.* Oxford: Oxford University Press.

Brody, Howard. 1987. *Stories of Sickness.* New Haven, Conn.: Yale University Press.

Brumberg, Joan. 1989. *Fasting Girls.* Cambridge, Mass.: Harvard University Press.

Camenisch, Paul F. 1979. The right to health care: A contractual approach. *Soundings* (Fall): 293–310.

Cassell, Eric J. 1986. The changing concept of the ideal physician. *Daedalus* 115 (2): 185–207.

Cassel, John. 1976. The contribution of the social environment to host resistance: The fourth Wade Hampton Frost lecture. *American Journal of Epidemiology* 104:107–23.

Cherlin, Andrew. 1992. *Marriage, Divorce, and Remarriage.* Cambridge, Mass.: Harvard University Press.

Churchill, Larry R. 1987. *Rationing Health Care in America.* Notre Dame, Ind.: University of Notre Dame Press.

Coale, Ansley J., and Paul Demeny. 1983. *Regional Model Life Tables and Stable Populations.* Princeton, N.J.: Princeton University Press.

Cole, Thomas R. 1992. *The Journey of Life: A Cultural History of Aging in America.* Cambridge: Cambridge University Press.

Conrad, Peter. 1988. Learning to doctor: Reflections on recent accounts of the medical school years. *Journal of Health and Social Behavior* 29 (4): 323–32.

Cornman, John M., and Eric R. Kingson. 1996. Trends, issues, perspectives, and values for the aging of the baby boom cohorts. *The Gerontologist* 36 (1): 15–26 (excerpt 19–23).

Crimmins, Eileen M., Yasuhiko Saito, and Dominique Ingegneri. 1989. Changes in life expectancy and disability-free life expectancy in the United States. *Population and Development Review* 15:235–67.

Daniels, Norman. 1985. *Just Health Care.* New York: Cambridge University Press.

Dressler, William W. 1993. Health in the African American community: Accounting for health inequalities. *Medical Anthropology Quarterly* 7:325–45.

Durkheim, Emile. 1951. *Suicide: A Study in Sociology.* Translated by John A. Spaulding and George Simpson. Glencoe, Ill.: Free Press.

Estes, Carroll L. 1993. The aging enterprise revisited. *The Gerontologist* 33:292–98.

Estes, Carroll L., and Elizabeth A. Binney. 1989. The biomedicalization of aging: Dangers and dilemmas. *The Gerontologist* 29:587–96.

Fabrega, Horatio. 1974. *Disease and Social Behavior.* Cambridge, Mass.: M.I.T. Press.

Faden, Ruth, and Tom L. Beauchamp, with Nancy M. P. King. 1986. *A History and Theory of Informed Consent.* New York: Oxford University Press.

Farmer, Paul. 1992. *AIDS and Accusation.* Berkeley: University of California Press.

Fausto-Sterling, Anne. 1985. *Myths of Gender: Biological Theories about Women and Men.* New York: Basic Books.

Flack, Harley E., and Edmund D. Pellegrino, eds. 1992. *African-American Perspectives on Biomedical Ethics.* Washington, D.C.: Georgetown University Press.

Fleck, Leonard, and Harriet Squier. 1995. Just caring: Facing the ethical challenges of managed care. *Family Practice Management* (October): 49–55.

Fleck, Leonard, and Marcia Angell. 1991. Case Studies: Please don't tell! *Hastings Center Report* 21 (6): 39–40.

Fox, Renée C. 1986. Medicine, science, and technology. In *Applications of Social Science to Clinical Medicine and Health Policy,* edited by Linda Aikin and David Mechanic. New Brunswick, N.J.: Rutgers University Press.

——. 1988. The Autopsy: Its place in the attitude learning of second year medical students. In *Essays in Medical Sociology,* 2nd ed. New Brunswick, N.J.: Transaction.

——. 1988. Is there a "new" medical student?: A comparative view of medical socialization in the 1950s and the 1970s. In *Essays in Medical Sociology,* 2nd ed. New Brunswick: Transaction.

——. 1988. Training for uncertainty. In *Essays in Medical Sociology,* 2nd ed. New Brunswick: Transaction.

Fries, James F. 1980. Aging, natural death, and the compression of morbidity. *New England Journal of Medicine* 303:130–35.

——. 1984. The compression of morbidity: Miscellaneous comments about a theme. *The Gerontologist* 24:354–59.

Fuchs, Victor. 1984. The "rationing" of medical care. *New England Journal of Medicine* 311:1572–73.

Geertz, Clifford. 1973. *Interpretations of Culture.* New York: Basic Books.

Gerber, Lane A. 1983. Specialness. In *Married to Their Careers: Career and Family Dilemmas in Doctors' Lives.* New York: Tavistock.

Gijsbers van Wijk, Cecile M. T., et al. 1992. Male and female morbidity in general practice: The nature of sex differences. *Social Science and Medicine* 35:665–78.

Good, Mary-Jo DelVecchio. 1995. *American Medicine: The Quest for Competence.* Berkeley: University of California Press.

Haan, Mary N., George A. Kaplan, and S. Leonard Syme. 1989. Socioeconomic status and health: Old observations and new thoughts. In *Pathways to Health: The Role of Social Factors,* edited by John Bunker et al. Menlo Park, Calif.: Henry J. Kaiser Family Foundation.

Hafferty, Frederick W. 1991. *Into the Valley: Death and the Socialization of Medical Students.* New Haven, Conn.: Yale University Press.

Hahn, Harlan. 1988. The politics of physical differences: Disability and discrimination. *Journal of Social Issues* 44:39–47.

Hawkins, Ann Hunsaker. 1993. *Reconstructing Illness: Studies in Pathology.* West Lafayette, Ind.: Purdue University Press.

Hunter, Kathryn Montgomery. 1991. *Doctors' Stories: The Narrative Structure of Medical Knowledge.* Princeton University Press.

James, Sherman. 1994. John Henryism and the health of African-Americans. *Culture, Medicine, and Psychiatry* 18:163–82.

Johansson, S. Ryan. 1991. The health transition: The cultural inflation of morbidity during the decline of mortality. *Health Transition Review* 1:39–68.

Jonsen, Albert, and Stephen Toulmin. 1988. *The Abuse of Casuistry.* Berkeley: University of California Press.

Kant, Immanuel. 1985. *Foundations of the Metaphysics of Morals.* Translated by Lewis White Beck. New York: Macmillan.

Kaplan, George A., et al. 1988. Social connections and mortality from all causes and from cardiovascular disease: Prospective evidence from eastern Finland. *American Journal of Epidemiology* 128:370–80.

Kass, Leon R. 1985. *Toward a More Natural Science: Biology and Human Affairs.* New York: Free Press.

Kitagawa, Evelyn M., and Philip M. Hauser. 1973. *Differential Mortality in the United States: A Study in Socioeconomic Epidemiology.* Cambridge, Mass.: Harvard University Press.

Klass, Perri. 1988. *A Not Entirely Benign Procedure: Four Years as a Medical Student.* New York: Putnam.

Kleinman, Arthur. 1980. *Patients and Healers in the Context of Culture.* Berkeley: University of California Press.

——. 1986. *The Social Origins of Distress and Disease.* New Haven, Conn.: Yale University Press.

——. 1988. *The Illness Narratives.* New York: Free Press.

Kleinman, Arthur, Leon Eisenberg, and Byron Good. 1978. Culture, illness, and care: Clinical lessons from anthropologic and cross-cultural research. *Annals of Internal Medicine* 88:83–93.

Konner, Melvin. 1987. *Becoming a Doctor: A Journey of Initiation in Medical School.* New York: Viking.

Kreiger, Nancy. 1994. Epidemiology and the web of causation: Has anyone seen the spider? *Social Science and Medicine* 39:887–903.

Kreiger, Nancy, and Mary Bassett. 1986. The health of black folk: Class and ideology in science. *Monthly Review* (July–August): 74–85.

Kreiger, Nancy, et al. 1993. Racism, sexism, and social class: Implications for the study of health, disease, and well-being. *American Journal of Preventive Medicine* 9 (Suppl. 2): 81–122.

Kriegel, Leonard. 1991. *Falling Into Life: Essays.* Minneapolis, Minn.: Northpoint Press.

Lang, Gretchen Chesley. 1989. Making sense about diabetes: Dakota narratives of illness. *Medical Anthropology* 11:305–27.

Lasker, Judith N., Brenda P. Egolf, and Stewart Wolf. 1994. Community social change and mortality. *Social Science and Medicine* 39:53–62.

LaVeist, Thomas A. 1994. Beyond dummy variables and sample selection: What health services researchers ought to know about race as a variable. *Health Services Research* 1:1–16.

LeBaron, Charles. 1982. *Gentle Vengeance: An Account of the First Year at Harvard Medical School.* New York: Penguin Books.

LeVay, Simon. 1993. *The Sexual Brain.* Cambridge, Mass.: M.I.T. Press.

Lock, Margaret. 1994. *Encounters with Aging.* Berkeley: University of California Press.

MacDonald, Michael. 1989. The medicalization of suicide in England: Laymen, physicians, and cultural change, 1500–1870. *Milbank Quarterly* 67 (Suppl. 1): 69–91.

MacIntyre, Alasdair. 1984. *After Virtue.* Notre Dame, Ind.: University of Notre Dame Press.

Macintyre, Sally, Kate Hunt, and Helen Sweeting. 1996. Gender differences in health: Are things really as simple as they seem? *Social Science and Medicine* 42 (4): 617–24.

McKeown, Thomas R. 1976. *The Role of Medicine: Dream, Mirage, or Nemesis.* London: Nuffield Provincial Hospitals Trust.

Macklin, Ruth. 1991. Artificial means of reproduction and our understanding of the family. *Hastings Center Report* 21 (1): 5–11.

Manton, Kenneth G. 1982. Changing concepts of mortality and morbidity in the elderly population. *Milbank Memorial Fund Quarterly* 60:183–244.

Marmot, M. G., M. Kogevinas, and M. A. Elston. 1987. Social/economic status and disease. *Annual Reviews of Public Health* 8:111–35.

Mechanic, David. 1962. The concept of illness behavior. *Journal of Chronic Disease* 15:189–95.

——. 1989. Socioeconomic status and health: An examination of the underlying processes. In *Pathways to Health:*

The Role of Social Factors, edited by John Bunker et al. Menlo Park, Calif.: Henry J. Kaiser Family Foundation.

Merton, Robert K. 1957. Some Preliminaries to a Sociology of Medical Education. In *The Student Physician,* edited by R. K. Merton, G. G. Reader, and P. L. Kendall. Cambridge, Mass.: Harvard University Press.

Mill, John S. 1957. *Utilitarianism.* New York: Liberal Arts Press.

Miller, Robert, and Harold Luft. 1994. Managed care plan performance since 1980. *Journal of the American Medical Association* 271:1512–19.

Mosely, William H., and Lincoln C. Chen. 1984. An analytical framework for the study of child survival in developing countries. In *Child Survival: Strategies for Research,* edited by W. H. Mosely and L. C. Chen. Cambridge: Cambridge University Press.

Mullan, Fitzhugh. 1976. Student of the body, captive of the system. *White Coat, Clenched Fist.* New York: Macmillan.

Murphy, Robert M. 1987. *The Body Silent.* New York: W. W. Norton.

Murray, Christopher J. L., and Lincoln C. Chen. 1992. Understanding morbidity change. *Population and Development Review* 18:481–504.

Myers, George C., and Kenneth G. Manton. 1984. Compression of mortality: Myth or reality? *The Gerontologist* 24:346–53.

National Academy of Social Insurance (NASI). 1994. *Rethinking Disability Policy: The Role of Income, Health Care, Rehabilitation and Related Services in Fostering Independence.* Preliminary Status Report of the Disability Policy Panel.

National Commission for the Protection of Human Subjects of Biomedical and Behavioral Research. 1978. *The Belmont Report: Ethical Principles and Guidelines for the Protection of Human Subjects of Research.* DHEW pub. no. (OS) 78-0012-78-0014. Washington, D.C.: U.S. Government Printing Office.

Navarro, Vicente. 1990. Race or class versus race and class: Mortality differentials in the United States. *Lancet* 336:1238–40.

Okojie, Christina E. E. 1994. Gender inequalities in the Third World. *Social Science and Medicine* 39:1237–48.

Osborne, Newton G., and Marvin D. Feit. 1992. The use of race in medical research. *Journal of the American Medical Association* 267:275–79.

Otten, Mac W., et. al. 1990. The effect of known risk factors on the excess mortality of black adults in the United States. *Journal of the American Medical Association* 263:845–50.

Pappas, Gregory et al. 1993. The Increasing Disparity in

Mortality between Socioeconomic Groups in the United States, 1960 and 1986. *New England Journal of Medicine* 329:103–9.

Parsons, Talcott. 1951. *The Social System.* New York: Free Press.

Pearson, Veronica. 1995. Goods on which one loses: Women and mental health in China. *Social Science and Medicine* 41:1159–73.

Preston, Samuel H. 1984. Children and the elderly in the U.S. *Scientific American* 251 (6): 44–49.

Price, Reynolds. 1994. *A Whole New Life.* New York: Atheneum.

Rapp, Rayna. 1993. Accounting for amniocentesis. In *Knowledge, Power, Practice,* edited by S. Lindenbaum and M. Lock. Berkeley: University of California Press.

Reilly, Phillip. 1987. *To Do No Harm: A Journey through Medical School.* Dover, Mass.: Auburn House.

Rosenberg, Charles. 1962. *The Cholera Years: The United States in 1832, 1849, and 1866.* Chicago: University of Chicago Press.

Sade, Robert. 1971. Medical care as a right: A refutation. *New England Journal of Medicine* 285:1288–90.

Scribner, Richard. 1996. Paradox as paradigm—The health outcomes of Mexican Americans. *American Journal of Public Health* 86:303–4.

Shryock, Henry S., and Jacob S. Siegel and Associates. 1980. *The Methods and Materials of Demography.* Washington, D.C.: U.S. Bureau of the Census.

Starr, Paul. 1982. *The Social Transformation of American Medicine.* New York: Basic Books.

Starr, Paul. 1994. *The Logic of Health Care Reform.* Revised and expanded edition. New York: Whettle Brooks.

Styron, William. 1990. *Darkness Visible: A Memoir of Madness.* New York: Random House.

Taussig, Michael. 1980. Reification and the consciousness of the patient. *Social Science and Medicine* 14B:3–13.

Thurow, Lester. 1984. Learning to say no. *New England Journal of Medicine* 311:1569–72.

Tong, Rosemarie. 1993. *Feminine and Feminist Ethics.* Belmont, Calif.: Wadsworth.

Townsend, Peter, and Nick Davidson. 1982. *Inequalities in Health: The Black Report.* New York: Penguin Books.

Veatch, Robert. 1981. *A Theory of Medical Ethics.* New York: Basic Books.

Verbrugge, Lois M. 1984. Longer life but worsening health? Trends in health and mortality of middle-aged and older persons. *Milbank Memorial Fund Quarterly/Health and Society* 62:475–519.

——. 1989. The twain meet: empirical explanations of sex differences and mortality. *Journal of Health and Social Behavior* 30:282–304.

Verbrugge, Lois M., and Deborah L. Wingard. 1987. Sex differentials in health and mortality. *Women and Health* 12:103–46.

Vladeck, Bruce, Nancy Miller, and Steven Clauser. 1993. The changing face of long term care. *Health Care Finance Review* 14 (4): 5–23.

Waldron, Ingrid. 1990. What do we know about causes of sex differences in mortality? A review of the literature. In *The Sociology of Health and Illness,* edited by P. Conrad and R. Kern. New York: St. Martin's Press.

Walzer, Michael. 1983. *Spheres of Justice: A Defense of Pluralism and Equality.* New York: Basic Books.

Wenneker, Mark B., and Arnold M. Epstein. 1989. Racial inequalities in the use of procedures for patients with ischemic heart disease in Massachusetts. *Journal of the American Medical Association* 261:253–57.

Wingard, Deborah L., et al. Sex differentials in morbidity and mortality risks examined by age and cause in the same cohort. *American Journal of Epidemiology* 130:601–5.

Wise, Paul H. 1993. Confronting racial disparities in infant mortality: Reconciling science and politics. *American Journal of Preventive Medicine* 9 (Suppl. 2): 7–16.

Wise, Paul H., et al. 1985. Racial and socioeconomic disparities in childhood mortality in Boston. *New England Journal of Medicine* 313:361–66.

Woolf, Virginia. 1986. On Being Ill. In *The Essays of Virginia Woolf, 1896–1941.* London: Hogarth Press.

World Bank. 1993. *1993 World Bank Development Report.* Washington, D.C.: World Bank.

Wright, Anne L., et al. 1993. Cultural interpretations and intracultural variability in Navajo beliefs about breastfeeding. *American Ethnologist* 20:781–96.

Zimmerman, Rick S., et al. 1994. Who is Hispanic? Definitions and their consequences. *American Journal of Public Health* 84:1985–87.

Acknowledgment of Copyrights

∎

Abraham, Laurie K., " 'Where Crowded Humanity Suffers and Sickens': The Banes Family and Their Neighborhood," from *Mama Might Be Better Off Dead: The Failure of Health Care in America.* © 1993. Reprinted by permission of University of Chicago Press and the author.

Adler, Nancy E., Boyce, W. Thomas, Chesney, Margaret A., Folkman, Susan, Syme, S. Leonard, "Socioeconomic Inequalities in Health: No Easy Solution," from *Journal of the American Medical Association,* vol. 269, no. 24. © 1993. Reprinted by permission of the publisher.

Andre, Judith, "Swapping Stories: A Matter of Ethics," from *Medical Humanities Report,* Winter 1992. © 1992 by the Center for Ethics and Humanities in the Life Sciences. Reprinted by permission of the author.

Angell, Marcia, "The Case of Helga Wanglie: A New Kind of 'Right to Die' Case," from *New England Journal of Medicine,* vol. 325, no. 7, 511–512. © 1991 by the Massachusetts Medical Society. Reprinted by permission of the publisher. All rights reserved.

Annas, George J., "Faith (Healing), Hope, and Charity at the FDA: The Politics of AIDS Drug Trials," from *Standard of Care: The Law of American Bioethics.* © 1993 by George J. Annas. Reprinted by permission of Oxford University Press, Inc.

Annas, George J., "Informed Consent, Cancer, and Truth in Prognosis," from *New England Journal of Medicine,* vol. 330, no. 3, 223–225. © 1994 by the Massachusetts Medical Society. Reprinted by permission of the publisher.

Annas, George J., "The Prostitute, the Playboy, and the Poet: Rationing Schemes for Organ Transplantation," from *American Journal of Public Health,* vol. 75, no. 2, 187–189. © 1985. Reprinted by permission of American Public Health Association and the author.

Asch, David A. and Parker, Ruth M., "The Libby Zion Case: One Step Forward or Two Steps Backward?" from *New England Journal of Medicine,* vol. 318, no. 12, 771–775. © 1988 by the Massachusetts Medical Society. Reprinted by permission of the publisher.

Balshem, Martha, "Cancer, Control, and Causality: Talking About Cancer in a Working-Class Community," from *American Ethnologist,* vol. 18, no. 1, 152–171. © February 1991. Reprinted by permission of the American Anthropological Association and the author. Not for further reproduction.

Basson, Marc D., Dworkin, Gerald, Cassell, Eric J., "Case Study: The 'Student Doctor' and a Wary Patient," from *The Hastings Center Report,* vol. 12, no. 1, 27–28. © 1982. Reprinted by permission of the Hastings Center and M. Basson.

Betts, Doris, "The Mother-in-Law," from *Beasts of the Southern Wild and Other Stories.* © 1973 by Doris Betts and HarperCollins Publishers, Inc. Reprinted by permission of Russell & Volkening as agents for the author.

Bloom, Amy, "Silver Water," from *Come to Me.* © 1993 by Amy Bloom. Reprinted by permission of HarperCollins Publishers, Inc. and the author.

Branch, William, Pels, Richard J., Lawrence, Robert S., Arky, Ronald, "Becoming a Doctor—Critical Events Reports from Third-Year Medical Students," from *New England Journal of Medicine,* vol. 329, no. 15, 1130–1132. © 1993 by the Massachusetts Medical Society. Reprinted by permission of the publisher.

Brewster, Abenaa, "A Student's View of a Medical Teaching Exercise," from *New England Journal of Medicine,* vol. 329, no. 26, 1971–1972. © 1993 by the Massachusetts Medical Society. Reprinted by permission of the publisher.

Callahan, Daniel, "What Do Children Owe Elderly Parents?" from *The Hastings Center Report,* vol. 15, no. 2, 32–37. © 1985. Reprinted by permission of the Hastings Center and the author.

Canin, Ethan, "We are Nighttime Travelers," from *Emperor of the Air.* © 1988 by Ethan Canin. Reprinted by permission of Houghton Mifflin Company. All rights reserved.

Carver, Raymond, "What the Doctor Said," from *A New Path to the Waterfall.* © 1989 by The Estate of Raymond Carver. Reprinted by permission of Grove/Atlantic, Inc.

Cassell, Eric J., "The Nature of Suffering and the Goals of Medicine," from *New England Journal of Medicine,* vol. 306, no. 11, 639–645. © 1982 by the Massachusetts Medical Society. Reprinted by permission of the publisher.

Chervenak, Frank A. and McCullough, Laurence B., "Justified Limits on Refusing Intervention," from *Hastings Center Report,* vol. 21, no. 2, 12–18. © 1991. Reprinted by permission of the Hastings Center and the authors.

Churchill, Larry R., "Bioethics in Social Context," from

Perkoff, Gerald T., "The Boundaries of Medicine," from *Journal of Chronic Diseases*, vol. 383, no. 3, 271–278. © 1985 Elsevier Science Inc. Reprinted by permission of the publisher.

Povar, Gail and Moreno, Jonathan, "Hippocrates and the Health Maintenance Organization: A Discussion of Ethical Issues," in *Annals of Internal Medicine*, vol. 109, 419–424. © 1988. Reprinted by permission of the publisher.

Quill, Timothy E., "Death and Dignity: A Case of Individualized Decision Making," from *New England Journal of Medicine*, vol. 324, no. 10, 691–694. © 1991 by the Massachusetts Medical Society. Reprinted by permission of the publisher.

Redmayne, Sharon and Klein, Rudolph, "Rationing in Practice: The Case of In Vitro Fertilisation," from *British Medical Journal*, vol. 306, 1521–1524. © 1993. Reprinted by permission of the publisher and S. Redmayne.

Reinhardt, Uwe E., "Reforming the Health Care System: The Universal Dilemma," from *American Journal of Law and Medicine*, vol. 19, no. 1, 21–36. © 1993 by Uwe Rheinhardt and *American Journal of Law and Medicine*. Reprinted by permission of the publisher and the author.

Relman, Arnold, "The Changing Demography of the Medical Profession," from *New England Journal of Medicine*, vol. 321, no. 22, 1540–1541. © 1989 by the Massachusetts Medical Society. Reprinted by permission of the publisher.

Relman, Arnold S., "Physicians and Business Managers: A Clash of Cultures," from *Health Management Quarterly*, vol. 16, no. 3, 11–14. © 1994 by Baxter Foundation. Reprinted by permission of the publisher.

Rhoden, Nancy K., "Cesareans and Samaritans," from *Law, Medicine and Health Care*, vol. 15, no. 3, 118–125. © 1987 by American Society of Law and Medicine. Reprinted by permission of the publisher and the author.

Seldin, Donald W., "Presidential Address: The Boundaries of Medicine," from *Transactions of the American Association of Physicians*, vol. 94, 75–84. © 1981 by Donald W. Seldin and American Association of Physicians. Reprinted by permission of the publisher and the author.

Surbone, Antonella, "Truth Telling to the Patient," from *Journal of the American Medical Association*, vol. 268, no. 13, 1661–1662. © 1992. Reprinted by permission of the publisher.

Szasz, Thomas S. and Hollender, Marc H., "The Basic Models of the Doctor-Patient Relationship," from *Archives of Internal Medicine*, vol. 97, 585–592. © 1956 by American Medical Association. Reprinted by permission of the publisher.

Weaver, Gordon, "Finch the Spastic Speaks," from *The Entombed Man of Thule*. © 1972 by Gordon Weaver. Reprinted by permission of Louisiana State University Press.

Williams, William Carlos, "The Last Words of My English Grandmother," from *The Collected Poems of William Carlos Williams, 1909–1939*, vol. I. © 1938. Reprinted by permission of New Directions Publishing Corporation.

Williams, William Carlos, "The Paid Nurse," from *The Doctor Stories*. © 1938. Reprinted by permission of New Directions Publishing Company.

Williams, William Carlos, "The Use of Force," from *The Doctor Stories*. © 1938. Reprinted by permission of New Directions Publishing Company.

Winkenwerder, William Jr., "Ethical Dilemmas for House Staff Physicians: The Care of Critically Ill and Dying Patients," from *Journal of the American Medical Association*, vol. 254, no. 24, 3454–3457. © 1995. Reprinted by permission of the publisher.

Wright, Lawrence, "One Drop of Blood," from *The New Yorker*, July 25, 1994, 46–55. © 1994 by Lawrence Wright. Reprinted by permission of The Wendy Weil Agency, Inc.

Zola, Irving, "Self, Identity, and the Naming Question: Reflections on the Language of Disability," from *Social Science and Medicine*, vol. 36, 167–173. © 1993. Reprinted by permission of Elsevier Science Ltd. and the author.

Zola, Irving, "Tell Me, Tell Me," from *Ordinary Lives*. © 1982 by Irving Zola. Reprinted by permission of the author.

Index to Authors

■

About the Editors

■

Gail E. Henderson is Associate Professor in the Department of Social Medicine, and Adjunct Associate Professor in the Department of Sociology, University of North Carolina School of Medicine and College of Arts and Sciences. She is author of *The Chinese Hospital: A Socialist Work Unit*. Her work focuses on health and inequality, equity in access to medical care, and cross-cultural issues in research ethics.

Nancy M. P. King is Associate Professor in the Department of Social Medicine, University of North Carolina School of Medicine and author of *Making Sense of Advance Directives*. Her scholarly interests include decision-making in health care and research, the relationship between law and ethics in medicine, and informed consent policy and practice.

Ronald P. Strauss is Professor in the Department of Dental Ecology and in the Department of Social Medicine, University of North Carolina Schools of Dentistry and Medicine. His recent publications have been on physician communication of "bad news" and on resource allocation, health policy, and craniofacial care. His scholarly interests focus on the social and ethical issues associated with stigmatizing health problems, chronic childhood illness, birth defects, and HIV/AIDS.

Sue E. Estroff is Professor in the Department of Social Medicine and Adjunct Professor in the Departments of Psychiatry and Anthropology, University of North Carolina School of Medicine and College of Arts and Sciences. She is author of *Making It Crazy: An Ethnography of Psychiatric Clients in an American Community*. Her recent work concerns the life and illness course of people with severe persistent mental illness, moral reasoning, and the production of qualitative research and public mental health policy.

Larry R. Churchill is Professor and Chair in the Department of Social Medicine, University of North Carolina School of Medicine. His chief interests are in health policy and the ethics of research with human subjects. His most recent books are *Self-Interest and Universal Health Care: Why Well-Insured Americans Should Support Coverage for Everyone* and *Rationing Health Care in America: Perceptions and Principles of Justice*.

Library of Congress Cataloging-in-Publication Data
The social medicine reader / Gail E. Henderson . . .
[et al.], editors.
Includes bibliographical references.
ISBN 0-8223-1957-8 (cloth : alk. paper). —
ISBN 0-8223-1965-9 (paper : alk. paper)
1. Social medicine.   I. Henderson, Gail, 1949–
[DNLM: 1. Social Medicine.   2. Sick Role.
3. Socioeconomic Factors.   4. Managed Care Programs.
5. Ethics, Medical.   WA 31 S67803   1997]
RA418.S6424   1997
306.4′61—dc21
DNLM/DLC for Library of Congress   96-50376 CIP